Textbook of
PRACTICAL PHYSIOLOGY

As per Competency-Based MCI Curriculum

Textbook of
PRACTICAL PHYSIOLOGY

FIFTH EDITION

G K Pal

MBBS, MD (Physiology), PhD, DSc, BNYT (Naturopathy and Yoga Therapy), MD (Alt. Medicine), MD (Yoga), MABMS, FABMS, FABAP, FSAB
Professor (Senior Scale) of Physiology, JIPMER, Puducherry
Program Director, Advance Center for Yoga, JIPMER, Former Dean, JIPMER (K), Puducherry
Dean, Faculty of Medicine, Pondicherry University
Honorary Professor, Sri Aurobindo International Center of Education, Sri Aurobindo Ashram, Pondicherry
Editor-in-Chief, International Journal of Clinical and Experimental Physiology

Pravati Pal

MBBS, MD (Physiology), BNYT, MD (Alt. Medicine), MABMS
Professor and Head, Department of Physiology
Jawaharlal Institute of Postgraduate Medical Education and Research (JIPMER), Puducherry

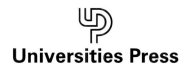

Universities Press

Textbook of Practical Physiology (Fifth Edition)

UNIVERSITIES PRESS (INDIA) PRIVATE LIMITED

Registered Office
3-6-747/1/A & 3-6-754/1, Himayatnagar, Hyderabad 500 029, Telangana, India
info@universitiespress.com; www.universitiespress.com

Distributed by
Orient Blackswan Private Limited

Registered Office
3-6-752 Himayatnagar, Hyderabad 500 029, Telangana, India

Other Offices
Bengaluru / Bhopal / Chennai / Guwahati / Hyderabad / Jaipur
Kolkata / Lucknow / Mumbai / New Delhi / Noida / Patna / Visakhapatnam

© Universities Press (India) Private Limited 2001, 2005, 2010, 2016, 2020

First published 2001
Reprinted 2003, 2004
Second edition 2005
Reprinted 2006, 2007, 2008, 2009
Third edition 2010
Reprinted 2010 (Twice), 2011 (Twice), 2012, 2013, 2014, 2015
Fourth edition 2016
Reprinted 2017, 2018, 2019
Fifth edition 2020

ISBN 978-93-89211-64-1

Cover and book design
© Universities Press (India) Private Limited 2001, 2005, 2010, 2016, 2020

Typeset in Minion Pro 11/13.5 pt *by*
ELITE Graphics, Hyderabad 500 039

501736

Illustrations by
RK Majumdar
New Delhi 110 092

Printed in India at
Rasi Graphics Pvt Ltd, Chennai 600 014

Published by
Universities Press (India) Private Limited
3-6-747/1/A & 3-6-754/1 Himayatnagar, Hyderabad 500 029, Telangana, India

Contents

*The manifestation of the Supramental upon earth is no more a promise but a living fact, a reality.
It is at work here, and a day will come when the most blind, the most unconscious,
even the most unwilling shall be obliged to recognise it.*

The Mother (of Sri Aurobindo Ashram)

Acknowledgements

It gives us great pleasure to see the timely publication of the fifth edition of the *Textbook of Practical Physiology* which has been thoroughly updated as per the new competency-based integrated curriculum prescribed by the Medical Council of India. Apart from the competency-based integration, this edition has also been brought up to date with revised human and clinical experiments and improved presentation of techniques in the hematology section.

Given our substantial administrative, academic and research responsibilities at the institute, the revision of this textbook seemed, at first, a daunting task. For making it less so, we thank Mr Madhu Reddy, Director, Universities Press and President, Orient Blackswan Pvt. Ltd. We express our sincere and heartfelt appreciation to Mr Reddy for his efforts to see the book through to completion and for giving it a fresh, contemporary look in four-colour. We profusely thank Dr Sudha Ganesan, Managing Consultant, Medical Publishing, Universities Press, for conceptualising such an attractive layout for the book and for supervising the work on this edition at every step of the way. We must also acknowledge the contribution of Mrs Parvath Radha, Editor, Universities Press, who worked tirelessly and meticulously with us all through the process of preparing the manuscript for the new edition; we sincerely thank her for getting this book ready despite the time constraints and the challenges presented by the COVID pandemic. We also thank Dr Alpa Agarwal, Senior Development Editor, for her immense help in the preparation of schematic diagrams for the book.

We express our sincere thanks to Ms M. Renugasundari, PhD scholar, for her technical support in the preparation of the practical demonstrations and for helping us in the proofreading of the manuscript. We are profoundly grateful to Mrs Bharathi Balakumar, Ms N Padmapriya and Mr S Bakthavachalam, the technical staff, for providing us logistic support in the demonstration of many of the experiments that are depicted in this book. We sincerely thank all our colleagues, viz. Dr G S Gaur, Dr S Velkumary, Dr Y Dhanalakshmi, Dr S Karthik, Dr B M Naik, Dr N Prabhu, Dr K Saranya, Dr R Rajalakshmi, all senior and junior residents and other PG and PhD students for their constant support in all our endeavours.

We are grateful to our friends from Sri Aurobindo Ashram, Pondicherry, the late Mr Narayan Mahapatra, Mr Chandramani, Ms Sujata Kar and Mr Vasanth for volunteering to act as subjects of our clinical examinations. Words cannot express our sincere appreciation for Mr Auroprakash Pal, Dr Auroprajna Pal, Dr Nivedita Nanda and Ms Sabita Nanda—the members of our family who have been inexhaustible repositories of inspiration and support. We are forever indebted to our parents, the late Mrutyunjay Pal, the late Dr Atratran Nanda, the late Anupama Nanda and Smt Malatimani Pal for instilling in us such a strong sense of discipline; we owe our place in society and our successes to them. We will always be grateful to all our teachers of the past and the present for imparting to us the knowledge that we are sharing with our readers today.

We are ever indebted to the infinite grace of the Divine Mother Sri-Ma and the Divine Master Sri Aurobindo without which we are certain none of these achievements would have come to pass.

G. K. Pal
Pravati Pal
Email: gkpalphysiology@gmail.com

All can be done if God-touch is there.

– Sri Aurobindo (in SAVITRI)

Preface to the Fifth Edition

We are pleased to present the fifth edition of the *Textbook of Practical Physiology*, which has been considered the most reliable book on practical physiology for medical students in India and abroad for over two decades. It has been our aim to provide medical students with a book that is up to date in all aspects of applied and clinical physiology as well as the requisite knowledge and skills in these areas. In light of the new competency-based integrated curriculum prescribed by the Medical Council of India in 2019, we have thoroughly revised various sections of this book including those on hematology, human experiments and clinical physiology.

The fifth edition of this book has been fortified with new chapters on body composition, basal metabolism, birth control methods, examination of higher functions, cardiac efficiency tests, the use of a handgrip dynamometer, blood pressure variability and baroreflex sensitivity. Numerous new flowcharts and tables have been added to facilitate the comprehension of various concepts. Animal experiments have been refined and restricted to the essential learnings. The viva voce questions at the end of each chapter, the OSPE and index of normal values have been revised entirely and updated.

The book is specially designed for step-by-step learning through practicals and experiments, which are vital to medical students seeking to develop expertise in clinical medicine. We are certain that the new, contemporary four-colour design of this edition will appeal to students and aid in reading and retention.

This fifth edition features numerous illustrations that have been meticulously revised, redrawn and re-represented to facilitate the easy assimilation of techniques. Several new colour photographs have been added across the book to demonstrate the methodology of conducting the practical tests. The learning objectives in each chapter have been divided into 'Must Know' and 'Desirable to Know' categories. The information on clinical examination has been grouped separately under one section to emphasise the growing need for clinical physiology in medicine.

It is our belief that the fifth edition of the *Textbook of Practical Physiology* is now a comprehensive practical textbook on the subject for undergraduate and postgraduate students of medicine. We hope that our readers will find that this book fulfils all the requirements of the current field of practical physiology. Any inputs and constructive criticisms our readers and well-wishers might have are welcome and will help us perfect this book further.

G K Pal
Pravati Pal
Email: gkpalphysiology@gmail.com

A drop of practice is better than an ocean of theories, advices and good resolutions.

—The Mother

Preface to the First Edition

This textbook of practical physiology covers all the aspects of the practicals in the subject. The authors hope that it will fulfil the needs of the medical student.

We have tried our best to provide high quality material in a precise and comprehensive form. Every effort has been made to incorporate all the aspects of practical physiology. Till now, students used to come to practical classes with a manual and a theory book. The manual helps them learn the techniques to perform the practical, and the theory book helps them understand the practical. Often, the theory books do not cover all the theoretical aspects of the practical. Therefore, in this book, we have made a sincere effort to provide the essential underlying principles of practical physiology, to help the student perform various practicals, and to learn and apply the knowledge of practical physiology in clinical medicine. This book is therefore meant to be a complete textbook of practical physiology.

The Medical Council of India (MCI) has recently suggested significant changes in the first MBBS curriculum. It has recommended an increase in the number of human practicals, reduction in experimental practicals, and more applied and clinically oriented teaching to provide an objective oriented learning. In view of this, more than seventy percent of this book contains human practicals, and experimental physiology has been described in a very compact (but essentially useful) form. Each practical in the book contains learning objectives, theoretical aspects of the practical, details of clinical oriented discussion and possible viva voce questions with answers. The unique feature of this book is the introduction of objective structured practical examination (OSPE). The 'General Introduction' describes OSPE and suggests how best the book could be used.

A book of this kind may be complete but is not perfect. Indeed, we visualise the book as a project in evolution that should be able to accommodate the constructive criticism and suggestions, and the fast-changing concepts and needs of the science. We welcome the reader's views and suggestions, to make future editions of the book as useful to the students as the current edition.

G K Pal
Pravati Pal

Special Features of This Book

Education is the process that brings about desirable changes in the behaviour of the learner in the form of acquisition of knowledge, proficiency in skills and development of attitudes. Knowledge and skill should grow simultaneously and harmoniously. Knowledge without skill is useless and skill without knowledge is dangerous. Therefore, to become a good physician, a medical student should have knowledge, skill and proper attitude.

Physiology is a vast subject. Knowledge of physiology is used in all branches of medicine, from biochemistry and pharmacology to gynecology and medicine. **A good physician is a good physiologist and a true physiologist is the best physician**. Knowledge of practical physiology is applied in clinical medicine to understand the pathophysiology of the disease, to explain the clinical manifestation of the disease, to provide the physiological basis of the diagnosis and treatment of the disease, and to assess the prognosis. In this book, we have tried to explain the clinical significance of the practicals, in addition to detailed descriptions of various physiological aspects of the topics. *This introduction will help you extract maximum benefit from the book.*

Each topic of this book has most of these sections: **learning objectives, introduction, methods (including observation and result), discussion, OSPE and viva.**

Learning objectives

Objectives are to a student (or teacher) what blueprints are to an architect. Learning objectives give the student an idea of the desired competence in the form of acquisition of knowledge and skill. Unless these competencies are clearly stated, it cannot be known whether they are properly acquired. Objectives help the students organise their efforts to obtain the desired knowledge and skill. Therefore, each topic, whether theory or practical, must have learning objectives. The objectives should be relevant, unequivocal, observable, measurable and feasible.

A set of 'Learning Objectives' has been given at the beginning of each topic. The student should go through these objectives before performing the practical. The objectives are intended to inform the students what they must know and what is desirable for them to know. Accordingly, the learning objectives are divided into two categories. The first set of MUST KNOW objectives provides what students must learn *(the minimum that they should learn)* by performing that practical and the second set of DESIRABLE TO KNOW objectives describes what they may know *(it is better to learn this too, though it is not mandatory)*. In the latest recommendation by the Medical Council of India, it has been emphasised that teaching should be clinically based with clearly outlined objectives of what students must know and what is desirable for them to know. For physiology practicals, the students should read the objectives *before* starting the practical and should again look at them *after* completing the practical, to assess whether they have achieved the required skill and knowledge. The objectives that are described in this book are basic in nature. The teacher can modify these objectives according to the needs and the instructions of the university teaching curriculum.

Introduction

It is desirable that the students have a basic knowledge of the topic before they perform the practical. It helps them understand the scientific basis and the importance of the practical. Every effort has been made to give a clear and concise theoretical explanation in this section. It introduces the topic and describes the important points of the methods. Therefore, the students should read this before they perform a practical.

Methods

Under "Methods", a detailed description has been given of the different methodologies that are used widely in different laboratories. Each method contains four to five sub-sections—Principle, Requirements, Procedure, Precautions, Observation and Result. A brief description of the "**Principle**" of the method is given at the beginning. In "**Requirements**", the equipment and chemicals required to perform the test are listed and a brief description is given about the important equipment and chemicals. A short description is also given about the *use* of the equipment. In "**Procedure**", a detailed and stepwise description of how to perform the practical is given. Important steps are followed by a "**Note**", which describes the significance of that particular step. A list of important "**Precautions**" are given following the procedure. The methods that are usually not used but are important from the examination point of view (likely to be asked in the viva voce) are described briefly. A practical, unless done properly following the proper procedure and precautions, is likely to yield erroneous results. Therefore, the student should read and understand the procedure and precautions thoroughly before performing the practical.

Discussion

"Discussion" gives details of the physiological and clinical significance of the practical. Only points that are pertinent to the practical have been included. Discussion of the result, merits and demerits of different methods, and practical implications of a specific test should be undertaken by the teacher only after the student has completed the practical and got the result. Therefore, the student should not read this section before performing the practical. However, *there must be discussion at the end of the practical* because only after a thorough and complete discussion does one gain complete practical knowledge.

OSPE

OSPE stands for **objective structured practical examination**. In this, a small but important component of the practical is evaluated in a stepwise manner as prefixed and described in the checklist. This is an objective method of assessment, where specific competencies are tested. In clinical examinations, it is called **OSCE**. This is a new concept of evaluation of the practical or clinical skill of medical students. Teachers have always been concerned about the reliability and uniformity of assessment of students. Traditionally, in examinations, students perform the practical and the examiner assesses their practical knowledge (not the skill) after they have already performed the test. The examiners do not evaluate the skill of the students, as they do not observe them while performing the practical. Therefore, the skill aspect of the practical, which is the most important aspect, remains under-evaluated. The skill improves and gradually attains perfection only when a practical is performed and evaluated with **specific structured objectives**. Therefore, at present, OSPE is the best way to determine the skill of the students, as it is transparent, reliable, valid and objective. OSPE is designed to overcome the deficiencies of conventional practical examinations. Since each practical is broken down into smaller components and each component has prescribed steps, a **greater degree of objectivity** is achieved. Marks are allotted for each component and for each step.

In OSPE, the students are required to perform an important component of the practical within a specified time. The examiners keep a checklist (the steps of OSPE) with them and observe whether the examinee performs the test in the proper sequence as described. The examiners *do not ask anything,* they only observe the stepwise performance by the student and enter marks against the corrected steps (for a detailed procedure on conducting the OSPE, see "Methodology of OSPE"). In this book, under OSPE, we have given a stepwise description (this serves as the checklist for the teacher) of all important practicals. Therefore, the student should practice the methods carefully as described under OSPE. It should be introduced in all medical colleges to bring about **uniformity, objectivity, validity, transparency and reliability in the evaluation** of the practical skill of the students.

Viva

The questions that are usually asked in viva voce are described under 'Viva'. Answers to many of the questions are already given in the text; therefore, **the answers are not repeated** in this section. *Answers to a few questions for which answers may not be found in the text are given in the viva section.* Therefore, students must read all the questions and answers in the viva section, otherwise they may miss some important points.

General Laboratory Instructions

A medical laboratory is the workshop that provides the knowledge and experience to develop practical skills and attitudes. To achieve this, the working atmosphere in the laboratory should be congenial to the teachers and students. For smooth and harmonious conduct of laboratory work, cooperation from the technical staff, attendants, students and teachers is of utmost importance.

Instructions for students

Desire to learn, dedication to study, sincerity and cooperation in work, and a caring attitude are essential qualities in a medical student. The student should keep in mind the following:

1. Wear a clean and well-ironed white coat and good looking shining shoes while working in the laboratory. Wear your official ID card, making sure that it is visible to others.
2. Bring the necessary equipment for hematology (disposable lancets, etc.), amphibian or experimental (dissecting instruments) and human practicals (stethoscope, knee hammer, etc.).
3. Have a basic theoretical knowledge of the concerned practical (the practical of that day). For this, read the introduction to each topic, before attending the instruction of the demonstrator or before performing the practical.
4. Pay due attention to the demonstration of the practical given by the instructor or teacher.
5. Check to see if the apparatus is working properly before starting the experiment.
6. Do not disturb the instruments that are not assigned to you or are not required for the practical.
7. For any technical assistance, take help from the appointed technician or the instructor without disturbing other students.
8. Handle the apparatus gently and carry out the experiment without damaging it.
9. Perform the practical step by step following the proper procedure and precautions. For this, refer to the method described for each practical.
10. After obtaining the observation, discuss with the teacher about the accuracy of the result, and about the physiological and clinical utility of the practical. For this, read the discussion section given under each topic.
11. Enter the observation and result in your practical record, and note the physiological and pathological variation in the parameters and also write the answers to the questions given.
12. After completing the practical, check whether you have achieved the minimum knowledge and skill prescribed. For this, refer to the list of learning objectives given for that practical.
13. Get the practical record checked by the teacher regularly.
14. Return the apparatus to the laboratory staff before leaving the laboratory.
15. Keep the practical record and book in good condition.

Instructions for demonstrators

A medical educator has a dual ethical obligation: to produce competent health professionals for the society, and to improve the standard of the student under care. Teachers of practical physiology have two important roles to play. First, they should familiarise themselves with the objectives (both essential and desirable objectives) and select what the student should learn, and second, they should help facilitate the learning of the student. Teachers (demonstrators) should:

1. Wear a white coat while taking practical classes for the students.
2. Give proper direction to the students to follow the laboratory discipline.
3. Practise, read and understand the practical, before taking classes for the students.
4. Do the demonstration confidently and clearly, without confusion.
5. Emphasise and explain the important steps of the practical.
6. Pay equal attention to all the students.
7. Not be seen sitting idle in the laboratory.
8. Encourage students to express their difficulties without fear.
9. Try to detect and solve the individual practical problems of the students.
10. Explain the physiological and clinical importance of the practical.
11. Check and evaluate the practical record of the students regularly.
12. Give feedback to the students for their improvement.

Methodology of OSPE

Conducting OSPE needs proper planning and organisation. **Planning for OSPE** includes setting down valid, appropriate and important questions, and preparing an accurate checklist suitable for evaluating the student's performance. **Organisation** includes arrangement of stations that contain all the materials required to perform the test and motivated subjects (if clinical practicals), and trained manpower to regulate the movement of the students during the practical.

OSPE can be used for evaluating performance in class examinations as well as in the final examination. During the examination, the students move around a number of stations spending a specific amount of time (3 to 5 minutes) in each. In each station they perform a specific practical within the stipulated time and then move to the next station in response to an auditory signal (say, ringing of a bell). In the final examination, since there are usually four examiners (two internal and two external), four OSPE stations can be kept. When students perform the OSPE, examiners sit beside each of them with the checklist, observe their performance, and grade them accordingly in the checklist. The examiners must carefully check each and every step of the practical without disturbing the candidate; they are just active observers and should not interfere in any way with the performance of the candidate. They are not supposed to ask any questions nor are they expected to respond to any query from the student.

It is better to have **non-skill stations between the OSPE (skill) stations**. Ideally, the non-skill stations should have the question related to the previous skill station, so that it reinforces the skill and knowledge of the student. For example, if the skill station has asked for the student to elicit a tendon jerk, the non-skill station can have any one of the following questions:

1. Draw a reflex arc.
2. List the five important differences between upper and lower motor neuron paralysis.
3. Name two conditions each in which the tendon reflexes are i) exaggerated and ii) depressed.

Likewise the questions can be framed according to the previous skill stations. In university examinations, eight stations (four skill and four non-skill) can be kept. The examiners evaluate the skill station on the spot and non-skill stations afterwards. This can replace conventional spotting-type examination (students write the answer according to the spotter given). After the OSPE is over, the student can perform the long and short practicals as they usually do in the university examination. Ideally, as per MCI recommendations, twenty students (not more than 25) should be evaluated for practical examination per day. In OSPE, the twenty students in eight stations (four skill and four non-skill) spending four minutes at each will not take more than 90 minutes. If the examination starts at 8.30 am, OSPE can be completed by 10.00 am and the remaining three hours can be used for other practicals and practical viva examination; the theory viva can be conducted in the afternoon. For routine class examinations, more stations (10–20) can be set up to include the maximum number of practicals. This may be done easily with the help of the junior teaching staff of the department. The students should be exposed to the OSPE at least two or three times before the final examination. OSPE should carry a weightage of 30–50 per cent of the total marks allotted for the practical.

Before the OSPE is conducted, it must be ensured that all the equipment (instrument, solution, gauze, cotton, spirit, etc.) is available in the station according to the question given. As only 3 to 5 minutes are given to each student, the students should not spend time searching for the equipment. It should also be ensured that as soon as the indication is given (ringing a bell), the student moves immediately to the next station. The OSPE questions too should be prepared in such a way that the student should be able to perform the practical (both in the skill and non-skill stations) within the stipulated time. For this, the question for **OSPE should contain only an important component of the practical**, not the whole of the practical. One of the problems in conducting OSPE, especially hematology practicals, is to supply adequate material during the examination. For example, if the question is 'Dilute the blood for total RBC count', adequate number of pipettes should be supplied, otherwise, a laboratory attendant should help throughout the examination to wash the used pipettes. Similarly in human practicals, the main problem would be to provide cooperative and motivated subjects. This will need to be planned in advance.

How to make a checklist

Question: *Examine the radial pulse of the subject and report your finding.*

Student number	1	2	3	4	5	6	7	8	9	10 20

Criteria of OSPE	**Group score**
1. Stands on the right side ...	
2. Places three middle fingers ...	
3. Counts for 1 min	
4. Checks the condition of the ...	
5. Compares with opposite side ...	
6. Checks for radio-femoral delay	
7. Reports properly	
Individual score	

Advantages of OSPE

1. Uniform evaluation of performance of all the students.
2. Methodical assessment of skill.
3. No examiner bias.
4. Evaluation is more transparent.
5. Evaluation is valid and reliable.
6. All the students are given the same practical and are allowed the same duration of time. Therefore, there is no candidate bias.
7. Provides direct feedback to the student as well as to the teacher. The students get feedback on a mistake in a particular step (feedback is given after the practical, usually in a group). If many students make the same error in a particular step of OSPE, it indicates that the step was probably not properly demonstrated or emphasised by the teacher.
8. Junior examiners can also be appointed.

Competency Mapping Table

No.	COMPETENCY The student should be able to:	Core Y/N	Chapter number	Page number
Topic: Hematology Number of competencies: (08) Number of procedures that require certification: (NIL)				
PY2.4	Describe RBC formation (erythropoiesis and its functions)	Y	7	46,47
PY2.5	Describe different types of anaemias and jaundice	Y	3, 51	19, 327
PY2.7	Describe the formation of platelets, functions and variations	Y	18	123, 124, 127
PY2.8	Describe the physiological basis of hemostasis and anticoagulants. Describe bleeding and clotting disorders (haemophilia, purpura)	Y	2, 17	8, 111, 119,120
PY2.9	Describe different blood groups and discuss the clinical importance of blood grouping, blood banking and transfusion	Y	15	99-107
PY2.11	Estimate Hb, RBC, TLC, RBC indices, DLC, Blood groups, BT/CT	Y	3, 7, 9, 8, 11, 15, 17	11–20, 46–54, 59–66. 55–58, 79–85, 99–107, 111–122
PY2.12	Describe test for ESR, Osmotic fragility, Hematocrit, Note the finding and interpret the test results, etc.	Y	14, 16, 4	93–98, 108–110, 21–25,
PY2.13	Describe steps for reticulocyte and platelet count	Y	18, 19	123–128, 129–133
Topic: Nerve and Muscle Physiology Number of competencies: (04) Number of procedures that require certification: (NIL)				
PY3.14	Perform ergography	Y	33	229-234
PY3.15	Demonstrate effect of mild, moderate and severe exercise and record changes in cardiorespiratory parameters	Y	30	206-214
PY3.16	Demonstrate Harvard Step test and describe the impact on induced physiologic parameters in a simulated environment	Y	30	213
PY3.18	Observe with Computer assisted learning (i) amphibian nerve-muscle experiments (ii) amphibian cardiac experiments	Y	59–72	444–487
Topic: Gastro-intestinal Physiology Number of competencies (01) Number of procedures that require certification(NIL)				
PY4.10	Demonstrate the correct clinical examination of the abdomen in a normal volunteer or simulated environment	Y	54	363–370
Topic: Cardiovascular Physiology (CVS) Number of competencies (05) Number of procedures that require certification: (03)				
PY5.12	Record blood pressure and pulse at rest and in different grades of exercise an postures in a volunteer or simulated environment	Y	27–30	180–214
PY5.13	Record and interpret normal ECG in a volunteer or simulated environment	Y	26	168–179
PY5.14	Observe cardiovascular autonomic function tests in a volunteer or simulated environment	N	36–38	248–274
PY5.15	Demonstrate the correct clinical examination of the cardiovascular system in a normal volunteer or simulated environment	Y	53	351–362
PY5.16	Describe and discuss arterial pulse tracing	N	27	180, 188
Topic: Respiratory Physiology Number of competencies (03) Number of procedures that require certification: (01)				
PY6.8	Demonstrate the correct technique to perform and interpret Spirometry	Y	23	145–157
PY6.9	Demonstrate the correct clinical examination of the respiratory system in normal volunteer or simulated environment	Y	52	335–350
PY6.10	Demonstrate the correct technique to perform measurement of peak expiratory flow rate in a normal volunteer or simulated environment	Y	23	150–151

Topic: Reproductive Physiology Number of competencies(03) Number of procedures that require certification (NIL)

PY9.6	Enumerate the contraceptive methods for male and female. Discuss their advantages and disadvantages	Y	50	320–323
PY9.9	Interpret a normal semen analysis report including (a) sperm count, (b) sperm morphology and (c) sperm motility, as per WHO guidelines and discuss the results	Y	48	313–315
PY9.10	Discuss the physiological basis of various pregnancy tests	Y	49	316–319

Topic: Neuropathy Number of competencies: (04) Number of procedures that require certification (NIL)

PY10.11	Demonstrate the correct clinical examination of the nervous system: Higher functions, sensory system, motor system, reflexes, cranial nerves in a normal volunteer or simulated environment	Y	55-57	371–434
PY10.12	Identify normal EEG forms	Y	35	238–247
PY10.19	Describe and discuss auditory and visual evoked potentials	Y	39, 40	275–283
PY10.20	Demonstrate (i) testing of visual acuity, colour and field of vision and (ii) hearing (iii) Testing for smell and (iv) taste sensation in volunteer/simulated environment	Y	43–47	291–312

Topic: Integrated Physiology Number of competencies: (03) Number of procedures that require certification; (NIL)

PY11.11	Discuss the concept, criteria for diagnosis of Brain death and its implications	Y	36	246–247
PY11.13	Obtain history and perform general examination in the volunteer/simulated environment	Y	51	324–334
PY11.14	Demonstrate Basic Life Support in a simulated environment	Y	24	159–161

CHAPTER 1

Introduction to Hematology

Learning Objectives

After studying this chapter, you will be able to (MUST KNOW):
1. Define hematology.
2. State the components of blood.
3. Explain the functions of each component.
4. Name the routine hematologic tests.

5. List the sources of collection of specimens used in a hematology laboratory.

You may also be able to (DESIRABLE TO KNOW):
1. Describe the appearance of a blood specimen after centrifugation.
2. Explain the significance of buffy coat.

INTRODUCTION

Hematology is defined as the branch of science that deals with the study of blood. The word "hematology" is derived from the Greek words *haima*, meaning blood, and *logos*, meaning study. It is primarily concerned with the study of formed elements of blood. Blood is the fluid constituent of the body that flows through the vascular channels. The total volume of blood in a 70 kg adult is about 5.5 litres or 8 per cent of the body weight. About 45 per cent of this amount is composed of formed elements. Plasma constitutes about 5 per cent of the body weight.

BLOOD COMPONENTS AND THEIR FUNCTIONS

Blood has two major components: cells and fluid (plasma).

The Cellular Component

The cellular component consists of red blood cells (erythrocytes), white blood cells (leucocytes) and platelets (thrombocytes). The thrombocytes are the smallest (2–4 μm), the erythrocytes are medium-sized (7–8 μm), and the leucocytes are the largest of all the cells with a wide range (8–20 μm) of size. The red blood cells constitute the highest number of formed elements in the circulation (4.5–6 million/mm^3 of blood) followed by platelets (1.5–4 lakhs/mm^3 of blood) and leucocytes

(4–11 thousand/mm^3 of blood). The **erythrocytes** help in transport of gases, that is, they carry oxygen from the lungs to the tissues and carbon dioxide from the tissues to the lungs. The **leucocytes** assist in the defence processes of the body. The **thrombocytes** assist in stoppage of bleeding (hemostasis). Development of blood cells is called **hemopoiesis**. In post-natal life (after birth), hemopoiesis occurs in the bone marrow.

The Fluid Component

The fluid component of the blood is known as **plasma** which consists of a soluble protein called **fibrinogen**. During the process of coagulation of blood, fibrinogen is removed from plasma as fibrin, and the clear fluid left behind is called **serum**. Therefore, to obtain plasma for diagnostic tests, blood should not be allowed to clot.

Plasma Plasma is the principal medium for transportation of materials from one part of the body to another through the blood vessels. Plasma carries various substances: nutrients, metabolites, waste products, hormones, chemicals and other substances. Plasma contains clotting factors that participate in blood coagulation.

Serum The serum contains most of the chemicals present in the plasma except fibrinogen and some clotting factors. Therefore, many investigations like estimations of glucose, proteins and lipids are performed in serum, which is collected by clotting the blood.

HEMATOLOGIC TESTS

Several hematologic tests are regularly performed as part of every patient's initial laboratory investigations. Many of these tests are considered routine and can be done by a technician with limited training. These routine hematologic tests include estimation of hemoglobin, total RBC count, total leucocyte count, ESR and differential count of leucocytes. These tests are performed mainly to study the patient's ability to fight diseases. These tests also aid in diagnosis of diseases and help in assessing the prognosis.

Performing accurate hematologic tests, however, requires repeated practice. Many of the techniques require adequate skill and experience, especially for using instruments. In recent years, especially in advanced laboratories, many of these tests are performed by automated methods. However, in most clinical and medical college laboratories, tests are performed mainly by manual techniques.

A student should acquire enough knowledge about the formed elements of blood, their enumeration and their characteristics, to perform and analyse these tests accurately. They should therefore be knowledgeable about the formation, structure and functions of blood cells, the basic principle of determination, the use and care of equipment, the preparation of reagents, and the calculation and interpretation of results.

SPECIMEN

Blood samples for hematologic study are usually obtained by finger puncture (capillary blood) or venipuncture (venous blood). Arterial blood sample is usually not needed for hematology practicals in Physiology.

Capillary Blood

Capillary blood can be used with good results for morphologic studies in hematology. Capillary blood is obtained from the fingertip, earlobe, heel or big toe. In newborns and infants, blood is usually obtained by heel puncture because blood supply in fingertips is limited, and removing blood by venipuncture would deplete too much of their blood. In adults, the tip of any of the middle three fingers is punctured to obtain a sample.

Venous Blood

It is not always advisable to obtain capillary blood, especially when a large quantity of blood is needed for hematologic tests. Venous blood is used for this purpose. Coagulation should be prevented as clotted blood cannot be used. For most hematologic studies, the anticoagulant used is EDTA (ethylenediamine tetra-acetic acid). This preserves the morphology of the cellular elements. It is important that the blood be mixed well with the anticoagulant immediately after it is collected to ensure proper anticoagulation. White cell count, microhematocrit, platelet count and sedimentation rates can be measured up to 24 hours after blood is collected in EDTA if it is refrigerated at 4°C. Immediately after collecting the blood, the sample should be gently mixed with anticoagulants by repeated inversion to ensure thorough contact of blood with the anticoagulant. The presence of even a tiny clot in a specimen may affect the result.

Appearance When the blood specimen has been properly drawn and preserved, the plasma will have its natural colour, a very light yellow or the colour of straw. In some diseased states, the plasma may have altered colour. But this can also result from improper handling of the specimen.

Two types of blood samples are **unsuitable for hematologic investigations**: (1) clotted samples and (2) samples that are hemolysed in the process of collection or handling.

If blood is collected, anticoagulated and allowed to settle or centrifuged, three layers will be observed (Fig. 1.1). The bottom layer will consist of packed red blood cells which make up 43–47 per cent of the total blood volume. On top of this layer is a thin whitish

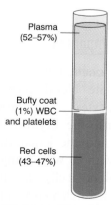

Plasma
(52–57%)

Bufty coat
(1%) WBC
and platelets

Red cells
(43–47%)

Fig. 1.1 Layers formed after centrifugation of a normal blood sample.

layer called **buffy coat**. This consists of leucocytes and platelets, and makes up about 1 per cent of the total volume. Abnormal cells like LE cells as found in SLE, and atypical mononuclear cells as found in malignant conditions are detected in smears made from buffy coat. Buffy coat preparation is also useful for detection of bacteria, fungi and parasites within the circulating leucocytes. The uppermost layer is the colloidal liquid called plasma, which makes up 52–57 per cent of the total blood volume.

VIVA

1. What is blood and what are its components?
2. What are the formed elements of blood and what are their functions?
3. What is the difference between plasma and serum?
4. How is the serum prepared in the laboratory?
5. What is the purpose of performing routine hematologic tests?
6. What are the types of specimens collected for hematologic tests?
7. Why are the middle three fingers preferred for skin puncture?
8. Why is venipuncture not used for collecting blood samples in newborns and infants?
9. Which is the ideal site for collecting blood in newborns and infants, and why?
10. Why is EDTA commonly preferred for collecting venous blood?
11. What is buffy coat and what is its significance?
12. Why should blood be properly mixed with anticoagulants immediately after collection?
13. What types of blood samples are unsuitable for hematologic tests and why?

CHAPTER 2

Collection of Blood Samples

Learning Objectives

After completing this practical, you will be able to (MUST KNOW):

1. List the general precautions for collecting blood.
2. List the methods of collection of blood sample.
3. Collect peripheral blood by finger prick method.
4. List the precautions observed during collection of blood by finger prick method.
5. Name the specific uses of commonly used anticoagulants in hematological procedures.

You may also be able to (DESIRABLE TO KNOW):

1. Collect blood by the venipuncture method.
2. List the precautions for the venipuncture method.
3. List the steps of collection of blood by the earlobe puncture and heel puncture methods.
4. Explain the mechanism of action and uses of various anticoagulants.

INTRODUCTION

Blood is one of the most common specimens used in laboratory determinations. Venous blood is preferred for most hematological examinations. Peripheral samples (capillary blood) can be used satisfactorily for many purposes if a free flow of blood is obtained, but this procedure should be avoided in patients who may be possible carriers of transmissible diseases. Capillary blood is used commonly for hemoglobin estimation, cell counts, blood grouping, bleeding and clotting time determination, and other investigations that use less blood, whereas venous blood is preferred for a comprehensive hematological investigation.

General Precautions

Because of the increasing risks of fatal transmissible diseases, the following precautions must be taken while collecting a blood sample from a patient. All aseptic procedures are followed for blood collection. The word **asepsis** refers to the state of being free from contamination by any infective organism. For this purpose, disposable or sterilised lancets or needles are used.

1. Care must be taken to prevent injuries while handling syringes and needles.
2. Disposable rubber gloves should always be used while collecting blood samples. The operator must wear disposable plastic/rubber gloves, especially if the patient is uncooperative and if the operator has any cuts, abrasions or skin breaks on the hands.
3. It should be ensured that there is no leakage from the specimens (if collected in bottles or bags).

METHODS OF COLLECTION

For physiology practicals, blood is often collected by pricking the tip of the finger. Therefore, collection of peripheral blood by finger puncture method (with details of steps and precautions) is described clearly in this chapter.

Principle

There are two general sources of blood for clinical laboratory tests: **peripheral (capillary) blood** and **venous blood**. For small quantities of blood for hematologic investigations, the specimen is obtained from the capillary bed by puncturing the skin. The tip of the finger is the most common site for puncture. For larger quantities of blood, a puncture is made directly into a vein (phlebotomy) using a sterile syringe-and-needle collection system.

Collection of Capillary (Peripheral) Blood

Capillary blood is often used for bedside investigations. But this blood is likely to give erroneous results if not collected properly; therefore, it should only be used when it is not possible to obtain venous blood. Free flow of blood is essential and only a gentle squeezing is permissible. Ideally, large drops of blood should exude slowly but spontaneously.

Source

Blood can be obtained from the earlobes or the **fingertips** of adults and older children, and from the heel or plantar surface of the big toe of infants. The earlobe is not ideal for puncture as the flow of blood is slow and the concentration of cells and of hemoglobin is more in earlobe.

Note: The blood obtained from the ear lobe contains a higher concentration of hemoglobin and more cells than from the fingertips or venous blood. Hence, it is not reliable for hemoglobin estimation and total leucocyte count. However, blood from the ear lobe is preferred for preparing blood films for differential count and to study leucocyte abnormalities, since larger cells are frequently trapped in the capillary bed of the ear lobe due to its slow circulation.

Requirements

- Disposable sterile lancet (or 24G needle)
- Alcohol
- Dry gauze
- Slides or pipettes

Various types of disposable lancets are used for skin puncture. Non-disposable lancets are not recommended because of the risk of transmission of infectious pathogens. 24G disposable needles can be used if lancets are not available. The **lancet is preferred** to a needle because the puncture (depth and size of the wound) is effectively performed and well controlled with lancets.

Procedure

For finger puncture

1. Assemble the necessary equipment (lancet device, alcohol, dry gauze, slides).
2. Make the subject sit comfortably.
3. Put on disposable rubber gloves.
4. Select the fingertip suitable for puncture.

Note: A fingertip free from calluses, infection, edema or cyanosis is ideal for puncture.

5. Warm the puncture site by rubbing it.

Note: Warming the skin before puncturing improves circulation and ensures free flow of blood. This must always be done if the fingertip is cold.

6. Clean the skin of the tip of the finger by using cotton or a gauze piece touched with alcohol.

Note: This removes dirt and makes the area relatively sterile.

7. Allow the area to dry. The subject can shake his finger in air to hasten drying.

Note: The finger should not be punctured until the tip of the finger is completely dry, because of the following reasons.

i) A blood drop does not form on the fingertip if it is not dry. Blood spreads sideways along with spirit. Formation of a spherical blood drop is essential for many procedures, especially for pipetting (sucking blood into the RBC, WBC or hemoglobin pipette).
ii) Sterilisation by alcohol is effective only after it dries on the fingertip.
iii) Blood cells are hemolysed when they come in contact with alcohol. Therefore, drying of the fingertip must be ensured for any investigation that requires study of cells.

8. Hold the finger firmly and make a quick puncture about 3–5 mm deep with the lancet (Fig. 2.1).

Note: The puncture should be at the middle of the tip, not too far down on the finger nor too close to the nail.

9. Wipe the first drop of blood using sterile dry gauze.

Note: The first drop is diluted with tissue fluid and interferes with laboratory results, therefore it should be discarded. The succeeding drops are used for tests.

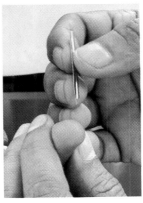

Fig. 2.1   Firmly holding the finger before finger prick using lancet.

10. Allow the blood to flow slowly and freely. If it does not come out spontaneously, apply pressure gently so that a spherical drop is formed (Fig. 2.2).

> **Note:** Squeezing (milking) the tip of the finger to draw blood must be strictly avoided, as it causes exudation of tissue fluid, which dilutes the blood.

11. Rapidly collect blood and use immediately for laboratory study to prevent coagulation.
12. Once the blood sample is collected, give the subject a sterile, dry piece of gauze or cotton to hold over the puncture site until the bleeding stops.
13. Remove gloves and wash hands.

Precautions

1. Sterile gloves should be always used when blood is collected from unknown subjects or patients.
2. The fingertip should be warmed by rubbing slightly as this improves circulation.
3. Disposable lancets should be used.
4. The tip of the lancet should not touch anything until it punctures the skin of the subject.
5. The fingertip should not be squeezed because this dilutes the blood with tissue fluid.
6. The first drop of blood should be discarded as it is diluted with tissue fluid.
7. It is preferable to puncture any of the middle three fingers, because the venous bursa (palmar fascia) of the thumb and the little finger are continuous with that of the limb, whereas the venous bursa of the middle three fingers are limited to the hand only. Therefore, if infection occurs following puncture it will be limited to the hands.

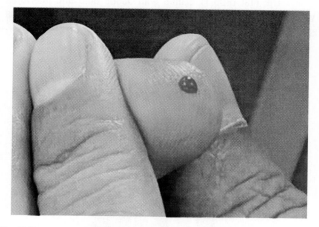

Fig. 2.2 Formation of a spherical drop of blood by finger prick method. Gloves must be used while performing finger prick of an unknown subject or a patient.

For earlobe puncture

1. Select and warm (by gentle rubbing) the puncture site.
2. Clean the earlobe with a cotton swab touched with spirit.
3. Make a quick puncture (to a depth of about 2 mm) of the earlobe with the help of a sterile lancet.
4. Collect blood as it drops down spontaneously.
5. Apply pressure to stop bleeding.

For heel puncture

1. Select, warm and clean the puncture site (Fig. 2.3).

> **Note:** Perform puncture only if the heel is really warm, otherwise it may need to be warmed in warm water.

2. Hold the heel firmly and puncture on the most medial or most lateral portions of the plantar surface.

> **Note:** The central plantar area and the posterior curvature should not be punctured in infants as this may cause injury to the underlying tarsal bones. The puncture should not be more than 2–4 mm deep.

3. Apply pressure to stop bleeding.

Collection of Venous Blood

Source

Venous blood is generally obtained by performing venipuncture of the veins of the forearm, wrist or ankle. This is best withdrawn from an antecubital (forearm) vein because the veins are larger and fuller than those in the wrist, hand or ankle. The wrist, hand and ankle veins are used only if the forearm site is not available. The median cubital vein is usually chosen for

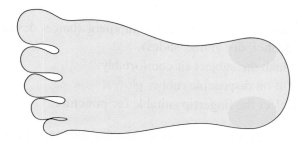

Fig. 2.3 Sites of heel puncture (shaded areas). Middle of the heel is spared.

venipuncture because it does not roll or slip beneath the skin (Fig. 2.4).

Requirements

1. Disposable syringe and needle
2. Alcohol
3. Sterile gauze or cotton
4. Collection bottle containing anticoagulant
5. Disposable gloves

Procedure

Venipuncture should be performed with proper care and skill. The veins have to be made prominent by applying a tourniquet in the arm just above the elbow and just tight enough to stop blood flow. The subject should also be instructed to clench the fist to aid in building up the blood pressure in the area of the puncture.

1. Assemble all the materials required for blood collection, like disposable syringe and needle, alcohol, gauze or cotton, collection bottle, and so on.
2. Decide on the total amount of blood to be collected; for example, if a total hemogram is required, 2 ml of blood will be sufficient. Keep the required anticoagulant (details described below) in the collection bottle.
3. Wash your hands and put on sterilised/disposable gloves.
4. Reassure the subject. Ask him to sit alongside the table, keeping his arm on the table with palm facing upwards.

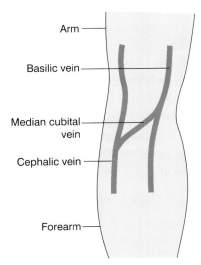

Fig. 2.4   Forearm veins. Median cubital vein is used for venipuncture.

Note: Never draw blood from a patient in standing posture.

5. Select the puncture site carefully after inspecting the arm. Using the index finger of your left hand, feel for the vein where you will introduce the needle.
6. Make the vein prominent by asking the subject to clench his fist. If necessary, apply a tourniquet above the elbow.
7. Clean the area with cotton touched with alcohol.
8. Remove the syringe and needle from the protective wrap. Assemble them and see that the needle is fixed tightly with the syringe. Do not touch the needle.

Note: Ensure that the needle is not blocked and the syringe does not contain air.

9. Grasp the elbow of the subject with your left hand and hold his arm fully extended. Anchor the vein with your thumb, drawing the skin tight over the vein to prevent it from moving.
10. Hold the syringe in the right hand and position the needle to keep the bevel upward, and then push it firmly and steadily into the centre of the vein. First enter the skin and then the vein, at a 30°– 40° angle.
11. Push the needle along the line of the vein to a depth of 1–1.5 cm.

Note: As the needle enters the vein, there occurs a sudden loss of resistance.

12. Look for blood appearing in the barrel. Slightly pull back the piston and fill the syringe with the required amount of blood.
13. Ask the subject to relax and release the tourniquet.

Note: Always remove the tourniquet before taking the needle out of the vein to prevent the formation of a hematoma.

14. Withdraw the needle from the vein in one rapid movement.
15. Ask the patient to press the site firmly with a cotton wool swab for 3–5 minutes.
16. Remove the needle from the syringe and gently expel the blood into the container. Mix the blood immediately and thoroughly but gently with anticoagulant to prevent clotting.
17. Immediately dispose the set (if disposable) or rinse the syringe and needle with water.

18. Before the subject leaves the laboratory, ascertain that the bleeding has stopped. Otherwise, ask him to continue to apply pressure until the bleeding stops.

Precautions

1. The collection bottle containing anticoagulant should be kept ready before collecting blood.
2. The subject should be seated comfortably and should be reassured.
3. Disposable gloves should always be used to prevent contamination.
4. A disposable syringe and needle should be used to draw the blood.
5. The puncture site should be cleaned with alcohol.
6. The vein should be made prominent before making a puncture.
7. The needle should be held at an angle of 30°–40° and introduced into the vein steadily and firmly.
8. The tourniquet if applied should be removed before taking the needle out of the vein to prevent hematoma formation.
9. The patient should be instructed to press the puncture site for 3–5 minutes with cotton wool to prevent bleeding.
10. To prevent clotting, the blood from the syringe should be immediately transferred to the bottle containing anticoagulant.

DISCUSSION

Causes of Misleading Results Related to Specimen Collection

It is essential to have standard procedure for collection and handling of blood specimen, as the constituents of blood may get altered due to faulty procedure of collection (Table 2.1).

Differences Between Capillary and Venous Blood

The constituents of capillary and venous blood are not identical (Table 2.2). Though the blood obtained by skin puncture (capillary blood) is mainly the capillary blood, it also contains some quantity of a mixture of blood from arterioles and venules, and also the

Table 2.1   Factors that may alter the results due to improper collection procedure.

A. Precollection factors
1. Physical activity like fast walking within 20 min.
2. Smoking within 1 hour
3. Drugs within 8 hours or dietary supplement
4. Food or water intake within 2 hours
5. Urination within 30 min.
6. Stress

B. Factors during collection
1. Excessive negative pressure when drawing blood into the syringe
2. Incorrect type of tube
3. Hemoconcentration due to prolonged application of tourniquet
4. Time of collection (Morning/Day/Evening/Night): diurnal variation
5. Posture (Standing/Sitting/Lying)
6. Capillary blood versus venous blood

C. Improper handling of specimen
1. Improper quantity (less or excess) of anticoagulant
2. Inadequate mixing of blood with anticoagulant
3. Delay in dispatch to laboratory
4. Inadequate specimen storage condition
5. Error in identification of patient
6. Error in identification of specimen

interstitial and intracellular fluid, whereas the blood of venipuncture is only the venous blood. Arterial blood is usually not required for tests performed in the hematology laboratory for I MBBS Physiology students.

Anticoagulants

Anticoagulants prevent blood from clotting. They are added to the blood sample, especially when blood is collected by venipuncture, and sent to the laboratories for investigation. Several anticoagulants are available, but some of the standard and commonly used anticoagulants in hematology are EDTA, trisodium citrate, double oxalate, sodium fluoride and heparin. EDTA is usually used in hematology while citrated blood is used for coagulation studies and in blood banks. Use of heparin and fluoride (oxalated) is limited to testing of blood gases (and pH) and plasma glucose respectively.

EDTA (Ethylenediamine Tetra-acetic Acid)

This is also known as sequestrene or versene. The sodium and potassium salts of EDTA are powerful anticoagulants.

Table 2.2   Differences between capillary and venous blood.

	Capillary blood	Venous blood
1. Collection procedure	Skin puncture of fingertip, earlobe, etc.	Venipuncture of superficial veins
2. Type of specimen	Capillary blood mixed with small quantity of blood from arterioles and venules	Venous blood
3. Contamination with tissue fluid	May contain tissue fluid, especially if the finger is squeezed to collect blood	Does not contain tissue fluid
4. Difference in counts	PCV, RBC and Hb concentration of capillary blood are slightly less than that of venous blood. TLC and neutrophil counts are higher by 8%, and monocyte count by 12%, especially in children.	Platelet count is higher in venous blood than in capillary blood. This may be due to adhesion of platelets to the site of skin puncture.
5. Preferred	When individual count or less number of counts are done	When more number of counts or complete hemogram is needed that requires more blood

Preparation

Prepare a 10 per cent solution of dipotassium salts of EDTA. Dissolve 10 g of salt in about 80 ml of water in a 100 ml volumetric flask and then make up the volume of the solution to 100 ml. Dipotassium salts of EDTA are preferred over disodium salts of EDTA as the former are more soluble.

Mechanism of action

EDTA acts by its chelating effect on the calcium molecules of the blood. Calcium is one of the important factors required in the coagulation process.

Effective concentration

To achieve the chelating effect, a concentration of 1.2 mg of the anhydrous salt per ml of blood is required. Excess of EDTA, irrespective of its salts, affects both red cells and leucocytes, causing shrinkage and degenerative changes. If the concentration of the anticoagulant is high, it causes distortion of cells. EDTA in excess of 2 mg/ml of blood may result in a significant decrease in packed cell volume (PCV) by centrifugation and increase in mean cell hemoglobin concentration (MCHC). The platelets are also affected. They swell and then disintegrate causing an artificially high platelet count, as the fragments are large enough to be counted as normal platelets. Therefore, care must be taken to ensure that the correct amount of EDTA is added, and by repeated inversions of the container, the blood is thoroughly mixed with the anticoagulant.

Uses

EDTA is suitable for all routine hematological investigations except coagulation studies.

Sodium Citrate

Trisodium citrate (32 g/l, $Na_3C_6H_5O_7 \cdot 2H_2O$) is the anticoagulant of choice in coagulation studies.

Preparation

It is prepared as a 0.106 M solution of trisodium citrate in distilled water and then sterilised.

Mechanism of action

Sodium citrate prevents coagulation by inactivating calcium ions (chelating effect).

Concentration

Nine volumes of blood are added to one volume of sodium citrate (9 : 1) solution for anticoagulation studies. If it is used in estimation of ESR (erythrocyte sedimentation rate), four volumes of venous blood are added to one volume of the sodium citrate (4 : 1) solution.

Uses

It is used for coagulation studies, including prothrombin times and partial thromboplastin tests, in blood banks, and in the estimation of ESR, especially by the Westergren method.

Double Oxalate

This is an anticoagulant containing ammonium oxalate and potassium oxalate. Therefore, it is called double oxalate. Potassium oxalate alone causes shrinkage of red cells whereas ammonium oxalate increases their volume. So, double oxalate is also called **balanced oxalate** as it preserves cell morphology.

Preparation

Double oxalate is prepared as a solution containing 1.2 per cent ammonium oxalate and 0.8 per cent potassium oxalate. Double oxalate solution 0.25–0.5 ml is delivered into penicillin bottles and evaporated in an oven (60°C) or incubator (37°C) and then kept for collecting blood.

Mechanism of action

The oxalates in the anticoagulant form an insoluble complex with the calcium in the blood, and thereby inhibit coagulation. When calcium ions are combined with oxalate and are therefore not available to participate in clotting, the blood does not clot.

Uses

This is used for estimation of ESR, PCV or investigations in which the volume of the cells should not be affected.

Sodium Fluoride

This anticoagulant is used mainly for preparing blood specimens for plasma glucose estimation. Fluoride is an inhibitor of glycolytic enzymes and thus prevents loss of glucose. However, fluoride is not a strong anticoagulant, and hence, it is mixed with the oxalate.

Oxalates

Oxalates of sodium, potassium, ammonium or lithium as dry additives act as anticoagulants. They form insoluble complexes with calcium and therefore calcium is not available to participate in clotting.

Heparin

Heparin is, theoretically, the best anticoagulant because it is a natural constituent of blood and introduces no foreign contaminants into the blood specimen.

Preparation

Sodium, lithium, potassium and ammonium salts of heparin are commercially available. Suitable concentration of stock solution is prepared and the required amount is taken in a penicillin bottle and dried at room temperature.

Mechanism of action

It prevents coagulation for approximately 24 hours by inhibiting the action of thrombin, thus preventing formation of fibrin from fibrinogen.

Concentration

Heparin is used at a concentration of 10–20 IU/ml of blood. In this concentration, it does not alter the size of red cells.

Uses

It is used for blood gas determination and pH assays. It is the best anticoagulant for the osmotic fragility test. It is inferior to EDTA for general use and should not be used for leucocyte count as it promotes clumping of the leucocytes. It is also not used for differential count as it gives a blue colour to the background.

VIVA

1. *Name the methods of blood collection.*
2. *Name the sites of skin puncture for collecting capillary blood.*
3. *What are the important precautions for fingertip puncture?*
4. *Why are middle three fingers preferred for fingertip puncture?*
5. *What are the advantages and disadvantages of earlobe puncture?*
6. *What are the indications for heel puncture?*
7. *Which are the veins that are preferred for venipuncture?*
8. *List the precautions for venipuncture.*
9. *List the factors that may alter the results of blood counts due to improper procedure of blood collection.*
10. *List the differences between capillary blood and venous blood.*
11. *Name some anticoagulants; give their mechanism of action and specific uses.*

CHAPTER 3

Estimation of Hemoglobin Concentration

Learning Objectives

After completing this practical, you will be able to (MUST KNOW):

1. Describe the clinical importance of estimation of hemoglobin.
2. Estimate hemoglobin by Sahli's acid hematin method.
3. List the precautions and sources of error of estimation of Hb.
4. List the advantages and disadvantages of Sahli's method.
5. Name the other methods for estimation of Hb.
6. Give the normal values of Hb in males and females and in different age groups.
7. List the functions of Hb.
8. List the common conditions of decreased and increased Hb concentration in the blood.
9. Define anemia.
10. List the common causes of anemia in developing countries.

You may also be able to (DESIRABLE TO KNOW):

1. Describe the synthesis and structure of Hb.
2. Classify Hb.
3. Describe different complexes and derivatives of Hb.
4. Explain the principle of other methods of Hb estimation.
5. Compare the merits and demerits of different methods.
6. Explain the variation of Hb concentration in different conditions.
7. Briefly describe different types of anemia.

INTRODUCTION

Hemoglobin (Hb) is a conjugated protein present in red blood cells. It carries O_2 from the lungs to the tissues, and CO_2 from the tissues to the lungs. It is made up of heme and globin. The heme group is an iron complex containing one iron atom. Iron is essential for the primary function of hemoglobin, i.e., the transport of oxygen. When reduced hemoglobin is exposed to oxygen at increased pressure, oxygen is taken up at the iron atom until each molecule of hemoglobin has bound four oxygen molecules, one molecule at each iron atom. This is not a true oxidation–reduction reaction, and therefore, the combination of hemoglobin with oxygen is known as oxygenation. When the Hb molecule is fully saturated with oxygen, that is, when four oxygen molecules combine with one hemoglobin molecule, it is called oxyhemoglobin. One gram of hemoglobin carries 1.34 ml of oxygen. Hemoglobin returning with carbon dioxide from the tissues is called reduced hemoglobin.

Synthesis and Structure of Hemoglobin

Hemoglobin is made up of two components: heme and globin. It is synthesised in the precursors of red cells during their development in the bone marrow.

It appears in the early normoblast stage and attains maximum concentration in the late normoblast stage (*for details, refer* Chapter 7).

Heme

Heme is a complex molecule, made up of a series of tetrapyrrole rings, terminating in protoporphyrin, with a central iron atom. After their normal lifespan (120 days), the red cells are destroyed by the reticuloendothelial cells especially in the spleen, and the components of hemoglobin undergo metabolic degradation. The iron part of heme is recycled and used up again in hemoglobin synthesis. The only component of Hb that cannot be recycled is protoporphyrin, which forms **bilirubin**. Bilirubin is finally converted to various bile salts and pigments.

Globin

Globin is a protein substance that consists of four chains of amino acids (polypeptides). Each polypeptide chain is attached to a heme moiety to form a single hemoglobin molecule. After the degradation of hemoglobin, the globin component breaks down into its amino acid constituents that are recycled for hemoglobin synthesis.

Types of Hemoglobin

Hemoglobins can be broadly divided into normal and abnormal types.

- ◆ **Normal Hb**   Adult Hb, fetal Hb and embryonic Hb.
- ◆ **Abnormal Hb** HbS, HbC, HbD, HbE and unstable hemoglobins.

Normal Hemoglobins

Adult hemoglobins

Hemoglobin A (HbA)   About 97 per cent of hemoglobins of adult red cells is HbA. It consists of two α and two β chains with the structural formula $\alpha_2\beta_2$. HbA is detected in small amounts in the fetus as early as the eighth week of intrauterine life. During the first few months of postnatal life, HbA almost completely replaces HbF and the adult pattern is fully established in six months.

Hemoglobin A_2 (HbA$_2$)   This is the minor hemoglobin in the adult red cell. It has the structural formula $\alpha_2\delta_2$. HbA$_2$ is present in very small amounts at birth and reaches the adult level of 3 per cent during the first year of life. Its concentration increases in some types of anemia.

Fetal hemoglobins

Fetal hemoglobin (HbF)   HbF is the major hemoglobin in intrauterine life. It has the structural formula $\alpha_2\gamma_2$. HbF accounts for 70–90 per cent of hemoglobins at term. It then falls rapidly to 25 per cent in one month, and 5 per cent in six months. The adult level of 1 per cent is not reached in some children until puberty. HbF concentration in adults increases in some types of anemia, hemoglobinopathies and sometimes in leukemia.

Hemoglobin Bart's (Hb Bart's)   This is the minor hemoglobin present in fetal life. It consists of four gamma (γ) chains, γ_4. Hb Bart's concentration increases in fetal life in thalassemia.

Embryonic hemoglobins

These hemoglobins are confined to the very early stages (the embryonic stage) of development. There are three embryonic hemoglobins:

1. **Hb Gower 1** (consisting of two zeta and two epsilon chains: $\zeta_2\varepsilon_2$),
2. **Hb Gower 2** (consisting of two alpha and two epsilon chains: $\alpha_2\varepsilon_2$), and
3. **Hb Portland** (consisting of two zeta and two gamma chains: $\zeta_2\gamma_2$).

Abnormal hemoglobins

There are four clinically important abnormal hemoglobins: HbS, HbC, HbD and HbE. These are present in different hereditary hemoglobinopathies. The most commonly encountered hemoglobin is HbS, which consists of $\alpha_2\beta_2$, but in the beta chain, valine is substituted for glutamic acid at the sixth position. HbS is present in sickle cell anemia.

Unstable hemoglobins are hemoglobin variants that undergo denaturation and precipitate in the red cells as **Heinz bodies**. Unstable hemoglobins are present in a type of congenital non-spherocytic hemolytic anemia.

Hemoglobin Complexes

Hb can combine with other substances besides oxygen, some normally and some abnormally. Some of these commonly encountered complexes are carbaminohemoglobin, carboxyhemoglobin, methemoglobin, sulfhemoglobin and cyanmethemoglobin.

Carbaminohemoglobin

When CO_2 combines with Hb, carbaminohemoglobin is formed. CO_2 combines with amino groups in the polypeptide chains of globin, not with heme. It helps in the transport of CO_2 from the tissues to the lungs.

Carboxyhemoglobin

When hemoglobins combine with carbon monoxide (CO), carboxyhemoglobin is formed. Hemoglobin has a much greater affinity for CO than for oxygen. Therefore, it readily combines with CO even when CO is present in low concentration. Fortunately the formation of carboxyhemoglobin is reversible, so, once CO is removed from the blood, the hemoglobin combines with oxygen. Carboxyhemoglobin is found in very low concentrations in normal persons, but in smokers, its concentration is in the range of 1–10 g/dl, which impairs transport of oxygen from the lungs to the tissues.

Methemoglobin

Methemoglobin is an abnormal Hb in which iron is oxidised from its ferrous state to ferric state. Therefore, it is incapable of carrying oxygen.

Normally, it is present in low concentration, but its formation increases in the presence of certain chemicals or drugs. The formation of methemoglobin is also reversible.

Sulfhemoglobin

This is an abnormal Hb complex formed by the action of some drugs and chemicals such as sulphonamides. Once it is formed, it is irreversible and remains in the carrier RBC. It is incapable of transporting oxygen.

Cyanmethemoglobin (Hemiglobincyanide)

This is formed by the action of a chemical called cyanide (for example, potassium cyanide, KCN). The combination is reversible. Hemiglobin is the hemoglobin in which the iron has been oxidised to the ferric state. Hemiglobincyanide is the methemoglobin bonded to cyanide ions.

> Note: To accurately measure the total Hb in the blood, it is essential to prepare a stable derivative that will contain all the Hb forms (complexes) that are present in the blood. All forms of circulating hemoglobin are readily converted to hemoglobincyanide (cyanmethemoglobin), except for sulfhemoglobin which is normally not present in the blood. Therefore, the cyanmethemoglobin method is the most accurate method for the determination of hemoglobin.

Hemoglobin Derivatives

When red blood cells are destroyed in the tissue macrophage system, hemoglobin is degraded into heme and globin. Globin returns to the body's metabolic pool where its amino acids are subsequently reutilised. The porphyrin ring of heme is cleaved by the microsomal enzyme, heme oxidase, yielding **biliverdin**. The biliverdin is further reduced to form **bilirubin** by biliverdin reductase.

Normal Values

Adult males   : 14–18 (16 ± 2) g/dl of blood
Adult females : 12–16 (14 ± 2) g/dl of blood

In newborns, hemoglobin concentration is normally 14–20 g/dl. It decreases to 9–14 g/dl by about two months of age. By ten years of age, the normal hemoglobin concentration will be 12–14 g/dl. There may be a decrease in hemoglobin level after 60 years of age.

Functions of Hemoglobin

Hemoglobin serves two important functions: the transport of gases and pH homeostasis. However, Hb also contributes to tissue blood flow.

1. It transports oxygen from the lungs to the tissues by forming oxyhemoglobin, and carbon dioxide from the tissues to the lungs by forming carbaminohemoglobin. When fully saturated, **1 g of hemoglobin carries 1.34 ml of oxygen.**

2. Hemoglobin acts as an important buffer in maintaining blood pH. In fact, Hb is an important non-bicarbonate buffer system of the body.

3. Hb to some extent contributes to regulation of tissue blood flow. Hb has sufficient affinity for another gas in the blood, nitric oxide (NO), which is a strong vasodilator. In the tissue, as Hb picks up NO, vasoconstriction occurs due to relative decrease in NO concentration, which in turn decreases tissue blood flow. In the lungs, Hb picks up super nitric oxide (SNO) and by altering SNO level, controls pulmonary blood flow. However, the role of Hb in the regulation of systemic blood volume, peripheral resistance and blood pressure is negligible.

METHODS

The different methods of estimation of hemoglobin can be classified under the following categories:
I. Visual methods
  1. Sahli's method
  2. Dare's method
  3. Haden's method
  4. Wintrobe's method
  5. Haldane's method
  6. Tallquist's method
II. Gasometric method
III. Spectrophotometric method
  1. Oxyhemoglobin method
  2. Cyanmethemoglobin method
IV. Automated hemoglobinometry
V. Non-automated hemoglobinometry
VI. Other methods
  1. Alkaline-hematin method
  2. Specific gravity method
  3. Comparator method

Visual methods are more commonly used than photometric methods. In Sahli's method, hemoglobin in the blood sample is converted to acid hematin which gives a brown colour. Since brown is more easily **matched** by the human eye than red (the colour of Hb), Sahli's method for testing hemoglobin is one of the most acceptable visual methods. However, the error in visual methods is higher. Therefore, visual methods are usually not recommended for hemoglobin estimation in research. But, because visual methods (especially Sahli's) are convenient and the cost of estimation is less, they are usually practised in clinical hematology laboratories and by students performing physiology practicals in medical colleges.

Sahli's Acid Hematin Method

Principle

Hemoglobin is converted to acid hematin by the action of HCl. The acid hematin solution is further diluted until its colour exactly matches that of the permanent standard of the comparator block. The hemoglobin concentration is read directly from the calibration tube.

Requirements

1. **Sahli's hemoglobinometer** This contains a comparator, hemoglobin tube, hemoglobin pipette and stirrer.

    Comparator At the middle there is a slot which accommodates the hemoglobin tube. Non-fading, standard, brown-tinted glass pieces are provided on either side of the slot for colour matching. An opaque white glass is fitted at the back to provide uniform illumination (Fig. 3.1).

    Hemoglobin tube It is graduated on one side in gram per cent (g%), from 2 to 24, and on the other side as percentage (%), from 10 to 140. This tube is called the Sahli–Adams tube.

    Hemoglobin pipette The pipette bears only one mark indicating 20 mm^3 (0.02 ml) (Fig. 3.2). There is no bulb in this pipette.

    Stirrer It is a thin glass rod used for stirring the solution.
2. N/10 HCl
3. Distilled water
4. Dropper
5. Materials for a sterile finger prick

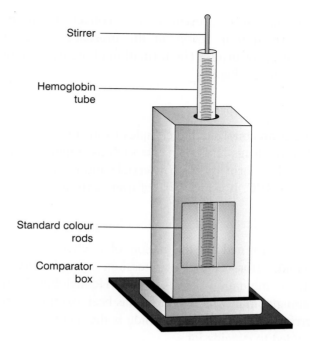

Fig. 3.1   Sahli's hemoglobinometer.

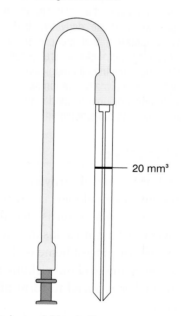

20 mm^3

Fig. 3.2   The hemoglobin pipette.

Procedure

1. Clean the hemoglobinometer tube and pipette and ensure that they are dry.
2. Fill the hemoglobinometer tube with N/10 HCl up to its lowest mark (10 per cent or 2 g%) with the help of a dropper.
3. Prick the finger observing all aseptic precautions, and discard the first drop of blood.

Note: The prick should be deep enough to enable spontaneous flow of blood. Do not squeeze the finger to bring out the drop of blood.

4. Allow a large drop of blood to form on the finger tip, then dip the tip of the hemoglobinometer pipette into the drop and suck blood up to the 20 cu. mm mark of the pipette (Fig. 3.3).

Note: While sucking blood into the pipette, care should be taken to prevent entry of air bubbles. This is done by not lifting the tip of the pipette out of the blood drop during pipetting. If an air bubble enters, remove and discard the blood and obtain another drop of blood to re-pipette. If blood is sucked above the 20 mm³ mark of the pipette, bring the blood column down to the mark by tapping the pipette against the finger, but not by using any absorbent material like cotton wool.

5. Wipe the tip of the pipette. Immediately transfer the 0.02 ml of blood from the pipette into the hemoglobinometer tube containing N/10 HCl by immersing the tip of the pipette in the acid solution and blowing out blood from the pipette. Rinse the pipette two to three times by drawing up and blowing out the acid solution. Withdraw the pipette from the tube.

Note: Make sure that no solution remains in the pipette.

6. Leave the solution in the tube in the hemoglobinometer, for about ten minutes (for maximum conversion of hemoglobin to acid hematin, which occurs in the first ten minutes).

7. After ten minutes, dilute the acid hematin by adding distilled water drop by drop. Mix it with the stirrer. Match the colour of the solution in the tube with the standards of the comparator.

Note: After addition of every drop of distilled water, the solution should be mixed and the colour of the solution should be compared with the standard. While matching, take care to hold the stirrer above the level of the solution. However, remember that at no stage should the stirrer be taken out of the tube (Fig. 3.4).

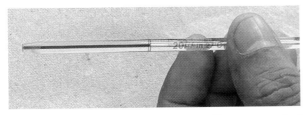

Fig. 3.3   Pipetting of blood exactly up to the 20 cu mm mark of the Hb pipette.

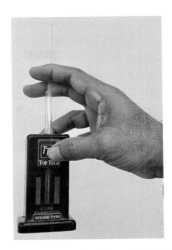

Fig. 3.4   Procedure of holding the stirrer. Note that it is kept above the Hb solution in the pipette, but never taken entirely out of the pipette.

8. If the colour of the test solution is darker, continue dilution till it matches that of the standard (Fig. 3.5).

9. Note the reading when the colour of the solution exactly matches the colour of the standard and express the hemoglobin content as g%.

Note: The reading of the lower meniscus of the solution should be noted as the result. One more drop of distilled water should be added and the colour should be observed to check the result. The colour will be lighter than the standard if the previous reading was accurate.

Precautions

1. A large volume of N/10 HCl (above the 20 per cent mark) should not be taken in the tube. This

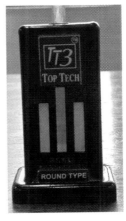

Fig. 3.5   Matching of the colour of Hb solution with that of the standard. The colour of the three bars should be the same and match exactly.

is because, in cases of severe anemia, the final colour produced will be lighter than that of the standard if more HCl is taken, and there is no way to concentrate the colour.

2. The pricking should be done boldly; the finger should not be squeezed as the tissue fluid comes out with the blood and gives a false low result.

3. The first drop of blood should be discarded as it is mixed with tissue fluid.

4. Blood should be sucked exactly up to the 20 mm^3 mark.

5. The tip of the pipette should be wiped before transferring blood from the pipette to the hemoglobinometer tube. Otherwise the extra blood adhering to the tip of the pipette will give a false high result.

6. Blood should be immediately transferred from the pipette into the tube containing HCl to prevent clotting in the pipette.

7. While transferring the blood, the pipette should be rinsed several times to remove all blood from the pipette.

8. A minimum of ten minutes after mixing blood with HCl should be given, for complete conversion of hemoglobin into acid hematin.

9. The colour of the acid hematin solution should be checked frequently (preferably after addition and mixing of every drop of distilled water), to prevent overdilution.

10. When the colour of the solution in the tube is compared with that of the standard, the stirrer should be kept above the solution but should not be taken out of the tube. If the stirrer is taken out of the tube, the solution sticking to the stirrer will be lost and will give a false low result. If the stirrer remains in the solution, the colour of the solution becomes lighter.

11. Comparison should always be done by holding the hemoglobinometer at eye level, at full arm length and against good light (Fig. 3.6). The tube should be placed in the comparator in such a way that the graduations on it do not lie directly in front, which may interfere with the matching of colour.

Sources of Error

A. Technical errors

i) Blood should be taken exactly up to the 20 mm^3 mark and the tip of the pipette should be wiped off

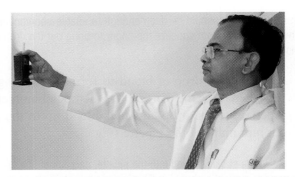

Fig. 3.6   Procedure of observing for matching the colour of Hb pipette with the standard. Note that the hemoglobinometer is held at arm-length, at eye-level and against a bright background.

before introducing the blood into the HCl taken in the hemoglobinometer tube.

ii) Ten minutes should be allowed for complete conversion of Hb into acid hematin.

iii) The solution should be diluted till the colour exactly matches that of the standard.

B. Errors inherent in the method

i) As it is a visual method, the matching of the colour may vary.

ii) It may not detect all types of hemoglobins in the blood.

iii) The colour of the standard may fade.

Reporting

As the hemoglobinometer tube has % markings on one side and g% markings on the other, the hemoglobin estimated can be reported as either of the values, that is, % of normal or g%. Usually, hemoglobin is reported as grams of hemoglobin per 100 ml of blood (g/dl or g%). Reporting hemoglobin as a percentage of the normal value is not satisfactory, because there are many methods and each method has its own standard of normal value. For example, 80 per cent of normal of one method may be 98 per cent of normal of another. The values for 100 per cent hemoglobin in five different testing methods are as follows:

Sahli	16.3 g/dl
Dare	16.0 g/dl
Haden	15.6 g/dl
Wintrobe	14.5 g/dl
Haldane	13.8 g/dl

Therefore, if it is reported as a per cent of the normal, the method by which it is estimated should also be mentioned.

Advantages

1. Sahli's method is easy to perform and convenient.
2. The cost is minimal.
3. It is not very time-consuming (maximum fifteen minutes).

Disadvantages

1. Being a visual method, error is very likely (about 5–10 per cent). Error can be reduced by taking the average of three readings; first, when the colour is slightly darker than the standard; second, when the colour exactly matches the standard; and the third, when the colour is slightly lighter than the standard.
2. The colour of the standard may not always be reliable, especially if an old apparatus was used.
3. Sahli's acid hematin method does not estimate all the hemoglobins. It estimates only oxyhemoglobin and reduced hemoglobins, but not the carboxyhemoglobin, methemoglobin and sulfhemoglobin.
4. The acid hematin is not a true solution. Some degree of precipitation may be present at times, which may interfere with colour matching.

Other Methods

Gasometric Method

The gasometric method of estimation of hemoglobin by using van Slyke apparatus is the **most accurate** method. But it is not used routinely in clinical laboratories because it is time-consuming and the process of estimation is complex. It is used as a reference method to obtain the hemoglobin concentration in blood samples used for standardisation of hemoglobin estimation procedures. This is the preferred method for research.

Spectrophotometric Method

These methods are rapid and give accurate results.

a) Oxyhemoglobin method

Ammonium hydroxide (0.04 ml/dl) is used to hemolyse the red cells and convert the hemoglobin to oxyhemoglobin for measurement in the spectrophotometer. This conversion is complete and immediate and the resulting colour is stable.

b) Cyanmethemoglobin method

Modified Drabkin's reagent is used in this method. Drabkin's reagent contains sodium bicarbonate, potassium ferricyanide and potassium cyanide. This reagent takes at least ten minutes for complete conversion of hemoglobin to cyanmethemoglobin. It also produces turbid solutions caused by protein precipitation or incomplete hemolysis. In modified Drabkin's reagent, potassium phosphate is used for sodium bicarbonate, which shortens the conversion time to three minutes, minimises turbidity and enhances red cell lysis.

Automated Hemoglobinometry

Various automated techniques have been employed to measure hemoglobin. Automatic pipettors and dilutors are used for pipetting and diluting blood in many procedures. Hemoglobin estimation by an automated instrument applies the same principle as that described for manual methods.

Non-automated Hemoglobinometry

Disposable, self-filling, self-measuring dilution micropipettes are commercially available for the determination of hemoglobin. One such system is the Unopette. These systems are easy to use and are available with a series of different diluting fluids for different purposes.

The Unopette system for hemoglobin determination consists of a self-filling, self-measuring pipette attached to a plastic holder. The pipette is filled with blood automatically by capillary action. A plastic container called a reservoir is filled with modified Drabkin's reagent. The pipette containing blood is inserted into the reagent reservoir, emptied and rinsed according to the manufacturer's instructions. The blood is mixed well with the reagent and is then ready to be read in the spectrophotometer.

Alkaline Hematin Method

The alkaline hematin method is a useful ancillary method, used under special circumstances as it gives a true estimate of total hemoglobin including methemoglobin and sulfhemoglobin. A true solution is obtained, and plasma proteins and lipids have little effect on the colour. The principle is to convert hemoglobin into alkaline hematin, which is in the true solution. There are two methods: the standard method, and the acid-alkaline method.

Specific Gravity Method

This method uses the principle that when a drop of whole blood is dropped into a solution of copper sulphate, which has a given specific gravity, the drop will maintain its own density for approximately 15 seconds. The density of the drop is directly proportional to the amount of hemoglobin in that drop. If that drop is denser than the specific gravity of the solution, the drop will sink to the bottom; if not, it will float on the surface. It is not a quantitative test. However, it is a quick, easy and reasonably accurate technique to screen blood donors for possible anemia. It is also used to detect hematocrit.

Comparator Method

This is a visual method similar to that of the acid hematin method, except that the diluent used is an alkali solution (ammonia solution 0.04 per cent). After mixing with dilute ammonia solution, the intensity of the colour of the hemolysed solution of red blood cells is compared against a standard colour disc in the comparator. This method carries all the disadvantages of Sahli's acid hematin method.

Tallquist Method

This method involves direct visual matching of the red colour of a drop of whole fresh blood on a filter paper with colour standards on a paper. This technique is totally unsatisfactory with a high degree of error, though it is one of the quickest methods.

Haldane Method

In this method, hemolysis of red cells is produced by mixing blood with a hypotonic solution like distilled water. Carbon monoxide is added to the mixture. The colour of the solution is compared with the standard one.

DISCUSSION

Physiological Significance

Hemoglobin is present in red blood cells and it forms more than 90 per cent of the dry weight of these cells. Erythrocytes appear red due to the presence of hemoglobin, which is a red pigment. The primary function of hemoglobin is to carry oxygen from the lungs to the tissues. Therefore, in conditions of hemoglobin deficiency, the tissues suffer from hypoxia. When hemoglobin is released into the plasma, as seen in hemolysis, it is filtered through the renal tubules and appears in the urine (hemoglobinuria). Hemoglobin casts block the renal tubules and cause acute tubular necrosis (acute renal failure). Hemoglobin in the blood (hemoglobinemia) exerts an osmotic effect and increases blood viscosity that affects cardiac output and alters the dynamics of blood flow.

Clinical Significance

Estimation of hemoglobin is the most frequently ordered laboratory test in clinical practice. It is done as part of routine investigation in outpatient departments and also as a bedside test in hospital patients. It is mandatory to check the hemoglobin status of a patient prior to any surgical intervention. Estimation of hemoglobin is usually done to detect anemia because it is convenient and less time-consuming than the total RBC count. Anemia is said to be present when the hemoglobin level in the blood is below the lower limit of the normal range for the age and sex of the individual. The value of hemoglobin must always be in the normal range appropriate for the age and sex of the individual.

Conditions That Alter Hemoglobin Concentration

Conditions That Decrease Hb Concentration

Physiological
1. Pregnancy (due to hemodilution).
2. Children have lower values than adults.
3. Women have lower values than men because the total RBC count is less in women. This is because estrogen inhibits erythropoiesis in females and there is cyclical loss of blood in women in the reproductive age group, while testosterone stimulates erythropoiesis in males.

Pathological
1. Different types of anemia.
2. Relative decrease in Hb concentration occurs in different pathological conditions that produce

hemodilution as for example, excess ADH secretion as seen in pituitary tumours.

Conditions That Increase Hb Concentration

Physiological
1. High altitude (due to hypoxia)
2. Newborns and infants
3. Excessive sweating (due to hemoconcentration)

Pathological
1. Conditions that produce hemoconcentration (due to loss of body fluid); for example, severe diarrhea, vomiting
2. Conditions that produce hypoxia; for example, congenital heart disease, emphysema
3. Polycythemia vera

Types of Anemia

Anemia is defined as decreased Hb content or RBC count below the range that is normal for the age and gender. Anemia is classified in two ways, morphologically (according to red blood cell indices) and etiologically (according to the cause).

Morphological Types

1. Hypochromic microcytic anemia

The values of MCV, MCH and MCHC are below normal. Such subnormal red cell indices correspond to microcytosis and hypochromia of red cells in the blood film. This is due to a defect in red cell formation in which hemoglobin synthesis is impaired to a greater extent than the synthesis of other cellular components. The most important examples are **iron deficiency anemia** in which there is inadequate iron for formation of the

heme component of the hemoglobin, and **thalassemia** in which the formation of the globin component of hemoglobin is defective.

2. Normochromic normocytic anemia

MCV, MCH and MCHC are within the normal range. The size and hemoglobin concentration of the red cells are normal in the blood film. It usually occurs:
i)   In substantial blood loss (**blood loss anemia**),
ii) In hemolysis (**hemolytic anemia**) and
iii) When red cell production is impaired by bone marrow failure, chronic kidney failure, chronic inflammation or infection (**aplastic anemia**).

3. Macrocytic anemia

The MCV is above the upper limit of the normal. It corresponds to macrocytosis of red cells in the blood film. MCH is also more. However, MCHC is normal or may be sometimes less. The red cells are usually normochromic. A classical example of this type of anemia is megaloblastic anemia, which occurs due to deficiency of vitamin B_{12} or folic acid.

Etiological Types

1. Blood loss
2. Impaired red cell production
   - Inadequate supply of nutrients (deficiency of iron, vitamins and proteins)
   - Aplastic anemia
   - Anemia associated with chronic diseases
   - Anemia associated with renal failure
   - Anemia due to inherited diseases (for example, thalassemia)
3. Excessive red cell destruction (hemolysis)

OSPE

Dilute the blood (from the given sample) for estimation of hemoglobin concentration.

Steps
1. Select the hemoglobin tube.
2. Take N/10 HCl up to the 10 mark.
3. Select the hemoglobin pipette.
4. Take a clean and dry pipette and tube (check dryness).
5. Thoroughly mix blood in the sample by shaking.
6. Suck blood in the pipette up to the 20 mm^3 mark.

7. Wipe the tip of the pipette.
8. Blow the blood into the acid solution in the hemoglobin tube. Wash out the blood from the pipette by repeated drawing in and blowing out of the diluting fluid (two to three times).
9. Note the time (the mixture is kept for ten minutes for conversion of Hb to acid hematin).

VIVA

1. *What is the normal value of hemoglobin in an adult?*
2. *Why is the hemoglobin content of blood lower in women?*
3. *What is the principle of hemoglobin estimation in Sahli's acid hematin method?*
4. *What difference would it make if N/10 HCl is taken above the 20 per cent mark?*

    Ans: If more HCl is taken, the colour of the undiluted solution may be lighter than the standard, especially if there is severe anemia.

5. *Can N/10 HCl be used for dilution?*

    Ans: Yes, because it will not change the colour of the solution. However, tap water should not be used as it causes turbidity and interferes with the colour of the solution.

6. *Why is the result preferably expressed in g/dl rather than in per cent?*
7. *What are the precautions to be observed during hemoglobin estimation?*
8. *Why should the stirrer be kept above the solution, but not taken out of the tube while matching the colour?*
9. *Why should the tip of the pipette be wiped before transferring blood from the pipette into the N/10 HCl in the tube?*
10. *Why should absorbent material not be used for adjusting the level to the 20 mm^3 mark, if more blood is sucked into the pipette?*
11. *Why should ten minutes be allowed before diluting the solution of blood and HCl?*
12. *What are the advantages and disadvantages of Sahli's acid hematin method? What are the possible errors in this method?*
13. *What are the other methods of hemoglobin estimation?*
14. *Which is the quickest method of hemoglobin estimation?*

    Ans: The quickest method is Tallquist's method as it only compares the colour of the blood with that of the standard. However, it is not an accurate method.

15. *Which method is more accurate for hemoglobin estimation, and why?*

    Ans: The most accurate method is the gasometric method using van Slyke apparatus. But because it is time-consuming and complicated, it is not routinely used in laboratories. Of the routinely used tests, the most accurate method is the cyanmethemoglobin method, because it detects all forms of hemoglobin including sulfhemoglobin and methemoglobin.

16. *What are the functions of hemoglobin?*
17. *What is the oxygen-carrying capacity of hemoglobin?*
18. *What are the types of hemoglobins?*
19. *What is the structure of normal adult hemoglobin (HbA)?*
20. *At what stage in erythropoiesis does hemoglobin appear in the red cells?*

    Ans: Hemoglobin appears in the early normoblast stage of erythropoiesis; then the concentration increases and attains its maximum in the late normoblast stage.

21. *What is the fate of hemoglobin in the body?*
22. *What is anemia? What are the types of anemia?*
23. *What is the most common cause of anemia in developing countries like India, and why?*
24. *Give a physiological cause for anemia. What is the physiological basis of anemia in this condition?*
25. *What is megaloblastic anemia and how is it produced?*
26. *What is pernicious anemia?*
27. *What is aplastic anemia?*

CHAPTER 4

Determination of Hematocrit

INTRODUCTION

Hematocrit literally means "blood separation." It measures the percentage of volume of packed red cells. Therefore, hematocrit is also known as **packed cell volume (PCV)**. Hematocrit is a reliable index of the red cell population in the blood. The manually estimated PCV is more reliable than the manually performed red cell count, because much less error is associated with determination of hematocrit. It provides valuable information about the red cells. Therefore, it should always be correlated with the number of red cells and their hemoglobin content. The hematocrit is used in the detection and classification of various types of anemias along with other parameters (hemoglobin and red cell count) of red cell indices.

Normal values

Adult male   : 46% (40–50%)
Adult female : 42% (37–47%)

METHODS

Two manual methods are used for determining hematocrit: the macrohematocrit method and the microhematocrit method. The microhematocrit method has the advantages of using less time and labour, and requiring less blood. The macrohematocrit method is known as the Wintrobe method. Hematocrit is also measured by automated techniques; these have virtually replaced the manual methods in advanced laboratories.

Macrohematocrit Method (Wintrobe Method)

Since a large volume of blood is needed in this procedure, only venous blood can be used.

Principle

Anticoagulated blood is taken in a Wintrobe tube, filled to the graduation mark and then centrifuged for the prescribed length of time. The volume of packed cells is read directly from the graduation mark on the Wintrobe tube.

Requirements

I. Apparatus

1. *Wintrobe tube* This is a 110-mm-long, narrow, thick-walled test tube with a 3 mm internal bore, graduated from 0 to 10 cm (100 mm) with graduations both in ascending and descending order on the two sides of the tube (Fig. 4.1). Thus, at the top, 0 and 10 cm coincide. The scale with the markings 0–10 from above downwards is used in ESR determination, while the scale with 0–10 from below upwards is used for hematocrit determination. It holds about 1 ml of blood.

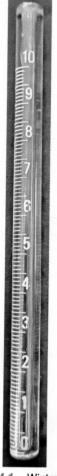

Fig. 4.1   Wintrobe tube.

2. *Centrifuge machine* The centrifuge should be capable of producing a force of 2300 g. A force of less than 2300 g will give a false high hematocrit reading; conversely, an excessive force may lead to false low values. The centrifuge should be standardised for speed and time by taking a reference blood sample and determining the time and speed necessary to obtain the reference value.

3. *Pasteur pipette* It is a 22-cm-long glass tube with a long thin nozzle about 13 cm in length. If Pasteur pipette is not available, a syringe with a Pasteur needle (needle with >13 cm nozzle) can be used. It is used to transfer blood from the container to fill the Wintrobe tube.

II. Blood sample   A sample of venous blood to which EDTA or double oxalate anticoagulant has been added is taken for the study.

Procedure

1. Carefully mix the blood specimen by repeated inversion. Collect blood in the Pasteur pipette or Pasteur needle carefully, ensuring that there is no entry of air bubble into the pipette or needle (Fig. 4.2).

2. Fill the Wintrobe tube with blood with the help of the Pasteur pipette to the 10 cm mark (which represents 100 per cent) (Fig. 4.3). If the level of blood crosses the mark, use a dropper to remove the extra blood. Do not use a cotton swab or blotting paper or any other absorbent material for this purpose. Otherwise, note the error from the top of the blood column, which can be deducted from the final result.

Note: Filling the Wintrobe tube requires special care since air bubbles may be trapped and cause damage to the red blood cells. To avoid this, place the tip of the pipette at the bottom of the Wintrobe tube and fill from the bottom, gradually withdrawing the pipette as the blood goes in. Try to keep the tip of the pipette under the rising column of blood to avoid foaming.

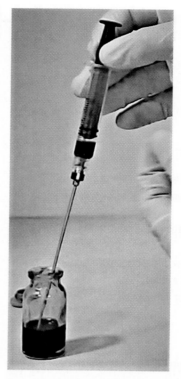

Fig. 4.2   Collection of blood for estimation of hematocrit by Wintrobe method. Syringe with a long nozzle needle (>13 cm length) is used. The tip of the needle should enter the blood column in the vial, so that air bubbles do not enter the syringe. Use of gloves is a must when a hospital sample is used for the purpose.

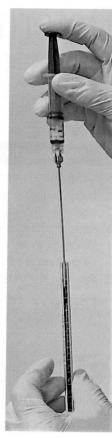

Fig. 4.3 Collection of blood in Wintrobe tube exactly up to the 10 mark.

3. Place the Wintrobe tube in one of the cups of the centrifuge, and place a Wintrobe tube containing water in the opposite cup of the centrifuge, to balance it.

4. Turn the centrifuge on to slow speed, then increase the speed gradually, and finally bring it up to the required speed.

5. Centrifuge for 30 minutes at 3000 rpm.

6. After 30 minutes, switch off the centrifuge and allow it to stop by itself. Do not use the brake. Take out the Wintrobe tube and read the PCV directly off the graduation given on the tube. If, for example, the red cell column is one division above the graduation mark of 4, the reading is 41, or the hematocrit is 41 per cent.

Note: A buffy coat (*refer* Fig. 1.1) is the thin grey-white layer of white cells at the top of the red cell column. Do not include this while reading the height of the red cell column.

Precautions

1. Hematocrit should be determined ideally within six hours of collection of blood.
2. Mix the blood thoroughly before taking the sample for hematocrit determination.
3. Do not use a hemolysed specimen. It will yield false low results.
4. A suitable anticoagulant should be used in proper concentration. The anticoagulant should not affect the size and shape of red cells.
5. If the blood is present above the graduation (10 cm) mark, do not remove the excess blood by cotton swab or blotting paper. Use a dropper for this purpose.
6. If air bubbles enter the tube while filling the tube with blood, the preparation should be discarded (blood should be removed totally) and the tube should be refilled.
7. Blood should be centrifuged for an adequate time.
8. While taking the reading, exclude the buffy coat.

Advantages

1. ESR (by Wintrobe method) can be determined simultaneously by using the same sample. For this, first the Wintrobe tube filled with blood is kept vertically in the Wintrobe rack for one hour (see Chapter 14) to record the ESR, following which the tube is centrifuged to determine the hematocrit.
2. It is not an expensive method.

Microhematocrit Method

This method requires only a small volume of blood. Therefore, it is ideal for a small specimen (for example, sample collected from pediatric patients and burn patients). It can be done with either free-flowing capillary blood from a finger puncture or EDTA-anticoagulated venous blood. Since the test is done with a high-speed centrifuge, it takes less time.

Principle

Anticoagulated blood is centrifuged in a sealed capillary tube, and the volume of packed red cells and percentage of whole blood (level of plasma) are determined by a special hematocrit reader.

Requirements

1. *Capillary hematocrit tubes* These tubes are approximately 75 mm in length, and have an internal diameter of approximately 1 mm. For anticoagulated venous blood, simple capillary tubes can be used. For blood collected by skin puncture, heparinised tubes should be used.

2. *Microhematocrit centrifuge* This is a special centrifuge that runs at high speed and is capable of producing a force of 12,000 *g*, and runs at a speed of about 12,000 rpm.

3. *Hematocrit reader* There are several hematocrit readers available. The simplest one is the card reader, which can be made by hand.

4. *Modelling clay* This is used to seal the end of the hematocrit tubes.

5. *Sterile skin puncture equipment* Disposable lancet, spirit and needle.

Procedure

1. Perform a sterile skin puncture and draw the blood sample into an appropriate capillary tube by capillary action.

> Note: Use a plain tube for anticoagulated venous blood, or a heparinised tube for skin puncture. The blood should flow freely in this case. Fill three-quarters of the tube.

2. The dry end of the tube is sealed with a specially manufactured plastic sealing clay. These tubes can also be heat-sealed.
3. Place the two sealed hematocrit tubes in the radial grooves of the centrifuge, with their heads opposite each other.
4. Turn the centrifuge on for 5 minutes at 12,000 rpm. Stop the centrifuge, take out the tubes, and read the PCV from the microhematocrit reader.

Precautions

1. The blood sample must be properly collected.
2. Anticoagulated venous blood should be used within six hours of collection.
3. The blood must not be clotted or hemolysed.
4. Centrifugation must be sufficient to yield packing of red cells.

Advantages

1. This procedure needs very little blood, so it can easily be done in pediatric patients and patients suffering from hemoconcentration or blood loss, like burns.
2. It is not a time-consuming test.
3. It can be used in mass surveys, because a large number of specimens can be handled simultaneously.
4. Capillary tubes are easy to fill.
5. The tubes are cheap and the replicates are easily obtainable.

Automated Method

Measurement of hematocrit by automated technique is done by using electronic cell counters. This result is computed from individual red cell volumes and not affected by the trapped plasma left in the red cell column of the manual hematocrit methods. Therefore, the hematocrit value obtained by automated cell counters is accurate and lower than the value obtained by manual methods.

DISCUSSION

Hematocrit or PCV is the percentage of packed red blood cells, following centrifugation. When blood is centrifuged in a tube, the red cells are packed together at the bottom of the tube by centrifugal force, as cells are heavier than the plasma. However, if the cells are deformed as in hereditary spherocytosis or sickle cell disease, more plasma remains between the packed cells, giving a false high result.

Physiological and Clinical Significance

1. Hematocrit is a reasonable index of red cell population or Hb content of blood (Fig. 4.4). Therefore, it is used to detect conditions in which red cell count increases (polycythemia) or decreases (anemia). The hematocrit measurement is more useful and reliable than the red cell count performed manually because less error is associated with it.
2. The value of hematocrit is used in determination of blood indices, especially MCV (mean corpuscular volume) and MCHC (mean corpuscular hemoglobin concentration). Blood indices help in the diagnosis and classification of various types of anemia.

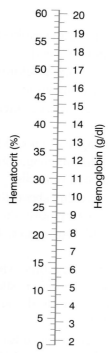

Fig. 4.4 Relationship between hematocrit and hemoglobin.

3. Hematocrit is an important factor that determines viscosity of blood. Increase in hematocrit increases blood viscosity, as observed in polycythemia. This increases peripheral resistance, which in turn decreases cardiac output as the afterload on the heart increases. Conversely, decrease in hematocrit, as seen in anemia, decreases the peripheral resistance that increases cardiac output. This also makes circulation hyperdynamic.

Conditions That Alter Hematocrit

Conditions that decrease hematocrit

Physiological
1. Pregnancy (due to hemodilution)
2. Excess water intake
3. Gender (lower in women)

Pathological
1. Various types of anemia
2. Conditions in which there is hemodilution and expansion of plasma volume; for example, hyperaldosteronism

Conditions that increase hematocrit

Physiological
1. High altitude (due to hypoxia)

2. Newborns and infants
3. Excessive sweating (due to hemoconcentration)

Pathological

1. Decreased oxygen supply to the tissues (hypoxia), for example, congenital heart disease and emphysema

2. Polycythemia
3. Conditions in which there is hemoconcentration, for example, severe vomiting and diarrhea (due to dehydration)

OSPE

Load the Wintrobe tube with the blood supplied for estimation of hematocrit.

Steps:

1. Select a Wintrobe tube.
2. Clean and dry the tube.
3. Mix blood thoroughly by swirling or by repeated inversions.
4. Take blood in the Pasteur pipette.
5. Fill the tube slowly by placing the tip of the pipette at the bottom, inside of the tube. Fill from the bottom by gradually withdrawing the pipette as blood goes in; at the same time, try to keep the tip of the pipette under the rising column of blood to avoid foaming.
6. Fill exactly up to the 0 mark. If blood is poured above the mark, remove the extra blood with the help of a dropper (not by using absorbent materials like cotton or gauze piece).
7. Place the Wintrobe tube in the cups of the centrifuge.

VIVA

1. *What is hematocrit? What is the significance of hematocrit?*
2. *What are the different methods of estimation of hematocrit?*
3. *What are the precautions and sources of error of the microhematocrit method?*
4. *What is the ideal anticoagulant to be used for hematocrit determination and why?*
5. *Why is an anticoagulant used in a recommended concentration for estimation of hematocrit?*
   Ans: The use of higher concentration of anticoagulant gives false low result, because excess EDTA may cause hemolysis.
6. *Why should the hematocrit ideally be determined within six hours of collection of blood?*
   Ans: If blood is kept for longer time, the change in metabolism of the red cells may cause a change in size and shape of the cells. Hemolysis starts after six hours of collection. Therefore, if the estimation of hematocrit cannot be done within six hours, the blood should be preserved in the refrigerator.
7. *What are the sources of error in the Wintrobe hematocrit method?*
   Ans: i) Improper mixing of blood   ii) Improper anticoagulant and improper concentration of anticoagulant
   iii) Inadequate centrifugation   iv) Reading of hematocrit with buffy coat
8. *What is the normal value of hematocrit in adults?*
9. *Why is the value lower in women?*
10. *What are the physiological and pathological conditions that alter hematocrit value?*
11. *Why is the hematocrit value of venous blood slightly higher than that of arterial blood?*
    Ans: Hematocrit value of venous blood is normally 3 per cent more than that of arterial blood because:
    i) Venous blood carries the blood that comes from tissues to the lungs. At the tissue, when one CO_2 molecule is added to the blood (to the red cell), there is an increase in one osmotically active particle that is either a bicarbonate ion or a chloride ion (because of chloride shift). Consequently, the red cells take up water and increase in size. This is the main cause of higher hematocrit in venous blood.
    ii) A small amount of fluid in arterial blood returns via the lymphatics, instead of the veins.

CHAPTER 5

Study of the Compound Microscope

Learning Objectives

After completing this practical, you will be able to (MUST KNOW):
1. Identify different parts of the compound microscope.
2. List the uses of different parts of the microscope.
3. Make microscopic adjustments for viewing the object under low-power, high-power, and oil-immersion objectives.
4. List the precautions to be taken while using the microscope.
5. Handle the microscope carefully.

You may also be able to (DESIRABLE TO KNOW):
1. Describe the principle of microscopy.
2. Explain the physical principles of construction of the compound microscope.
3. Provide the solutions for common problems encountered in microscopy.
4. Explain the basic principles of working of other types of microscopes.

INTRODUCTION

The microscope is usually used in physiology to study the morphology of blood cells and for making different cell counts. Therefore, a physiologist should be competent in microscopy and a student of physiology should learn the basic principles of microscopy. To obtain the best performance from a microscope, one needs to understand the optical principles, the basics of the construction of the microscope, and the scientific basis of routine care and maintenance of the instrument.

A microscope magnifies the image of an object and in simple terms, it is a magnifying glass. The modern compound microscope (light microscope) is one of the most frequently used equipment in medical laboratories for students. Improper use of the microscope leads to loss of clarity of the image, which results in loss of definition. Therefore, it must be kept in excellent condition, optically and mechanically.

Microscopes designed by different manufacturers differ greatly in details of their construction and mode of operation. Therefore, the manufacturer's manual and instructions for operating the microscope must be followed properly before using the instrument.

Physical Terms

The compound microscope consists of two magnifying lenses: the objective and the eyepiece. It is used to magnify an object to a point where it can be seen with the human eye. Before a student learns microscopy, he should understand a few physical terms fundamental to microscopy—the resolution, the working distance and the numerical aperture.

1. Resolution   The limit of useful magnification of a microscope is set by its resolving power, that is, its ability to reveal closely adjacent structural details as separate and distinct. Resolution, therefore, describes how small individual objects can lie close to each other and still be recognisable. Generally, the human eye can separate (or resolve) dots that are 0.25 mm apart; the light microscope can separate dots that are 0.25 mm apart; and the electron microscope can separate dots that are 0.5 nm apart.

> Note: 1 nanometre (nm) = 0.001 micrometre (μm)
> = **0.000 001** mm

The resolving power is expressed quantitatively as the microscope's **limit of resolution (LR)**, that is, the minimum distance between two visible bodies at which they are seen as separate and not in contact with one another. The LR is determined according to the following formula:

$$LR = \frac{0.61 \times W}{NA}$$

where, W is the wavelength of the light rays, and NA is the numerical aperture of the objective in use.

For example, if green light (wavelength 0.55 μm) and oil-immersion objective (NA 1.3) are used, the LR will be 0.25 μm (0.61 × 0.55 / 1.3 = 0.25 μm).

2. Working distance Working distance is the distance between the objective and the objective slide. The working distance decreases with increasing magnification. It is 0.15–1.5 mm in the case of the oil-immersion objective, 0.5–4 mm in the case of high-power, and 5–15 mm in the case of low-power objective.

3. Numerical aperture (NA) The numerical aperture of a lens is the ratio of the diameter of the lens to its focal length. Any particular lens has a constant numerical aperture and this value is dependent on the radius of the lens and its focal length (the distance from the object being viewed to the lens or the objective).

NA of a lens is an index of the resolving power. As the NA increases, the resolution (or distance from each other at which objects can be distinguished) decreases. That means the greater the NA, the greater is the resolving power. The NA for low-power, high-power and oil-immersion objectives are 0.30, 0.65 and 1.30 respectively. The NA is also described as an index of the light-gathering power of a lens, that is, the amount of light entering the objective. The NA can be decreased by decreasing the amount of light that passes through a lens. Therefore, the illumination has also to be increased in the same order when the objectives are changed from low-power to high-power.

PARTS OF THE COMPOUND MICROSCOPE

There are two commonly used compound microscopes: monocular and binocular. Basically, they are the same except that the monocular microscope has one eyepiece (ocular) whereas the binocular microscope has two eyepieces. The structure of the compound microscope can be discussed under four main systems:

1. The support system (the framework)
2. The illumination system
3. The magnification system
4. The adjustment system

The Support System

The support system is the framework of the microscope that holds its components. The framework consists of several units (Fig. 5.1).

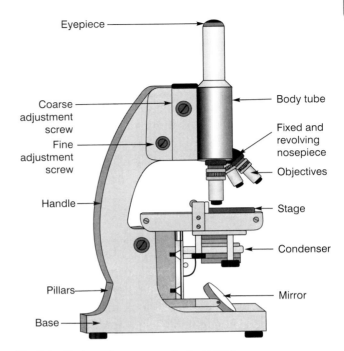

Fig. 5.1 Parts of the compound microscope.

1. Base The base supports the microscope and is horseshoe-shaped to provide maximum stability.

2. Pillars Two upright pillars project upwards from the base, and the handle of the microscope is hinged to the pillars.

3. Handle (arm) The arm supports the magnifying and adjusting systems. It is also the handle by which the microscope can be carried without damaging the delicate parts. It is curved and the microscope can be tilted at the hinged joint when desired.

4. Body tube The body tube is the part through which the light passes to the eyepiece. The length of the tube is usually 160 mm. This is the tube that actually conducts the image.

5. Stage The fixed stage is the horizontal platform on which the object being observed is placed. The centre of the stage has an aperture centre through which the converging cone of light passes. Most microscopes have a mechanical stage which makes it much easier to manipulate the objects being observed. It is calibrated and fitted on the fixed stage. There is a spring-mounted clip to hold the slide or the counting chamber in position, and two screws for moving these transversely, or forwards and backwards.

6. Nosepiece The fixed nosepiece is attached to the lower end of the body tube and the revolving nosepiece is mounted under it. The revolving nosepiece carries the objective lenses of different magnifying powers.

The Illumination System

A microscope cannot function optimally without proper illumination. The illumination system provides uniform and soft-bright illumination of the entire field viewed under the microscope. The illumination system is, therefore, an important part of the compound light microscope.

There are six types of illumination systems based on which the microscopes work:

1. Bright-field or light microscope   This uses white light, either external sunlight or internal tungsten filament lamp, as the source of illumination. When viewed under the microscope, objects look dark or coloured, contrasted against a lighted background.

2. Dark-field microscope   A special dark-field condenser is used that lights up the object, like stars against a dark sky.

3. Fluorescent microscope   This uses a special ultraviolet lamp as the source of illumination. A fluorescent dye is attached to the object through laboratory procedures; this glows when exposed to ultraviolet radiation.

4. Polarising microscope

5. Phase-contrast microscope

6. Interference-contrast microscope

The illumination system of a compound microscope consists of a light source, condenser and iris diaphragm.

Light Source

The illumination system begins with a source of light. This may be internal or external.

Internal source   In most modern compound microscopes, there is a built-in light source with an electric lamp, which provides better control of illumination. The lamp housing has a frosted tungsten lamp, which is placed directly under the stage.

External source   In the students' compound microscope there is no in-built light source. These microscopes use an external source of light. This can be from an electric lamp housed in a lamp box with a window, or from the sun. The rays of light are reflected by a mirror towards the object. The mirror is located at the base of the microscope. It has two surfaces, plane and concave.

The plane mirror is used for the oil-immersion objective whereas the concave mirror is used for the low- and high-power objectives.

Condenser

The condenser focuses the rays of light reflected from the mirror onto the object under examination and also helps in resolving the image. It is mounted below the stage of the microscope with a rack and pinion mechanism for adjusting its focus. Microscopes generally use a substage Abbe-type condenser. This Abbe condenser is composed of two lenses uncorrected for spherical and chromatic aberration. Therefore, for better microscopic examination, a good quality **achromatic condenser** should be used. The condenser can be raised and lowered beneath the stage by means of an adjustment knob. It must be correctly positioned to focus the light properly on the object being viewed, because, being a lens, it has a fixed numerical aperture. The numerical aperture of the condenser should be equal to or slightly less than the numerical aperture of the objective being used. Changing the position of the condenser can vary its numerical aperture. Therefore, the position of the condenser must always be adjusted with each objective used, to get the maximum focus of light and the accurate resolving power of the microscope.

When a low-power objective is used, the condenser is positioned at the lowest level; with a high-power objective, it is raised optimally; and with an oil-immersion objective, it is raised fully. Most modern microscopes do not need a condenser adjustment; the condenser is placed at the highest position and the illumination is adjusted primarily by opening or closing the iris diaphragm.

Iris Diaphragm

The iris diaphragm regulates the amount of light that passes through the material under observation. It is located at the bottom of the condenser. It has a central aperture, which can be opened for more light or closed for less light, according to necessity, by means of a lever provided with a shutter. The size of the aperture regulates the amount of light that passes to the field under observation. Regulation of the light by such means affects the numerical aperture of the condenser. By reducing the field size with the help of the iris diaphragm, the numerical aperture of the condenser is decreased. Thus, proper illumination procedure includes a combination of light intensity regulation, light source position, condenser position, and field size regulation.

The Magnification System

The magnification system plays an extremely important role in the use of a microscope because it magnifies the image of the object under view. The compound microscope consists of two magnifying lenses, the eyepiece and the objective. The total magnification provided by a compound microscope is the product of the magnification contributed by the objective and that by the eyepiece. The eyepiece forms a virtual magnified image of the real magnified image formed by the objective.

Eyepiece

The eyepiece or the ocular is a lens that magnifies the image formed by the objective. It fits into the top of the body tube. Most microscopes are provided with two eyepieces, 5× and 10×, with magnifying powers of 5 and 10 respectively. However, 2×, 8× and 20× eyepieces are also available. Most microscopes have a provision to fit one eyepiece and these are called monocular microscopes (Fig. 5.2), whereas some microscopes have a provision for fitting two eyepieces at a time and these are called binocular microscopes (Fig. 5.3). The magnification produced by the eyepiece

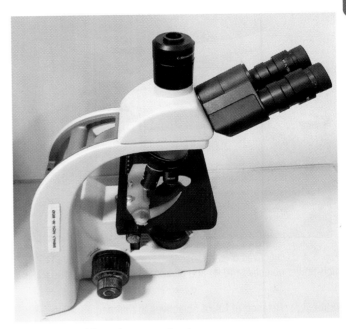

Fig. 5.3 The binocular research microscope.

multiplied by the magnification produced by the objective gives the total magnification of the object being viewed.

Objectives

Objectives are the most important part of the magnification system. Usually, three objectives are screwed into the revolving nosepiece in a compound microscope. The nosepiece is a pivot that ensures a quick change of objectives. The three objectives are (a) 10×: low-power objective, (b) 40× or 45×: high-power objective, and (c) 90× or 100×: oil-immersion objective (Fig. 5.4).

Low-power objective The low-power objective is usually 10×, which magnifies the image 10 times. This objective is used for initial focusing and observation. Some microscopes also have very low-power objectives (3× or 4×), the scanning objectives. These are used in initial scanning of histologic sections.

The numerical aperture (NA) of the low-power objective is always less than that of the condenser in most microscopes. Therefore, to achieve focus, the numerical apertures must be more closely matched by reducing the light to the specimen. This can be achieved by lowering the condenser and by closing the iris diaphragm (iris slightly opened). NA of objectives is related to the magnification capacity of microscope (Table 5.1).

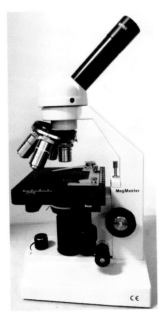

Fig. 5.2 The monocular microscope.

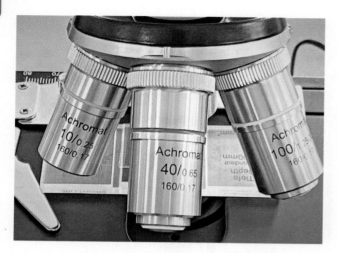

Fig. 5.4 Objectives of a microscope. Low-power objective (10×), high-power objective (40×) and oil-immersion objective (100×).

Table 5.1   Relation of NA of objectives to the magnification.

Objective	NA	Magnification		
		Objective	Eyepiece	Total
Low-power	0.30	10	10	100
High-power	0.65	45	10	450
Oil-immersion	1.30	100	10	1000

High-power objective It is usually a 40× or 45× magnification lens. It magnifies the image 40 or 45 times. This objective is used for more detailed study, as the total magnification (with a 10× eyepiece) is usually 400 or 450 times. It is used for a broad view of blood films or histologic sections prior to their examination under the oil-immersion objective. The numerical aperture of the high-power objective is almost close to (or slightly less than) that of most commonly used condensers. Therefore, the condenser should be slightly raised and the iris be partially opened to achieve maximum focus.

Oil-immersion objective The oil-immersion objective is generally a 90× or 100× lens, which magnifies the image 90 or 100 times. The objective lens almost rests on the slides when in use (Fig. 5.5). It requires a special type of oil called immersion oil, which is placed between the objective and the slide. The most commonly used immersion oil is cedar wood oil. Oil is used to increase the numerical aperture and thus the resolving power of the objective. Light travels through air at a greater speed than through glass; through the immersion oil, light travels at the same speed as through glass. Therefore, the oil is used to decrease the speed at which light travels to increase the effective numerical aperture of the objective. It also decreases the defraction of light rays.

Since the numerical aperture of the oil-immersion objective is always greater than that of the condenser, the condenser should be placed at the highest position and the iris diaphragm should be fully open (Table 5.2). The oil-immersion lens gives a total magnification of 1000 times or 900 times with a 10× eyepiece. Therefore, it is generally used for detailed morphologic examination of blood films or histologic slides.

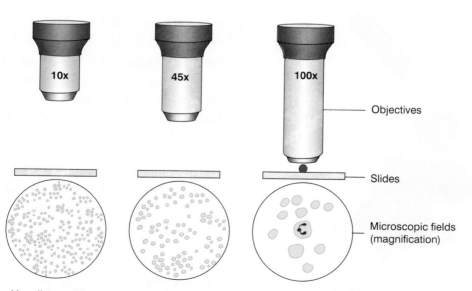

Fig. 5.5   Distance (working distance) between the objective lenses and the object in the three types of objectives. Note the magnification obtained under the three objectives.

Table 5.2 Adjustments in the microscope for using different objectives.

Objective	Mirror	Condenser position	State of iris diaphragm
Low-power	Concave	Lowest	Partially closed
High-power	Concave	Slightly raised	Partially opened
Oil-immersion	Plane	Fully raised	Fully opened

The Adjusting System

The adjusting system consists of two adjustment systems: the coarse adjustment system and the fine adjustment system. The coarse adjustment system is used to obtain an approximate focus whereas the fine adjustment system is used to obtain the exact focus of the object after prior coarse adjustment.

Coarse Adjustment System

Two **coarse adjustment screws** are used for making coarse adjustments. These screws are mounted on the top of the handle by a double-sided micrometer mechanism, one on each side. If one screw is rotated, its member on the opposite side also rotates at the same time. Therefore, there is no need to operate the adjustment screws from both sides simultaneously. If the left hand is used for handling the adjustment screw, the right hand can be used for manipulating the body tube or the mechanical stage. The body tube or stage can be raised or lowered quickly with the coarse adjustment screw.

Fine Adjustment System

Two **fine adjustment screws** are used for making fine adjustments. Usually these screws are mounted on the handle below the coarse adjustment screws by double-sided micrometer mechanisms, one on each side. These screws are operated for fine adjustment and exact focusing of the object.

METHODS

Method of Use of the Microscope

Principle

In the compound microscope, a focused beam of light scans the specimen or object placed on a glass slide on the stage of the microscope. Parts of the specimen that are optically dense, have a high refractive index or are coloured with a stain, cast a potential image like a shadow which is magnified in different stages as it passes up the microscope to the eye.

Requirements

1. Microscope
2. Light source
3. Blood film

Procedure

The microscope should be handled carefully. Before using the microscope, examine it thoroughly. The student should follow the steps given below while using a compound microscope.

1. Place the microscope on the working table in the upright position and adjust the height and position of your chair so that you are comfortable and prepared for prolonged viewing. The eyepieces of the microscope should level with and be close to your eyes while you are sitting upright (Fig. 5.6). Keep your forearms on the table so that you can easily handle the adjustment screws. You need not remove your glasses if you use them constantly.

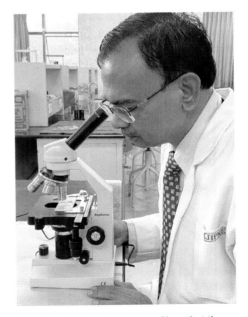

Fig. 5.6 Working with the microscope. Note that the eye position should be at the level of the eyepiece in the upright sitting position; an examiner using spectacles should wear them while viewing through the eyepiece. (*Courtesy:* Physiology Department, Hematology Laboratory, JIPMER, Puducherry, India.)

Note: Observers who wear glasses may be able to dispense with them when using a microscope; if not, they must take care to prevent their spectacles touching and scratching the lenses of the eyepieces.

2. Check that the eyepieces and objectives are free from dust and oil. Use a fresh lens tissue for this purpose.

Note: Only benzol or xylol should be used to remove hardened oil.

3. Provide adequate illumination. If you have to use the external lamp, place it about 20 cm away from the microscope, switch on the lamp and allow the light to fall on the mirror. If you have to use natural light, place the microscope near the window for maximum illumination.

4. Select and adjust the mirror for optimal illumination according to the objective to be used. Direct the path of light to pass through the hole of the stage with maximum intensity while setting the mirror (look from the side to check illumination).

5. Place the slide with the object on the stage, such that it is held by the stage clips and pressed at both ends so as to be in close contact with the surface of the stage.

6. Make various microscopic adjustments to view the object under low-power objective (the correct procedure is to first view the object in low-power). The steps are:
   - Bring the low-power objective (10×) into position by revolving the nosepiece (the objective must click into place).
   - Adjust the illumination to improve contrast. Use the concave mirror, place the condenser at the lowest position, and slightly open the iris.

Note: For low-power, the illumination is cut down to the minimum by reducing the aperture size.

   - Use the coarse focusing adjustment to focus the specimen on the slide.

Note: Never use the fine focusing adjustment until the specimen has been made visible and brought nearly into focus with the coarse adjustment.

   - Use the fine adjustment only to obtain and maintain exact focus. Put one hand on the focusing knob (coarse or fine, one at a time)

and the other on the screw to move the stage.
   - Bring the object of interest to the centre.

7. After preliminary screening under low-power objective, proceed to examine the film under high-power objective. The steps are:
   - Bring the high-power objective (40× or 45×) into position by rotating the nosepiece; make sure that the objective clicks into place.
   - Use the concave mirror, raise the condenser slightly, and check that the iris diaphragm is partially open so that the illumination is properly centred. Increase the illumination as needed.
   - Repeat the process of focusing as described earlier by using the coarse adjustment knob and the fine adjustment knob in sequence.

Note: As the high-power objective does not normally touch the slide (check carefully the distance between the slide and the high-power objective at its lowest position), the use of the coarse and fine adjustment knobs may not be so critical and they can be switched freely.

8. After screening under the low-power and examining under the high-power, use the oil-immersion objective to obtain greater details of the object. The steps are:
   - Swing away the high-power objective and put a tiny drop of immersion-oil on the slide over the path of light.
   - Change the mirror to the plane side.
   - Raise the condenser to maximum (to place below the stage) and open the iris fully to obtain maximum illumination.
   - Turn the nosepiece and set the oil-immersion objective in position; make sure that the objective has clicked into place.
   - Use the fine adjustment knob to get the object in focus. If this fails, look from the side, keep the eye level with the slide and lower the objective carefully with the coarse adjustment knob until the oil-immersion objective touches the oil. Lower the objective further down and stop when the oil-immersion objective touches the slide (caution: avoid pressing hard on the preparation). First, focus the object with the coarse adjustment knob while increasing the gap between the slide and the objective. Finally, focus the object with the help of the fine adjustment knob.

Precautions

1. The microscope should be placed on the working table in a stable position.
2. The height of the observer's chair should be raised to a position that allows for comfortable handling of the microscope.
3. Objectives and eyepieces should be free from dust and oil. Xylol or benzol should be used to remove hardened oil. Lenses should never be touched with the fingers.
4. If natural light is used, the microscope should be kept near the window; if the lamp is used, it should be kept about 20 cm from the microscope, to prevent heating of the microscope.
5. The mirror, the position of the condenser and the aperture of the iris should be checked in order to get proper illumination.
6. While changing the objective, it should be noted that the objective clicks into its proper position. Otherwise the objective may not remain in position.
7. Never bring down the objective with the coarse adjustment while looking through the microscope. You should look from the side.
8. Examination of the specimen under low and high power should always precede examination under the oil-immersion objective.
9. The stage of the microscope should always be brought down before bringing the oil-immersion objective into position. Otherwise it may damage the preparation.
10. The distance between the slide and the objective should always be checked while using the coarse adjustment screw, especially for high-power and oil-immersion objectives.
11. The stage should be always kept clean and not be soiled with specimen material, stain, oil or water.
12. The microscope should be kept covered when not in use.

DISCUSSION

The common difficulties in microscopy and the solutions to these, tips for routine care and maintenance of microscopes, and other types of microscopes are discussed here.

Common Difficulties in Microscopy

A number of difficulties may be encountered by beginners. The following tips are given to overcome them.

1. *Inability to achieve focus or obtain a clear image.*
   i) The failure to find focus may be due to the slide not being brought close enough to the objective to remain within its focal distance, or there may be no visible material on that small area of the slide within the field of the objective. First, move the slide so that the focus material is brought into the field. This procedure will ensure that there is visible material to focus on. Then, with the eyes level with the stage, use the coarse adjustment to raise the slide until it again comes as close as possible to the objective without touching it. Finally, apply the eyes to the eyepieces and use the coarse adjustment to move the objective away from the slide until the specimen is seen in focus.
   ii) Check that no dirt or dried oil has adhered to the objective lens. If so, clean it thoroughly.
   iii) Check that the slide carrying the object has not been placed upside down on the stage. If so, reverse it.
   iv) Check that the immersion oil has not become sticky. If so, wipe off the old oil and replace.
   v) Check whether the specimen is covered with a layer of dried oil or dirt (left on it by a previous viewer). If so, clean it with a lens paper moistened with benzol or xylol.
   vi) Check whether the coverslip placed on the specimen is too thick or whether the mountant is so thick that the objective cannot reach close to the specimen to bring it within its focal length.
   vii) If none of the above steps improve the performance of the microscope, you should consider the possibility that the objective may be faulty. Exchange the objective with one from another good microscope and if a sharp image is obtained, discard the faulty one.

2. *A dark shadow in the field resulting in loss of definition of the image.*
   i) This is usually due to a dirty eyepiece. If the shadow moves when the eyepiece is rotated, remove the eyepiece and clean it.

ii) It may also be due to the presence of an air bubble in the immersion oil. It is better to remove the oil from the slide and put fresh oil on it.

3. *Poor illumination.*

   i) Check whether the condenser is appropriately positioned, that is, racked fully upwards. Sometimes it slips downwards in its mounting ring. It should be pushed up so that it can be racked up to within 1 mm below the specimen slide, for the oil-immersion objective.

   ii) Check whether the iris is kept fully open while using an oil-immersion objective.

   iii. Check that the illumination is properly centred. Ensure that the concave surface of the mirror faces the light while using the low- and high-power objectives and the plane surface faces the light while using the oil-immersion objective, and that it is in the correct position to reflect light centrally into the condenser.

4. *Presence of unclear image under the oil-immersion objective.*

   i) It suggests a problem in the slide or with the objective. First check the slide to see whether it contains dirt. If so, clean it with benzol.

   ii) Check the objective, and if required, clean it properly.

   iii) Check for air bubbles in the specimen by holding the slide against the light.

5. *Object not coming into focus even when the objective is in the lowermost position (and the fine adjustment screw not bringing the objective any closer to the slide).* This happens when the fine adjustment screw reaches the end of the thread before the object is brought to focus. To correct this, turn back the fine adjustment screw in the reverse direction for several turns and then focus the object carefully with the coarse adjustment knob to find the focus. Finally, sharpen the focus by turning the fine adjustment knob.

Note: It is a good practice to keep the fine adjustment knob in the middle position. To check the position, turn the fine adjustment knob to either extreme end, then turn back, counting each turn until the knob reaches the midpoint.

6. *The field of view looking oval.* Check if the objective is placed in the correct position. Note that whenever the objective is changed, it must click into position.

Routine Care and Maintenance of the Microscope

A microscope if properly maintained can be used for many years. Fungal growth and scratches (caused by dust particles) on the lens damage microscopes in a short time.

The following points must be noted carefully for routine use of the microscope:

1. Whenever the microscope is to be transported, carry it by holding its arm with one hand and keeping the other hand under the base.

2. When not in use during the day, the microscope should be covered, preferably with a plastic cover. At the end of the day, blow off the dust particles from the surface and store the microscope in a warm and dry place. Do not store the microscope in its wooden box.

3. Remove oil from the oil-immersion objective immediately after use by wiping with a clean lens paper.

4. Clean the eyepiece frequently because it is vulnerable to dirt as it is placed at the top of the microscope and usually comes in contact with the observer's eye. An air syringe can be used for this purpose.

5. Do not remove the eyepiece from the microscope for a long duration; otherwise dust will enter the body tube and will be deposited on the rear lens of the objectives.

6. While working with the oil-immersion objective, do not pull out the specimen-slide from the stage without lowering down the stage or swinging out the objective; the slide may scratch the objective. Also remember that you should not push the oil-immersion objective on the slide; it may damage both the slide and the objective.

7. While handling the fine and coarse adjustments to achieve focus, if the screws offer unusual resistance, do not use force to overcome it, as it may damage the screw and the pinion mechanism. It is better to contact the mechanic.

8. Before storing the microscope after work, clean the lenses.

9. *Cleaning of lenses* Lenses should never be touched with fingers. Lenses are cleaned with special care to avoid dust scratch. If the lens is taken out for cleaning (eyepiece or objective), keep it on a clean

surface. The eyepiece is pulled out from the tube while the objective is unscrewed from the nosepiece. First, blow off the dust particles from the surface of the lens with the help of an air syringe or a rubber bulb or a paint brush, followed by gentle rubbing with a lens paper. For cleaning the lens, breathe on it through the mouth but do not clean it by spitting or blowing on it. The oil-immersion objective requires proper cleaning. Use clean tissue paper for removing oil by repeated gentle rubbing on the surface. Move the cloth across and not circularly.

Note: Do not use organic solvents like ethanol and xylene frequently because the solvent may dissolve the cement holding the lens in the socket.

OTHER TYPES OF MICROSCOPES

There are other types of microscopes that are not routinely used in laboratories but these microscopes are specially designed and have some advantages over compound microscopes. They are based on different illumination systems. the character of light delivered to the specimen in different systems varies.

Dark-Field Microscope

A special condenser is used in this microscope, which allows light waves to cross on the specimen rather than pass through the specimen. Therefore, the field in view looks dark, as light does not pass from the condenser to the objective. However, if an object is placed on the stage, light is deflected as it hits the object and passes through the objective which is seen by the viewer. Thus, the object under study appears light against a dark background. This microscope is usually used in the microbiology laboratory to study spirochetes in exudates from leptospiral or syphilitic infections.

Fluorescence Microscope

Certain compounds when irradiated by short wavelengths, say ultraviolet light, absorb the radiation and then re-emit light energy of longer wavelength, that is, visible light. This phenomenon is called fluorescence. In fluorescence microscope, the material in the specimen that fluoresces becomes visible. The fluorescence microscope is a dark-field microscope, which has been modified by incorporating two special filters. The condenser is preceded by an **exciter filter** that allows only shorter wavelength light to pass through the specimen. If the specimen contains an object that fluoresces, it absorbs the short wavelength light and emits light of a longer wavelength. A **barrier filter** is placed in the microscope tube or eyepiece, which filters only the wavelength of emitted light for the particular fluorescent system. The fluorescence microscope is usually used in immunology laboratories to study fluorescent antibodies.

Polarising Microscope

A polarising microscope differs from an ordinary microscope in that it has two polarising devices, a polariser and an analyser. The polariser (the filter) absorbs light waves radiating in all directions and allows light waves from a particular direction to pass through the filter. The polariser is placed usually between the light source and the specimen and the analyser is placed between the objective and the eyepiece. The polariser and the analyser are rotated until the two are at right angles to each other. This causes disappearance of light through the microscope because light waves are cancelled when they are at right angles to each other. However, some objects have the property of **birefringence**, that is, the ability to rotate (polarise) light. These objects bend light and can be seen in this microscope. they appear light under a dark background.

Phase-Contrast Microscope

An important property of light is its phase. If two light waves are completely in phase, they show interference, the resultant amplitude is greater and brighter light is seen. When an object is seen without staining, the indirect waves passing through the object are retarded. The principle of phase-contrast microscope lies in further retardation of these indirect waves. This is achieved by inserting a phase plate within the objective lens. Since some diffracted light passes through the grooves of the plate, a halo appears around the object. The advantage of this microscope is that the cells or the organisms in wet preparations (without prior dehydration or staining) can be observed. As the name of the system indicates, the structures observed show added contrast compared with the bright-field microscope. The retardation of the speed of light makes the system sensitive to differences in refractive index. Objects with differences in refractive index show added differences in the intensity and shade of light passing through them. Therefore, one can observe unstained wet preparations with good resolution and detail. This microscope is used in hematology for counting platelets, by using a direct method.

Interference-Contrast Microscope

This microscope yields a three-dimensional image of the object. A special beam-splitting prism is added to the condenser. The two split beams are then polarised; one passes through the specimen, which alters the amplitude of the light wave, and the other (which serves as a reference) does not pass through the specimen. The two dissimilar light beams then pass separately through the objective and are recombined by a second prism. This recombination of light waves provides the three-dimensional image. It is very useful for wet preparations such as urinary sediments, showing finer details without the need for special staining.

Electron Microscope

The electron microscope uses a beam of electrons instead of light rays. The magnified image is visible on a fluorescent screen and can be recorded on a photographic film. The magnification obtained is very high. It gives the image on the photographic plate, at a magnification of about 5000 to 20,000 times. The negative is then enlarged to about 10 times thus enabling a total magnification of about $120,000\times$ or more. In this microscope, electromagnetic fields are used in place of lenses. This is usually used for the study of finer details of organisms, cells or tissues.

OSPE

I. **Make microscopic adjustments for focusing a film under a low-power objective.**

Steps

1. Change to concave mirror.
2. Slightly open the iris diaphragm.
3. Bring the low-power objective into position.
4. Use the fine adjustment screw for final focusing.
5. Bring the condenser to the lowest position.
6. Place the slide on the stage of the microscope.
7. Make coarse adjustments to focus the image.

II. **Make microscopic adjustments for focusing a film under a high-power objective.**

Steps

1. Change to concave mirror.
2. Partially open the iris diaphragm.
3. Bring the high-power objective into position.
4. Use the fine adjustment screw for final focusing.
5. Slightly raise the condenser.
6. Place the slide on the stage of the microscope.
7. Make coarse adjustments to focus the image.

Note: To get the focus easily under a high-power objective, it is better to focus the film first in a low-power objective.

III. **Make microscopic adjustments for focusing a film under an oil-immersion objective.**

Steps

1. Change to plane mirror.
2. Open the iris diaphragm fully.
3. Place a drop of oil at the centre of the smear.
4. Move the slide on the stage of the microscope to bring the centre of the slide under view so that the objective touches the oil.
5. Make coarse adjustments to focus the image.
6. Bring the condenser to the highest position.
7. Place the slide on the stage of the microscope.
8. Bring the oil-immersion objective into position.
9. Use the fine adjustment screw for final focusing.

Note: To get the focus easily under an oil-immersion objective, it is better to examine the films first in low- and high-power objectives.

VIVA

1. Who invented the compound microscope?
2. What is the principle of microscopy?
3. What do you mean by resolution?
4. What is the use of the terms numerical aperture (NA) and working distance in microscopy?
5. How are different adjustments made in the microscope while using different types of objectives?

Ans:

Objective	Mirror	Condenser position	State of iris diaphragm
Low-power	Concave	Lowest	Partially closed
High-power	Concave	Slightly raised	Partially opened
Oil-immersion	Plane	Fully raised	Fully opened

6. What are the functions of the condenser and iris diaphragm?
7. How is the NA of objectives related to magnification?

Ans:

Objective	NA	Magnification		
		Objective	Eyepiece	Total
Low-power	0.30	10	10	100
High-power	0.65	45	10	450
Oil-immersion	1.30	100	10	1000

8. Why is a special grade of oil (immersion oil) used in the oil-immersion objective?
    Ans: Immersion oil (cedar wood oil or liquid paraffin) is used to increase the NA and thus the resolving power of the objective. Light travels through air at a greater speed than through glass. Thus, to increase the effective NA of the objective, oil is used to slow down the speed at which light travels (speed of light is measured in terms of the refractive index), increasing the gathering power of the lens and decreasing the diffraction of light rays. The refractive indices of air, glass and immersion oil are 1.00, 1.515 and 1.515, respectively.
9. Why should the eyepiece, objective and condenser lenses never be cleaned with paper tissue, gauze or ordinary cloth?
    Ans: These optical lenses are softer than ordinary glass. Therefore, cleaning with paper tissue, gauze or ordinary cloth will scratch the lens. To clean the lenses of the microscope, a lens paper is used. Before polishing with a lens paper, care must be taken to see that nothing is present on the surface that will scratch the optical glass in the polishing process. Potentially abrasive dust or dirt is blown away using an air syringe before polishing.
10. Why should the oil be removed from the oil-immersion objective immediately after use?
    Ans: Oil is removed from the oil-immersion objective by wiping with a clean lens paper immediately after use. If it is not removed, it may dry on the outside surface of the objective or may seep inside the lens and damage it.
11. What microscopic adjustments are made when the field of view is not clear?
12. What is the cause of dark shadows in the field of view, and how can this be prevented?
13. What microscopic adjustments are made if the image is not clear in the oil-immersion objective?
14. What is the cause of oval field of view, and how do you correct it?
15. In microscopy, what does the term parfocal mean?
    Ans: It means that if one objective is in focus and a switch is made to another objective, the focus will not be lost. Thus the microscope can be focused under low-power and then switched to the high-power or oil-immersion objective and it will still be in focus except for fine adjustment. Usually, after focusing in low-power if you switch to high-power, one complete rotation of the fine adjustment screw (which adjusts about one micron) brings the object into clear focus.

CHAPTER 6

Hemocytometry

Learning Objectives

After completing this practical, you will be able to (MUST KNOW):

1. Identify RBC and WBC pipettes.
2. Focus RBC and WBC squares of the chamber under low-power and high-power objectives of the microscope.
3. Dilute the blood in the pipette for RBC and WBC counts.
4. List the precautions for diluting blood.
5. Charge the Neubauer's chamber.
6. List the precautions for charging the chamber.
7. Calculate the area and volume of RBC and WBC squares.

You may also be able to (DESIRABLE TO KNOW):

1. Explain the possible sources of error and their effects in diluting the blood in pipettes.

INTRODUCTION

The formed elements of blood are counted by hemocytometry. The apparatus used is called the hemocytometer, consisting of diluting pipettes and counting chambers. The procedures used for enumeration of blood cells include the manual method of hemocytometry and the use of electronic counting devices. The cells counted in routine practice are red cells, white cells and platelets. Manual techniques lend themselves to enumeration of all small separate bodies such as spermatozoa, eosinophils and cells in the cerebrospinal fluid. In the manual method, the hemocytometer is used for counting, whereas in electronic methods, automated electronic counting devices are used. The electronic counting device bypasses the element of human error and is also statistically more accurate because it can count many more cells.

Units for Reporting

Since the enumerated constituents are to be reported in units per litre of blood, the number of cells actually counted must be converted to the number present per litre of blood. The alternative method is units of cells per cubic millimetre (mm^3) or microlitre (μl), since 1 μl is essentially equal to 1 mm^3. Though the report is usually expressed per cubic millimetre of blood, the reporting unit of choice is cells per litre of blood.

$$1 \ mm^3 = 1 \ \mu l = 10^{-6} \ l$$

$$1 \ \mu l \times 10^6 = 1 \ litre$$

METHODS

Hemocytometry includes pipetting (diluting the blood in the pipette) and charging (charging the Neubauer's chamber with diluted blood).

Pipetting

Principle

A measured unit of blood is diluted quantitatively with diluents by using special measuring devices (pipettes).

Requirements

1. Pipettes   To ensure proper dilution of the sample to be used for counting blood cells, the blood can be precisely measured and diluted with specially designed pipettes. For counting the blood cells, two types of pipettes are used: RBC pipettes and WBC pipettes (Fig. 6.1). In hematology, the hemoglobin pipette is used for estimation of hemoglobin (not for counting cells).

⬥ **RBC pipette**   This is used for counting red cells. It has a stem, bulb, rubber tube and mouthpiece. The stem has two markings, 0.5 and 1. The stem widens

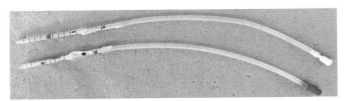

Fig. 6.1 RBC pipette and WBC pipette. Note that the RBC pipette has a red bead in the bulb and a red mouthpiece and the WBC pipette has a white bead in the bulb and a white mouthpiece.

into a bulb with a red bead in it (Fig. 6.2). The bead helps in identifying the pipette and mixing the fluid with blood in the bulb of the pipette. The capacity of the bulb is 100 parts (from 1 to 101 mark). The bulb narrows above ('101' is marked just above the bulb) and to this end, a rubber tubing which ends in a mouthpiece is attached (Fig. 6.3). The mouthpiece is red in colour. As the lumen diameter in the stem of the RBC pipette is less compared to

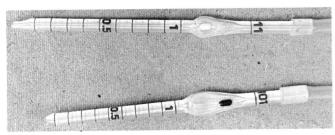

Fig. 6.2 The stem part of RBC pipette and WBC pipette. Note that the RBC pipette has a red bead in the bulb and a 101 mark after the upper part of the bulb, and the WBC pipette has a white bead in the bulb and a 11 mark after the upper part of the bulb.

that of the WBC pipette, sometimes the RBC pipette is called a slow-speed pipette.

⬥ **WBC pipette** This is used for counting white blood cells. It is similar to the RBC pipette except that the capacity of the bulb is less (10 parts) and the bulb contains a white bead. The marking above the bulb is '11' (Fig. 6.4). The mouthpiece is white in colour. In the WBC pipette, the lumen diameter in the stem is more than that of RBC pipettes (Table 6.1). Hence, sometimes the WBC pipette is called a fast-speed pipette.

2. Diluents (diluting fluids) Different varieties of diluting fluids are used for counting different types of cells. Diluting fluids are described with each cell count.

Procedure

1. Clean the pipette and ensure that it is dry.
2. Collect the diluting fluid in a watch glass from a stock bottle.
3. Prick the fingertip (as described in Chapter 2) with all aseptic precautions to obtain free flow of blood.
4. Discard (wipe off) the first drop of blood.
5. Let a large drop of blood accumulate on the fingertip (Fig. 6.5).
6. Hold the pipette tilted at an angle of about 60° (Fig. 6.6) or horizontally (Fig. 6.7) and dip its end into the drop of blood. Blood enters into the pipette by capillary action, or suck gently on the

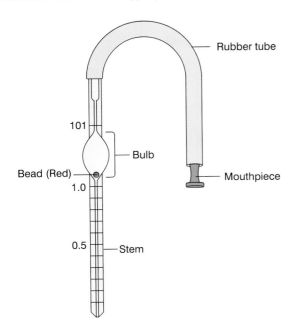

Fig. 6.3 RBC pipette.

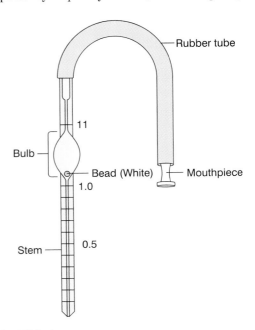

Fig. 6.4 WBC pipette.

Table 6.1 Differences between RBC and WBC pipettes.

		RBC pipette	WBC pipette
1.	Calibrations	0.5 to 1.0 in the stem, 101 above the bulb	0.5 to 1.0 in the stem, 11 above the bulb
2.	Bulb	Larger, capacity 100 parts, contains red bead	Smaller, capacity 10 parts, contains white bead
3.	Mouthpiece	Red	White
4.	Stem lumen diameter	Less	More
5.	Dilution	0.5 in 100, or 1 in 200	0.5 in 10, or 1 in 20

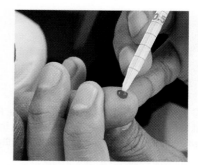

Fig. 6.6 Dipping the pipette into the drop of blood from one side, keeping the pipette at about 60° position.

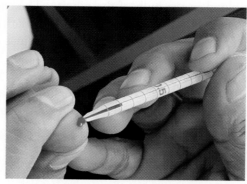

Fig. 6.7 Pipetting of blood. By keeping the pipette in the horizontal position, blood usually enters into the pipette by capillary action. If blood does not enter into the pipette automatically, blood may be gently sucked into it.

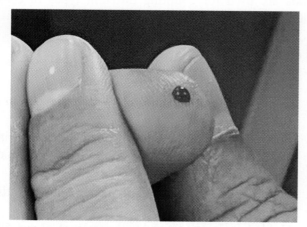

Fig. 6.5 Forming a drop of blood by finger prick for pipetting.

mouthpiece to draw blood up to the required mark (0.5) on the stem of the pipette. If more than the required amount of blood is drawn into the pipette, tap it gently onto the fingernail or palm, or touch the tip with a non-absorbent material keeping the pipette horizontal, in order to bring the blood to the desired 0.5 mark (Fig. 6.8).

Note: Do not blow out the extra blood or use absorbent material like cotton wool.

7. Wipe off the tip of the pipette to remove the extra blood sticking to it.
8. Maintain the blood level at the 0.5 mark, and place the tip of the pipette in the diluting fluid well below the surface of the liquid.

Note: Do not directly draw the fluid from the stock bottle as it may contaminate the solution with the cells.

9. Using constant suction, draw the diluting fluid into the pipette (Fig. 6.9). Draw the mixture exactly to

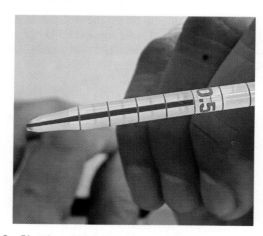

Fig. 6.8 Pipetting of blood exactly up to the 0.5 mark.

the top mark ('101' or '11') above the bulb. While the bulb is being filled, you may tap the pipette with a finger to knock the bead down below the surface of the solution in the bulb to prevent the formation of bubbles.

10. Maintain the level of the mixture exactly to the mark by closing the pipette tip with the index finger. Holding the pipette in the horizontal position is also important.

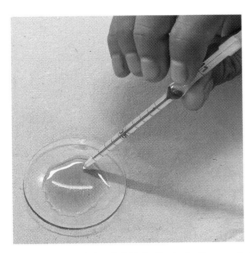

Fig. 6.9 Pipetting of diluting fluid into the bulb. Ensure that the tip of the pipette is inside the fluid level; otherwise air bubble enters into the pipette.

11. Mix the contents of the bulb thoroughly for 2–3 minutes by rotating the pipette with its tip pressing against the palm of the left hand (the rubber tube may be removed to facilitate mixing).

> **Note:** The contents may also be mixed by holding and rotating the pipette between the palms, but there is some risk of leakage, especially if it is not held horizontally.

12. Place the pipette on a horizontal surface. The pipette is now ready for charging.

Precautions

Cell counts are performed by determining the number of cells in the diluted sample, and converting the number of cells counted in the diluted sample to the final result, i.e., the number of cells in 1 litre or in 1 ml of whole blood. Blood cell counts are performed on minute quantities taken from small samples of an individual's blood. Errors are inherent even in the best methods. Therefore, the steps in the procedure must be followed as carefully as possible to reduce the variation of the final result from the actual or true count.

1. Pipettes should be clean, dry and without chipped or broken tips.
2. The puncture should be deep enough for free flow of blood. The first drop should be discarded as it contains tissue fluid.
3. A large drop of blood should have formed on the fingertip to provide adequate blood to fill up to the 0.5 mark of the pipette at a time.

4. The tip of the pipette should dip into the blood drop, otherwise while sucking blood into the pipette, air bubbles also enter along with blood.
5. Blood should be taken exactly up to the 0.5 mark. If blood is present above the mark, absorbent material, such as gauze or cotton, should not be used to adjust the blood level because these materials absorb the water content of the blood and cause blood to concentrate.
6. The tip of the pipette should be wiped off. Otherwise, the extra blood attached to the tip enters the pipette along with diluent when the diluting fluid is sucked in.
7. Blood in the pipette should be diluted immediately, otherwise it will clot.
8. Contaminated diluting fluids should not be used. Blood should not be allowed to get into the diluent because this will affect subsequent cell counts with the same diluent. Therefore, the diluent should not be drawn into the pipette directly from the bottle. Rather, the fluid should be taken in a watch glass from where it should be drawn into the pipette.
9. The tip of the pipette should dip inside the diluting fluid throughout the process of filling the bulb, otherwise air bubbles enter the pipette.
10. The upper dilution mark on the pipette should not be exceeded by more than 1 mm; and the mixture should not be corrected back to the top mark if overdiluted because this would cause the cells from the bulb to be forced to enter into the lower stem of the pipette.
11. If blood is to be used from a blood sample, the preserved blood sample should not be hemolysed nor should it contain a fibrin clot. It should be mixed (preferably by gentle shaking) before use.

Charging the Chamber

Principle

A mixture of blood and diluting fluid is released smoothly onto the central platform of the chamber beneath a coverslip.

Requirements

1. Counting chamber
2. Pipette containing the mixture
3. Coverslip

Counting chamber

The counting chamber in common use is the Improved Neubauer Chamber. This consists of a thick glass slide divided into two central platforms by an H-shaped groove (Fig. 6.10). The central platform is slightly lower than the sides; i.e., when a coverslip is placed, it covers the central platform and rests on the side platforms. The depth, i.e., the distance between the undersurface of the coverslip and the central platform is 1/10 mm (Fig. 6.11). When the chamber is charged with diluted blood, a thin film of fluid of known volume is spread on the central platform, and this is used for performing the cell counts.

The counting grid On the central platforms are engraved ruled squares used for various cell counts. The ruled area on each central platform is called counting grid. The ruled area is a square measuring 3 mm × 3 mm (Fig. 6.12). This area is divided into nine large squares, each having an area of 1 mm² (1 mm × 1 mm). The four large corner squares are used for WBC count, while the large 1 mm square in the centre is used for RBC count.

Each WBC square is further subdivided into 16 smaller squares, each measuring 1/16 mm². The 1 mm² central RBC square is divided into 25 medium-sized squares by means of triple lines (the Old Neubauer's chamber has central 16 medium-sized squares). Each medium-sized square measures 1/5 mm in length and has an area of $1/5 \times 1/5 = 1/25$ mm². The medium-sized squares of the four

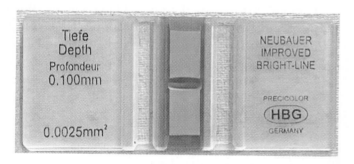

Fig. 6.10 Improved Neubauer's chamber (Brightline).

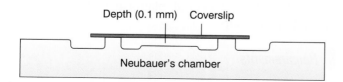

Fig. 6.11 Side view of Neubauer's chamber showing the space between the undersurface of the coverslip and the surface of the platform (0.1 mm deep).

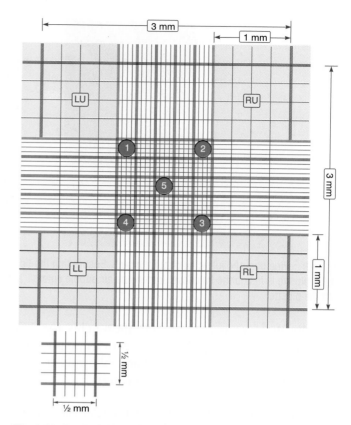

Fig. 6.12 Improved Neubauer's chamber (LU: Left upper; RU: Right upper; LL: Left lower; RL: Right lower WBC squares; 1, 2, 3, 4 and 5: RBC squares).

corners and the central medium-sized square are used for the RBC count. The area of the five medium-sized squares is $1/25 \times 5 = 1/5$ mm². Since the depth of the chamber is 1/10 mm, the volume of the five medium-sized squares is $1/5 \times 1/10 = 1/50$ mm³ (Fig. 6.12).

Each medium-sized square is further divided into 16 small squares, that is, $25 \times 16 = 400$ small squares. The side of the smallest RBC square measures 1/20 mm. Therefore, the area of the smallest RBC square is $1/20 \times 1/20 = 1/400$ mm². Since the depth under the coverslip is 1/10 mm, the volume of the smallest RBC square is $1/400 \times 1/10 = 1/4000$ mm³. The red cells are counted in 80 small squares (5 medium-sized squares); the volume of 80 small-sized RBC squares is $1/4000 \times 80 = 1/50$ mm³.

Other counting chambers Other counting chambers are Thoma's chamber and old Neubauer chamber. Presently, both these chambers are not in use. In Thoma's chamber, the central platform is depressed and circular. The grid is only 1 mm², consisting of 25 groups of 16 smaller squares each. The corner 1 mm squares are absent. The Old Neubauer chamber has nine 1 mm squares. The four larger corner squares of 16 squares each are meant for WBC counting, and the central 1 mm^2 area has 16 groups of 16 squares each, meant for RBC counting. In the improved Neubauer chamber, 25 groups of 16 smallest squares are available for RBC counting. However, in both the chambers, medium squares are separated by triple lines.

Procedure

1. Clean the Neubauer's chamber and the coverslip.
2. Place the coverslip on the central platform of the chamber (Fig. 6.13).
3. Mix the contents of the bulb thoroughly.

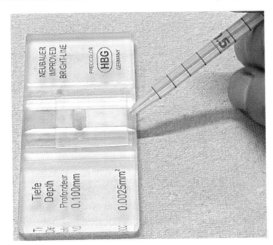

Fig. 6.13   Placing the coverslip at the central platform of the Neubauer's chamber so that it remains mainly on the desired counting chamber.

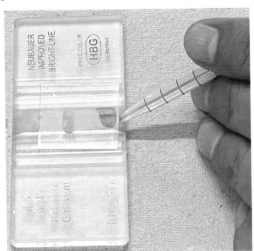

Fig. 6.14   Charging (in progress) of the Neubauer's chamber. The tip of the pipette is kept at the edge of the coverslip at a 45° angle and the fluid from the pipette is released under control beneath the coverslip.

4. Discard the first two drops of fluid from the pipette as it contains only the diluting fluid.
5. Place the tip of the pipette on the surface of the chamber touching the edge of the coverslip at an angle of 45°. Allow the diluted blood to flow under the coverslip by capillary action (Fig. 6.14). Remove the pipette quickly from the edge of the coverslip as soon as the counting platform is filled with the diluted blood. Take care to avoid entry of air bubbles and overflow of the fluid into the gutters.

Note: The mixture should completely cover the platform, but should not enter the gutters (Fig. 6.15). If air bubbles enter the platform or fluid enters the gutters, discard the specimen and recharge.

6. Allow the cells to settle for 2–3 minutes before placing the charged chamber on the stage of the microscope for counting.

Precautions

1. The chamber and the coverslip should be properly cleaned.
2. The contents of the bulb must be thoroughly mixed before charging.
3. Two drops of fluid must be discarded from the pipette before charging as the stem of the pipette contains only diluting fluid.
4. Air bubbles should not enter the platform of the chamber while charging.

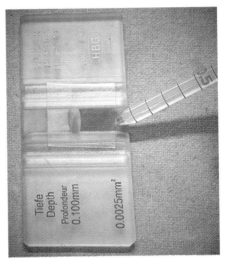

Fig. 6.15   Completion of charging of the Neubauer's chamber. Note that the fluid remained on the platform, and there was no entry into the gutter.

5. The chamber should not be overcharged (overflow of fluid into the gutters) or undercharged (fluid does not spread on the entire central platform). If the chamber is overcharged, the cells may enter the gutter and settle there, which gives false low results. If the chamber is undercharged, the cells may not be found in the peripheral squares (Fig. 6.16).

DISCUSSION

Students should practise pipetting and charging repeatedly. But, before learning this, they should learn to focus the RBC and WBC squares of the chamber under the low-power and high-power objectives of the microscope. While focusing the chamber, especially in the high-power objective, care should be taken not to break the chamber. In fact, before charging the chamber, the chamber should have been focused earlier under the low-power microscope, so that focusing becomes easier after the charging.

Beginners would find it difficult to directly bring to focus a charged chamber. Therefore, they should first bring to focus the uncharged chamber to locate the desired squares and then take out the chamber from the stage of the microscope for charging without disturbing the setting of the microscope. After charging the chamber, they can place the charged chamber on the platform of the microscope and easily bring it into focus using the fine adjustment screws.

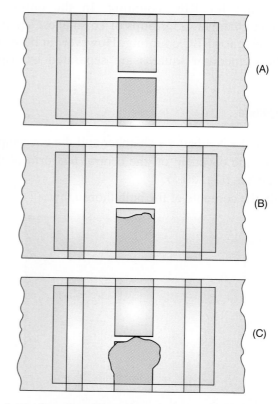

Fig. 6.16 Charging of Neubauer's chamber (only the central part of the chamber is shown). (A) Normal (ideal) charging; (B) Undercharging; (C) Overcharging.

OSPE

I. **Dilute the given sample of blood for RBC count.**

Steps
1. Select the pipette.
2. Clean and dry the pipette.
3. Take diluting fluid in a watch glass.
4. Shake the blood sample to mix it properly.
5. Place the tip of the pipette deep into the blood and suck blood exactly up to the 0.5 mark. If blood is sucked above the mark, adjust the level by tapping the tip of the pipette against a fingernail or by touching the tip of the pipette with non-absorbent material.
6. Wipe the tip of the pipette.
7. Maintaining the blood level at the 0.5 mark, place the tip of the pipette in the diluting fluid and suck fluid exactly up to the 101 mark. Take care to prevent entry of air bubbles into the pipette.
8. Mix the contents of the bulb of the pipette by rotating the pipette with its tip pressed against the fingers.
9. Place the pipette on a horizontal surface.

II. **Dilute the given sample of blood for WBC count.**
1. Same as OSPE 1 except that the student uses the WBC pipette and WBC diluting fluid.

III. **Charge the Neubauer's chamber with the diluted blood from the supplied pipette.**

Steps
1. Clean the Neubauer's chamber and the coverslip.
2. Place the coverslip on the central platform of the chamber.
3. Mix the contents of the bulb thoroughly.
4. Discard the first two drops of fluid from the pipette.
5. Place the tip of the pipette on the surface of the chamber touching the edge of the coverslip at an angle of 45° and allow the diluted blood to flow under the coverslip by capillary action.
6. Remove the pipette quickly from the edge of the coverslip as soon as the counting platform is filled with the diluted blood. Take care to prevent overcharging or undercharging of the chamber.
7. Place the charged chamber on a flat surface.

VIVA

1. *What are the uses of the hemocytometer in hematology?*
2. *How do you identify the RBC and WBC diluting pipettes?*
3. *What are the steps for diluting the blood for various cell counts?*
4. *What are the precautions taken for pipetting?*
5. *How do you bring down the level of blood if the blood is sucked above the 0.5 mark of the pipette?*
6. *Why is the fluid not sucked directly from the stock bottle?*
7. *How do you prevent the entry of air bubbles into the pipette while diluting the blood?*
8. *How do you calculate the area and volume of RBC and WBC squares?*
9. *What are the steps for charging the Neubauer's chamber?*
10. *What are the precautions taken for charging the chamber with diluted blood?*
11. *Why are the contents of the bulb mixed thoroughly before charging?*
12. *Why are the two drops of fluid discarded from the pipette before charging?*
13. *What do the terms overcharging and undercharging mean and what is their significance?*

CHAPTER 7

Total RBC Count

Learning Objectives

After completing this practical, you will be able to (MUST KNOW):

1. Describe the importance of performing RBC count in practical physiology.
2. Identify the RBC diluting pipette.
3. Suck blood up to the 0.5 mark of the pipette.
4. Dilute the blood in the pipette.
5. Charge the Neubauer's chamber.
6. Perform the total RBC count.
7. Calculate total RBC count to express the result in mm³ of blood.
8. List the precautions taken for performing RBC count.
9. Describe the composition and function of each constituent of the RBC diluting fluid.
10. List the steps and factors involved in the regulation of production of red cells.

11. Enumerate the functions of red cells.
12. List the normal value of RBC count in adults.
13. Define polycythemia and anemia.
14. Name the common causes of alteration in RBC count.

You may also be able to (DESIRABLE TO KNOW):

1. State the name, composition and advantages of other RBC-diluting fluids.
2. Explain the principle of automated methods of red cell count.
3. Classify polycythemia and anemia.
4. Explain the physiological basis of alteration of red cell count in different conditions.
5. Describe the stages and regulation of erythropoiesis.
6. Explain the causes and mechanism of polycythemia and anemia.

INTRODUCTION

The human red cell is normally a circular, non-nucleated, biconcave disc. The red blood cells (erythrocytes) contain hemoglobin. The surface area of the red cell is much greater than that of a sphere of the same size. Thus the exchange of oxygen and carbon dioxide is maximal with the biconcave configuration. This shape also helps it to withstand osmotic lysis and to easily pass through narrow capillaries.

Red Cell Dimensions

Shape   : Biconcave disc
Size   : 7.5 (7 to 8) μm in diameter
Thickness   : 2.0 μm
Surface area : 140 μm²

Formation

The development of red cells is known as **erythropoiesis**. In postnatal life, erythropoiesis takes place in the bone marrow. In children, cells are produced in the marrow cavities of all the bones. By the age of 20, the marrow in the cavities of the long bones, except for the upper humerus and femur, becomes inactive. The active cellular marrow is called the red marrow; the inactive marrow that is infiltrated with fat is called the yellow marrow. During fetal life, erythropoiesis occurs in the spleen, liver, thymus and bone marrow. After birth, it is confined to the red marrow.

The **stages of erythropoiesis** are as follows:

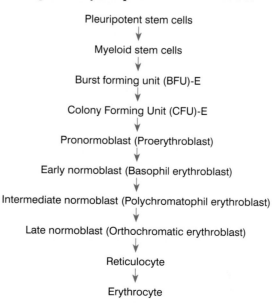

Pleuripotent stem cells
↓
Myeloid stem cells
↓
Burst forming unit (BFU)-E
↓
Colony Forming Unit (CFU)-E
↓
Pronormoblast (Proerythroblast)
↓
Early normoblast (Basophil erythroblast)
↓
Intermediate normoblast (Polychromatophil erythroblast)
↓
Late normoblast (Orthochromatic erythroblast)
↓
Reticulocyte
↓
Erythrocyte

As the cell matures in the bone marrow, its diameter decreases and the nucleus becomes denser and smaller and finally disappears from the cell. While this occurs, the hemoglobin concentration increases and the cytoplasm progressively changes from blue to orange in appearance, on a stained blood film. The whole sequence of maturation from the early precursor to a circulating red cell takes 3–5 days.

Erythropoiesis is subject to feedback control. It is inhibited by a rise in the circulating red cells and is stimulated by decreased red cell count. This alteration is mediated by a number of factors that influence the secretion of erythropoietin, a hormone secreted by the kidney. Interleukins (IL1, IL3, IL6) and GM-CSF also affect the development of red cells.

Functions

The main function of RBCs is to carry oxygen from the lungs to the tissues of the body. Red cells also transport carbon dioxide from the tissues to the lungs. Red cells contribute to blood viscosity and therefore to peripheral resistance of blood. Viscosity of blood is less in anemia and more in polycythemia.

Lifespan and Fate

The average lifespan of red cells is about 120 days. The bone marrow releases new red cells into circulation every day. The dead red cells are broken down by the reticuloendothelial system. They break down globin to amino acids which are returned to the protein storage pool of the body. They are also essential for the retention and reuse or storage of iron, which is needed for hemoglobin synthesis.

Normal Values

In adults:
Males   : 5.2 (4.5–6.0) million per mm^3 of blood
Females : 4.7 (4.0–5.5) million per mm^3 of blood
RBC count is higher in newborns (6–8 million per mm^3 of blood). The count rapidly decreases thereafter, and is lowest at about two to four months of life (3–4 million per mm^3). The count slowly increases from one year of life to reach 5 million per mm^3 at about ten years.

METHODS OF COUNTING

Red cells are counted by two methods: non-automated (manual) and automated. Manual cell count is less accurate but is still widely used in developing countries as automated counting is expensive.

Manual Method

Principle

The blood specimen is diluted (usually 200 times) with the diluting fluid, which does not remove the white cells, but allows the red cells to be counted in a known volume of fluid. Finally, the number of cells in undiluted blood is calculated and reported as the number of red cells per mm^3 of whole blood.

Requirements

I. Apparatus
1. Microscope
2. Hemocytometer (RBC diluting pipette and counting chamber)
3. Equipment for sterile finger prick
4. Watch glass
5. Coverslip

II. RBC diluting fluid
The red cell diluting fluid is isotonic; therefore, it prevents hemolysis. Of the different diluting fluids used for red cell count, the most frequently used is Hayem's fluid.
1. **Hayem's fluid**
   Composition
   Sodium chloride : 0.5 g
   Sodium sulphate : 2.5 g
   Mercuric chloride : 0.25 g
   Distilled water : 100 ml
   Dissolve thoroughly with a stirrer, in a beaker.

   Function of each component
   • Sodium chloride—maintains osmolarity.
   • Sodium sulphate—prevents aggregation of RBC.
   • Mercuric chloride—acts as a preservative (it is antifungal and antibacterial)
   • Distilled water—acts as a solvent.
2. **Dacie's fluid**   This is an alternative to Hayem's fluid.
   Composition
   Trisodium citrate : 3.13 g
   Commercial formaldehyde (37% formalin) : 1.0 ml
   Distilled water : 100 ml

Dissolve thoroughly with a stirrer, in a beaker.

Caution Formaldehyde is corrosive, and should be handled carefully.

Advantages Dacie's fluid is preferred in some laboratories because of the following advantages:

- It is simple to prepare.
- It keeps well and does not need to be sterilised.
- Red cells maintain their normal disc-like form and do not agglutinate.

Cells are well-preserved and counts may be performed several hours after the blood has been diluted.

3. **Isotonic saline** If the above two diluting fluids are not available, isotonic saline may be used. The counting should commence immediately following dilution as it does not contain any agent to prevent aggregation of red cells.

Procedure

1. Assemble all equipment needed for the practical and ensure that the pipettes, coverslip and Neubauer's chamber are thoroughly clean and dry.
2. Take adequate RBC diluting fluid in a watch glass.
3. Prick the finger under aseptic conditions (as described in Chapter 3) to make a medium-sized blood drop (Fig. 7.3) and suck blood into the pipette (*refer* Figs. 6.6–6.8) and dilute it following the step-by-step procedure as described in Chapter 6 (procedure of pipetting).
4. Hold the pipette horizontally and close both ends, then gently mix the contents of the bulb. For mixing, shake the pipette at right angles to its long axis for a few seconds. The red bead in the pipette should move from one side to the other during the mixing.
5. After mixing, keep the pipette in a horizontal position to prevent any loss of its contents until the cell count is performed.
6. Discard the first two drops of fluid from the pipette.
7. Charge the Neubauer's chamber as described in Chapter 6 (*refer* Figs. 6.13–6.15) and allow two minutes so that the cells settle down.
8. Place the charged chamber on the stage of the microscope and adjust the microscope for observation under low power.
9. Focus the central square of the Neubauer's chamber under the low-power objective, and check for uniform distribution of cells. If the cells

are not uniformly distributed (Fig. 7.1), clean the Neubauer's chamber and recharge it.

10. Focus the RBC squares under the high-power objective. Count the cells in five medium RBC squares in sequence as described in Fig. 7.2A (four corner and the central medium-sized RBC squares) that is $16 \times 5 = 80$ small RBC squares.

> **Note:** Care should be taken not to count the same cells again. To avoid this, Rules of Counting should be followed, according to which the red cells present in the square and on its left and lower lines are counted, and those on its right and upper lines are ignored. This is called 'L pattern' counting, as demonstrated in Fig. 7.2B. However, 'inverted L pattern', i.e., counting cells present on the left and upper lines of the square, and avoiding those present on the right and lower lines, can also be followed. But, 'L pattern' for few squares and 'inverted L pattern' for other squares should not be practised. Only one pattern should be followed for the entire counting, and preferably the same should be practised by all the students of the class to maintain uniformity and to avoid confusion.

11. Draw the RBC squares in your notebook and enter the observation. Calculate the final result.

Dilution Obtained

The volume of the bulb is 100 ($101 - 1 = 100$). The stem of the pipette (from the tip of the pipette to mark 1) contains diluting fluid that does not take part in dilution.

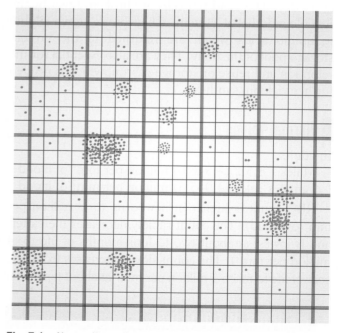

Fig. 7.1 Non-uniform distribution of red cells (as seen under low power). Note that cells are clumped at a few places and sparse at other places.

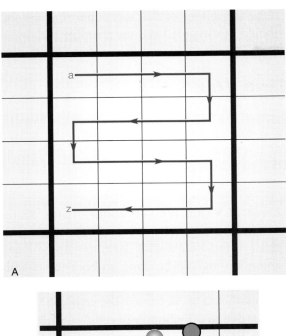

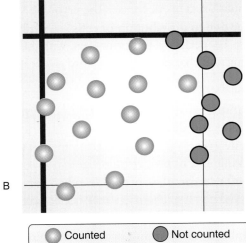

○ Counted   ● Not counted

Fig. 7.2   Pattern of counting red cells in a medium RBC square. (A) Direction of counting as indicated by arrow; (B) Cells to be counted as shown in a small square.

Dilution (mixing of blood with diluting fluid) occurs only in the bulb. Thus 100 volumes of diluted blood (in the bulb) contain 0.5 volumes of blood and 99.5 volumes of diluting fluid, resulting in a dilution of 0.5 in 100. Thus, the dilution obtained is 1 in 200 or 200 times.

▌ Calculation

Area of 5 medium-sized squares $= 1/25 \times 5 = 1/5$ mm^2.
Volume of 5 medium-sized squares $= 1/5 \times 1/10 = 1/50$ mm^3 (1/10 is the depth).
Dilution factor $= 1 : 200$
Let us say the cells in $1/50$ mm^3 volume of diluted blood is n.

Therefore, cells in 1 mm^3 volume of diluted blood $= n \times 50$
Therefore, cells in 1 mm^3 volume of undiluted blood $= n \times 50 \times 200$
$= \boldsymbol{n \times 10{,}000}$ where n is the total number of cells counted in 5 medium-sized RBC squares.

▌ Precautions

1. The pipette, coverslip and Neubauer's chamber should be thoroughly clean and dry.
2. The puncture should be deep enough to allow spontaneous flow of blood (*refer* Fig. 6.5). Blood should not be squeezed, as squeezing expresses tissue fluid. If blood is taken from a sample, it should be mixed properly prior to pipetting.
3. The first drop of blood should be wiped off, as it is mixed with tissue fluid.
4. The tip of the pipette should gently touch the blood drop (Fig. 7.3) and blood should be drawn exactly up to the 0.5 mark (Fig. 7.4). The blood

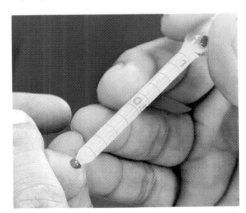

Fig. 7.3   Obtaining a medium-sized blood drop for RBC count by finger pricking. The tip of the pipette should gently touch the drop from the side.

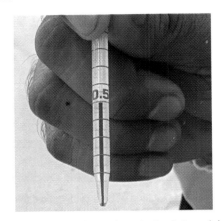

Fig. 7.4   Pipetting of blood exactly up to the 0.5 mark in the stem of the RBC pipette.

column (from the tip of the pipette to the 0.5 mark) should not be fragmented, nor should it contain air bubbles. If blood is drawn above the mark, it is gently tapped against the fingertip or nail bed to bring to the level. Absorbent material should never be used for this purpose as it absorbs water from the blood and makes the blood concentrated.

5. The tip of the pipette should be wiped clean before diluting the blood. This should always be done; otherwise the extra blood sticking to the tip of the pipette will be sucked into the bulb along with the diluing fluid and will give a false high result.

6. Blood in the pipette should be diluted quickly but steadily (Fig. 7.5); otherwise blood clots will be formed in the pipette.

7. The RBC diluting fluid is sucked exactly up to the 101 mark. If the fluid is drawn much above the mark (more than 1 mm), it should not be adjusted back to the mark as it forces cells in the bulb to enter into the stem of the pipette. This affects the dilution and cell concentration in the bulb. Therefore, it is better to discard this, clean the pipette and restart the procedure.

8. Before charging the chamber, the contents of the bulb are gently mixed.

9. The first two drops of fluid are discarded as fluid in the stem does not contain cells.

10. The chamber should neither be overcharged nor undercharged. If it is overcharged, the contents should be discarded, the chamber cleaned and then recharged.

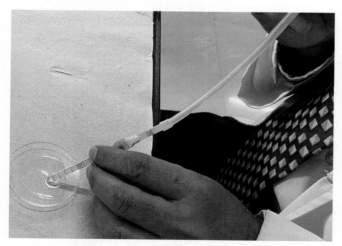

Fig. 7.5   Process of pipetting of RBC diluting fluid into the bulb of the pipette. Ensure that the sucking of the fluid is done steadily with the tip of the pipette dipped in the fluid in the watch glass, so that air bubbles do not enter the pipette.

11. If the distribution of cells is not uniform, the contents should be discarded and the chamber recharged.

12. Counting the same cells twice should be avoided.

Sources of Error

The error in manual total RBC count is 15–30 per cent. It can be reduced by counting more cells. The possible sources of error may be errors inherent in the method or technical errors.

A. Errors inherent in the method

1. **Error of visual red cell count**   Error decreases with increased total number of cells counted. Both sides of the Neubauer's chamber can be charged, and counting can be done on both the chambers. The average of these can be taken for final calculation. This decreases the error.

2. **Error due to distribution of cells**   Distribution can never be perfectly uniform even with near-perfect mixing and charging, and therefore gives rise to error.

B. Technical errors

1. **Dilution error**   Improper volume measurement of blood and diluent

2. **Pipette error**   Use of defective pipettes (improper marking and improper bulb size)

3. **Chamber error**   Use of defective chambers (counting grid and depth of chambers may not be accurate)

4. **Charging error**   Improper charging of the chamber (overcharging or undercharging)

5. **Counting error**   Improper counting (few cells are not counted or few cells are counted twice)

6. **Calculation error**   Wrong calculation

Automated Methods

There are two automated methods: (1) impedance counting and (2) light scattering technology. As these methods are not usually practised in Indian students' laboratories, only the basic principles of the methods are described here.

Impedance Counting

This was first described by Wallace Coulter in 1956. Impedance counting depends on the fact that red cells are poor conductors of electricity, whereas certain diluents are good conductors. Blood is highly diluted in a buffered electrolyte solution. An external vacuum initiates movement of a mercury siphon, which causes a major volume of the sample to flow through an aperture tube of specific dimension. By means of a constant source of electricity, a direct current is maintained between two electrodes, one in the sample beaker or the chamber surrounding the aperture tube, and the other inside the aperture tube. When a blood cell is carried through the aperture, it displaces some of the conducting fluid and increases the electrical resistance. This produces a corresponding change in potential between the electrodes which lasts as long as the red cells pass through the aperture. The height of the pulses produced indicates the volume of the cells passing through. The pulses can be displayed on an oscillograph screen. The height of the pulses is used to determine the volume of the red cells.

Light Scattering Technology

Red cells are counted by means of electro-optical detectors. A diluted cell suspension flows through an aperture so that the cells pass in single file, in front of the light source; light is scattered by the cells passing through the light beam. Scattered light is detected by a photomultiplier or photodiode, which converts it into electrical impulses which are accumulated and counted. The amount of light scattered is proportional to the surface area and, therefore, the volume of the cells, so that the height of the electrical pulses can be used to estimate the cell volume.

DISCUSSION

Clinical Significance

The total RBC count is performed to assess the red cell mass in the blood. The change in erythrocyte number is frequently detected in clinical practice by ordering estimation of hemoglobin rather than total RBC count, as estimation of hemoglobin is easy and less expensive. Moreover, total RBC count by the manual method is more likely to be erroneous (more than 20 per cent). The total RBC count is still performed in some conditions to detect the red cell population, especially if the count is expected to be very high, as in polycythemia.

Conditions That Alter Total RBC Count

Conditions That Decrease RBC Count

Physiological
1. Pregnancy (due to hemodilution).
2. Children have lower values than adults.

3. Women have lower values than men. RBC count is higher in men because male sex hormones stimulate erythropoiesis. It is lower in women because estrogen inhibits erythropoiesis and there is cyclical loss of blood during reproductive life.

Pathological
1. Different types of anemia.
2. Relative decrease in RBC count occurs in different pathological conditions that produce hemodilution, for example, excess ADH secretion as occurs in posterior pituitary tumours.

Conditions That Increase RBC Count

Physiological
1. High altitude (due to hypoxia).
2. Newborns have a high count.
3. Excessive sweating (due to hemoconcentration).

Pathological
1. Conditions that produce hemoconcentration (due to loss of body fluid), for example, severe diarrhea and vomiting.
2. Conditions that produce chronic hypoxia, for example, congenital heart disease and emphysema.
3. Polycythemia vera.

Polycythemia

The term polycythemia, strictly speaking, implies elevated levels of all the cellular elements of blood, though it is usually used to describe the increase in the red cell count alone. Polycythemia may result from an increase in the total number of red cells in the body (true polycythemia) or from a reduction in the plasma volume relative to the volume of the red cells (relative polycythemia). True polycythemia may be due to a primary disorder of the hemopoietic tissue which produces excess of red cells (polycythemia vera) or may be secondary to excessive stimulation of erythropoiesis by erythropoietin (secondary polycythemia).

Causes

I. True polycythemia
1. Polycythemia vera
2. Secondary polycythemia
    a) Secondary to tissue hypoxia
        i) High altitude

ii) Congenital heart disease

iii) Chronic pulmonary disease

b) Secondary to inappropriately increased erythropoietin production

   i) Kidney tumours

   ii) Liver tumours

   iii) Pheochromocytoma

   iv) Virilising ovarian tumour

II. Relative polycythemia

1. Dehydration

2. Redistribution of body fluids

Anemia

Decrease in number of red cells or Hb content below normal is known as anemia (*refer* Chapter 3 *for a detailed account*).

OSPE

I. Dilute the blood (from the given sample) for total RBC count.

Steps

1. Select the RBC pipette and ensure that it is clean and dry.
2. Mix blood thoroughly.
3. Pipette blood exactly up to the 0.5 mark.
4. If blood is drawn above the mark, remove the extra blood by tapping with a finger nail (not by touching with absorbent material).
5. Wipe the tip of the pipette.
6. Suck diluting fluid up to the 101 mark. While drawing the fluid, avoid entry of air bubbles.
7. Gently mix the contents of the bulb and keep the pipette on the table.

II. Charge the Neubauer's chamber for total RBC count.

Steps

1. Clean the coverslip and Neubauer's chamber.
2. Place the coverslip on the platform of the Neubauer's chamber.
3. Mix the contents of the bulb of the RBC pipette.
4. Discard two drops of the fluid from the pipette.
5. Touch the tip of the pipette with the edge of the coverslip.
6. Slowly release fluid from the pipette (fluid moves by capillary action) in such a way that the fluid spreads just beneath the coverslip and does not spill into the gutters or contain air bubbles.

VIVA

1. *What is the composition and function of each component of Hayem's fluid? What other fluid can be used as RBC-diluting fluid?*

2. *What are the advantages of using Dacie's diluting fluid?*

3. *What are the precautions to be taken for RBC count?*

4. *What are the functions of the red bead in the bulb of the pipette?*

   Ans: The red bead has two functions. It helps in mixing the contents of the bulb and in quick identification of the RBC pipette.

5. *What is the significance of different markings present on the RBC pipette?*

   Ans: There are three markings on the RBC pipette: 0.5, 1 and 101. The 0.5 mark is the mark up to which blood is sucked and the 101 mark is the mark up to which the diluting fluid is sucked to get a dilution of 1 in 200. In cases of polycythemia, dilution may have to be increased and in case of anemia, dilution may have to be decreased. The 1 mark is used for pipetting blood in conditions of severe anemia where more blood is taken for dilution. In such conditions, blood is sucked up to the 1 mark and then diluted up to the 101 mark, giving a dilution of 1 in 100.

6.   *When is the RBC pipette used for white cell counting? What are the other uses of the RBC pipette?*

   Ans: An RBC pipette is used for counting WBC in leukemia where leucocytes are counted not in thousands but in lakhs or millions per mm^3 of blood. In leukemia, blood is sucked up to mark 1 in the RBC pipette and then diluted to 101 mark giving a dilution of 1 in 100. The RBC pipette is also used for sperm count and platelet count.

7.   *Why are the two drops of the solution from the pipette discarded before charging the Neubauer's chamber?*

8.   *Why is the dilution obtained 1 in 200, not 1 in 202?*

9.   *What are the sources of error in RBC count?*

10.   *What happens to WBCs in the RBC count?*

   Ans: WBCs are not lysed, and hence can be seen along with red cells. But the normal ratio of RBC to WBC is 700 : 1. Therefore, hardly any WBC is counted, as total red cells counted in 5 medium RBC squares are usually less than 700. So WBCs do not affect RBC count.

11.   *How do you remove a blood clot from the pipette?*

   Ans: First the clot is dissolved and removed by a strong acid or H_2O_2; then the pipette is cleaned with distilled water. The pipette can be rinsed with alcohol or ether for rapid drying.

12.   *What is the use of coverslip for charging and counting?*

   Ans: Coverslip, due to its flat and smooth surface, facilitates uniform spread of diluted blood on the chamber beneath the coverslip. By surface tension, it holds the diluted blood on the platform and prevents its spillage into the gutter.

13.   *Should both sides of the chamber be charged? Why?*

   Ans: Preferably, both sides of the chamber should be charged. If the distribution of cells is not uniform or the counting on one side of the chamber is not successful, counting on the other side can be done immediately. Moreover, counting should ideally be done on both sides to assess the accuracy of the result. Charging both sides simultaneously may keep the chamber in balance and uniformly deep.

14.   *How do you differentiate red cells from debris or dust particles?*

   Ans: Debris particles are irregular, having different shapes and sizes. Red cells are round and uniform, having a central halo-like appearance due to thinness. Therefore, counting is done using high-power objective to distinguish between red cells and debris/dust particles.

15.   *Why should the 'Rules of counting' be followed?*

   Ans: Rules of counting are followed to prevent counting the same cells again. For this, either 'L pattern' (count the red cells present in the square and those present on its left and lower lines and ignore those on its right and upper lines) or 'inverted L pattern' (count cells on the left and upper lines and ignore those on the right and lower lines of the square) can be followed. But, pattern' for few squares and 'inverted L pattern' for other squares should not be practised. Only one pattern should be followed for the entire counting.

16.   *What is the value of normal red cell count in adults and why is there a sex difference?*

17.   *What are the functions of red cells?*

18.   *What are the sites of red cell formation before and after birth?*

   Ans:

   I.   **Before birth (fetal life)**   During fetal life, erythropoiesis takes place in three stages:

   i)   *Mesoblastic stage*   In the early embryo, blood formation takes place first in the mesoderm of the yolk sac (the area vasculosa), and later in the body of the fetus. The mesoderm consists of the syncytium (nucleated mass of protoplasm) which later gives rise to a network of capillary vessels. Erythropoiesis takes place intravascularly. This is the only example of intravascular hemopoiesis.

   ii)   *Hepatic stage*   After the third month of fetal life, the spleen and the liver are the most important sites of blood formation. Erythropoiesis occurs mainly in the liver. Therefore, it is called the hepatic stage. Red cells develop from the mesenchyme between the blood vessels and the tissue cells.

   iii)   *Myeloid stage*   From about the middle of fetal life (5th month), the bone marrow begins to form red cells. Slowly, the erythropoiesis in the liver decreases and finally towards term, the marrow becomes the sole region of erythropoiesis.

   II.   **After birth**   After birth, blood cells are actively produced in the marrow cavities of all the bones. By the age of 20, the marrow in the cavities of the long bones, except for the upper humerus and femur, becomes inactive. In adults, erythropoiesis is limited to the bone marrow of the femur, humerus and membranous bones like the sternum. This is called medullary hematopoiesis. Sometimes, because of increased demand, erythropoiesis takes place in the liver and spleen. This is called extramedullary hematopoiesis.

19. *What are the stages of erythropoiesis?*

20. *What are the factors that regulate erythropoiesis?*

Ans: The factors involved in regulation of erythropoiesis can be classified as follows.

i)   **Environmental**   Hypoxia

ii) **Hormonal**   Erythropoietin, Androgens, ACTH, thyroid hormones, TSH, growth hormone, estrogen (All these hormones stimulate erythropoiesis except estrogen, which inhibits it.)

iii) **Hemolysates (products of hemolysis)**   Products of red cell destruction stimulate erythropoiesis.

iv) **Vitamins**   Vitamin B12, folic acid, ascorbic acid

v)   **Metals**   Iron, cobalt, copper, iodine

vi) **Proteins**   Albumin

21. *What are the conditions that alter RBC count?*

22. *What is anemia?*

23. *What is the most common cause of anemia in developing countries? What are the types of anemia?*

24. *What is polycythemia and what are its causes?*

25. *What is the fate of red cells?*

26. *What is stem cell therapy and stem cell harvesting?*

Ans: Stem cell therapy is the transplantation of stem cells from the bone marrow of normal persons to the bone of patients suffering from leukemias or other bone marrow abnormalities. Recently, stem cells are collected (harvested) from umbilical cords or blastocysts of embryos in large numbers, cultured, and used in the treatment of various diseases such as Parkinson's disease, Alzheimer's disease, diabetes, cardiomyopathy, etc.

CHAPTER 8

Determination of Red Blood Cell Indices

Learning Objectives

After completing this practical, you will be able to (MUST KNOW):

1. Explain the importance of calculating red cell indices in clinical hematology.
2. Calculate different red cell indices.
3. State the normal values of MCV, MCH and MCHC.

4. Name the common conditions in which these indices are altered.

You may also be able to (DESIRABLE TO KNOW):

1. Correlate the change in red cell indices in different clinical conditions.
2. Explain the physiological basis of these changes.

INTRODUCTION

From the estimated hemoglobin content, PCV (packed cell volume) and red cell count, it is possible to derive other values which indicate the red cell volume, hemoglobin content and concentration in the red cells. These values are commonly referred to as the red blood cell indices. They are mean corpuscular volume (MCV), mean corpuscular hemoglobin (MCH) and mean corpuscular hemoglobin concentration (MCHC). The MCV defines the volume or size of the average RBC, the MCH defines the weight of hemoglobin in the average RBC, and the MCHC defines the hemoglobin concentration or colour of the average RBC.

Another quantitative measurement of red cells, the mean corpuscular diameter (MCD), is made directly. A derived measurement determined electronically is the red cell distribution width (RDW). This is a measurement of red cell variability.

Determination of these indices is of considerable clinical importance and is widely used in the classification of anemia. When the red cell indices are calculated from manually determined values for hemoglobin, hematocrit and red cell count, the major disadvantage results from the errors associated with manual counts. If electronic counting devices are used, the error is significantly reduced. Indices calculated directly by electronic methods have been found to be more accurate. In recent years, electronic counting of indices is routinely practised in advanced laboratories.

It is important to verify all indices against observations of stained films. When the red cell indices are used in conjunction with an examination of the stained blood film, a clear picture of red cell morphology is obtained. Since red cells are very small and the amount of hemoglobin in a single cell is minute, the units in which the red cell indices are expressed are picograms (pg) and femtolitres (fl).

METHODS

Red cell indices are determined by two methods: 1) indirectly by calculating the indices from PCV, hemoglobin and red cell count and 2) directly by automated counting.

Calculation of Red Cell Indices

Mean Corpuscular Volume (MCV)

MCV is the average volume of a red cell expressed in femtolitre or cubic micrometre (1 fl = 10^{-15} l = 1 μm^3).

$$MCV\ (fl) = \frac{Hematocrit\ (per\ cent) \times 10}{RBC\ cout\ in\ millions/mm^3}$$

where the factor 10 is introduced to convert the hematocrit reading (in per cent) from volume of packed red cells per 100 ml to volume per litre.

For example, if the hematocrit reading is 45 per cent, and the red cell count is 5 million/mm^3 of blood, then the MCV will be 90 fl.

$$MCV = \frac{45 \times 10}{5} = 90 \text{ fl}$$

Normal value The MCV in normal adults is 78–96 fl.

Derivation of the formula

45 percent = $45/100 = 45 \times 10/1000 = 45 \times 10 \times 10^{-3}$
5 million/mm^3 = $5 \times 106/10^{-6}$ l = $5 \times 10^{12}/$ l [since
1 million = 10^6, 1 mm^3 = 10^{-6} l]

$$MCV = \frac{45 \times 10 \times 10^{-3}}{5 \times 10^{12}/\text{l}}$$

$$= \frac{45 \times 10}{5} \times 10^{-3} \times 10^{-12} \text{ l}$$

$$= \frac{45 \times 10}{5} \; 10^{-15} \text{ l} = 90 \text{ fl}$$

Manual estimation of red cells is less reliable; so is the determination of MCV. Automated electronic counting devices measure the electrical impedance caused by each red cell when it passes through the counting devices. The extent of impedance provides an accurate indication of the volume of each cell. Such machines not only indicate the profile of distribution of the volume of red cells, but also provide a highly reproducible value for the MCV. Therefore, the MCV derived by this means provides a reliable index of the average size of red cells.

Mean Corpuscular Hemoglobin (MCH)

The MCH is the average weight of hemoglobin content in a red cell expressed in picograms (1 pg = 10^{-12} g).

$$MCH \text{ (pg)} = \frac{Hb \text{ (g/dl)} \times 10}{RBC \text{ count in millions/mm}^3}$$

For example, if the hemoglobin content is 14 g/dl, and the RBC count is 5 million/mm^3,

$$MCH = 14 \times 10/5 = 28 \text{ pg}$$

Normal value The normal range for MCH is 27–33 pg. It may be as high as 50 pg in macrocytic anemia, or as low as 20 pg or less in hypochromic microcytic anemia.

Derivation of the formula

14 g/dl = 14 g/100 ml = 14×10 g/1000 ml = 14×10 g/l
5 million/mm^3 = $5 \times 10^6/10^{-6}$ l = $5 \times 10^{12}/$ l [since
1 million = 10^6, 1 mm^3 = 10^{-6} l]

$$MCH = \frac{14 \times 10}{5 \times 10^{12}/\text{l}} \text{ g/l} = \frac{14 \times 10 \text{ g/l}}{5} \times 10^{-12} \text{ l}$$

$$= \frac{14 \times 10}{5} \; 10^{-12} \text{ g} = 28 \text{ pg}$$

Mean Corpuscular Hemoglobin Concentration (MCHC)

The MCHC is an expression of the average hemoglobin concentration per unit volume of packed red cells. It is expressed as g/dl or per cent.

$$MCHC \text{ (per cent)} = \frac{Hb \text{ (g/100 ml)}}{PCV/100 \text{ ml} \times 100}$$

For example, if the hemoglobin content is 15 g/dl and hematocrit is 45 per cent,

$$MCHC = 15/45 \times 100 = 33.3 \text{ per cent.}$$

Normal value The normal range of MCHC is 30–37 g/dl (or per cent).

An MCHC above 40 per cent indicates errors in the instrument or in the calculation of the manual measurements used, since an MCHC value of 37 per cent is near the upper limit for hemoglobin solubility. Therefore, this limits the physiologic upper limit of the MCHC. MCHC is a more reliable index than other indices as it does not involve RBC count for its calculation. Therefore, the error associated with RBC count is excluded in MCHC.

In hypochromic anemias, the hemoglobin concentration is reduced and values as low as 20–25 per cent are not uncommon.

Colour Index (CI)

This is the ratio of hemoglobin per cent and RBC per cent.

$$CI = \frac{Hb \text{ per cent}}{RBC \text{ per cent}}$$

$$= \frac{\text{Estimated Hb }/100 \text{ per cent of Hb}}{\text{Calculated RBC count}/100 \text{ per cent of RBC}}$$

100 per cent of Hb = 14.8 g/100 ml

100 per cent of RBC = 5 million/mm^3

For example, if estimated Hb = 12 g/100 ml and calculated RBC count is 4 million/mm^3,

$$CI = \frac{12/14.8}{4/5} = \frac{12}{14.8} \times \frac{5}{4} = 1.01$$

Normal value   The normal range of CI is between 0.85 and 1.10.

CI less than 0.85 indicates hypochromic anemia.

DISCUSSION

MCV

The MCV indicates whether the RBCs are microcytic, normocytic or macrocytic. If the MCV is less than 80 fl, the red cells are microcytic. If it is greater than 96 fl, the red cells will be macrocytic. If it is within the normal range, the red cells will be normocytic. The main source of error in the MCV is the considerable error in the manual red cell count.

Microcytosis

Definition   When the MCV is subnormal, the condition is called microcytosis.

Causes   Microcytosis occurs due to decreased synthesis of hemoglobin. Hemoglobin deficiency can be caused by either iron deficiency or by a defect in the formation of the globin component of hemoglobin.
1.   Iron deficiency (as in iron deficiency anemia)
2.   Globin deficiency (as in thalassemia)
Microcytosis frequently occurs in anemia due to hypoproteinemia and iron deficiency.

Macrocytosis

Definition   When MCV is elevated the condition is called macrocytosis.

Causes   Macrocytosis occurs due to a number of diseases, the most important being megaloblastosis of the bone marrow due to vitamin B12 or folate deficiency.

MCH

MCH indicates the mean amount of hemoglobin per red cell. A subnormal MCH occurs in microcytosis, but MCH is significantly less when microcytosis is associated with hypochromia (decreased concentration of hemoglobin in red cells). This is seen in iron deficiency and thalassemia minor.

MCHC

MCHC reflects a parameter entirely different from MCH. It indicates the average hemoglobin concentration per unit volume of packed red cells.

Decreased MCHC

A subnormal MCHC indicates the abnormality where interference with hemoglobin formation is more than that of other constituents of red cells. This is commonly seen in iron deficiency or thalassemia.

Increased MCHC

Increased MCHC reflects dehydration of the red cells. This is commonly seen in spherocytosis.

Colour Index (CI)

CI is the ratio of Hb per cent to the RBC per cent. CI decreases if Hb per cent is low and increases if RBC per cent is low. The CI indicates the Hb content of RBC. It is not a good index of hemoglobin content because when the Hb per cent and the RBC per cent change proportionately, the CI may not change as it is calculated as the ratio of both these parameters.

Red Cell Distribution Width (RDW)

RDW is a quantitative measure of anisocytosis.

RDW = Standard deviation + Mean cell volume) × 100

Normal value 11.5 to 14. 5 %
Significance RDW is used in differentiating anemia due to iron deficiency anemia (IDA) and thalassemia.

It is increased in IDA (along with low MCV) and also in megaloblastic anemia (with high MCV). In thalassemia trait, RDW is normal with low MCV.

VIVA

1. What are the different red cell indices?
2. What is the practical utility of red cell indices in clinical hematology?
3. Define MCV, MCH and MCHC.
4. How do you calculate MCV, MCH and MCHC?
5. What is the significance of calculating MCV?
6. What are macrocytosis and microcytosis? What are their causes?
7. What does MCH indicate? What is the significance of calculating MCH?
8. What does MCHC represent? What is the significance of calculating MCHC?
9. Why is MCHC more reliable than other indices?
10. Why does MCHC have a physiological upper limit?

   Ans: Because red cells cannot possess hemoglobin beyond a limit (metabolic limit), anemia can never be hyperchromic.

11. Why is the colour index not a good indicator of hemoglobin content of the red cells?
12. Classify anemia based on blood indices.

   Ans: Described in Chapter 4.

13. What is red cell distribution width (RDW) and what is its significance?

CHAPTER 9

Total Leucocyte Count

INTRODUCTION

Leucocytes (white blood cells) are nucleated cells that are involved in the defence mechanism of the body. White cells use the bloodstream primarily for transportation to their place of function in the body tissues. Leucocytes are classified as granulocytes and agranulocytes. Neutrophils, eosinophils and basophils are granulocytes, and lymphocytes and monocytes are agranulocytes.

Formation of Leucocytes

Development of leucocytes is called leucopoiesis. In the embryo, white blood cells develop in the mesoderm and migrate secondarily in the blood vessels. After birth, granulocytes develop exclusively in the bone marrow. The lymphocytes and monocytes also develop from the stem cells in the bone marrow. In adults, lymphocytes are produced primarily in the lymphoid tissue (lymph nodes and spleen) and secondarily in the bone marrow. Leucocytes develop from two types of stem cells: myeloid stem cells forming granulocytes and monocytes, lymphoid stem cells forming lymphocytes (Fig. 9.1).

The number of circulating leucocytes is very precisely controlled. Though there is no definite feedback control system like that for red cells, a

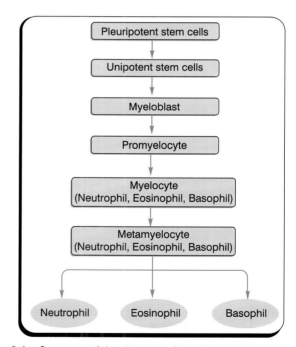

Fig. 9.1   Sequence of development of granulocytes.

number of chemical substances released from the site of destruction of leucocytes affect the development of the cells. The substances that regulate the development of leucocytes are loosely called leucopoietins or leucocyte-promoting factors. These substances are various types of interleukins (produced by monocytes, macrophages and endothelial cells), colony-stimulating factors (produced by monocytes and T lymphocytes), prostaglandins (produced by monocytes), other cytokines and lactoferrin.

Functions of Leucocytes

The granulocytes act as phagocytic scavengers. They engulf and destroy invading microorganisms, and clear the body of unwanted particulate materials such as dead or injured tissue cells. The neutrophils are said to be the first line of defence against acute bacterial invasion. They kill organisms by phagocytosis. The monocytes are also phagocytes and are thought to be the second line of defence against microbial invasion. The monocytes enter the tissues where they form tissue macrophages (mononuclear phagocyte system) and phagocytose microorganisms in the tissues. Lymphocytes and plasma cells act as immunocytes and maintain the body's immunity. Plasma cells are not normally found in blood, but they are formed from B lymphocytes under specific immunologic stimulation. Plasma cells produce antibodies that destroy or inactivate antigens.

Life History of Leucocytes

Radioactive labelling has shown that the entire maturation process, from myeloblast to neutrophil, takes about three days. The leucocytes, especially the granulocytes that circulate in blood, are marginated on vessel walls (margination) and sequestered in closed capillaries. Neutrophils have a half-life of about six hours in the circulation. After their immigration into the tissues, they never return to the bloodstream, and survive in the tissues for a few days. The lifespan of granulocytes is about four to eight days. Their entire population turns over about two and half times each day. Thus, over 100 billion cells are produced by the bone marrow each day. Lymphocytes survive for about 80 to 100 days. Monocytes, after their activities in circulation for few hours, enter different tissues of the body where they transform themselves into tissue macrophages, and stay in the tissues for a long time (a few months or years).

The life history of leucocytes has three phases: marrow phase, circulation phase and tissue phase.

Marrow phase This is the phase of development of leucocytes. In this phase there are two pools: mitosis pool (development of myeloblast to myelocyte) and maturation pool (development of metamyelocytes to matured cells).

Circulation phase Many leucocytes, especially neutrophils stick to the endothelial margin of blood vessels (margination pool) and remaining circulate in the blood (active circulation pool).

Tissue phase After activities in circulation, leucocytes enter the tissues (tissue pool). Monocytes in the tissue form the mononuclear phagocyte system (previously known as reticuloendothelial system)

Normal Count

Adults	:	4000–11,000/mm^3 of blood
Newborns	:	10,000–25,000/mm^3 of blood
Infants	:	6000–18,000/mm^3 of blood
Children	:	5000–15,000/mm^3 of blood

There is no gender difference.

METHODS OF COUNTING

White blood cells are counted by two methods: non-automated (manual) and automated. The manual cell count is less accurate, but is still used widely in developing countries, especially in laboratories of medical colleges.

Manual Method

Principle

Blood is diluted with an acid solution that removes red cells by hemolysis and accentuates the nuclei of white cells. The counting of the white cells then becomes easy. Counting is done using a microscope under low-power objective, and with knowledge of the volume of fluid examined and the dilution of the blood obtained, the number of white cells per mm^3 of undiluted whole blood is calculated.

Requirements

I. Apparatus

1. Microscope
2. Hemocytometer (WBC diluting pipette and counting chamber)
3. Equipment for sterile finger prick
4. Watch glass
5. Coverslip

II. WBC diluting fluid Also known as Türk's fluid (Fig. 9.2).

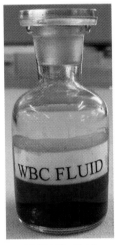

Fig. 9.2 WBC diluting fluid (Türk's fluid).

Composition

1. 1% glacial acetic acid solution
2. Gentian violet stain or aqueous methylene blue (0.3 per cent w/v)
3. Distilled water

Function of each constituent

◈ Acetic acid—causes destruction of red cells (hemolysis).
◈ Gentian violet—stains the nuclei of leucocytes.
◈ Distilled water—acts as a solvent.

Procedure

1. Clean and dry the pipette, watch glass, coverslip and Neubauer's chamber thoroughly.
2. Take enough WBC diluting fluid in a watch glass.
3. Prick the finger under aseptic conditions and wipe off the first drop of blood. Allow a good-sized blood drop to form on the fingertip spontaneously (do not squeeze).
4. Touch the blood drop with the tip of the pipette (*refer* Fig. 6.6) and suck blood exactly up to the 0.5 mark (Fig. 9.3A). If blood is drawn above the 0.5 mark, bring the blood column to the 0.5 mark by tapping the tip of the pipette on the palm or finger, or by using non-absorbent material. Do not use gauze or cotton for this adjustment, because the liquid portion of the sample inside the stem will be drawn into the absorbent material, leaving a higher concentration of cells inside the stem.
5. Wipe the tip of the pipette and maintain the blood level at the 0.5 mark by holding the pipette in a horizontal position.

6. Dip the tip of the pipette into the diluting fluid (in the watch glass) well below the surface of the liquid (Fig. 9.3B).
7. Suck WBC diluting fluid exactly up to the 11 mark. While the bulb is being filled, you may tap the pipette with a finger to knock the bead down below the surface of the solution in the bulb. This will help prevent the formation of bubbles.
8. While removing the pipette from the diluent, maintain the level of the mixture at the 11 mark by closing the pipette tip with the index finger.
9. Hold the pipette horizontally and close both ends of the WBC pipette, then gently mix the contents of the bulb. For mixing, shake the pipette at right angles to its long axis for a few seconds. The glass bead in the pipette should move from one side to the other.
10. After mixing, place the pipette in a horizontal position (Fig. 9.4) to prevent any loss of its contents until the cell count is completed.
11. Discard the first two drops of fluid from the pipette as the fluid in the stem does not contain cells.
12. Charge the Neubauer's chamber as described in Chapter 6 and allow two minutes for the cells to settle down.

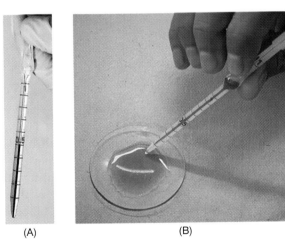

(A)   (B)

Fig. 9.3 (A) Pipetting of blood up to the 0.5 mark; (B) Process of pipetting of WBC diluting fluid into the bulb of the pipette. Ensure that the sucking of fluid is done steadily with the tip of the pipette dipped in the fluid in the watch glass, so that air bubbles do not enter the pipette.

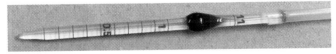

Fig. 9.4 Horizontal placement of the WBC pipette containing the fluid mixture, after completion of pipetting. Note that the upper level of the fluid mixture is at the 11 mark.

13. Place the charged chamber on the stage of the microscope and adjust it for observation under low power.

14. Focus the Neubauer's chamber under the low-power objective and check for uniform distribution of cells in the WBC squares. If the cells are not uniformly distributed, clean the Neubauer's chamber and recharge it.

15. Count the total number of WBCs in the four corner squares under the low-power objective. To avoid counting the same cells again, follow the 'Rules of Counting'. Using the 'L pattern' counting, count the white cells present in the square and those on its left and lower lines. Ignore those on its right and upper lines. 'Γ (inverted L) pattern' counting may also be followed, i.e., count cells on the left and upper line of the square, in addition to cells in the square. But, 'L pattern' for few squares and 'Γ pattern' for other squares should not be practised. Only one pattern should be followed for the entire counting, and preferably the same should be practised by all the students of the class.

> **Note:** WBCs appear similar to clumped red cell debris or stained particles. They are identified as clear, nucleated and refractile bodies.

16. Draw the WBC squares in your notebook and enter the observation. Calculate the final result.

Dilution Obtained

The volume of the bulb is 10 (11 − 1 = 10). The stem of the pipette (from the tip of the pipette to mark 1) contains diluting fluid that does not take part in the dilution. Dilution (mixing of blood with diluting fluid) occurs only in the bulb. Thus 10 volumes of diluted blood (in the bulb) contain 0.5 volumes of blood and 9.5 volumes of diluting fluid, giving a dilution of 0.5 in 10. Thus, the dilution obtained is 1 in 20, or 20 times.

Calculation

Area of 4 WBC squares = $4 \times 1 = 4$ mm^2
Volume of 4 WBC squares = $4 \times 1/10 = 4/10$ mm^3
Dilution factor = 1 : 20
Cells in 4/10 mm^3 volume of diluted blood = n
Therefore, cells in 1 mm^3 volume of diluted blood = $n \times 10/4$
Therefore, cells in 1 mm^3 volume of undiluted blood = $n \times 10/4 \times 20 = \mathbf{\mathit{n} \times 50}$

Precautions

(Same as precautions taken for RBC count; *for details see* Chapter 7.)

1. The pipette, coverslip and Neubauer's chamber should be dry and thoroughly cleaned.
2. The prick should be at least 3 mm deep. Do not squeeze to get blood.
3. Wipe off the first drop of blood.
4. Draw blood exactly up to the 0.5 mark
5. Wipe the tip of the pipette.
6. Suck the WBC diluting fluid exactly up to the 11 mark.
7. Air bubbles should not enter while pipetting the fluid.
8. Before charging the chamber, gently mix the contents of the bulb of the pipette.
9. Discard the first two drops of fluid.
10. Do not overcharge or undercharge.
11. Do not allow air bubbles to enter the chamber.
12. Once the counting chamber is filled (charged), complete the counting as early as possible before the fluid begins to dry.
13. If the distribution of cells is not uniform, discard and recharge.
14. Avoid counting the same cells twice.

Sources of Error

Fortunately, error in the leucocyte count is not as critical as error in the red cell counts. Even an error of 20 per cent does not affect the result much. The possible sources of error may be the errors inherent in the method or technical errors.

A. Errors inherent in the method

1. **Error of visual count** One potential error is mistaking dirt or clumped red cell debris for leucocytes. This error decreases by making a second count in the Neubauer chamber of the opposite side.

2. **Error due to distribution of cells** Distribution can never be perfectly uniform even with thorough mixing and charging. If there is clumping of leucocytes, recharge the chamber.

B. Technical errors

1. **Dilution error** Improper volume measurement of blood and diluent
2. **Pipetting error** Use of defective pipettes
3. **Charging error** Improper charging of the chamber

4. **Counting error**   Improper counting
5. **Calculation error**   Wrong calculation

Additional Information

In case of a very high leucocyte count, as seen in leukemia, dilution may have to be increased to 100 times or more. The RBC pipette can be used for this purpose. Blood is sucked up to mark 1 of the RBC pipette and then diluted 100 times. Calculation is done according to the dilution.

Automated Method

Automated cell counting is done either by impedance counting or by light scattering technology. The principle is the same as that described in Chapter 7.

DISCUSSION

Physiological Significance

Total leucocyte count is performed to assess the subject's ability to defend his body against microbial invasions. The leucocytes are a part of the body's defence system that provides protection against infections. The leucocytes constitute the **mobile defences of the body.** They can pass through the vascular endothelium and enter the tissues by means of diapedesis. Leucocytes migrate to the site of injury in response to chemical substances released by the microorganisms, or by the injured or infected cells. The process of migration is called chemotaxis and the substances that promote migration are called chemoattractants. The white cells, once they reach the site of invasion, engulf and digest the foreign substances (phagocytosis). All granulocytes, especially neutrophils, and monocytes kill the organisms by **phagocytosis.** Lymphocytes are the principal cells of the body's immune system.

Clinical Significance

Total leucocyte count is a part of the routine hematologic investigation used to assess the nature and severity of an infection, extent of spread of the disease and the body's defence capability. In some diseases, alteration in leucocyte count alone may be diagnostic, but frequently the leucocyte count is ordered with other investigations, especially with the differential leucocyte count, to aid in diagnosis. When the total leucocyte count increases above the normal, the condition is called leucocytosis, and when the count decreases below normal, it is called leucocytopenia.

Conditions That Alter Total Leucocyte Count

Leucocytosis

Physiological

1. **Newborns and infants**   Count is as high as 15,000–20,000/mm^3.
2. **Physical exercise**   During physical exercise, circulation becomes more dynamic, which causes disruption of margination of the leucocytes along the vascular endothelium. Therefore, leucocytes are shifted from their margination pool into the circulation pool (into general circulation). This is called **shift leucocytosis.** Leucocytosis does not occur due to increased formation of cells.
3. **After food intake**   Following food intake, the body's metabolism increases; this increases the body's temperature. Because of this, circulation improves. This causes disruption of margination of leucocytes and results in leucocytosis.
4. Exposure to sun and increased environmental temperature.
5. **Pregnancy**   Leucocytosis occurs in spite of hemodilution. The exact cause of leucocytosis in pregnancy is not known, but it may possibly be due to the action of hormones on leucopoiesis.
6. **Parturition**   Leucocytosis occurs due to the combined effects of tissue injury, hemorrhage and severe exertion.
7. Pain, nausea and vomiting
8. Menstruation
9. Emotion and anxiety

Pathological

1. **Acute bacterial infection**   Infection with pyogenic bacteria (localised or generalised) is the commonest cause of leucocytosis. Examples of bacterial infections are boils, abscess and pneumonia. But, there are a few bacterial infections in which leucocyte count decreases. One of the typical examples of leucocytopenia in acute bacterial infection is typhoid fever.
2. **Chronic bacterial infection**   An example is tuberculosis.
3. Tissue injury

Infarction

Burns

Surgery

4. Hemorrhage
5. Neoplasia
6. Stress states and hyperactivity

Convulsions

Severe colic

7. Inflammatory disorders

Certain collagen diseases

Rheumatic fever

8. Metabolic disorders such as diabetic ketoacidosis
9. Corticosteroid therapy
10. Viral infections, e.g., infectious mononucleosis

Leucocytopenia

Physiological Physiological decrease in leucocyte count is very rare. Exposure to severe cold may sometimes decrease the total WBC count.

Pathological

1. Infections

Typhoid fever

Paratyphoid fever

Early phases of many viral infections such as infectious hepatitis

2. **Overwhelming sepsis** In severe sepsis, consumption of neutrophils exceeds production.
3. Replacement of hemopoietic tissue in the bone marrow by neoplastic infiltrative cells:

Acute leukemia

Lymphoma

Multiple myeloma

Myelofibrosis

4. **Aplastic anemia** Hypoplasia of bone marrow decreases all the cell counts.
5. **Cytotoxic therapy** Treatment of malignant diseases by cytotoxic drugs
6. Drugs (especially in sensitive individuals):

Chloramphenicol

Sulpha drugs

Aspirin

7. Hypersplenism
8. Starvation and malnutrition
9. Radiation

Leucocytopenia usually occurs due to neutropenia.

Leukemia

Leukemia is a cancerous disease of the blood-forming tissues. Uncontrolled proliferation of one or more of the various hematopoietic cells occurs, and these progressively displace the normal cellular elements.

Definition

Leukemia is a malignant neoplasia of hemopoietic cells in which there is abnormal proliferation of leucocytes and their precursors. It results in appearance of abnormal and immature cells with very high leucocytosis in the peripheral blood, and infiltration of tissues by leukemic cells. There is increased infiltration of bone marrow by the proliferating cells. The total leucocyte count is usually very high, except in the subleukemic or aleukemic form of leukemia. Usually, the proliferation involves the leucocytic series; occasionally, erythroid precursors or megakaryocytes may also be involved in the disease process.

Causes

The exact cause of leukemia is not known. Some of the probable causes are:

1. Heredity and genetic predisposition
2. Environmental factors, especially exposure to gamma radiation producing genetic mutation or chromosomal aberration
3. Various chemicals and drugs
4. Some viral infections

Classification

Leukemia is broadly classified into two main categories: myeloid (myelocytic) and lymphocytic leukemia. These two types are again classified into acute and chronic forms on the basis of the clinical course and the number of blast cells present.

Acute lymphoblastic leukemia (ALL)

ALL is primarily a disease of children and young adults. This constitutes 80 per cent of childhood acute leukemias. It rarely occurs in adults and the elderly. The most common mode of presentation is with symptoms of anemia or hemorrhage, infective lesions of the mouth and pharynx, fever, prostration, headache and malaise. There is generalised lymphadenopathy, splenomegaly and hepatomegaly. The typical blood picture consists of anemia, thrombocytopenia and moderate or marked increase in leucocytes, the majority of which are blast cells (lymphoblasts; 60–80 per cent).

Acute myeloblastic leukemia (AML)

This primarily affects adults between the ages of 15 and 40 years. It constitutes only 20 per cent of childhood leukemias. The presentation is like that of ALL, but lymphadenopathy and hepatosplenomegaly is not common. Blood picture presents anemia, thrombocytopenia and moderate-to-high leucocytosis. More than 60 per cent of leucocytes in the peripheral blood are blast (myeloblast) cells.

Chronic myeloid leukemia (CML)

This form of leukemia accounts for about 20 per cent of all cases of leukemia. It is primarily a disease of adults of 30–60 years with peak incidence in the fourth and fifth decades of life. Onset is usually slow with non-specific features like anemia, weight loss, weakness and easy fatigability. Splenomegaly is the outstanding physical sign. Hepatomegaly may be present, but lymph node enlargement is rare. Markedly elevated total leucocyte count, usually more than one lakh cells per mm^3 of blood, is seen. Neutrophils and metamyelocytes constitute most of the circulating cells. Blast cells are rarely present except in the blastic crises.

Chronic lymphocytic leukemia (CLL)

CLL is the most indolent of all leukemias. It occurs typically in persons over 50 years of age. Men are affected twice as frequently as women. Patients present non-specific symptoms. Lymphadenopathy is the outstanding physical sign. Hepatosplenomegaly may be present. Mild to severe increase in leucocyte count is seen. More than 90 per cent of leucocytes are lymphocytes.

Leukemoid and Leukoerythoblastic Reactions

Leukemoid Reaction

This is a condition in which the leucocyte count is very high, and may be more than 50,000 per mm^3 of blood. This occurs rarely in severe infections, especially in children and may occur in acute hemolysis, acute hemorrhage and malignant diseases such as carcinoma of breast, lungs and kidney. Few immature cells may be seen in peripheral blood. This is not leukemia, but blood picture resembles chronic leukemia. Therefore, it is called leukemoid reaction. This is differentiated from leukemia by demonstrating high leucocyte alkaline phosphatase (LAP) in blood, which is depressed in CML.

Leukoerythoblastic Reaction

This is similar to that of leukemoid reaction, but in addition, nucleated red cells (erythroblasts) are seen in blood smear, indicating that erythrocytic series is involved in the process. This may occur in severe hypoxia, severe anemia and malignancies infiltrating bone marrow.

Leukostasis

When leucocyte count is above 100,000 per mm^3 of blood, sometimes thrombus consisting mainly of leucocytes are lodged in brain, lung and heart. This is called leukostasis. The risk of leukostasis is high when blood is transfused before TLC is reduced in conditions of high leucocytosis.

OSPE

I.   Dilute the blood (from the given sample) for total leucocyte count.

   Steps
   1.   Select the WBC pipette and ensure that it is dry and clean.
   2.   Take adequate diluting fluid in the watch glass.
   3.   Mix blood thoroughly by gently shaking the sample.
   4.   Suck blood exactly up to the 0.5 mark. If blood is drawn above the mark, the extra blood is removed by tapping with a finger tip (not by touching with absorbent material).
   5.   Wipe the tip of the pipette.
   6.   Suck diluting fluid up to the 11 mark. While drawing the fluid, avoid entry of air bubbles.
   7.   Gently mix the contents of the bulb and keep the pipette on the table.

II. Charge the Neubauer's chamber for total WBC count.

Steps

1. Clean the coverslip and Neubauer's chamber.
2. Place the coverslip on the platform of the Neubauer's chamber.
3. Mix the contents of the bulb of the WBC pipette.
4. Discard two drops of the fluid from the pipette.
5. Touch the tip of the pipette with the edge of the coverslip.
6. Slowly release fluid from the pipette (fluid moves by capillary action) in such a way that the fluid spreads just beneath the coverslip and does not spill into the gutters and does not contain air bubbles.

VIVA

1. *Which diluting fluid is used for determining total leucocyte count and what is its composition? What is the function of each component?*
2. *Why are two drops of blood discarded from the pipette before charging the Neubauer's chamber?*
3. *Why is the dilution obtained 1 in 20, and not 1 in 22?*
4. *In which condition is the RBC pipette used for white cell counting?*
5. *What are the precautions for performing total leucocyte count? What are the possible sources of error in total leucocyte count?*
6. *What are the functions of the white bead present in the WBC pipette?*
7. *What are the functions of leucocytes?*
8. *What is the physiological significance of performing a total leucocyte count?*
9. *What are the causes of physiological leucocytosis?*
10. *What is the mechanism of leucocytosis in physical exercise?*
11. *What are the pathological causes of leucocytosis and leucocytopenia?*
12. *What is leukemia? What are the types of leukemia?*
13. *What are the most frequently occurring leukemias in children and in adults?*
14. *What is the principle of bone marrow transplantation (BMT) and what are the indications?*

    Ans: BMT is the intravenous transfusion of red bone marrow from a healthy donor to the recipient. Usually, the marrow is taken from ileac crest. However, the donor's marrow should match with the recipient's. The stem cells of the donor settle in the recipient's marrow, proliferate and produce cells of different cell lines. This is usually indicated in some form of leukemia, malignancies, severe hemolytic anemia, genetic disorders and severe combined immunodeficiency diseases.

15. *What is leukemoid reaction and leucoerythroblastic reaction?*
16. *How are leucocytes produced (give broad steps of leucopoiesis)?*
17. *How is leucopoiesis regulated and what are the leucopoietic growth factors (leucopoietins)?*
18. *What is the lifespan of leucocytes?*
19. *What is the fate (different phases in the life history) of various leucocytes?*
20. *What is mononuclear phagocyte system, and what are its components?*

    Ans: Monocytes after entering the tissue become tissue macrophages that are combinedly called mononuclear phagocyte system (MPS). They kill microbes by phagocytosis. The cells of MPS in different tissues are:

    A. In blood
       - Monocytes
    B. In bone marrow
       - Monoblasts, Promonocytes
    C. In tissues
       - Kupffer cell in liver
       - Osteoclasts in bone marrow
       - Alveolar macrophages in lungs
       - Histiocytes in connective tissue
       - Microglia in brain
       - Red pulp macrophages in spleen
       - Macrophages in lymph nodes and thymus
       - Mesangial cells in kidney
       - Dendritic cells/histiocytes in skin

CHAPTER 10

Preparation and Examination of Blood Smear

INTRODUCTION

Microscopic examination of peripheral blood smear is performed as a routine hematologic investigation. It is done by preparing, staining and examining a thin film of blood on a glass slide. The blood film is often called peripheral blood smear. The cellular components of blood are noted while examining a blood smear under a microscope.

The unique feature of a blood smear is that it can be retained and preserved as an original record in the laboratory to recheck for errors or to evaluate the progress in the clinical status of the patient, or to assess the response of the patient to treatment. Thus, it can be reused after days, months or years. No other routine hematologic test can be reassessed. Therefore, a peripheral smear is a permanent record. A peripheral smear made for differential count of leucocytes not only provides information regarding them but also about the other cellular elements of blood. It is used to study the morphology of red cells and platelets, and to detect the presence of various parasites like malarial parasites and microfilaria. Peripheral blood smear is also used to verify hemoglobin status, hematocrit and the red cell count of the subject. Because the blood film has many uses, a smear must be carefully prepared and studied.

METHODS OF PREPARATION OF A SMEAR

The blood smear is prepared in two stages:
1. Making a blood smear
2. Fixing and staining the blood smear

Making a Blood Smear

A blood smear can be made by three methods:
1. Glass slide (wedge) method
2. Cover glass method
3. Centrifugal method
    The glass slide method is commonly practised.

Wedge or Glass Slide Method

The wedge method is so called because the smear resembles a wedge.

Principle

Spreading a drop of blood on the glass slide makes a thin film.

Requirements

1. Glass slides

2. **Spreader** These are specially designed glass slides with a smooth edge, the breadth is slightly less than that of usual glass slides. If spreaders are not available, a glass slide with a smooth edge can be used.

3. Equipment for sterile finger puncture

Procedure

1. Take four clean and grease-free glass slides and select one as a spreader.
2. Clean the tip of the middle finger with alcohol, allow the finger to air-dry and prick the fingertip with a sterile lancet.
3. Discard the first drop of blood.
4. Place a drop of blood on one end (say the right end) of a slide, in the middle, about 1 cm from the end, in such a way that only the top of the blood drop touches the slide. Ensure that the skin of the tip of the finger does not touch the slide.

Note: If the finger touches the slide, moisture or oil from the skin of the finger may spoil the smear.

5. Place the specimen slide on the flat surface of the table, and hold it in position at the left end of the slide (the end opposite the blood drop) with the middle or index finger and thumb of the left hand.
6. Place the smooth clean edge of the spreader slide on the specimen slide just in front of the drop of blood (Fig. 10.1A). There should be an approximate angle of 30°– 45° between the two slides.
7. Using the right hand, draw the spreader back until it touches the drop of blood. Let the blood run along the edge of the spreader (Fig. 10.1B). The spreader can be slightly shaken sideways to facilitate the spread of blood along the edge of the spreader.
8. When the blood has spread evenly across the edge of the spreader slide, push the spreader to the other end of the slide with a smooth, quick and controlled movement.

Note: All the blood should be used up before you reach the other end of the slide.

Keep the angle of the spreader constant throughout the process. As the spreader is moved, a thin film of blood will be deposited behind it. The blood film should cover half to three-fourths of the slide when properly prepared (Fig. 10.1C). It should also be noted that no blood is left at the end of the smear (all blood should be completely used in making the smear), otherwise distribution of cells becomes unequal (*for explanation, see* Precaution 8).

9. Turn the spreader slide over (this gives another clean edge) and prepare a second blood film using the same procedure.

Note: A third smear can also be prepared. At least two films should be made for the same blood specimen.

10. Dry the blood smears quickly by waving them in the air, or if the moisture is too high, as occurs in the rainy season, dry the films by waving them rapidly about 5 cm above the flame of a spirit lamp. Never bring the smear close to the flame as excess heat may damage it.

Note: If the smears are not dried quickly, the blood cells will shrink and appear distorted.

Never put the slide directly over the flame. However, adequate drying is essential to preserve the quality of the film. Hence, before staining the slide, make sure that the film is completely dry. It is also observed that if the smear is not dry, it washes off when the slide is washed after staining.

Precautions

1. The glass slides must be scrupulously cleaned. Dirty slides do not give an even smear.
2. The first drop of blood is discarded as it contains tissue fluid and is rich in neutrophils.
3. The drop of blood should not be obtained by squeezing. The puncture should be deep enough to form the blood drop spontaneously.
4. A medium-sized blood drop should be used. If the drop is small, the size of the smear decreases, and if it is too large, some blood will be left at the tail end of the smear.
5. A smear is made immediately after placing the drop of blood on the slide. A delay will cause uneven distribution of white cells on the film. Rouleaux formation by the red cells and clumping of platelets occurs if the blood is not spread immediately. The blood may also clot.
6. The spreader slide must be moved steadily and confidently with a single, quick and smooth movement. Loss of contact between the spreader

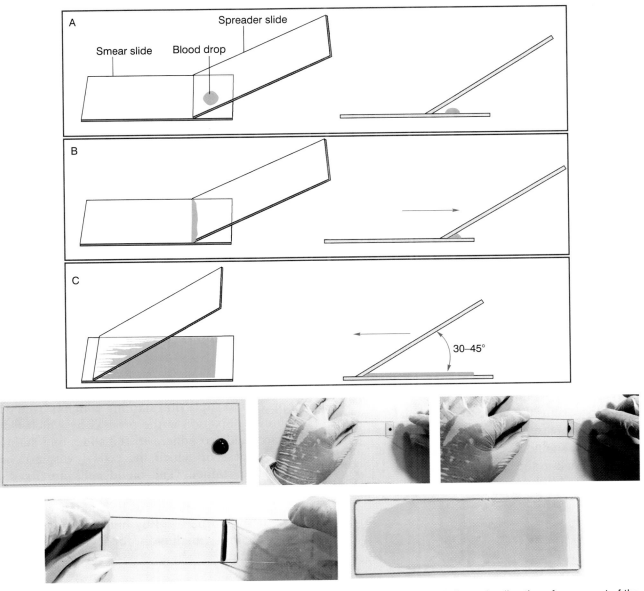

Fig. 10.1 (A–C) Schematic representation of steps in the preparation of blood smear (arrows indicate the direction of movement of the spreader slide). The lower five slides demonstrate the five major steps in making a blood smear.

slide and smear slide yields poor smears. Pressing too much on the spreader slide results in accumulation of white cells and platelets at the end of the smear. Pushing the spreader slide with an uneven movement results in thicker and thinner areas in the body of the smear (Fig. 10.2C). The smear should not be made very fast or slow. The smear becomes thick if made very fast or thin if made slow. With practice, the student will learn the optimum speed.

7. Before the smear is made (before the spreader slide is moved), it should be ensured that the blood has spread uniformly along the edge of the

spreader; otherwise a thick narrow smear results (Fig. 10.2B).

8. The entire amount of blood taken on the slide should be used in making the film. The film should gradually fade away at the feather edge and no blood should be left at the tail end of the smear (Fig. 10.2A). A defined border at the end of the smear indicates that most of the white cells have piled up at the end. When this occurs, the heavier neutrophils accumulate at the end to a greater extent than the other white cells, resulting in uneven distribution of white cells in the body of the smear. Platelets also tend to accumulate at the end of the

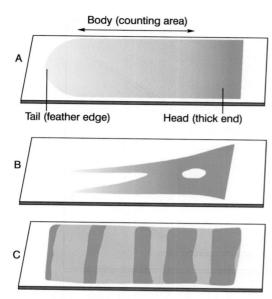

Fig. 10.2   (A) Good smear; (B and C) Bad smears.

smear if some blood is left (not used in the smear), decreasing the number in the body of the smear.

9. The angle between the spreader slide and the glass slide should be about 45°. The angle of holding the spreader slide contributes to the thickness of the film. Increasing the angle yields a thicker smear, whereas decreasing it gives a thin smear.

10. The smear should be completely dry. A wet smear will not stick to the slide when staining. The cells are distorted if the smear takes a long time to dry.

Cover Glass Method

▌ *Principle*

A drop of blood is spread between two cover glasses as they are pulled in opposite directions.

▌ *Disadvantages*

1. It is a time-consuming method. It takes more time than the wedge method.
2. It is difficult to learn and perform correctly.
3. The preparation has to be handled carefully.

Centrifugal Blood Smear Method

With the use of a cytocentrifuge, a monolayer of cells can be prepared. These centrifuges facilitate rapid spreading of the cells across a slide.

▌ *Principle*

A drop of blood is spun from a central point creating an evenly dispersed monolayer of cells. The blood spreads across the slide by virtue of the high torque and low inertia of motion.

▌ *Advantages*

1. Only a small volume of a sample of blood is used.
2. Cellular destruction and artifacts present in the glass slide method are eliminated.
3. Cells are evenly distributed and less distorted.
4. A smear of single-layer thickness is easily obtained.

▌ Fixing and Staining a Smear

Method of Fixing and Staining a Smear

▌ *Principle*

The staining method for blood films fixes dead cells, as opposed to supravital staining which is used with living cells. Fixation is the process by which blood cells are made to adhere to the slide, and staining is the process by which the cells (cytoplasm and nuclei) are stained. The blood cells are fixed by methanol. It is advisable to stain the smear soon after making it. If it cannot be stained within few hours, it should be fixed by immersion in absolute methyl alcohol (methanol) for 2–3 seconds, and then air-dried.

▌ *Requirements*

1. Leishman stain   This is a mixture of methylene blue and eosin in acetone-free methyl alcohol.
- **Methylene blue**   Stains the acidic part of the (basic dye) cell, that is, the nuclei (DNA) and cytoplasm (RNA) of WBCs and granules of basophils.
- **Eosin (acidic dye)**   Stains the basic part of the cell—eosinophilic granules and Hb of red cells.
- **Methyl alcohol**   Fixes the smear to the slide. It is acetone-free because acetone causes lysis of the cell (breaks cell membrane).

Other stains that can be used in place of the Leishman stain are the following:
- **Wright stain**   This is a modified Romanowsky stain, very similar to the Leishman stain. It

produces the same colour reaction with the cellular components of blood as the Leishman stain.

◆ **May–Grunwald and Giemsa stain**   The slide is first stained with the May–Grunwald stain for 5 minutes, and then replaced by the Giemsa stain for 10 minutes. Staining of the cells is similar to that of the Leishman stain.

◆ **Field stain**   It was originally introduced for thick films for malarial parasites in field study. Staining is rapid and convenient. It is used for rapid screening of blood smears.

2. Staining rack   This consists of two glass rods placed in parallel, about 5 cm apart, on a tray. The glass rods hold the slides and the tray holds the stain and water poured on the slides.

3. Distilled water
4. Pasteur pipette
5. Blood smears

Procedure

1. Place the slides on the staining rack with the blood smear (dull side of the slide) facing up. If the staining rack is not available, place two glass rods over a tray to hold the slide.
2. Pour 8–12 drops of Leishman stain on the slide. The stain should just cover the smear.
3. Note the time and leave it for 1½ to 2 minutes.

> Note: During this period, the alcohol in the stain fixes the cells (fixation time).

4. Add double the amount of distilled water on the smear, with the help of a dropper, taking care that the water does not spill.
5. Mix the stain and the water evenly by blowing gently or by blowing air through a Pasteur pipette.

> Note: A metallic shiny layer (greenish scum) should form on the top of this mixture.

6. Note the time and leave it for 7–10 minutes.

> Note: This is the time when staining occurs (staining time). Staining time may have to be adjusted according to the reaction of the stain. Reduce the time if it is overstained, and increase the time if it is poorly stained.

7. Pour off the stain, and wash the slide gently and thoroughly under tap water.

> Note: Make sure that the stream of water does not fall directly on the smear. While pouring off the stain, it should be ensured that the greenish scum does not stick to the surface of the smear.

8. Shake off all water adhering to the slide and set the slide in an upright position in a drying rack.

> Note: Keep the smeared surface of the slide face down. This prevents dust from settling on the smear.

Precautions

1. The smear should dry completely before staining. Unless completely dry, the smear will not stick to the slide and is removed while washing.
2. Adequate quantity (8–10 drops) of stain should be poured on the smear and the stain should cover the entire smear. Do not pour excess stain (it should just cover the smear).
3. Adequate fixing time should be allowed (check the recommended time of fixation for the given sample of stain).
4. The distilled water should just cover the slide. Care should be taken to prevent spill-over of the mixture of water and stain.
5. It is important that the staining rack be kept on a level surface so that the stain is uniform throughout the film and the mixture does not spill over.
6. Water and stain should be mixed by gentle blowing. Mixing should be done immediately after pouring the distilled water.
7. Exact timing for staining should be followed (check the recommended time).
8. When the mixture of stained water is poured off the slide, care should be taken to prevent deposition of scum on the smear.
9. While washing, it should be ensured that the smear is not directly under the stream of water.

EXAMINATION OF A STAINED BLOOD SMEAR

After the initial preparation of the smear, it is examined under the low-power and high-power objectives, and then under the oil-immersion objective. Examination under the low-power and high-power objectives includes:

◆ Evaluation of the quality of the smear
◆ Rough estimation of the red cell and leucocyte numbers

- Distribution of the cells in the smear
- A scan of the film

Examination under the   oil-immersion objective includes:
- Examination of the erythrocytes for alterations and variations in morphology
- Evaluation of platelet numbers and morphology
- Differential count of leucocytes

Steps of Examination

Examination of a smear takes place in three steps: general scanning, selection of the site for examination, and identification and count of cells.

General Scanning

First, examine the stained blood smear under low-power objective for screening. This allows you to scan the entire slide of blood smear quickly. Note the background colour and distribution of white cells. In an ideal stained smear, three zones can be identified (Fig. 10.2A):
i)   the thick area or the 'head' of the smear
ii)   the 'body' of the smear
iii)   the thin end or 'tail' of the smear

Towards the tail end, the red cells lie singly, and neutrophils and monocytes predominate, while in the body, the red cells overlap each other to a certain extent and the lymphocytes predominate. Towards the head end, the red cells considerably overlap and eosinophils predominate. This non-uniform distribution of various types of leucocytes is inherent to the smear prepared by the glass slide method. Therefore, the smear should be examined in a zigzag

fashion (*refer* Fig. 11.1) across the length of the smear but not along the breadth of the smear, to get an accurate differential count. If the scanning indicates very irregular distribution of leucocytes (neutrophils and monocytes are fully concentrated in the tail), the smear will give an inaccurate differential count. In this case, make a new smear. The scanning of the entire slide also gives an opportunity to detect the presence of large abnormal cells like megakaryoblasts, and parasites like microfilariae.

Selection of Site for Examination

If the smear is an ideal one (one-cell thickness), it should be examined throughout its length excluding the extreme, thin portion of the tail and the very thick portion of the head. But, if the smear is not an ideal one (which often happens in practice) select the portion of the blood smear where the red cells just touch each other or slightly overlap but are not piled on top of one another. This area is usually found near the feather edge (between the body and tail) of the film. Place a drop of immersion oil on the slide (do not place on a coverslip) directly on the smear. Now switch to the oil-immersion objective. Ensure that the objective makes contact with the oil. Look through the microscope and increase the light by opening the iris as needed.

Identification of Cells

Identify various types of cells on the basis of the following characteristics as a result of staining with the Leishman stain. Even if the smear is not properly stained, the shape and size of the cells provide sufficient clues for their identification (Fig. 10.3).

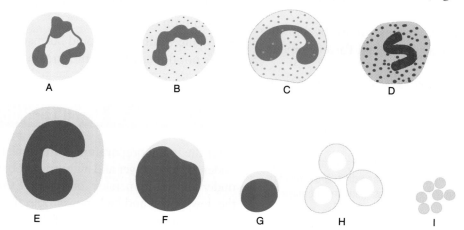

Fig. 10.3   Cells observed in a normal peripheral smear. (A) Segmented neutrophil; (B) Band neutrophil; (C) Eosinophil; (D) Basophil; (E) Monocyte; (F) Large lymphocyte; (G) Small lymphocyte; (H) Red cells; (I) Platelets.

1. Red blood cells

Appearance : Red cells appear as round bodies containing no nucleus, granules or discrete materials.

Staining : Stain orange-red. The red colour is darker at the edge of the cell than in the centre (giving the appearance of a central halo). This variation is caused by the biconcave shape of the cells which contains less hemoglobin in its (thinner) centre.

Size : The diameter of the cells is about 7.2 μm.

2. Platelets

Appearance : Under high power, they look like dirt and stain deposits. Under oil-immersion, they look like pin heads. They contain no nuclei. On fine adjustment, platelets look refractile; this is a characteristic feature that distinguishes them from deposited stained particles.

Staining : Stain mauve-pink.

Distribution : Usually they are present in groups or aggregates (many platelets lying close to each other), but presence of a single (isolated) platelet is not unusual.

Size : They are the smallest cells in the peripheral smear. The diameter of the platelets is 2–4 μm.

3. Leucocytes

i) **Neutrophils** (Fig. 10.4)

Size : 10–14 μm

Nucleus : Multilobed (2–6 lobes), lobes are connected by thin strands. In band-form, the nucleus is sausage-shaped (also called stab form).

Cytoplasm : Looks pale pink, contains fine pink granules.

ii) **Eosinophils** (Fig. 10.5)

Size : 10–14 μm

Nucleus : Usually bilobed, lobes are connected by a thick strand, giving the appearance of spectacles (spectacle-shaped nucleus).

Cytoplasm : Stains faint pink containing coarse brick-red or red-orange granules. The cytoplasm is usually not visible as it is obscured by granules.

iii) **Basophils**

Size : 10–14 μm

Nucleus : Usually bilobed or trilobed, but lobes are usually not distinctly visible because the cell is studded with granules (Fig. 10.6).

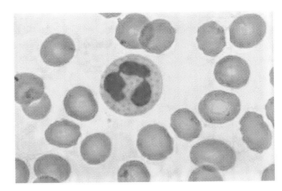

Fig. 10.4   Neutrophil.

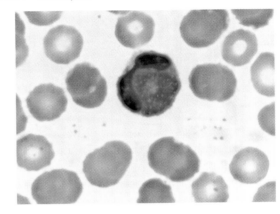

Fig. 10.5   Eosinophil.

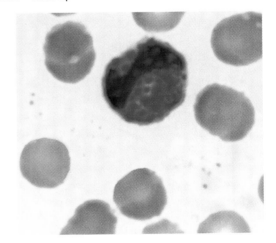

Fig. 10.6   Basophil.

Cytoplasm : Contains numerous coarse granules. Granules are blue-black and fill the cells and obscure the nucleus.

iv) **Large lymphocytes** (Fig. 10.7)

Size : 10–14 μm

Nucleus : Occupies 80–90 per cent of the cell. It is eccentrically placed and oval or round with or without a dent. It is homogeneous (compact) and violet in colour.

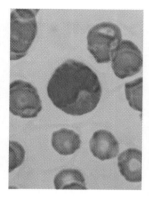

Fig. 10.7 Large lymphocyte.

Cytoplasm : Clear blue cytoplasm; usually contains no granules.

v) Small lymphocytes (Fig. 10.8)

Size : 6–9 μm (same as or slightly larger than red cells)

Nucleus : Occupies almost the whole cell. It is homogeneous (compact) and deep violet in colour.

Cytoplasm : May not be present or sometimes there may be a thin rim of clear blue cytoplasm present at the periphery. There are no granules.

vi) Monocytes (Fig. 10.9)

Size : 12–24 μm, the largest leucocytes

Nucleus : Occupies 50 per cent of the cell, centrally or slightly eccentrically placed. It is usually kidney-shaped or horseshoe-shaped, but may be round, oval, dumb-bell shaped, or irregular. Non-homogeneous (spongy) in appearance and pinkish violet in colour

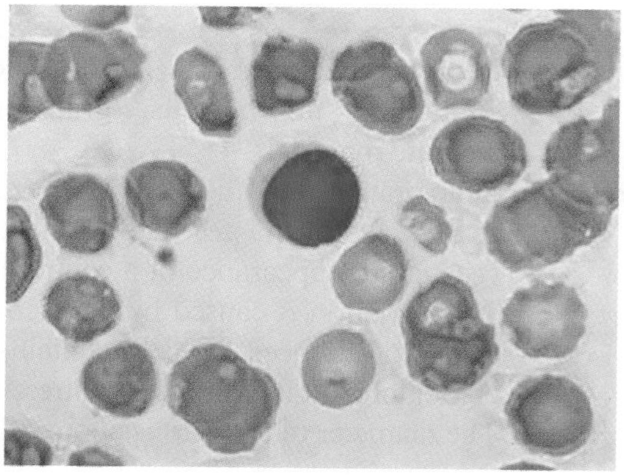

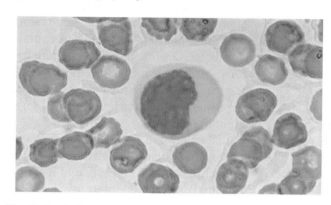

Fig. 10.8 Small lymphocyte.

Fig. 10.9 Monocyte.

Cytoplasm : Ground-glass (hazy, turbid) appearance
– grey-blue in colour
– usually contains no granules, but sometimes (15–30 per cent of monocytes) fine granules may be present.

The differences in structure and function of leucocytes are summarised in Table 10.1.

Table 10.1 Structure and functions of various leucocytes.

Leucocytes	% in DLC	Structure	Functions
Neutrophils	50–70%	10–14 μm diameter; nucleus is multilobed, connected by thin strands of chromatin; cytoplasm has fine, pink granules.	Phagocytosis of organisms (first line of defence against bacterial infection)
Eosinophils	1–4%	10–14 μm diameter; nucleus is bilobed; coarse brick-red granules in cytoplasm	Combat the effects of histamine in allergic reactions, kill parasitic worms
Basophils	0–1%	10–14 μm diameter; nucleus is bilobed or irregular in shape; large cytoplasmic granules are deep blue-purple	Release heparin, histamine, and serotonin in allergic reactions that promote overall inflammatory response
Lymphocytes	20–40%	Small lymphocytes are 6–9 μm in diameter; large lymphocytes are 10–14 μm in diameter; nucleus is round or slightly indented; cytoplasm forms a clear rim around the nucleus	Mediate immune responses
Monocytes	2–8%	12–25 μm diameter; nucleus is oval or kidney-shaped or horseshoe-shaped; cytoplasm turbid in appearance	Phagocytosis (second line of defence) (more phagocytic after transforming into tissue macrophages)

DISCUSSION

A bad smear results from lack of sincerity and interest in making the smear. If all the steps for preparing and staining the smear are properly followed, the smear will definitely be a good one. The smear may be prepared well but improper staining may spoil it completely.

Staining Defects

The following staining defects are frequently observed.

1. **Presence of more precipitated stained particles** This occurs due to either improper washing or using an old stain that has not been properly filtered. Improper washing means inadequate washing of metallic scum. It can be corrected by using a freshly prepared or adequately filtered stain or by correcting the washing procedure. The smear should be washed for about one minute.

2. **Excessively red appearance** This occurs due to understaining, overwashing or use of a highly acidic stain or water (for staining). It can be rectified by increasing the fixing and staining time, and properly washing the smear. Buffered water (pH 6.8) or distilled water should be used for staining.

3. **Excessively blue appearance** This results from overfixing, overstaining, inadequate washing or use of a highly alkaline stain or water (for staining). It can be rectified by decreasing the fixing and staining time, proper washing of the smear and using proper stain and water.

4. **Faded appearance of the cells** This results from overwashing, understaining, underfixing or from an improperly made stain.

Morphological Differences in Leucocytes

Usually, students confuse neutrophils with eosinophils, and large lymphocytes with monocytes. The important points that help to differentiate between these cells are given in Table 10.2.

Criteria of an Ideal Smear

1. A good blood smear should cover one-half to three-quarters of the length of the slide.
2. It should be thickest at the origin and gradually thin out rather than having alternate thick and thin areas. The thin end of the smear should have a good feather edge, that is, the film should fade away without a defined border at the end. It should be tongue-shaped.
3. There should be no streaks or gaps in the smear.
4. It should be one-cell thick (of red cells), that is, the red cells should not overlap each other nor should they remain far away from each other. If a film is thick, the cells pile up.

   Thickness of the film is determined by:
   i) **Size of the drop of blood used**—a thick film results when the drop of blood is large and a thin film from a small drop of blood.
   ii) **The speed of the stroke used to move the spreader slide**—a thick film results from fast

Table 10.2 Differences between neutrophils and eosinophils, and large lymphocytes and monocytes.

		Neutrophils	Eosinophils
1.	Size	Double the size of red cells	Double the size of red cells
2.	Nucleus	Multilobed (2–6 lobes), lobes connected by thin strands	Usually bilobed, lobes connected by a thick strand (gives spectacular appearance)
3.	Cytoplasm	Contain fine pink granules	Contain coarse brick-red granules
		Large lymphocyte	**Monocyte**
1.	Size	About double the size of red cells	Triple the size of red cells, or more
2.	Nucleus	i) Oval or round, usually with a dent ii) Compact (homogeneous) iii) Eccentric iv) Occupies 80–90 per cent of the cell	Kidney or horse-shoe shaped nucleus. But may be round, oval or dumb-bell shaped Spongy (non-homogeneous) Centrally placed Occupies 50 per cent of the cell
3.	Cytoplasm	Clear, sky blue, contains no granules	Hazy, ground glass in appearance, sometimes (15–20% monocytes) may contain fine granules
4.	Nuclear-Cytoplasmic ratio	80 : 20	50 : 50

spreader movement and a thin film from slow movement.

iii) **The angle at which the spreader slide is moved**—a thick film results when the angle is greater than 45° and a thin film results when the angle is less than 30°.

5. It appears salmon pink to the naked eye if stained properly.

6. It should not contain precipitated stained particles.

7. When examined microscopically, the background or space between the cells should be clear, the red cells should appear light red-orange, the platelets should look pink, and the leucocytes should have the proper colour for the nucleus, cytoplasm and granules.

Preparation of Thick and Thin Smears

Thick smears are mainly prepared for detection of microfilariae in the peripheral blood. A drop of blood is placed at the centre of the slide and spread with the corner of another slide. The film is allowed to dry for 30 min. at 37°C and then stained. The entire film is scanned using a low-power objective.

OSPE

I. Prepare a smear from the given sample of blood.

Steps

1. Clean four slides.
2. Select a spreader.
3. Mix the blood thoroughly.
4. Place a drop of blood at one end of a slide.
5. Hold the opposite end of the slide with the middle or index finger, and thumb of the left hand.
6. Place the spreader in front of the drop of blood at an angle of 30°– 45°, and then draw the spreader back until it touches the drop of blood. Wait for spread of blood along the edge of the spreader or slightly shake the spreader to facilitate spreading.
7. Push the spreader with a steady, smooth, and quick movement to the other end of the slide to make an ideal smear (examiner to look for thickness and size of the smear).

Immediately dry the smear by waving the slide in the air.

II. Stain the supplied smear for DLC.

Steps

1. Select an ideal smear.
2. Place the slide horizontally across the two glass rods on the staining tray.
3. Select Leishman stain.
4. Put 8–12 drops of stain on the smear (the stain should be adequate to cover the smear) and note the time.
5. After 1½ minutes, add distilled water, and double the amount of stain on the smear, taking care not to spill the mixture.
6. Mix the stain with water by blowing gently or with the help of a Pasteur pipette. Take care to prevent spill-over of mixture.

III. Focus a neutrophil in the given smear under the oil–immersion objective.

Steps

1. Select an ideal smear.
2. Place the slide on the stage of the microscope and scan the smear under the low-power objective by making necessary microscopic adjustments (concave mirror, condenser at lowest position and iris partially closed) and select the proper site for further examination under the oil-immersion objective.
3. Place a drop of oil on the chosen site and change to the oil-immersion objective.
4. Make other microscopic adjustments (change to plane mirror, raise the condenser to maximum height, and open the iris fully) for examination under the oil-immersion objective.
5. Focus on the neutrophil and make fine adjustments to get a clear picture of the cell.

IV. Focus an eosinophil in the given smear under the oil–immersion objective.

Steps are the same as for OSPE 3 except that the student focuses on the eosinophil.

V. Focus a large lymphocyte in the given smear, under the oil-immersion objective.

Steps are the same as for OSPE 3 except that the student focuses on the large lymphocyte.

VI. Focus a monocyte in the given smear, under the oil-immersion objective.

Steps are the same as for OSPE 3 except that the student focuses on the monocyte.

VIVA

1. *What are the methods of making a blood smear?*
2. *Why is the glass slide method called the wedge method?*
3. *What are the advantages of making a smear by the centrifugal method?*
4. *How is a spreader selected for making a smear?*
5. *Why should the angle between the spreader and the specimen slide be between 30° and 45°?*
6. *Why should the smear be dried quickly after preparing it?*
7. *What is the method of drying the blood smear?*
8. *What are the precautions to be taken while preparing a blood smear?*
9. *Why is the smear immediately made after placing the drop of blood on the slide?*
10. *Why is the smear made by a steady and smooth movement of the spreader?*
11. *Why should the initial drop of blood be fully used in making a smear?*
12. *Name the factors that determine the thickness of a smear.*
13. *Why is the fixing done immediately after making a smear?*
14. *What is the method of fixing a smear if staining is to be delayed?*
15. *Which is the stain usually used in staining the blood smear? What are its constituents and what are the functions of each constituent?*
16. *Why is the alcohol present in the Leishman stain acetone-free?*
17. *Why is distilled water added to the stain after fixation?*

    Ans: In the first two minutes, methanol in the stain causes fixation of cells. Distilled water is added after that to cause ionisation of the stain (ionisation of methylene blue and eosin). Stains work only in their ionised form. Therefore, distilled water is added to the stain after fixation has taken place.

18. *Why is water not used as a solvent for the Leishman stain?*

    Ans: Staining of cells is done only after they are fixed, by adding distilled water. Water opposes fixation of cells.

    If water is present in the stain, the cells will stain but will not fix to the smear. Therefore, stain is water-free. Water also enhances rouleaux formation of red cells, but this rarely happens after the smear is made.

19. *Why is buffer water preferred to distilled water for staining?*

    Ans: Ionisation of stain particles occurs maximally at pH 6.8. The pH of buffer water is 6.8. Tap water is not used as it contains impurities.

20. *Name the other stains that can also be used for staining the smear.*
21. *In which special circumstances is the Field stain used?*
22. *What are the precautions for staining a smear?*
23. *Why is the stain diluted with distilled water after 1½ to 2 minutes and not earlier?*
24. *What is the significance of the appearance of scum on the staining fluid after addition of distilled water?*

    Ans: It indicates that the staining has been done properly. If the greenish scum does not float on the diluted stained surface, this indicates that the scum is deposited on the surface of the smear. In that case, the cells look hazy when examined under a microscope.

25. *Why is the smear examined under low-power objective before being examined under an oil-immersion objective?*
26. *What is the purpose of general scanning of the smear prior to DLC?*
27. *Which is the most ideal area of the smear for DLC and why?*
28. *What are the uses of a blood smear?*

Ans: A blood smear is used for:

i)   DLC and detection of abnormalities of leucocytes if present, for example, immature and abnormal leucocytes as seen in different leukemias.

ii) Study of red cell morphology (size, shape, hemoglobin content).

iii) Rough estimation of red cells and PCV.

iv) Determination of indirect platelet count and morphology of platelets.

v)   Detection of the presence of parasites, for example, malarial parasite, microfilariae and so on.

vi) Sex can be differentiated by identifying the presence of Barr body in the nucleus of neutrophils (it needs special staining).

29. *How do you identify red blood cells and platelets in a smear?*

30. *How will you differentiate neutrophils from eosinophils and large lymphocytes from monocytes?*

31. *What are the criteria of an ideal smear?*

32. *What are the causes of deposition of precipitated stains in the smear and how do you prevent it?*

33. *What are the causes of excessive red or blue appearance of the smear and how do you prevent it?*

34. *What are the causes of the faded appearance of the cells in the smear and how do you prevent it?*

35. *What is punctate basophilia (basophilic stippling) and what does it indicate?*

Ans: Punctate basophilia or basophilic stippling is the presence of numerous basophilic granules in red cells. It indicates disturbed rather than increased erythropoiesis. It occurs in thalassemia, megaloblastic anemia, infections, liver disease, poisoning by lead and heavy metals, unstable hemoglobins and pyrimidine 5'-nucleotidase deficiency.

36. *What are Dhol bodies, and what do they indicate?*

Ans: Dhol bodies are small, round or oval, pale blue-grey bodies usually found in the periphery of neutrophils. They consist of ribosomes and endoplasmic reticulum. Their presence indicates bacterial infections. But they are also seen in tissue damage, inflammation and pregnancy.

CHAPTER 11

Differential Leucocyte Count

After completing this practical, you will be able to (MUST KNOW):
1. Describe the importance of performing DLC in practical physiology.
2. Select a good spreader slide.
3. Prepare a good smear for making DLC.
4. Identify the leucocytes.
5. Perform a differential count within the stipulated time.

6. Describe the structure and functions of various leucocytes.
7. List the common causes of increase or decrease in different leucocytes.

You may also be able to (DESIRABLE TO KNOW):
1. Explain the functions of different leucocytes.
2. State the physiological basis of alteration in cell counts in different clinical conditions.

INTRODUCTION

The types and numbers of each type of leucocyte counted are traditionally reported as percentages. Determination of percentage distribution of leucocytes in peripheral blood is known as differential leucocyte count (DLC). Increase or decrease in individual cell lines are reported separately and give more meaningful information to the physician regarding the status of the leucocytes in the blood. Five types of leucocytes are encountered in normal peripheral blood. They are divided into granulocytes and agranulocytes. Neutrophils, eosinophils and basophils are **granulocytes**, and lymphocytes and monocytes are **agranulocytes**. In 15–30 per cent of monocytes, fine granules are seen. However, since this is not a constant feature, monocytes are classified under agranulocytes.

The size of the cells, whether small, medium or large, cannot be directly measured in the smear in the microscopic field but can easily be compared with the size of the surrounding normal red blood cells in the same field, which are approximately 7.5 μm in diameter. The various characteristics of the nucleus and the cytoplasm of the cells are considered for identifying leucocytes. The features of the nucleus include the shape and size compared to the rest of the cell, and the pattern of chromatins in the nucleus. The features of the cytoplasm include the presence or absence of granules, the nature of granules and their

staining characteristics and colour, and the relative amount of cytoplasm.

STRUCTURE AND FUNCTIONS OF LEUCOCYTES

Neutrophils

Neutrophils are the commonest leucocytes. They constitute 50–70 per cent of the total leucocytes. Typically, there are two types: segmented and band neutrophils.

Segmented Neutrophils

Structure

The diameter of neutrophils (Fig. 10.4) varies from 10 to 14 μm, and the nucleus forms a relatively small part of the cell. The nucleus can assume various shapes, but its usual configuration is lobular (a series of lobes connected by narrow strands of chromatin filaments). It usually contains 2–5 lobes, but sometimes may contain more. No nucleoli are visible in the nucleus. The cytoplasm has a faint pink colour and contains a large number of fine pink granules. About two-thirds of the granules are specific neutrophilic granules, while the remaining one-third are azurophilic granules.

Functions

Neutrophils are **actively phagocytic** (Table 10.1, Chapter 10). The granules have many hydrolytic enzymes and appear to be lysosomal in character. Phagocytosis occurs through a series of events, which include opsonisation, chemotaxis, ingestion and degranulation. During phagocytosis, a number of chemicals are released, such as hydrogen peroxide, and hypochlorite and hydroxyl radicals, all of which are strongly bactericidal. Neutrophils form the **first line of defence** against acute bacterial infections.

Band Neutrophils

These neutrophils are younger neutrophils. The relative band neutrophil count in adults is 2–5 per cent (of the total neutrophils).

Structure

Band neutrophils resemble segmented neutrophils except for the shape of their nucleus. The nucleus may be rod- or band-shaped. There may be slight indentations, but without definite lobes. The number of granules in band neutrophils is more than in segmented neutrophils.

Functions

The functions are the same as that of segmented neutrophils except that the cells are more active (phagocytic).

Eosinophils

Structure

Eosinophils (Fig. 10.5) are slightly larger than neutrophils. Their diameter is 10–14 μm. The nucleus usually has 2 lobes (sometimes 3). The lobes are plumper. No nucleoli are visible. The cytoplasm is packed with brick-red coarse granules. The cytoplasm is pale blue, but is usually obscured by granules. The granules are hard, firm bodies that are not easily damaged. Eosinophilic granules are also highly refractile, a feature that is often valuable in distinguishing them from neutrophilic granules.

Functions

Eosinophils are involved in **defending the body from allergic reactions** (Table 10.1). Eosinophil granules contain a number of chemicals like MBP (major basic proteins), protein X, ECF-A (eosinophil chemotactic factor of anaphylaxis) and lysozymes that neutralise allergens and are also larvicidal and parasiticidal.

Basophils

Basophils are the rarest leucocytes, constituting 0.5 per cent of the total leucocyte population in peripheral blood.

Structure

They are about the same size as neutrophils. The nucleus occupies a relatively greater portion of the cell. The nucleus is often irregular in shape. The cytoplasm is colourless and contains coarse granules. The nucleus and cytoplasm are very often totally obscured by granules which are large, deeply stained and blue-black or deep brown in colour (Fig. 10.6).

Functions

Basophils mediate allergic reaction. Basophil granules contain heparin, histamine and a slow-reacting substance (SRS). The cells are phagocytic. They contribute to the prevention of minute intravascular clot formation. After their activities in the blood, they enter the tissue.

Monocytes

Monocytes constitute 2–8 per cent of the total leucocytes.

Structure

Monocytes (Fig. 10.9) are the largest leucocytes, 12–25 μm in diameter. The nucleus is large and occupies 50 per cent of the cell. The nucleus is frequently kidney-shaped or horseshoe-shaped, but it may be oval, lobular, notched or polymorphic. It never undergoes segmentation. Nuclear chromatins are sharply segregated and distributed in a linear arrangement of delicate strands which gives the nucleus a stringy appearance. The cytoplasm is abundant and is ground-glass or muddy blue in appearance. Sometimes, it contains extremely fine pink granules. The granules are azurophilic.

Functions

Monocytes are actively phagocytic (Table 10.1). They remain in circulation for a few hours and then migrate into the tissues and transform themselves into tissue macrophages. They are the second line of defence of the body. They protect the body against bacteria, viruses, fungi and parasites. They also participate in immunity. They act as the antigen-presenting cells, and also secrete a number of cytokines that mediate various immunologic responses.

Lymphocytes

Lymphocytes constitute 20–40 per cent of leucocytes in adults. But the count is slightly higher in infants and children, who have more lymphocytes and less neutrophils.

Structurally, lymphocytes are of two types—small and large. The majority (80 per cent) of the circulating lymphocytes are small. Only 20 per cent of lymphocytes are large.

Small Lymphocytes

The size of small lymphocytes (Fig. 10.8) is the same as or slightly bigger than the red cells. Their diameter ranges from 7 to 10 µm. The cells are mainly occupied by the nucleus. The nucleus is round or slightly notched. Almost the entire nucleus stains deep purple. The cytoplasm may not be present, but there may be a thin rim of cytoplasm to one side at the periphery.

Large Lymphocytes

Large lymphocytes (Fig. 10.7) are of the same size as or slightly larger than neutrophils. Their diameter varies from 10 to 16 µm, but may be as much as 20 µm. A large lymphocyte is confused with monocytes. The nucleus is large and occupies about 90 per cent of the cell. The nucleus contains homogeneous chromatin with some clumping at the nuclear periphery. This gives the nucleus of lymphocytes a compact appearance in contrast to the spongy appearance of the nucleus of monocytes. The cytoplasm is clear and navy blue in colour, in contrast to the hazy or turbid cytoplasm of monocytes. The cytoplasm contains no granules, but on very rare occasions, a few fine azurophil granules may be seen.

Functions

Lymphocytes mediate the immunologic responses of the body (Table 10.1). Functionally, lymphocytes are divided broadly into two categories: T lymphocytes and B lymphocytes. The majority (80 per cent) of the circulating lymphocytes are T lymphocytes. **T lymphocytes mediate cellular immunity,** which is concerned with viral and fungal infections, parasitic infestation, cancer cells, transplant rejection and rejection of tumour cells. **B lymphocytes mediate humoral immunity** by producing antibodies concerned with protecting the body against bacterial and other infections. B lymphocytes do not directly synthesise antibodies, which are produced by plasma cells. B cells, on specific immunologic stimulation, transform themselves into plasma cells. Therefore, plasma cells are not normally found in the blood.

Normal Count

For a differential leucoctye count, a minimum of 100 cells should be counted, though ideally, 200 or more cells should be counted to find out the more accurate percentage of each type of leucocyte. The percentage distribution of cells in a normal leucocyte count in adults is:

Neutrophil : 50–70 per cent
Eosinophil : 1–4 per cent
Basophil : 0–1 per cent
Lymphocyte : 20–40 per cent
Monocyte : 2–8 per cent

Infants and children have fewer neutrophils (40–60 per cent) and more lymphocytes (25–55 per cent).

METHODS

Method of Counting Leucocytes

Principle

A blood film stained with Leishman stain is examined under an oil-immersion objective and the different types of white blood cells are identified. The percentage distribution of these cells is then determined.

Requirements

1. Glass slides
2. Leishman stain
3. Microscope
4. Distilled water
5. Pasteur pipette

Procedure

1. Prepare blood smears and stain the smears with Leishman stain as described in Chapter 10.
2. First, examine the smear under a low-power objective for general scanning and assessing the quality of the smear, and for studying the distribution pattern of the cells.
3. Place a drop of cedar wood oil on the smear at the feather edge. Bring the oil-immersion objective into position and make the lower end of the objective touch the drop of oil. Using the fine adjustment screw, adjust the objective and focus the cells.
4. For counting cells, start from one end of the smear and move the slide in a zigzag manner (Fig. 11.1).

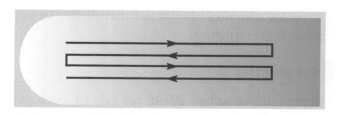

Fig. 11.1 Zigzag way of counting leucocytes for differential count. Arrows in the blood smear indicate the direction of counting.

Count individual white cells that you come across and enter your observation in a table (as described below) in your rough notebook. Continue counting until 100 cells are counted.

5. Calculate the percentage of each leucocyte and report your observation.

Observation and Result

Different leucocytes are placed in groups of 5, five lines indicating five cells (four vertical lines and one oblique line placed over the four lines indicates the fifth cell). In this way, 100 cells are counted. An example of such type of counting is shown below.

Neutrophils	⊬⊓	⊬⊓	⊬⊓	⊬⊓	⊬⊓	⊬⊓	⊬⊓	⊬⊓	⊬⊓	⊬⊓	⊬⊓	=	55	cells
Eosinophils	⊬⊓	⊬⊓	⊬⊓									=	15	cells
Basophils												=	nil	
Lymphocyte	⊬⊓	⊬⊓	⊬⊓	⊬⊓	⊬⊓							=	25	cells
Monocytes	⊬⊓											=	5	cells
												Total =	**100 cells**	

Neutrophils : 55 per cent
Eosinophils : 15 per cent
Basophils   : 0 per cent
Lymphocytes : 25 per cent
Monocytes   : 5 per cent

Alternatively, a table of 100 small squares can be drawn and each cell counted can be entered in the small squares of the table, till 100 cells are filled. On the right side of the table, against each row, the number of different leucocytes present in that row can be entered in separate columns and finally, the percentage can be taken as shown below.

N	N	N	L	L	N	N	N	E	M
N	L	L	N	L	E	E	N	N	N
N	N	N	L	E	N	E	M	N	N
N	L	L	E	N	N	N	L	N	N
N	N	N	L	L	L	N	E	N	E
N	N	N	L	L	N	N	N	N	M
N	L	L	N	E	E	N	L	E	N
N	N	N	L	L	N	E	M	N	N
N	L	L	E	E	N	M	L	N	N
N	N	N	L	L	L	N	E	N	N

N	E	B	L	M
6	1	0	2	1
5	2	0	3	0
6	2	0	1	1
6	1	0	3	0
5	2	0	3	0
7	0	0	2	1
4	3	0	3	0
6	1	0	2	1
4	2	0	3	1
6	1	0	3	0
55	**15**	**0**	**25**	**5**

Precautions

All the precautions described in the previous chapter are applicable to this practical. In addition, the following precautions should be observed:

1. The quality of the smear should be assessed before starting the count. The smear should be discarded if it is not good and a fresh smear should be prepared.
2. Cells should be counted throughout the length of the smear, except the extreme ends of head and tail.
3. Counting should be done in a zigzag pattern to prevent double counting of a cell.
4. A minimum of 100 cells should be counted.
5. The slide should be preserved for future rechecking of the result.

Inference

There is moderate eosinophilia of 15 per cent. Other leucocytes are in the normal range.

DISCUSSION

Differential count is a frequently ordered investigation in clinical medicine. Usually it is done along with other hematologic tests, like total leucocyte count, to assess the ability of the subject to defend the body from microbial invasion, and also to assist in diagnosing the disease.

Clinical Significance

Differential count is vital for the diagnosis of a number of blood-related diseases involving leucocytes or red cells. Its primary use is to identify changes in the distribution of white cells, which may be related to a particular disease like a specific infection (for example, typhoid) or a malignant condition (like leukemia). Clinical terms like increase in specific white cells (neutrophilia, eosinophilia, lymphocytosis and monocytosis) or their decrease (neutropenia, eosinopenia, lymphocytopenia and monocytopenia) are based on the result of the differential count. In addition, a study of the blood smear reveals morphological abnormalities of blood cells, the presence of abnormal cells, and the presence of blood parasites. Differential count also helps in the approximate estimation of other cells (RBCs and platelets). Morphological studies of red cells enable a physician to recognise the hemoglobin status and types of anemia, and also help to check reports on blood indices.

Conditions That Alter Different Cell Counts

I. Neutrophilia

Physiological
1. Exercise
2. Pregnancy
3. Parturition
4. Food intake
5. Emotional stress
6. Exposure to cold

Pathological
1. Acute pyogenic infections, for example, tonsillitis, pneumonia
2. Non-infective inflammations, for example, rheumatic fever
3. Non-inflammatory conditions, for example, myocardial infarction, pulmonary embolism
4. Acute hemorrhage
5. Muscle trauma, for example, following surgery
6. Leukemia, for example, chronic myeloid leukemia
7. Toxic conditions, for example, uremia, hepatic coma
8. Corticosteroid therapy

II. Neutropenia

Physiological Physiological neutropenia is very rare. Sometimes, it occurs after chronic exposure to severe cold.

Pathological
1. Starvation and debility
2. Typhoid and paratyphoid fever
3. Aplastic anemia (bone marrow failure)
4. Parasitic infections, like malaria, kala azar
5. Viral infections like measles, influenza, viral hepatitis
6. Hypersplenism
7. Drug-induced neutropenia

III. Eosinophilia
1. Allergic conditions
   − Bronchial asthma

- Urticaria
- Food allergy
- Hay fever
2. Parasitic infestations
   - Hookworm
   - Filariasis
   - Hydatid disease
3. Skin diseases
   - Psoriasis
   - Pemphigus
4. Collagen diseases
   - Periarteritis nodosa
5. Hodgkin's disease
6. Addison's disease
7. Certain leukemias

IV. Eosinopenia

1. ACTH therapy
2. Cushing's disease
3. Acute pyogenic infections
4. Aplastic anemia

V. Basophilia

1. Chronic myeloid leukemia
2. Polycythemia

VI. Basophilopenia

It occurs rarely, as seen in severe septicemia or aplastic anemia.

VII. Lymphocytosis

1. Chronic infections
   - Tuberculosis
   - Pertussis (whooping cough)
   - Syphilis
   - Brucellosis
2. Infectious mononucleosis
3. Lymphocytic leukemia
4. Lymphomas
5. Viral infections

VIII. Lymphocytopenia

1. Immunosuppressive therapy
2. ACTH therapy
3. Hodgkin's disease
4. Bone marrow failure

IX. Monocytosis

1. Protozoan diseases
   - Malaria
   - Kala azar
2. Hodgkin's disease
3. Monocytic or myelomonocytic leukemia
4. ACTH therapy

X. Monocytopenia

1. Bone marrow failure
2. Aplastic anemia
3. Septicemia

OSPE

⬥ The OSPE discussed in the previous chapter is also applicable to this chapter.

VIVA

All the 36 questions listed in the previous chapter are suitable for this chapter also. The following are some additional questions:

37. *What are the functions of neutrophils, eosinophils and basophils?*
38. *What are the functions of lymphocytes and monocytes?*
39. *What is the normal percentage distribution of different leucocytes in peripheral blood?*
40. *What is the clinical significance of performing DLC?*
41. *What are the conditions that increase or decrease the different types of leucocytes?*
42. *How do you calculate the absolute count of each type of leucocyte by using the value of TLC and DLC?*

   Ans: Absolute count of a cell is equal to the number of that cell counted in DLC divided by 100 × TLC

For example, if TLC = 7000/mm^3 of blood, DLC is as follows:

Neutrophils : 55 per cent

Eosinophils : 15 per cent

Basophils   : 0 per cent

Lymphocytes : 25 per cent

Monocytes   : 5 per cent

Absolute count of the various leucocytes is as follows:

Neutrophils = (55/100) × 7000 = 3850/mm^3 of blood

Eosinophils = (15/100) × 7000 = 1050/mm^3 of blood

Lymphocytes = (25/100) × 7000 = 1750/mm^3 of blood

Monocytes   = (5/100)   × 7000 =   350/mm^3 of blood

CHAPTER 12

Arneth (Cooke-Arneth) Count

Learning Objectives

After completing this practical, you will be able to (MUST KNOW):
1. Identify neutrophils of various stages.
2. State the percentage distribution of neutrophils in various stages.
3. Perform the Arneth count.
4. List the precautions taken while doing the Arneth count.

5. List the functions of neutrophils.
6. Explain the meaning and causes of 'shift to right' and 'shift to left'.

You may also be able to (DESIRABLE TO KNOW):
1. Explain the clinical significance of the Arneth count.
2. Explain the mechanism of 'shift to right' and 'shift to left' that occur in various conditions.

INTRODUCTION

Arneth count (also called Cooke–Arneth count) is the determination of the percentage distribution of different types of neutrophils on the basis of the number of their nuclear lobes. Joseph Arneth, a German physiologist classified neutrophils into five types (stages) according to the number of lobes of their nuclei (Fig. 12.1).

N1 (Stage 1) : The nucleus is unilobed. This is called band neutrophil because the nucleus is rod- or band-shaped. There may be slight indentations, but distinct lobes (clearly separated lobes by thin strands) are not found. In some of the neutrophils, the nucleus may be U-shaped (these are called stab neutrophils.)

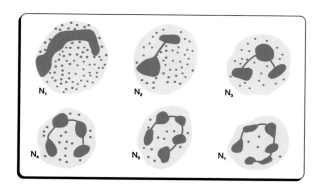

Fig. 12.1 Stages of neutrophils. Note that with maturation, the number of nuclear lobes increases but the number of granules and cell size decrease.

N2 (Stage 2) : The nucleus is bilobed (two lobes, separated by a thin strand).

N3 (Stage 3) : The nucleus is trilobed (three lobes, separated by thin strands).

N4 (Stage 4) : The nucleus is tetralobed (four lobes, separated by thin strands).

N5 (Stage 5) : The nucleus is pentalobed (five lobes, separated by thin strands).

Rarely, **N6** (six lobes) and **N7** (seven lobes) may be encountered.

This staging of neutrophils is based on the degree of maturity. The younger neutrophils contain fewer nuclear lobes than the older ones.

Sometimes it is difficult to stage neutrophils, especially when the lobes of the nucleus are folded. In such situations, two other parameters may be considered: (1) the number of granules and (2) the cell size. The younger cells contain more granules. As the cells participate in physiologic activities, they lose their granules (degranulation), and therefore, the older cells contain less granules. The neutrophils of Stage 6 or 7 contain very few or no granules. The size of the cell also decreases as the age advances. In older cells (N5, N6 and N7), the nucleus may also exhibit the features of degeneration in the form of fragmentation (of lobes) and pyknosis.

Normal count

N1 : 2–10 per cent
N2 : 20–30 per cent
N3 : 40–50 per cent

N4 : 10–15 per cent

N5 : 2–5 per cent

METHODS

Method for Arneth Count

Principle

Neutrophils are grouped into different stages based on their nuclear lobes. The percentage distribution of different stages of neutrophils is determined by examining a stained smear under an oil-immersion objective.

Requirements

Same as for differential leucocyte count (Chapter 11).

Procedure

1. Prepare blood smears and stain with Leishman stain as described under DLC.
2. Examine the smear under a low-power objective to assess the distribution of cells.
3. Count neutrophils under an oil-immersion objective as N1, N2, N3, N4 and N5 for neutrophils of Stages 1, 2, 3, 4 and 5, respectively.

> Note: For counting the cells, start from one end of the smear and proceed in a zigzag manner as described under DLC.

4. Count at least 100 neutrophils and enter your observation in a tabular format (in 100 small squares).

Observation

Note the percentage distribution of various stages of neutrophils and plot a graph (Fig. 12.2).

Precautions

1. The smear should be one-cell thick.
2. Staining should be proper.
3. Lobes of the neutrophil should be counted accurately. If there is confusion in staging a neutrophil, the number of granules and the size of the cell should be considered.
4. At least 100 neutrophils should be counted.

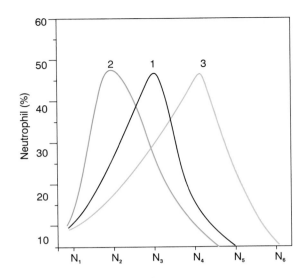

Fig. 12.2   Arneth curve (1: Normal count; 2: Shift to left; 3: Shift to right).

DISCUSSION

Neutrophils are active phagocytic cells in the blood. They are the first line of defence against acute bacterial infections. They are actively mobile; therefore, they migrate immediately to the site of infection and kill the organisms. In acute infections, the neutrophil count increases in the blood proportionate to the degree of assault.

Clinical Significance

Arneth count is not usually ordered in clinical practice, but in some clinical conditions, it is used to determine the number of younger or older neutrophils in circulation. When there are more younger cells, the change is called shift to left; and when there are more older cells, the change is called shift to right. In shift to left, the total cells counted in N1 and N2 are more than 50 per cent, and in shift to right, the total cells counted in N4 and N5 are more then 20 per cent. As Arneth count reveals the production of neutrophils, it indirectly reflects the activity of the bone marrow.

Shift to Left

This indicates that the bone marrow is hyperactive, therefore the circulating neutrophils are mainly N1 and N2. This occurs due to the active response of the bone marrow to different stimuli to form and release more neutrophils into the circulation. The band forms increase in number, which may sometimes be accompanied by the presence of immature neutrophils. If immature neutrophils are present with the younger neutrophils, the condition is called a **leucoblastotic reaction**. Toxic changes may manifest in neutrophils in the form of **basophilic stippling**, deep blue staining of the neutrophil granules like that of basophil granules (basophilic stippling is seen in red cells in lead poisoning). Because the shift to left occurs due to increased production of cells, this is also called **regenerative shift**.

Shift to Right

This indicates the presence of older cells in the circulation. It occurs due to decreased production of cells by the bone marrow (inadequate hematopoiesis) as occurs in aplastic anemia. Sometimes, neutrophils of Stage 6 or 7 may also appear in the blood. Neutrophils may undergo toxic changes in the form of presence of basophilic granules (dark blue granules that resemble basophilic granules), vacuolisation of cytoplasm, hypersegmentation (more than five lobes) of nucleus, and degeneration and pyknosis of the nucleus. As shift to right occurs due to hypofunction of the bone marrow, this is also called **degenerative shift**.

Conditions That Affect Arneth Count

Shift to Left

1. Acute pyogenic infections
2. Tuberculosis (In tuberculosis, lymphocytosis occurs. However, in Arneth count, a shift to left is observed. This may be due to increased destruction of older neutrophils)
3. Hemorrhage
4. Irradiation (exposure to radiation)—Low-dose irradiation stimulates the bone marrow and increases production of cells. However, exposure of bone marrow to a high dose of irradiation causes shift to right as the bone marrow is suppressed.

Shift to Right

1. Megaloblastic anemia
2. Aplastic anemia
3. Septicemia
4. Uremia

OSPE

Focus a neutrophil of Stage 3 in the supplied slides under an oil–immersion objective.

Steps

1. Select an ideal smear.
2. Place the slide on the stage of the microscope and scan the smear under a low-power objective by making necessary microscopic adjustments (concave mirror, condenser at lowest position and iris partially closed). Select the appropriate site in the smear for further examination under an oil-immersion objective.
3. Place a drop of oil on the chosen site and change to the oil-immersion objective.
4. Make other microscopic adjustments (change to plane mirror, raise the condenser and open the iris fully) for examination of the slide under the oil-immersion objective.
5. Place in focus a neutrophil of Stage 3 and make fine adjustments to get a clear picture of the cell.

VIVA

All questions of Chapters 10 and 11 are suitable for this chapter also.
1. *What are the functions of neutrophils?*
2. *What is the half-life of neutrophils in circulation and how long do they survive in tissues?*
3. *What is the normal percentage distribution of neutrophils in different stages of Arneth count?*
4. *What is the relationship between the lobes and age of the neutrophils?*
5. *What is 'shift to left' and what is its clinical significance?*
6. *What is 'shift to right' and what is its clinical significance?*

CHAPTER 13

Absolute Eosinophil Count

Learning Objectives

After completing this practical, you will be able to (MUST KNOW):

1. Describe the importance of performing absolute eosinophil count (AEC) in practical physiology.
2. Describe the structure and functions of eosinophils.
3. State the normal value of AEC.
4. Count eosinophils by using the principle of hemocytometry.
5. List the precautions taken for AEC.
6. Explain the composition and function of each constituent of the Pilot solution.

7. List the common causes of eosinophilia and eosinopenia.

You may also be able to (DESIRABLE TO KNOW):

1. Explain the principle of indirect absolute eosinophil count.
2. Describe other diluting fluids used for eosinophil count.
3. Name the chemicals present in the granules of eosinophils and list their functions.
4. State the physiologic basis of alteration of eosinophil count in different conditions.

INTRODUCTION

Differential count of leucocytes yields the relative number of eosinophils in the leucocyte population. It is possible to find the absolute number of eosinophils in circulation by performing direct and indirect absolute counts. The direct method of absolute eosinophil count (AEC) is done by using the principle of hemocytometry. Indirect AEC is done by calculating the number of eosinophils as a percentage of the total leucocytes present in the circulation. Therefore, for indirect count, two tests should be performed: the differential count and the total count of leucocytes. The sources of error are greater in the indirect count as it multiplies the error of both the methods. The direct count on the other hand is more accurate. The staining properties of eosinophils make the direct count possible.

Structure and Development of Eosinophils

Eosinophils have the same size as that of neutrophils (10–14 μm), but usually have bilobed nuclei. In a stained preparation, the granules take on a deep red or brick-red colour (Fig. 13.1). Eosinophils are distinguished from neutrophils primarily on the basis of granules rather than the number of lobes in the nuclei. In absolute count, other leucocytes and red cells are destroyed, making it easy to distinguish eosinophils.

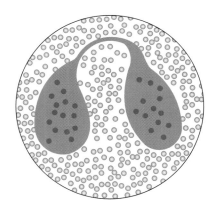

Fig. 13.1   Structure of eosinophil. Note the presence of brick red coarse granules.

Development of eosinophils occurs along the same lines as that of other granulocytes (as described in Chapter 9). Production of eosinophils is regulated by GM-CSF and interleukins IL3 and IL5.

Life History

Once released into the bloodstream, most eosinophils migrate within 30–60 minutes into extravascular tissues where they survive for 8–12 days. Like neutrophils, eosinophils are mobile cells whose movement is directed by chemotactic factors derived from a variety of sources including mast cells and lymphocytes.

Functions

1. Eosinophils are present in large numbers in parasitic infestations in which they appear to serve an important defence function. The granules of eosinophils contain a number of chemicals. Some of these chemicals directly kill the larvae of the parasites (larvicidal) and also the adult parasites (parasiticidal).

   Granular contents The granules of the eosinophils contain the following chemicals.

   Major basic protein (MBP) The MBP makes 50 per cent of the mass of the granules. It is a potent tissue toxin that kills larvae and adult parasites.

   Eosinophilic cationic proteins (ECP) The ECP is a bactericidal and larvicidal agent.

   Eosinophil peroxidase This enzyme participates in inflammatory activities.

   Aryl sulphatase B This enzyme inactivates leukotrienes that are involved in hypersensitivity reactions. It also inactivates the slow-releasing substance A.

   Lysophospholipase This is a membrane-bound enzyme that causes hydrolysis of intracellular lipoproteins.

   Histaminase It causes degradation of histamine.

2. Eosinophil count also increases in patients suffering from allergic diseases in which exposure to abnormal exogenous or endogenous antigens leads to an immunologic reaction. In these allergic conditions, eosinophils dampen the host's response by limiting the antigen-induced release of mediators of inflammation.

3. Eosinophils are also phagocytic and destroy organisms through oxidative mechanisms similar but not identical to those of neutrophils. Eosinophils can phagocytose bacteria, fungi and inert particles, but are less efficient than neutrophils.

Normal Count

The normal range is 40 to 440 per ml of blood. There is no sex and age variation.

METHODS OF COUNTING

Absolute count of eosinophils is done by two methods: (1) directly by using the principle of hemocytometry and (2) indirectly by studying the smear and total leucocyte count.

Direct Method

Principle

Blood is diluted 10 times in a WBC pipette with a special diluting fluid, which removes red cells and stains the eosinophils. The diluted blood specimen is then charged in a counting chamber and the cells are counted under a high-power objective. The population of eosinophils is then calculated for the undiluted blood.

Requirements

I. Equipment

1. Microscope
2. Hemocytometer (WBC pipette and counting chamber). Three counting chambers are commonly used.
   i)   Fuchs–Rosenthal counting chamber
   ii) Neubauer counting chamber
   iii) Speir counting chamber

   Fuchs–Rosenthal counting chamber is preferred because it is specially designed for the eosinophil count. It has a depth of 0.2 mm to accommodate more diluting fluid.

   The **Speir chamber** is very similar to the Fuchs–Rosenthal counting chamber.

   However, as these chambers are not usually available, the Neubauer chamber is commonly used in our laboratories.
3. Materials for sterile finger puncture
4. Watch glass
5. Filter paper
6. Petri dish

II. Reagents (diluting fluids)

There are three diluting fluids available for eosinophil count: Pilot solution, Randolph solution and Dunger solution.

Pilot solution This is the most frequently used diluting fluid.

Composition

i) Phloxine B (1% solution in water)	: 10 ml
ii) Propylene glycol	: 50 ml
iii) Sodium carbonate solution (10% solution in water)	: 1 ml
iv) Heparin	: 100 units
v) Distilled water	: 40 ml

Function of each constituent

◆ Phloxine—stains eosinophil granules.
◆ Propylene glycol—lyses the red cells.
◆ Sodium carbonate—lyses all white cells except (with water) eosinophils.
◆ Heparin—prevents coagulation.

Heparin is usually not added to the solution as red cells are lysed by propylene glycol. However, to prevent clumping of red cell fragments, heparin should be added to the solution.

Randolph solution This is very similar to the Pilot solution except that methylene blue is added to help in differentiating other leucocytes (blue) from eosinophils (orange-red).

Dunger solution

Composition

i)   Aqueous eosin (1%) : Stains eosinophil
ii) Acetone   : Fixes white cells
iii) Distilled water   : Lyses red cells

This solution does not remove other white cells, which appear as grey bodies.

III. Specimen

Capillary blood or EDTA-anticoagulated venous blood is used.

Procedure

1. Clean the watch glass, coverslip, WBC pipette and Neubauer's chamber thoroughly and ensure that these are dry.
2. Take adequate Pilot fluid in a watch glass.
3. Prick the fingertip under aseptic conditions.
4. Suck blood exactly up to the 0.5 mark and clean the tip of the pipette.
5. Suck Pilot fluid up to the 11 mark.
6. Shake the pipette for at least 2 minutes to mix the blood thoroughly with the diluting fluid.
7. Keep the pipette for 15 minutes under the cover of a petri dish lined with moist filter paper.
8. After 15 minutes, take out the pipette, mix the solution by gently shaking the pipette and discard 2–3 drops of the solution from the pipette.
9. Charge the Neubauer's chamber (as described in Chapter 6).
10. Count eosinophils in four WBC squares under the high-power objective of the microscope.
11. Enter the observations in your rough notebook in similarly drawn squares.

Calculation

Dilution is 1 in 20. Therefore, the number of eosinophils counted per mm^3 of blood will be $n \times 50$ (*for details see* Chapter 9) where n represents the total number of cells counted.

Precautions and Sources of Error

All the precautions observed for pipetting and charging the chamber (described in Chapter 6) should be followed for this experiment too. In addition, the following precautions should also be observed.

1. Counting with capillary blood gives a higher result (about 10–20 per cent more) than with venous blood.
2. Counting should be done within 30 minutes of charging the chamber because eosinophils slowly disintegrate in the diluting fluid.
3. For mixing the contents of the pipette, shake gently to avoid undue rupture of the eosinophil membranes.
4. After diluting the blood, the pipette should be kept under the cover of a petri dish lined with moist filter paper, for 15 minutes (staining time) to prevent evaporation.
5. Use the indirect counting method simultaneously to check the result of direct counting.

Indirect Method

This is one of the ways to check the result of the absolute eosinophil count. It should tally with the value obtained in the differential leucocyte count (relative count). In the indirect method, the value of the total leucocyte count is required in addition to the value of the eosinophil percentage of the differential count.

$$AEC = \frac{\text{Differential count}}{100} \times \text{Total leucocyte count}$$

For example, if the eosinophil percentage in DLC is 4 and the TLC is 7000/mm^3 of blood, then the AEC = (4/100) × 7000 = 280/mm^3 of blood.

> **Note:** If the results of the direct and indirect methods differ significantly, the absolute count of eosinophils by the direct method should be repeated.

DISCUSSION

Absolute count of eosinophils by the direct method is not a routine hematologic test. In clinical practice, the absolute count of eosinophils is usually done using the indirect method. However, sometimes, it becomes mandatory to determine the number of eosinophils in a particular volume of blood because this gives an accurate result.

Clinical Significance

The number of eosinophils in the blood is altered significantly in different allergic diseases and parasitic infestations. The eosinophil count is also taken as an index of ACTH activity in the blood. If ACTH is injected intramuscularly in a subject with normal adrenocortical function, it results in the reduction of the total number of circulating eosinophils. This effect has been used as a test of adrenocortical function. This is called the Thorn test. It is not a specific test and the value of the test is limited. Therefore, with the availability of superior methods, the Thorn test is not usually used for assessment of adrenocortical function.

The condition in which the eosinophil count increases is called eosinophilia and the condition in which the count decreases is called eosinopenia.

Conditions That Alter Eosinophil Count

Eosinophilia

1. Allergic diseases
   - Bronchial asthma   – Hay fever
   - Food allergy
2. Parasitic infestations
   - Hookworm   – Roundworm
   - Tapeworm   – Filaria
3. Skin diseases
   - Eczema   – Pemphigus
   - Dermatitis herpetiformis
4. Tropical pulmonary eosinophilia and Loeffler's syndrome
5. Malignant neoplasia
   - Eosinophilic leukemia
   - Lymphoproliferative disorders, for example, Hodgkin's disease
   - Secondary carcinomas
6. Addison's disease

Eosinopenia

1. Cushing syndrome
2. Aplastic anemia
3. ACTH therapy

VIVA

1. What are the methods of absolute eosinophil count?
2. What are the other counting chambers used for absolute eosinophil count in addition to Neubauer's chamber, and what are their advantages?
3. What are the different diluting fluids used for absolute eosinophil count?
4. What is the composition of Pilot solution and what are the functions of each constituent?
5. After diluting the blood, why is the pipette kept under the cover of a petri dish lined with moistened filter paper?
6. Why should the counting be performed within half an hour of diluting the blood?
7. Why is the blood with the diluting fluid in the pipette mixed gently?
8. What are the precautions for absolute eosinophil count?
9. How are eosinophils counted by the indirect method?
10. Why is the direct count preferred to the indirect count for obtaining the absolute value of eosinophils?
11. What is the structure of an eosinophil and what are the chemicals present in the eosinophil granules?
12. What is the half-life and fate of eosinophils?
13. What are the functions of eosinophils?
14. What is the normal eosinophil count?
15. What is the clinical significance of this investigation?
16. Name the conditions that alter eosinophil count.
17. What is the Thorn test? What is its significance?

CHAPTER 14

Determination of Erythrocyte Sedimentation Rate

Learning Objectives

After completing this practical, you will be able to (MUST KNOW):
1. Explain the importance of determining ESR in practical physiology.
2. Explain what ESR is and how it differs from PCV.
3. List the factors that affect ESR.
4. List the methods of determination of ESR.
5. Identify the Westergren pipette and Wintrobe tube.
6. Load the ESR tubes with blood.

7. List the precautions and sources of error in the determination of ESR.
8. State the normal value of ESR in males and females with each method.
9. Name the common conditions in which there is alteration of ESR.

You may also be able to (DESIRABLE TO KNOW):
1. Explain the role of fibrinogen and other factors in determining ESR.
2. Explain the physiological basis of variation in ESR in different physiological and pathological conditions.

INTRODUCTION

Sedimentation of the red cells occurs when anti-coagulated blood is allowed to settle. The rate at which the red cells fall is known as the erythrocyte sedimentation rate (ESR). Students should not confuse ESR with PCV. In the case of hematocrit, the packing of red cells is accomplished by centrifugation, while in ESR, the column of red cells settles by gravity. Sedimentation of red cells occurs due to **rouleau (singular rouleaux) formation**. Rouleaux is the piling up of red cells, so they look like a stack of coins. When the red cells form rouleau, the cells (together) become heavier as they sit on one another. Sedimentation is faster when the size and number of rouleau are large. Therefore, any factor that facilitates rouleaux formation increases ESR and any factor that inhibits it decreases ESR.

Factors Affecting ESR

ESR mainly depends on four factors: (1) the size of the rouleau, (2) plasma factors, (3) the shape and number of red cells and (4) technical and mechanical factors.

Size of the Rouleau

The ESR primarily depends on the size or mass of the falling particles, that is, the rouleaux. The larger the particle, the faster is the fall. The size of the falling particles depends on the formation of **red cell aggregates**, that is, rouleaux formation.

Plasma Factors

1. Plasma proteins   The size of the rouleaux depends on the presence of certain factors in the plasma, especially its **fibrinogen and globulin** content. Normally, red cells tend to repel each other, as they are negatively charged (zeta potential) due to the negative electrostatic charges imparted by sialic acid moieties on the cell membrane. Fibrinogen neutralises the charges on the red cells and makes them sticky. Therefore, when the fibrinogen concentration increases in the plasma, the repelling force on the red cells is removed; this facilitates rouleaux formation. In some pathological conditions, in addition to fibrinogen, other plasma factors called **acute-phase reactants** increase in the blood. These phase reactants also neutralise the charges on the red cell surface and facilitate rouleaux formation. A rise in **C-reactive protein** in the plasma in acute rheumatic fever is an example of such acute phase reactants.

2. Viscosity   When the medium in which red cells settle becomes thick (more viscous), the rate of sedimentation decreases and conversely when the medium becomes thin (less viscous), the rate of sedimentation increases. Thus, in the conditions in which the viscosity of blood increases, the ESR decreases, and in which viscosity decreases, ESR increases. Viscosity of blood increases in polycythemia and decreases in anemia. Therefore, **ESR is low in polycythemia and high in anemia.**

Shape and Number of Red Cells

Red cells are biconcave discs. This shape favours rouleaux formation. A change in the shape of red cells opposes rouleaux formation. Therefore, in **sickle cell disease and hereditary spherocytosis, the ESR is low** in spite of anemia. Polycythemia lowers ESR and anemia raises ESR.

Technical and Mechanical Factors

Some technical and mechanical factors also affect ESR:

1. Temperature   The rate of sedimentation increases with temperature. Increase in temperature increases ESR by decreasing the viscosity of blood.

2. Position of the pipette   ESR pipettes are kept vertical in the rack. Slanting of the tubes in the rack facilitates ESR.

Normal Values

Wintrobe method
    Males   :   0–9 mm/h
    Females   :   0–20 mm/h
Westergren method
    Males   :   3–5 mm/h
    Females   :   5–12 mm/h

METHODS OF DETERMINATION

There are two traditional methods for determining ESR: the Westergren method and the Wintrobe method. The Westergren method is more sensitive and provides more accurate values than the Wintrobe method, because the former uses longer and narrower tubes for ESR measurement.

Westergren Method

Principle

Anticoagulated blood is taken in a pipette and left undisturbed in a vertical position. The level of the column of red cells is noted in the beginning (0 h) and after 1 and 2 hours. The distance (mm) the column moves is noted as the ESR (mm/h).

Requirements

I. Apparatus required

1. *Westergren pipette*   The Westergren pipette is an open-ended tube. It is 300 mm in length with an internal bore of 2.5 mm. It is graduated from 0–200 mm along the lower two-thirds of its length. The graduated volume of the pipette is 1.0 ml. The pipettes are held vertically in the Westergren rack after filling with blood, and the rack is provided with rubber pads at the lower end and metal clips at the upper end (Fig. 14.1).

2. *Westergren rack*   This is a special rack designed to hold Westergren pipettes in a vertical position. It is constructed in such a way that the rubber stoppers attached to springs close the open ends of the tubes when they are placed in the rack (Fig. 14.1).

II. Blood sample   Anticoagulated blood is taken for the study. Sodium citrate solution (3.8%) is the preferred anticoagulant. The ratio of blood to the anticoagulant is 4 : 1, that is, 4 parts blood (say 2.0 ml) is mixed with 1 part anticoagulant (0.5 ml). EDTA can also be used.

Procedure

1.   Mix the blood thoroughly by inversion or swirling.

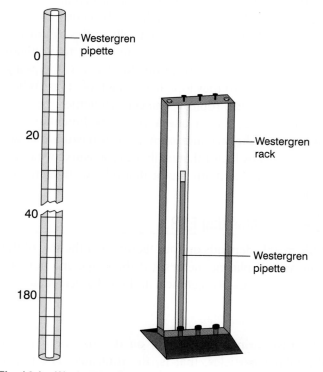

Fig. 14.1   Westergren pipette and rack.

2. Fill the citrated blood into the Westergren pipette up to the 0 mark, making sure that there is no air bubble in the blood column drawn through the tube. The Westergren pipette can either be filled by mouth suction (not usually recommended) or by means of a rubber bulb if available.

3. Immediately close the upper end of the Westergren tube to prevent the blood from running down.

Note: The upper level of the blood column should coincide with the 0 mark of the pipette. If a difference exists, it should be noted and adjusted accordingly with the final result.

4. Place the Westergren tube in the rubber pad of the Westergren rack and fix it vertically with the metal clips provided on the rack (Fig. 14.2).

5. Note the time and allow the tube to stand for 1 hour.

6. Record your observations (note the level to which the red cell column has fallen) after 1 hour.

Note: Ideally, observations should also be recorded at the end of the second hour.

Precautions

1. Concentration of anticoagulant should be appropriate.
2. Blood should be properly mixed before pipetting.
3. The pipette should be clean and dry.

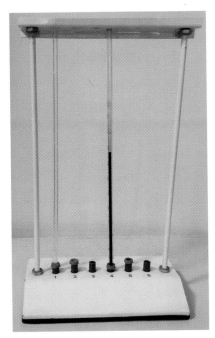

Fig. 14.2   Westergren pipette kept in the rack after filling the pipette (This filled pipette has been kept for one hour). An empty pipette is kept in the rack to the left.

4. Blood should be filled exactly up to the 0 mark and should not contain air bubbles. If the upper level of the blood is above the 0 mark (say 2 mm), care must be taken to add the additional distance travelled by the blood column (2 mm) in the final report. This means that if the reading is 12 mm after 1 hour, report it as 14 mm/1st h.

5. The tube should be kept vertically in the rack.

6. The reading should be taken at the end of 1 hour and 2 hours.

Sources of Error

1. The concentration of anticoagulant affects the ESR value. A false low value is reported in case of higher concentration of anticoagulant.

2. Be accurate about timing. Do not take a reading after 30 minutes and report it as a one-hour reading by multiplying by two. The rate of sedimentation is slow in the beginning and fast after about 45 minutes. A one-hour reading gives the final picture. Therefore, the reading should be taken only after one hour.

3. Temperature directly affects ESR. High temperatures lead to false high values; conversely, low temperatures give false low values. Therefore the specimen must be brought to room temperature before setting up the test.

4. Tilting of the tube increases the ESR.

Wintrobe Method

This method is not usually followed for the determination of ESR in clinical practice. It is used in some laboratories, because it provides two results simultaneously from the same sample, that is, ESR and hematocrit. The ESR reading is taken in the first hour, then the tube is centrifuged for hematocrit value. The Wintrobe tube is made in such a way that both the readings are available on two different graduations marked on the tube. However, the ESR result by this method is not as accurate as that of the Westergren method.

Principle

The principle is the same as that of the Westergren method.

■ Requirements

I. Apparatus required

1. *Wintrobe tube*   The Wintrobe tube is a thick-walled cylindrical tube, 11 cm in length with an internal bore of 3 mm. The tube is graduated in mm in both directions from 0 to 10 cm. The marking 0–10 from above downwards is used for reading ESR. The marking 0–10 from below upwards is used for reading hematocrit (Fig. 14.3A and B).

2. *Wintrobe rack*   This is a wooden rack with holes at the top for holding Wintrobe tubes (Fig. 14.4).

3. *Pasteur pipette*   This is a pipette with a long neck used for filling Wintrobe tubes.

II. Blood sample
Fresh EDTA-anticoagulated blood is used for this method. Note that blood is not diluted in this method. Double oxalate is also preferred as anticoagulant.

■ Procedure

1. Mix the blood thoroughly by inversion or swirling for at least 2 minutes.

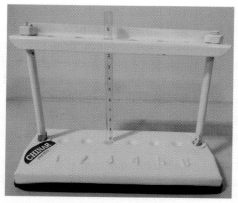

Fig. 14.4   Wintrobe tube kept in the Wintrobe rack.

2. With a long-necked Pasteur pipette or with a special syringe, fill the Wintrobe tube to the 0 mark. For this, the tip of the pipette should be introduced right down to the bottom of the Wintrobe tube and the blood slowly forced out of the pipette into the tube from below upwards (Fig. 14.5). While filling, draw out the pipette tip as the tube is filled with blood. This will prevent air bubble formation.

3. Place the Wintrobe tube in an exactly vertical position in the rack (Fig. 14.6). Note the time.

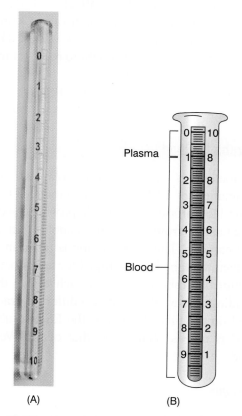

Fig. 14.3   (A) Wintrobe tube; (B) Schematic diagram of Wintrobe tube filled with blood.

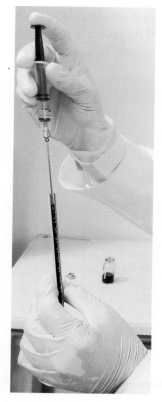

Fig. 14.5   Loading blood in the Wintrobe tube. Note that the tip of the long needle has to be kept below the rising column of blood in the pipette to prevent entry of air bubble.

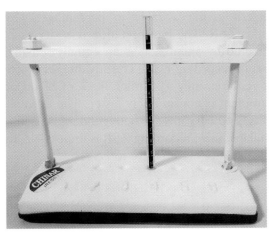

Fig. 14.6   Wintrobe tube kept vertically in the rack just after filling the pipette. Note that the blood is filled exactly up to the zero mark.

4. Note the reading of the erythrocyte column at the end of one hour and report ESR as mm/1st hr.

Precautions

1. The Wintrobe tube should be very clean and dry.
2. Hemolysed blood should not be used.
3. Blood should be mixed properly before pipetting.
4. Blood should be filled exactly up to the 0 mark. If blood is drawn above the mark, absorbent material should not be used to adjust the level. Instead, a dropper is used for this purpose.
5. The blood column should not contain air bubbles or blood clots.
6. The tube should be kept vertical in the rack.
7. The reading should be taken after an hour.
8. While filling the pipette, the tip of the pipette should be kept below the level of blood.

Sources of Error

1. The timing should be accurate. A reading taken after 30 minutes should not be reported as a one-hour reading by multiplying by two. The rate of sedimentation is slow in the beginning and fast after about 45 minutes. A one-hour reading gives the final picture. Therefore the reading should be taken only after one hour.
2. Temperature directly affects ESR. High temperatures lead to false high values; conversely, low temperatures give false low values. Therefore, the specimen must be brought to room temperature before setting up the test.

3. Tilting of the tube increases the ESR rate.

DISCUSSION

Clinical Significance

ESR is a non-specific test to **detect inflammation**. ESR increases in inflammatory conditions, be it infective or non-infective. A **rise in plasma fibrinogen** as occurs in acute infections (pneumonia), a **rise in plasma globulin** as seen in chronic infections (like tuberculosis), and a **rise in phase reactant** as seen in non-infective inflammations (like rheumatoid arthritis)—all these conditions increase ESR. ESR also increases in **malignant diseases** like carcinoma and leukemia. ESR is the index of inflammatory activity in the body. It increases with an increase in the rate of inflammation and decreases with a decline in inflammatory activity. Thus, ESR gives a clue to the physician regarding the progress of the disease and the response of the disease to treatment. Sometimes ESR remains elevated long after the clinical manifestations have disappeared, indicating that the defence mechanism of the body continues to be more active than normal.

Conditions That Alter ESR

I. Increased ESR

Physiological
1. Pregnancy (due to increased fibrinogen and globulin)
2. After a meal (therefore, blood for ESR measurement is collected early in the morning on an empty stomach).

Pathological
1. Acute infection (e.g., pneumonia)
2. Chronic infection (e.g., tuberculosis)
3. Acute non-infective inflammation (e.g., gout)
4. Collagen vascular disease (e.g., rheumatoid arthritis, systemic lupus erythematosus, etc.)
5. Malignant disease (e.g., carcinoma of breast, leukemia)
6. Anemia

II. Decreased ESR
1. Polycythemia
2. Afibrinogenemia
3. Sickle cell anemia
4. Hereditary spherocytosis

Zeta Sedimentation Ratio (ZSR)

Blood in special capillary tubes is spun in the vertical position for four 45-second cycles in a centrifugal device, called the Zetafuge. This leads to rapid compaction of red cells, allowing rouleaux to form and sediment in just three minutes. The capillary tube is then read like a microhematocrit. The value obtained is referred to as zetacrit. The true hematocrit is divided by zetacrit giving a value in percentage, which is known as ZSR. The interpretation is easier as ZSR is not affected by anemia. It is an equally sensitive test like that of recording ESR. The advantages of ZSR are that it requires only 100 microlitres of blood and its measurement is considerably faster. The normal value in adults is 40% to 50% for both genders. As zetafuge is not available now, recording ZSR is impossible, though it is a satisfactory alternative to ESR.

OSPE

I. Load the Wintrobe tube with the supplied blood for determining ESR.
    Steps
    1. Select and clean the tube.
    2. Mix the blood.
    3. With the help of a Pasteur pipette, fill the Wintrobe tube (starting from the bottom) with blood up to the 0 mark taking care to avoid air bubble formation.
    4. Place the Wintrobe tube vertically on the stand.
    5. Note the time.

II. Load the Westergren pipette with the supplied blood for determining ESR.
    Steps
    1. Mix the blood.
    2. Pipette blood up to the 0 mark taking care to avoid air bubble formation.
    3. Immediately close the upper end of the pipette.
    4. Observe the upper end of the blood column. Note the difference, if any, with the 0 mark.
    5. Place the pipette on the rubber pad of the stand and fix it vertically with the metal clips provided on the rack.
    6. Note the time.

VIVA

1. What is ESR? How does it differ from hematocrit?
2. What are the factors that affect ESR?
3. What is the role of plasma fibrinogen in ESR?
4. What are the methods of determining ESR?
5. Why should the anticoagulant concentration be appropriate for ESR estimation?
6. What are the precautions and sources of error in the Wintrobe method?
7. What are the precautions and sources of error in the Westergren method?
8. Why is the Westergren method more accurate than the Wintrobe method?
9. What is the clinical significance of determining ESR?
10. Why is the blood collected on an empty stomach for determining ESR?
11. What are the physiological conditions of increased ESR?
12. What are the diseases in which ESR increases? What are the diseases in which ESR decreases?
13. What is ZSR?

CHAPTER 15

Determination of Blood Group

Learning Objectives

After completing this practical, you will be able to (MUST KNOW):

1. Describe the clinical significance of determination of blood group.
2. Name the blood groups of the ABO and Rh systems.
3. State the physiological significance of the ABO and Rh systems.
4. Define Landsteiner's law.
5. State the principle of determination of blood groups.
6. Determine blood groups by using anti-A and anti-B antisera.
7. List the precautions taken while determining the blood group.
8. List the common indications of blood transfusion.
9. List the common hazards of transfusion.
10. Name the diseases transmitted by blood transfusion.
11. Explain universal donor and universal recipient.

12. Explain the importance of cross-matching.

You may also be able to (DESIRABLE TO KNOW):

1. Name and explain the importance of other blood group systems.
2. State the physiological basis of development of blood groups.
3. Explain the physiological basis of major and minor cross-matching.
4. List and explain all the effects of mismatched transfusion.
5. Explain the procedure of storage of blood in the blood bank.
6. Explain the physiological changes in red cells during storage and after transfusion.
7. List the cause, features, treatment and prevention of erythroblastosis fetalis.
8. Name the diseases associated with different blood groups.

INTRODUCTION

There are more than 30 blood group systems containing about 400 antigens. Fortunately, most of these antigens are not significant immunologically. Moreover, many of them have cold antibodies that do not react at body temperature. The antigens that are involved in blood groups are called agglutinogens and the antibodies that are produced against these antigens are called agglutinins. Clinically, the important blood group systems are: (1) the ABO system and (2) the Rh system. The MN system is important from the medico-legal point of view.

The ABO System

The ABO blood group system is the most important of all blood group systems because of the presence of natural A and B antibodies in individuals, from birth, who lack corresponding antigen on their red cells. In addition, transfusion of incompatible ABO blood groups immediately leads to serious consequences.

In this system, there are two antigens, antigen A and antigen B. Based on the presence or absence of these antigens, blood groups are classified as:

Group A   :   Antigen A is present
Group B   :   Antigen B is present
Group AB :   Both antigens A and B are present
Group O   :   Neither antigen A nor B is present

The A antigen is of two types, A and A1. Therefore, Group A is further divided into two subgroups:

Group A1 :   Containing A and A1 antigens.
Group A2 :   Containing the A antigen only.

Similarly, the AB blood group is subdivided into the A1B and A2B blood groups.

The antibodies in the ABO system are of two types, anti-A (α) and anti-B (β). These antibodies are naturally occurring and are present in the blood of individuals in whom the respective antigens are absent. Thus, Group A (having A agglutinogen on the red cell membrane) will have anti-B and Group B (having B agglutinogen on the red cell membrane) will have anti-A agglutinins in their plasma. The AB group will have no antibody and Group O will possess both the antibodies.

A and B agglutinogens are complex oligosaccharides that differ in their terminal sugars. On the RBC membrane, they are glycolipids, and in tissues and body fluids, they are soluble glycoproteins. H antigen is the fucose-containing antigen, which is found in all individuals. Usually, H antigen has no antigenic activity. Therefore, an individual with blood group O having no antigens of the ABO system, has no antigenic activity at all, and hence, identified as 'O'.

Distribution

In the Indian population, the distribution of the ABO blood group is as follows:

A   : 28 per cent
B   : 22 per cent
AB : 5 per cent
O   : 45 per cent

In the A blood groups, the distribution of A1 group is 75 per cent and that of A2 is 25 per cent.

Landsteiner's Law (Karl Landsteiner, 1900)

This law states that **if an agglutinogen is present on the red cell membrane, the corresponding agglutinin must be absent in the plasma**. If the agglutinogen is absent in the red cells, the corresponding agglutinin must be present in the plasma. The second half of the definition may not be applicable to all blood group systems. For example, in Rh-negative individuals, absence of Rh agglutinogen in the red cells is not accompanied by the presence of anti-Rh agglutinin in the serum.

The Rh (Rhesus) System

This system was first discovered in Rhesus monkeys; hence it is called the Rh system. In this system, there are six antigens, but there are no naturally occurring antibodies. The antigens are C, D, E, c, d and e. Of these six antigens, immunologically, D is the most significant. Therefore, the Rh system has two blood groups:

Rh-positive : D antigen present
Rh-negative : D antigen absent

The antibody in this system is called anti-D antibody and is produced only when an Rh-negative individual receives the Rh-positive blood. These antibodies develop slowly in the first encounter, but rapidly in subsequent encounters.

In the Indian population, 95–98 per cent are Rh-positive and 2–5 per cent are Rh-negative.

The MN System

In this system, there are three blood groups: M, N and MN. This system is usually required for paternity tests.

It can only determine who is not the father of a baby but cannot confirm who is. For example, if the baby's blood group is M and the suspected father's is N, then it can definitely be said that N is not the father of M. But, it can never specifically be said who the father of the baby is. Determination of other blood groups assists in establishing paternity.

MN groups are also useful for anthropological and genetic studies.

The Lewis System

The antigens of the Lewis system are Lea and Leb. These are not really red cell antigens because they are produced in the plasma and are then absorbed into the red cells. The antibodies are of the IgM type. They do not cross the placental barrier and, therefore, do not cause hemolytic disease of the newborn.

The Ii System

There are two antigens in the Ii system, I and i. This system differs from other blood groups in several ways:

1. At birth, the I antigen is poorly developed, but red cells of the fetus and neonates are rich in i antigens.
2. There occurs a gradual changeover from i to I in the first two years of life.
3. In conditions like hemoglobinopathies, red cells show increased i antigen without any decrease in the I antigen.

The Duffy System

There are two blood group antigens in this system, the Fya and the Fyb antigens. This system has three blood groups: Fya, Fyb and Fyab. A close relationship between the Duffy blood group and malaria has been well established. The Fyab blood groups are resistant to *Plasmodium vivax*, whereas Fya and Fyb are susceptible to vivax malaria. This is because the Fya and Fyb antigens, if present separately on the red cell membrane, increase the entry of the malarial parasite into the red cells.

The Kell System

In this system, there is only one antigen called the K antigen. People with K-positive blood group (containing K antigen on the red cell membrane) are susceptible to chronic granulomatous diseases.

METHODS

Determination of Blood Group

Principle

Red cells contain different types of agglutinogens while plasma contains agglutinins. The red cells of the subject are allowed to react with commercially made agglutinins. The presence or absence of the clumping of red cells in different agglutinins determines the blood groups.

Requirements

1. Anti-A serum (containing anti-A agglutinin), anti-B serum (containing anti-B agglutinin) and anti-D serum (Fig. 15.1). Usually, anti-A serum is blue in colour and the the cap of the bottle is blue, anti-B serum is yellow in colour and the the cap of the bottle is yellow, anti-D serum is straw coloured and the the cap of the bottle is black.
2. Test tubes
3. Slides
4. 0.9 per cent saline
5. Microscope
6. Equipment for sterile finger prick
7. Capillary pipette
8. Glass-marking pencil
9. Glass rods

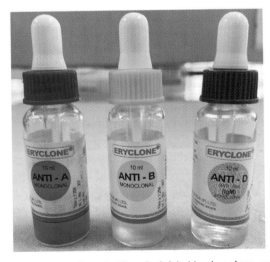

Fig. 15.1   Three antisera bottles. Anti-A is blue in colour and the cap of the bottle is blue. Anti-B is yellow in colour and the cap of the bottle is yellow. Anti-D is straw-coloured and the cap of the bottle is black.

Procedure

1. Take 2 ml of 0.9 per cent saline solution in a test tube.
2. Make a sterile finger prick and collect a large drop of blood into the test tube containing the saline solution.
3. Mix the solution to obtain red cell suspension.
4. On one of the slides, place a drop of anti-A serum on its left half and label it 'anti-A' with the help of the glass-marking pencil (Fig. 15.2). On the left half of another slide, place a drop of anti-B serum and label it 'anti-B'. On the left half of one more slide, place a drop of anti-D serum and label it as 'anti-D'.
5. Place a drop of saline on the right half of each slide and mark it as control (C).
6. To each of these drops, add a drop of red cell suspension by using a capillary pipette.
7. Mix the red cell suspension with the sera using separate glass rods or by gently shaking the slides. Wait for 5–10 minutes.
8. Observe the serum-cell mixtures for agglutination (clumping). Compare it with the cells in the saline controls (Fig. 15.3).
9. Confirm your findings under the low-power objective.

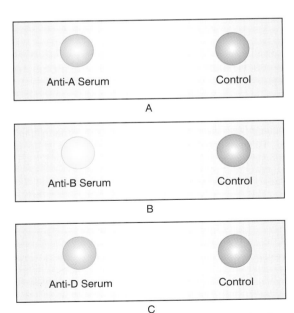

Fig. 15.2   Placement of antisera and control fluid (red cell suspension in normal saline) on testing slides. (A) Anti-A serum and control; (B) Anti-B serum and control; (C) Anti-C serum and control.

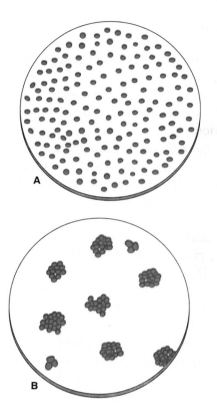

Fig. 15.3   Confirmation of blood grouping under low-power microscope. (A) No agglutination (cells are uniformly distributed); (B) Agglutination present.

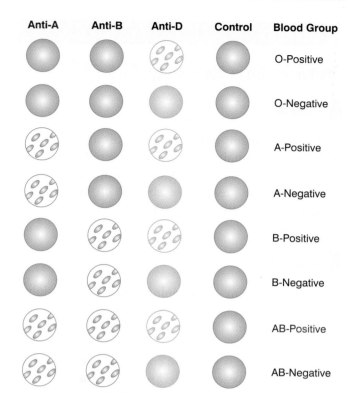

Fig. 15.4   Determination of blood group. Agglutination is marked by clumping of red cells and non-agglutination by absence of clumping (uniform distribution of RBC).

Note: The serum–cell mixture should be examined before it dries up to differentiate clumping (actual agglutination) from rouleaux formation of red cells.

10. Record the presence or absence of agglutination in each slide and interpret the result as follows (Fig. 15.4).

Note: A **false positive** result if present should be excluded by comparing with the control (control will also show clumping of cells). **False negative** results may occur because of decreased immmunocompetence of antisera which may occur due to use of improperly stored antisera.

Precautions

1. The slides must be labelled correctly.
2. While mixing the red cell suspension with antisera, care must be taken not to mix anti-A and anti-B sera with the same glass rod.
3. If there is no clumping in either of the slides, wait for at least 15 minutes.
4. The observations should finally be checked under the microscope.

Anti-A serum	Anti-B serum	Agglutinogens (on RBC)	Blood group
+	–	A	A
–	+	B	B
+	+	AB	AB
–	–	Nil	O

+: agglutination   – : no agglutination

5. A control should always be used to exclude false positive results.
6. Blood should always be diluted for blood grouping test. Use of undiluted blood may give false positive results (rouleaux formation may be confused with clumping). Dilution of blood decreases rouleaux formation.
7. Cell-sera suspension should be examined for clumping before the preparation dries up.

DISCUSSION

To be able to donate or receive blood, an individual should know his or her blood group. This may be required in many medical emergencies. Therefore, the blood group is always noted on the identity card of a person. The blood group is always determined prior to any surgical intervention.

Physiological and Clinical Significance

Uses of Blood Grouping

The uses of blood groups are to:
1. Ensure compatible blood transfusion
2. Eliminate hemolytic disease of the newborn due to Rh incompatibility
3. Solve paternity disputes
4. Detect susceptibility to various diseases
5. Detect personality

Blood Transfusion

Indications

1. **Acute blood loss**   Whole blood is preferred.
2. **Chronic anemia**   Packed red cells are preferred.
3. **Bone marrow failure**
   • Leukemia
   • Aplastic anemia
   • Bone marrow infiltration by neoplastic cells
   In bone marrow failure, fresh blood and specific blood components are required. Red cells are administered along with granulocytes to fight infections.
4. **Purpura**   Platelet transfusion is preferred (so blood grouping may not be necessary).
5. **Clotting factor deficiencies**   Fresh frozen plasma is preferred. In hemophilia, cryoprecipitate (rich in factor VIII and fibrinogen) is given.

Procedure

Blood grouping and cross-matching are always done before blood transfusion to ensure a safe and compatible transfusion. A satisfactory compatibility procedure should include:
i)   ABO and Rh typing
ii) Cross-matching
iii) Antibody screening of the patient (to detect the presence of clinically significant antibodies)

Cross-Matching

There are two types of cross-matching (i) major cross-matching and (ii) minor cross-matching.

Major cross-matching   The cells of the donor are directly matched against the plasma of the recipient. It is important to ensure that antibodies present in the recipient's plasma do not harm the donor's red cells.

Minor cross-matching   The donor's plasma is checked against the red cells of the recipient. It is called minor cross-matching because it is not very important, as the small volume of the donor's plasma is diluted in a large volume of the recipient's plasma. Therefore, the titre of antibodies present in the donor's plasma falls to such a low level after transfusion that they are quite unlikely to damage the red cells of the recipient.

Universal Donor and Recipient

Universal Donor

Persons with blood group O-negative are considered to be universal donors because the red cells contain no antigens. Therefore, their blood can be given safely to anyone.

Universal Recipient

Persons with blood group AB-positive are considered to be universal recipients because their plasma contains no antibodies. Therefore, they can receive blood from anyone.

Though technically this concept is true, its use sometimes may lead to mismatched transfusion due to the presence of various other minor blood groups. Therefore, prior to transfusion, blood should always be cross-matched to eliminate the possibilities of mismatch. However, in emergency conditions, this concept may be used in selecting the donor.

Hazards of Blood Transfusion

I. Due to Mismatched Transfusion

When an incompatible blood group is transfused, reactions occur primarily due to agglutination of the donor's red cells. This results in hemolysis. The severity of the reaction depends on the degree of hemolysis. The complications of mismatched transfusion are:
1. Shivering and fever
2. Hemoglobinemia and hemoglobinuria
3. Jaundice
4. Acute renal failure, which occurs due to:

- Hemoglobin casts blocking the renal tubules and damaging the tubes
- Release of toxic substances from the lysed red cells causing renal vasoconstriction
- Circulatory shock

5. Hyperkalemia (due to release of potassium ions from red cells) that causes cardiac problems

II. Due to Faulty Techniques of Giving Blood

1. Thrombophlebitis This is a common complication in those who receive repeated transfusions.

2. Air embolism Air enters the venous circulation and lodges at the outlet of the right ventricle and blocks the flow of blood to the lungs. Death may occur in severe cases. The use of plastic bags has reduced this complication.

III. Due to Massive Transfusion

This occurs when more than 10 units of blood are given within 24 hours or when the total blood volume is exchanged within 24 hours. Cardiac arrhythmias or cardiac arrest may occur due to high potassium levels in the stored blood.

IV. Febrile Reaction

The patient feels cold and may develop rigour due to raised body temperature. This occurs mainly due to the presence of pyrogens in the transfusion apparatus.

V. Allergic Reactions

This is less frequent and is characterised by itching, erythema, nausea, vomiting and, in severe cases, anaphylactic reactions.

VI. Transmission of Diseases

1. Hepatitis
2. Malaria
3. AIDS
4. Syphilis

Rh Incompatibility

If an Rh-negative individual receives Rh-positive blood, there will be no immediate reaction because Rh-negative individuals do not normally have anti-Rh antibodies. However, the donor's red cells induce an immune response in the recipient to synthesise anti-Rh antibodies. These take about 2–4 months to reach a significant titre, but by that time the donor's red cells die a natural death. The anti-Rh antibody cannot cause any harm to the recipient's red cells because the recipient's red cells contain no Rh antigens. But, if the same Rh-negative person receives a subsequent Rh-positive transfusion, the anti-Rh antibodies are synthesised in large amounts immediately by the memory cells, causing a mismatch reaction.

Erythroblastosis Fetalis

Etiopathogenesis

This is a hemolytic disease of the newborn which occurs due to Rh incompatibility, when an Rh-negative mother carries an Rh-positive fetus. Usually, no reaction occurs in the first pregnancy. However, if the mother has received transfusion of Rh-positive blood earlier, reaction may occur in the first pregnancy. A small amount of blood leaking into maternal circulation at the time of delivery induces formation of anti-Rh agglutinins in the mother. In subsequent pregnancies, the mother's agglutinin crosses the placenta to the fetus and causes hemolysis in the fetus.

Clinical features

If the hemolysis is severe, the fetus may die in utero or if the fetus is born alive, he may have the following features.

1. Anemia
2. Jaundice
3. Edema (hydrops fetalis)
4. **Kernicterus** This is a neurologic syndrome that occurs due to the deposition of bile pigments in the basal ganglia. Bile pigments cannot cross the blood-brain barrier (BBB) in adults but can do so in fetuses and infants because the BBB is not fully developed.
5. Presence of erythroblasts (nucleated red cells) in the blood.

Treatment

The best treatment is to carry out an exchange transfusion soon after birth.

Prevention

The disease is prevented by administering a single dose of anti-Rh antibodies in the form of Rh immunoglobulin during the postpartum period following the first delivery. The disease can also be prevented by passive immunisation of the mother with a small dose of Rh immunoglobulins during pregnancy.

Storage of Blood for Transfusion

Procedure

Blood is stored in the blood bank at 4°C. Disodium hydrogen citrate is used instead of trisodium citrate as anticoagulant, because this favours the fall of pH, which is required for survival of red cells. Stored blood should ideally be used within two weeks of storage. Blood should not be used if it is stored for more than four weeks, because gross hemolysis occurs after this period.

Red Cell Changes During Storage

Red cells undergo rapid changes during storage in simple citrate solutions even at 4°C. During cold storage, the changes that occur are mainly due to reduction of metabolism of cells. They are:

1. Increase in sodium and decrease in potassium concentration in the red cells. This occurs due to decreased active transport of ions across the cell membrane. There is mainly a decrease in Na^+–K^+ pump activity. This results in net increase in the total base and water of the cell.

2. Cells swell and become more spherocytic. This results in spontaneous hemolysis.

3. The ATP content in the cell decreases and inorganic phosphate concentration increases. This is due to an imbalance between the phosphorylation and dephosphorylation processes in the cells.

Changes in Stored Blood After Transfusion

Within 24 hours of transfusion, the cell metabolism greatly increases; consequently, the sodium is extruded from the cells and the potassium is drawn back into the cells. The volume, shape and fragility of the red cells revert to normal within 24–48 hours. Red cells show 80 per cent survival 24 hours after transfusion if the transfusion is given within 14 days of storage of the blood. But the survival rate greatly decreases if the blood is stored for more than two weeks. Therefore, it is ideal to use blood within 14 days of storage.

Diseases Associated With Blood Groups

Different blood groups are prone to different diseases.

Group A   : Carcinoma of stomach
O   : Duodenal ulcer
Fya and Fyb : Vivax malaria
K   : Chronic granulomatous diseases
Rh-negative : Autoimmune hemolytic anemia
Li   : Hemoglobinopathies

VIVA

1. *What is the physiological basis of determination of blood groups?*
2. *What are the precautions taken for determination of ABO blood groups?*
3. *How will you confirm the clumping (agglutination) of red cells?*
4. *What is the mode of inheritance of blood groups?*
   Ans: Blood groups are genetically determined. In general, the presence of a blood group antigen is a codominant characteristic. Therefore, the antigen is present in the phenotype regardless of the genotype (whether homozygous or heterozygous). However, the homozygous or heterozygous state determines the type of contributions the individual can make to the progeny. This is why the blood group of a child may be different from that of both parents.
5. *What is Landsteiner's law and what are the exceptions to this law?*
6. *What is a 'universal donor' and a 'universal recipient'?*
7. *What is cross-matching of blood and what is its clinical significance?*
8. *Why is minor cross-matching usually not done for blood transfusion?*
9. *What is Rh incompatibility and how does it differ from ABO incompatibility?*
   Ans: When an Rh-negative person receives blood from an Rh-positive person, there is a reaction. This is called Rh incompatibility. This differs from ABO incompatibility in terms of the speed with which the transfusion reactions develop. In ABO incompatibility, the reaction develops immediately, but Rh incompatibility reaction may not occur at all in the first exposure. Though the reaction does not occur in the first transfusion, the donor's red cells induce an immune response in

the recipient as a result of which anti-Rh agglutinins are slowly formed in the recipient's plasma. When the same individual receives a second transfusion of Rh-positive blood, the transfusion reaction occurs immediately.

10. *What is erythroblastosis fetalis and how can it be prevented?*

11. *How is blood stored in the blood bank?*

Ans: Blood is collected from the donor in a labelled plastic bag or glass bottle. Disodium hydrogen citrate is used as anticoagulant because it favours survival of red cells by decreasing the pH.

Blood is stored in the blood bank at 4°C.

12. *What are the physiological changes that occur in the red cells during storage?*

13. *What is the cause of hemolysis of stored blood?*

14. *What are cold and warm antibodies for blood group antigens? What are the differences among them?*

Ans: The terms 'cold' and 'warm' antibodies are applied to the antibodies of the ABO system and Rh systems of blood group, respectively. Their important features and differences among them are:

	Antibodies of ABO system	Antibodies of Rh system
i)	These are larger molecules, of the IgM type; cannot cross the placenta.	They are of the IgG type; can easily cross the placenta.
ii)	React with the antigens best at low temperature between 5–20°C. Hence called 'cold' antibodies.	React with antigens best at body temperature. Hence called 'warm' antibodies.
iii)	ABO incompatibility between a mother and fetus does not occur.	Rh incompatibility occurs.

15. *What is the importance of using a control on each side of the 3 test slides? What are false positive and false negative results?*

Ans: The control sample for blood group testing in each case is only a suspension of red cells in normal saline. Its purpose is to avoid 'false positive' and 'false negative' results?

False Positive Reaction: It means that though there is no actual agglutination, the reaction appears to be so. Formation of large rouleaux (this may happen if undiluted blood is used) may give a false impression of agglutination, but the cells will quickly disperse on tilting the slide a few times. Bacterial contamination of an antiserum, or of normal saline, may show agglutination in all tests or in all controls.

False Negative Reaction: It may occur due to loss of potency of the antisera because of faulty storage. All tests will come out negative with such an antiserum.

16. *What is zone phenomenon?*

Ans: For agglutination to occur, the concentration of agglutinogens and agglutinin should be approximately the same. This is called zone phenomenon. With a gross difference in these concentrations, the agglutination may not be significant.

17. *What is autologous transfusion and pre-donation?*

Ans: In addition to receiving blood from a donor, an individual may also receive one's own stored blood, i.e., during elective surgery on him in the future. The blood is collected much before surgery and the same blood is transfused during surgery. This is called autologous transfusion. This is also called predonation. The benefit of this procedure is that it avoids transmission of diseases such as AIDS, hepatitis, etc. as well as risk of transfusion reaction.

Predonation (Predeposit) is a form of autologous transfusion in which a course of iron tablets is given and after that two units of blood are collected (first unit 16 days before and second unit 8 days before surgery). An important technical innovation is the cell-saver machine which sucks up blood from the wound during the operation, recycles it, and returns it to the patient's body.

18. *What is blood doping and what is its advantage?*

Ans: Blood 'doping' is the athletic mispractice, in which one or two units of an athlete's blood (or red cells) is removed and stored 2 weeks before the athletic event. The blood is re-injected in 2 sessions just few days before the event. Since oxygen delivery to active muscles is the limiting factor, increased red cell count enhances their performance in marathon events. This practice is banned by the International Athletic and Olympic Committees.

19. *Which blood substitute is preferred if suitable blood donor is not available?*

Ans: Whole blood is ideal to replace lost blood as occurs in hemorrhage as it replaces cells and plasma in physiological ratio. But in a situation where it may not be available, an intravenous drip of a crystalloid or colloid solution is immediately started.

Crystalloid solutions: In clinical practice, the commonly used one is intravenous fluid of glucose saline, i.e., 6% glucose in 0.9% sodium chloride. As crystalloids leave the circulation in a short time, the restoration of the volume is temporary.

Colloid solutions: The colloid substitutes are plasma expanders, such as human albumin, dextrose and dextrose with NaCl, and a polymer from degraded gelatin. Plasma separated from donated blood can be stored in a liquid form (fresh frozen plasma) for many months. It can be dried and kept still longer, which is reconstituted with distilled water just before use.

Blood substitutes: Sometimes, especially if there is a chance of volume overload, instead of whole blood or plasma, a blood component is used to avoid circulatory overload and lower the risk of transfusion. The blood substitutes include packed red cells, WBC concentrates, immunoglobulins, and clotting factor concentrate.

20. *What is the speciality of Bombay blood group?*

Ans: The Bombay blood type is a rare variety in which the H antigen is absent. Since there is no H antigen, there is no antigen A or antigen B on the red cells. However, the plasma contains anti-A, anti-B and anti-H antibodies. Therefore, such a person can receive blood only from a person having Bombay blood group.

21. *What are forward and reverse blood typing?*

Ans: In blood grouping or typing, the red cells of a donor or a person whose blood type is to be determined are tested against anti-A and anti-B sera. This is called blood typing or forward blood typing.

In reverse blood typing, (also called serum typing or backward blood typing), the serum of the recipient is tested against red cells containing known antigens, i.e., red cells from persons with blood types A, B, AB, and O. If agglutination occurs with A and AB red cells, the blood type is B; if agglutination occurs with B and AB red cells, the blood type is A; if agglutination occurs with A, B, and AB red cells, the blood type is O and if there is no agglutination in any RBCs, the blood type is AB.

For blood transfusion in leukemic patients, serum typing is done along with blood typing as an extra precaution, because in leukemias, the RBC antigens may become considerably weak. This is also performed in pseudomonas infection, since in these infections, RBCs become agglutinated by all antisera due to unmasking of hidden antigens.

22. *What is the MN system and what is its clinical use?*

23. *Why does mismatching of blood of the Lewis system not cause hemolysis?*

24. *What is the clinical significance of the li system?*

25. *Which disease is closely associated with the Duffy system and why?*

26. *What is the clinical use of the Kell system?*

27. *What are the different diseases associated with different blood groups?*

28. *What is Bombay blood group and what is its significance?*

Ans: Bombay blood group is a rare occurrence, in which H antigen is not expressed. Due to absence of H antigen, agglutinogens A and B are absent on the membrane of red cells. However, in spite of absence of these three blood group agglutinogens, anti-A, anti-B and anti-H agglutinins are present in the plasma. Therefore, a person having Bombay blood group can receive blood only from a person having Bombay blood group, and not from others.

CHAPTER 16

Osmotic Fragility of Red Cells

Learning Objectives

After completing this practical, you will be able to (MUST KNOW):
1. Describe the utility of this practical in clinical physiology.
2. Prepare saline solutions of different percentage.
3. Perform the osmotic fragility test.
4. Explain the mechanism of hemolysis when red cells are exposed to hypotonic solutions.
5. List the precautions taken for the osmotic fragility test.

6. Define and explain osmotic fragility.
7. List the conditions that alter the osmotic fragility of red cells.

You may also be able to (DESIRABLE TO KNOW):
1. Correlate the applicability of this practical in different clinical conditions.
2. Explain the physiological basis of alteration in osmotic fragility in different diseases of red cells.

INTRODUCTION

Osmotic fragility of red cells is defined as the ease with which the RBCs are ruptured (hemolysed) when they are exposed to hypotonic solutions. It assesses the integrity of the membrane of red cells.

The osmotic fragility test helps in the diagnosis of anemia in which the physical properties of the red cells are altered. This test detects whether or not the red cells can be easily hemolysed. The red cell membrane allows water to pass through while restricting solutes. This is called osmosis. Red cells shrink due to exosmosis when they are placed in a solution that is more concentrated than the concentration of the solute inside. On the other hand, red cells absorb water by **endosmosis**, when kept in a hypotonic solution like water which results in **hemolysis due to swelling and rupture of the cells**. In an isotonic solution, that is, solution of equal concentration as the red cell content (e.g., 0.85% NaCl), the red cells stay intact.

The test of osmotic fragility attempts to determine the concentration of solute inside the red cells by placing the cell in different concentrations of sodium chloride and observing hemolysis in a hypotonic solution. When red cells are introduced into a hypotonic solution of sodium chloride, they take up water and swell until a critical volume is reached and then rupture. When the critical volume is reached, the cells become spherical. As the cells take up water, they become more fragile.

The **red cells that are already spherical**, as seen in hereditary spherocytosis, have **increased osmotic fragility** in hypotonic solutions because they can swell only a little before they burst. Conversely, the cells that are biconcave or flat have decreased osmotic fragility in hypotonic solutions because they can swell considerably before they reach the spherical shape and burst. The osmotic fragility is thus a measure of the rate of hemolysis of the red cells when exposed to hypotonic solutions of sodium chloride.

METHODS

Osmotic Fragility Test

Principle

When the red cells are suspended in a hypotonic solution of sodium chloride, they take up water and swell until a critical volume is reached and hemolysis occurs. As the cells take up water, they become increasingly fragile. Thus, the intracellular solute concentration, as reflected by red cell fragility, can be helpful in establishing the functional state of the red cells.

Requirements

I. Apparatus
1. Clean test tubes

2. Test tube rack
3. Distilled water
4. 1% NaCl solution
5. Dropper

II. Specimen   Freshly drawn heparinised or defibrinated venous blood is prepared for this test. The test should be carried out within two hours of blood collection. Heparin is frequently used as an anticoagulant because it causes less distortion of the red cells.

Procedure

1. Arrange the test tubes in the rack and number them serially from 1 to 12.
2. Prepare solutions of increasing hypotonicity by mixing the required number of drops of 1 per cent sodium chloride solution and distilled water in the test tubes serially from 1 to 12, as given in Table 16.1. Use one dropper for all saline solutions and another for distilled water.

   Note that the first tube contains saline, which is nearly isotonic and the last tube is filled with only distilled water (tonicity nil).
3. Shake the tubes thoroughly and add a drop of blood in each tube.

4. Invert each tube gently once to mix the blood with saline, and then place them in a rack.
5. After 30 minutes, observe the tubes against a white background without disturbing the tubes. Note the number of the first tube that shows partial hemolysis and the number of the tube in which hemolysis is complete. A tube with partial hemolysis shows an upward supernatant fluid with pink colour proportionate to the degree of hemolysis and a lower layer of sedimented red cells at the bottom of the tube. A tube with complete hemolysis shows a clear, uniformly pink solution in the absence of red cells at the bottom. A tube with no hemolysis shows a clear, straw-coloured supernatant fluid with few red cells settled at the bottom (Fig. 16.1).

Observation

Beginning of hemolysis: (in per cent saline).
Completion of hemolysis: (in per cent saline).

Express the result, giving the range from the beginning of hemolysis to its completion.

Normal Value

Normally, osmotic fragility begins at 0.45 to 0.50 and completes at 0.30 to 0.33 per cent saline.

Table 16.1   Demonstration of osmotic fragility test of red cells

Test tube no.	1	2	3	4	5	6	7	8	9	10	11	12
Distilled water drops	3	9	10	11	12	13	14	15	16	17	18	25
1 per cent saline drops	22	16	15	14	13	12	11	10	9	8	7	0
% saline soln. obtained	0.88	0.64	0.60	0.56	0.52	0.48	0.44	0.40	0.36	0.32	0.28	0

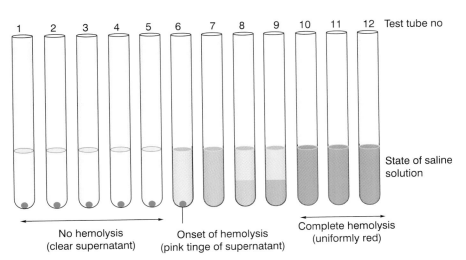

Fig. 16.1   Osmotic fragility test. Note that hemolysis starts in the sixth tube (slight pink tinge of the supernatant) and is completed in the tenth tube (solution is uniformly red). No hemolysis is observed in test tubes 1 to 5 (clear supernatant with red cell clumps at the bottom).

Precautions

1. Separate droppers should be used for pouring the drops of distilled water and 1% saline into the test tubes.
2. Drops should be counted exactly as recommended in the table.
3. A minimum time of 30 minutes should be allowed for hemolysis to occur.
4. Hemolysis should be checked against a white background by placing a white paper behind the tubes.
5. The tubes should not be disturbed while recording the observation.

DISCUSSION

When the rate of hemolysis of the red cell is increased, the osmotic fragility is increased, and when the rate of hemolysis is decreased, the osmotic fragility is decreased. Increased osmotic fragility of red cells denotes decreased resistance of these cells to rupture. Osmotic fragility is related to the **shape of red cells**. The shape of red cells is dependent on the volume, surface area and functional state of the red cell membrane. As the resistance of the red cell membrane to rupture is related to its geometric configuration, red cells which are **spherical (spherocytes) demonstrate increased hemolysis**, while the cells that are **flat (sickle cell or target cells) demonstrate decreased hemolysis.** Hypochromic red cells (as seen in iron deficiency anemia) are very thin and contain less hemoglobin; therefore, they can swell to a greater extent before they rupture.

Conditions That Alter Fragility of RBC

Diminished Fragility

1. Iron deficiency anemia
2. Thalassemia
3. Sickle cell anemia
4. Obstructive jaundice
5. After splenectomy
6. Variety of anemias where target cells are seen in the peripheral blood

Increased Fragility

1. Hereditary spherocytosis
2. Congenital hemolytic anemia
3. Other conditions in which spherocytes are found in the blood

VIVA

1. What do you mean by osmotic fragility of red cells? What are the factors that determine this?
2. What is the principle of the osmotic fragility test of red cells?
3. What is the normal range of osmotic fragility of red cells?
4. What are the conditions in which there is alteration in osmotic fragility of red cells?
5. What is the physiological basis of the increased fragility of red cells in hereditary spherocytosis and decreased fragility in sickle cell disease?

CHAPTER 17

Determination of Bleeding Time and Coagulation Time

Learning Objectives

After completing this practical, you will be able to (MUST KNOW):

1. Describe the importance of determining BT and CT in clinical physiology.
2. List the steps of blood coagulation.
3. Determine BT by the Duke method.
4. Determine CT by capillary tube method.
5. Give the normal values of BT and CT.
6. List the precautions taken for determination of BT and CT.
7. Name the diseases in which BT and CT are prolonged.

8. List the tests to determine platelet function and to assess the efficiency of intrinsic and extrinsic pathway of blood coagulation.

You may also be able to (DESIRABLE TO KNOW):

1. Explain the mechanism of intrinsic and extrinsic pathway of blood coagulation.
2. Describe the role of platelets in blood coagulation.
3. Explain the principle and clinical significance of different tests for investigation of bleeding disorders.

INTRODUCTION

Bleeding and clotting times are determined to assess the integrity of hemostatic mechanisms. Hemostasis is the stoppage of bleeding. It is a complex process that involves three major steps in sequence: (1) vasoconstriction, (2) platelet plug formation and (3) coagulation or clot formation. Bleeding time (BT) depends on the effectiveness of vasoconstriction and platelet plug formation whereas clotting time (CT) mainly depends on the effectiveness of the clotting mechanism. BT is the time from onset of bleeding till the stoppage of bleeding and CT is the time from onset of bleeding till clot formation.

Vasoconstriction

Vascular response is the immediate response of blood vessels to injury. The response is vasoconstriction. This decreases the loss of blood and assists in the process of platelet plug formation. The contraction of the smooth muscles of the blood vessels in response to injury is the immediate cause of vasoconstriction. It is potentiated by the release of chemicals like serotonin from the platelets aggregated at the site of injury.

The effectiveness of vascular response is detected by the capillary fragility test, but vascular response cannot

be clearly separated from platelet response. Therefore, determination of bleeding time and capillary fragility test is necessary to measure the integrity of both the responses.

Platelet Plug Formation

Platelet plug (temporary hemostatic plug) formation occurs due to three properties of platelets: adhesion, aggregation and release reaction. BT is the time from onset of bleeding to temporary hemostatic plug formation that stops bleeding. The response of platelets in hemostasis includes change in shape, increase in surface adhesiveness and the tendency to aggregate with other platelets to form a plug. Platelets adhere to the injured vessel wall. Adhesion is followed by aggregation of platelets, which are activated to release a number of chemicals (release reaction) that cause vasoconstriction and temporary hemostatic plug formation (see Chapter 18).

The effectiveness of platelets in hemostasis can be assessed by:

◈ Bleeding time
◈ Platelet count
◈ Platelet aggregation studies
◈ Platelet adhesiveness test
◈ Clot retraction test
◈ Prothrombin consumption test

Coagulation or Clot Formation

Blood coagulation occurs in **three stages**: (1) activation of Stuart–Prower factor, (2) formation of thrombin from prothrombin and (3) formation of fibrin from fibrinogen (Fig. 17.1). CT is the time from the onset of bleeding to the clot (definitive hemostatic plug) formation.

Activation of Stuart–Prower factor   The tissue extract (tissue thromboplastin or factor III) enters the blood through the site of injury and combines with factor VII and calcium (factor IV). This is called the extrinsic system. It originates outside the blood vessels and includes factor III, IV and VII. In the meantime, there is activation of the intrinsic system when factor XII is activated by its contact with the negatively charged surface of the collagen fibres of the injured vessel walls. The intrinsic system originates inside the blood vessels and includes factors XII, XI, IX, VIII, and calcium (IV). Finally, both extrinsic and intrinsic systems follow a common pathway, which results in the formation of active Stuart–Prower factor (Xa).

Any defect in the intrinsic system of stage 1 is recognised by the activated partial thromboplastin time (PTT).

Formation of thrombin from prothrombin   In stage 2, prothrombin (factor II) is activated by Xa in the presence of Va, calcium and platelet phospholipid, the end product of stage 1. This results in the formation of thrombin. Any defect in this stage results in prolongation of prothrombin time.

Formation of fibrin from fibrinogen   This is the final stage of the coagulation process. Fibrin is formed from fibrinogen

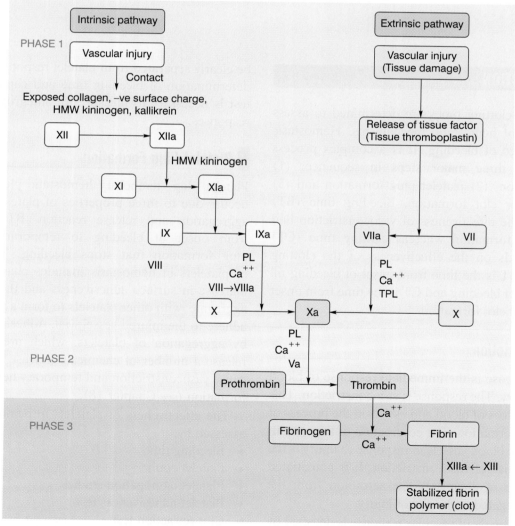

Fig. 17.1   Mechanism of blood coagulation. Note the three stages (phases) of blood clotting.

by thrombin, the end product of stage 2. First, fibrin monomers are formed, then polymerisation of fibrin takes place with the help of activated factor XIII, to form the fibrin clot.

Thrombin time is prolonged if there is a defect in the formation of fibrin from fibrinogen.

METHODS OF DETERMINATION OF BLEEDING TIME

Bleeding time (BT) is usually determined by **two methods**: (1) Duke method and (2) Ivy method.

Duke Method

The Duke method is the more frequently used method to determine BT in clinical laboratories as it is easy to perform and requires minimal equipment and laboratory skill.

▌ *Principle*

A deep skin puncture is made and the length of time required for bleeding to stop is recorded. It determines the function of the platelets and the integrity of the capillaries.

▌ *Requirements*

1. Equipment for sterile finger puncture
2. Blotting paper or filter paper
3. Stopwatch

▌ *Procedure*

1. Assemble all necessary material and provide proper instructions to the subjects (this can be done by the student).
2. Clean the fingertip or the ear lobe of the subject with alcohol, and allow the skin to dry completely.

Note: Though the ear lobe is a good site for this test, the fingertip is more convenient.

3. Make a deep puncture (blood should flow freely to form a moderate sized drop of blood) with the help of a sterile lancet and hold the finger firmly without squeezing hard or milking (Fig. 17.2).
4. Immediately start the stopwatch, as soon as bleeding starts.

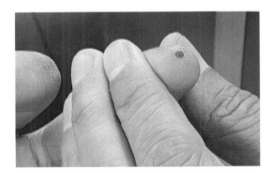

Fig. 17.2   Bleeding of fingertip for estimation of bleeding time. Hold the finger firmly, but ensure that blood oozes spontaneously without squeezing. Wear gloves if you are bleeding an unknown subject or a patient.

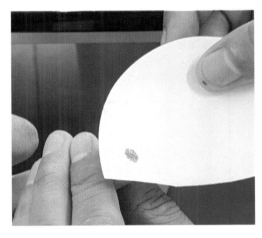

Fig. 17.3   Blotting of blood on the filter paper or blotting paper. Note that the blotting paper is just touched on the blood drop, but not pressed on it.

5. Blot the drop of blood coming out of the incision every 30 seconds by using the blotting paper or circular filter paper (Fig. 17.3). Place each subsequent drop a little further along the side of the filter paper.

Note: Do not allow the filter paper to press on the bleeding spot. Note that the drops become progressively smaller.

6. Stop the stopwatch as soon as bleeding ceases.
7. Count the number of drops on the filter paper and multiply it by 30 seconds, or the time can be noted on each drop of blood (Fig. 17.4). In some hospitals, blotting of drop of blood is done every 15 seconds; hence, noting the time on top of the marked spot of the blood drop is ideal.

Note: If the bleeding does not stop in 10 minutes, discontinue the test and apply pressure to the spot to stop bleeding.

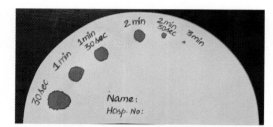

Fig. 17.4 Recording of bleeding time on the filter paper or blotting paper. Note that the size of blood drop decreases gradually. The time can be written on top of each drop and the name and hospital number of the subject/patient should also be noted.

Precautions

1. Gather all the necessary materials before starting the test.
2. Do not rub too much while cleaning the skin as rubbing increases blood flow and alters BT.
3. The skin should dry completely before pricking.
4. The puncture should be deep (about 4 mm).
5. Do not squeeze. Blood should flow freely.
6. Blot the blood exactly every 30 seconds.
7. Do not allow the filter paper to press on the bleeding spot as it may interfere with bleeding.
8. If bleeding continues for more than 10 minutes, discontinue the test and ask the subject to apply pressure to the wound.

Normal Value

The normal range of BT by the Duke method varies from 1 to 5 minutes.

Clinical Significance

Prolongation of BT is found in thrombocytopenia, thrombasthenia and von Willebrand disease. It occurs when platelet count is less than 50,000/ml of blood. Thrombasthenia is the condition of platelet dysfunction in which platelet count remains normal, but the platelets are functionally abnormal. In von Willebrand disease, platelet defect is combined with factor VIII deficiency.

Ivy Method

The Ivy method is more reliable than the Duke method, but it is more painful to the subject. Skill is required for using a sphygmomanometer. Therefore, the Duke method is commonly preferred in clinical laboratories.

Principle

A standard incision is made on the forearm under a standardised condition, and the length of time required for bleeding to cease is recorded.

Requirements

1. Sphygmomanometer
2. Sterile lancet, capable of making an incision 1 mm wide and 3 mm deep
3. Blotting paper
4. Alcohol
5. Cotton wool

Procedure

1. Explain the procedure to the subject.
2. Tie the sphygmomanometer cuff on the patient's arm above the elbow.
3. Raise the cuff pressure to 40 mm Hg, and maintain it for the entire period.
4. Select an area approximately 5 cm below the cubital fossa on the anterior aspect of the forearm and clean with alcohol.
5. Hold the skin tightly by grasping the underside of the forearm firmly and make two separate punctures 5 cm apart in quick succession using the sterile lancet. Start the stopwatch.
6. Blot the blood from each incision site on a separate piece of blotting paper, every 30 seconds.
7. When the bleeding stops, stop the watch and release the pressure from the sphygmomanometer cuff.
8. Record the bleeding time of both the punctures. The longer of the two bleeding times is more accurate than the average of the two.
9. If the bleeding continues for more than 15 minutes, discontinue the test and apply pressure to the puncture to stop bleeding, and report as BT more than 15 minutes.

Precautions

1. The procedure should be explained to the subject.
2. The area selected for puncture should be properly cleaned.
3. Two incisions should ideally be made for determination of BT by this method.

4. A constant pressure of 40 mmHg should be maintained throughout the procedure.
5. The incision should be made deep into the skin.
6. The longer of the two bleeding times (rather than the average) should be taken for the result.

Normal Value

The normal range of BT by the Ivy method varies from 5 to 11 minutes.

Clinical Significance

The clinical significance is the same as that of the Duke method. Though the Duke method is commonly followed, the Ivy method should be the method of choice, as it is more reliable.

METHODS OF DETERMINATION OF CLOTTING TIME

Clotting time (CT) is usually determined by two methods: (1) capillary tube method and (2) Lee–White (venipuncture) method. The capillary tube method is routinely used in clinical laboratories to determine CT.

Capillary Tube Method

Principle

A standard incision is made in the skin of the patient and blood is taken into a capillary glass tube. The length of time that it takes for the blood to clot (as detected by the appearance of fibrin string) is reported as CT.

Requirements

1. Materials for sterile finger prick
2. Capillary tubing (10–15 cm in length and 1.5 mm in diameter) without anticoagulant

Procedure

1. Explain the procedure to the subject.
2. Make a sterile finger puncture by using the lancet to a depth of 3 mm.
3. As soon as blood is visible, start the stopwatch.

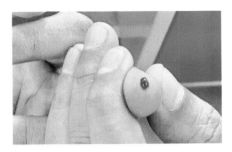

Fig. 17.5 Collection of blood drop on the fingertip for estimation of clotting time. Ensure that a large drop of blood is formed so that blood enters a larger length of capillary tube in one go without opportunity for air bubble to enter.

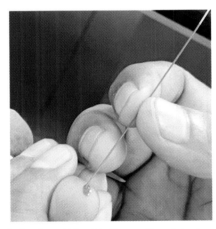

Fig. 17.6 Collection of blood in the capillary tube for estimation of CT. Note that blood enters the capillary tube automatically by capillary action.

4. Wipe off the first drop of blood. Allow the next drop of blood to form a drop of larger size (Fig. 17.5).

Note: If the size of blood drop is small, the blood may not be adequate enough to fill a larger length of the tube, and doing it again may allow air bubble to enter the tube.

Then allow the blood to flow into the capillary tube by introducing one end of the tube into the drop (Fig. 17.6). Usually blood enters the capillary tube automatically by capillary action, and if blood does not enter automatically, it can be done by holding the other end of the capillary tube at a lower level (Fig. 17.7). Blood enters into the capillary tube by capillary action.

5. Hold the capillary tube filled with blood between the palms so as to maintain it at body temperature.
6. After 2 minutes, break off the capillary tubing 1–2 cm from one end every 30 seconds and look for appearance of a thread of fibrin.

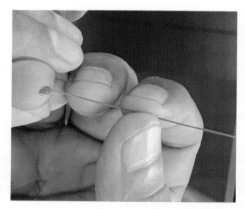

Fig. 17.7 Collection of blood in the capillary tube by lowering the other end of the capillary tube.

7. When a thin string of fibrin is seen between the broken ends (Fig. 17.8), stop the watch and note the time.
8. In the report, mention the use of the capillary method.

Precautions

1. Explain the procedure to the subject.
2. The fingertip should be cleaned with alcohol before pricking.
3. The puncture should be deep and blood should flow spontaneously.
4. Immediately after filling, the capillary tube should be held between the palms to maintain its temperature. External temperature affects clotting.
5. With each break of the capillary tube, appearance of the fibrin string should be looked for (Fig. 17.8).

Normal Value

The normal range of CT by capillary glass tube method is 2–8 minutes.

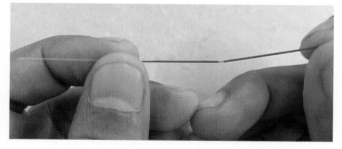

Fig. 17.8 Demonstration of fibrin string (thread of clot) by gently breaking the capillary tube and lightly separating the two broken ends little apart. Note the thread of clot between the broken ends of the capillary tube.

Clinical Significance

CT is prolonged in diseases in which clotting factors are deficient. If the CT is more than 10 minutes, the patient should be subjected to detailed investigations to identify the missing coagulation factors.

Lee–White Method

This is more reliable and sensitive than the capillary method, but it needs special arrangements for venipuncture and a temperature-controlled water bath.

Principle

Venous blood is collected in a clean glass tube without any anticoagulant. The time taken by blood to clot at 37°C is noted as clotting time.

Requirements

1. Materials for drawing blood by venipuncture
2. Test tubes
3. Water bath at 37°C
4. Stopwatch

Procedure

1. Explain the procedure to the subject.
2. Collect over 2 ml of venous blood by making a sterile venipuncture. Start the stopwatch as soon as the blood enters the syringe.
3. Remove the needle from the syringe and fill each of the two tubes to the 1 ml mark.
4. Plug the tubes with non-absorbent cotton wool and place them in the water bath at 37°C.
5. After 3 minutes, remove the first tube from the water bath and tilt the tube gently to 45° to check whether the blood has clotted. If not, return the tube to the water-bath and examine every 30 seconds to check the appearance of a clot.
6. When blood clots, the tube can be tilted through an angle of 90° without spilling the contents. As soon as the blood is clotted, examine the second tube. The blood in the second tube usually clots as soon as blood clots in the first tube.
7. Stop the stopwatch and note the time.

8. The CT is the clotting time of the second tube.

Precautions and Sources of Error

1. One important source of error is inappropriate volume of blood taken for the test (less than 1 ml gives a shorter CT).
2. The temperature of the tubes should be maintained at 37°C.
3. While collecting blood, air bubbles should not enter the syringe. Presence of air bubbles shortens the CT.

Normal Value

The normal range of CT by the Lee–White method is 5–12 minutes.

Clinical Significance

This method is more reliable than the capillary tube method. The clinical significance of this method is the same as that of the capillary tube method.

OTHER TESTS FOR BLEEDING DISORDERS

There are many other tests that are performed to detect the nature and degree of various bleeding disorders. As these tests are not routinely carried out in physiology laboratories but asked in viva, the basic principle and clinical significance of each test are described.

Capillary Fragility Test

Principle

This is also called Capillary Fragility Test of Hess or Tourniquet test. This test measures the ability of the capillaries to withstand increased stress. Petechiae appear in the forearm of the subject when the blood pressure cuff in the arm is inflated to a maximum pressure of 100 mm Hg for about 5 minutes.

Clinical Significance

Normally, 0–10 petechiae appear. More than 10 petechiae indicates capillary weakness, thrombocytopenia or both.

Platelet Aggregation Test

Principle

An aggregating agent is added to a suspension of platelets in plasma and the response is measured turbidometrically as a change in the transmission of light by an instrument called the aggregometer.

Clinical Significance

Measurement of platelet aggregation is an essential part of the investigation of any patient with suspected platelet dysfunction.

Platelet Adhesiveness Test

Principle

This test measures the ability of platelets to adhere to a glass surface. When anticoagulated blood is allowed to pass at a constant rate through a plastic tube containing glass beads, some platelets adhere to the glass beads. The percentage difference of the platelet count prior to and after passing through the glass bead column indicates the functional status of platelets.

Clinical Significance

The normal range is 75–95 per cent of platelet retention. The platelet adhesiveness test is non-specific. The results are abnormal in several platelet functional disorders.

Clot Retraction Time

Principle

Blood clots when collected in a glass tube without any anticoagulant. The clot begins to retract (after blood has clotted) within 30 seconds, and is about 50 per cent at the end of 1 hour. At the end of 18–24 hours the clot should have retracted completely.

Clinical Significance

Abnormal clot retraction is reported when less than 50 per cent retraction occurs at 1 hour. Clot retraction is primarily dependent on platelet function. Hematocrit and fibrinogen levels also affect it. Poor clot retractability is usually seen when platelet count is less than 1,00,000.

Clot Lysis Time

Principle

The clot is lysed due to fibrinolysis, which is a natural process. Due to lysis, the clot becomes fluid and red cells sink to the bottom of the test tube.

Clinical Significance

The lysis time for the normal clot is about 72 hours. If lysis is seen within 24 hours, fibrinolysis is considered to be abnormal.

Prothrombin Consumption Test

Principle

This test determines the amount of prothrombin present in the serum after clot formation.

Clinical Significance

Normally, in the coagulation process, more than 95 per cent of prothrombin is used up as it is converted to thrombin. The presence of more than 5 per cent of prothrombin in the serum indicates a quantitative or qualitative platelet deficiency.

Prothrombin Time (PT)

Principle

A preparation of rabbit brain emulsion (which contains tissue thromboplastin) is added to plasma in the presence of calcium. This, in the presence of factor VII, triggers stage 2 of the coagulation mechanism, and the clotting time is recorded after the addition of calcified thromboplastin to the plasma.

Normal Value

The normal value is 12–16 seconds.

Clinical Significance

Prolonged PT suggests the possibility of deficiency of factors II, V, VII and X. In stage 2, prothrombin is converted to thrombin which triggers the transformation of fibrinogen to fibrin. Abnormal prothrombin time suggests a stage 2 defect.

Partial Thromboplastin Time (PTT)

Principle

The platelet substitute, in the form of partial thromboplastin, is prepared from rabbit brain as chloroform extract. When mixed with test plasma containing excess of calcium, it leads to clot formation.

Normal Value

The normal value is 60–80 seconds.

Clinical Significance

PTT is prolonged when there is a deficiency of one or more clotting factors XII, XI, IX, VIII, X, V, II and I. Abnormal PTT indicates a stage 1 defect and the absence of one or more of the intrinsic factors.

Activated Partial Thromboplastin Time (APTT)

Principle

The platelet substitute, in the form of partial thromboplastin, is prepared from rabbit brain. This is incubated with a contacting agent (kaolin) to provide optimal activation of the intrinsic coagulation factors. The clotting time is determined after the addition of excess of calcium.

Normal Value

The normal value is 25–40 seconds.

Clinical Significance

APTT is prolonged in deficiencies of factors XII, XI, X, IX and VIII. APTT is a more reliable test than PTT. When used in conjunction with PT, it provides a simple method for differentiating between stage 1 intrinsic defects and other factor deficiencies. APTT is mainly determined in hemophilias that involve the deficiency of factors VIII, IX or XI.

Thrombin Time (TT)

Principle

Thrombin (commercially available) is added to the plasma along with calcium and the clotting time is determined.

Normal Value

The normal value is 15–20 seconds.

Clinical Significance

Thrombin time detects the effectiveness of stage 3 of coagulation in which fibrinogen is converted to fibrin. Prolonged TT is considered to be due to either a decrease in fibrinogen concentration or the presence of dysfunctional fibrinogen.

Plasma Recalcification Time (PRT)

Principle

When excess of calcium is added to the citrated plasma, clotting occurs. Because platelet factor III is also involved in clotting through the intrinsic pathway of coagulation, the clotting occurs in a shorter time in platelet-rich plasma than in platelet-poor plasma.

Normal Value

Platelet-rich plasma	:	100–150 seconds
Platelet-poor plasma	:	135–240 seconds

Clinical Significance

This is an easy screening test that detects deficiency of the factors of the intrinsic pathway, that is, factors XII, XI, IX, VIII, X, V and II (all coagulation factors except VII and XIII).

DISCUSSION

Bleeding occurs when a blood vessel is injured and stops by a process called hemostasis. Abnormal bleeding occurs spontaneously or following trauma, due to the derangement of hemostasis which warrants investigation. Patients prepared for surgery must be routinely checked for bleeding disorders to ensure normal hemostasis during the procedure.

Clinical Significance

Laboratory investigations for bleeding disorders are required for patients who have a history of spontaneous bleeding or excessive bleeding following injury or surgery. Hemorrhagic disorders are broadly classified into inherited and acquired defects. Acquired defects are more common than inherited defects. The platelet defects are more common than the coagulation defects. Deficiencies of factor VIII (hemophilia) and factor IX (Christmas disease) are more common inherited coagulation defects. The common acquired defects are thrombocytopenia, vitamin K deficiency, disseminated intravascular coagulation and liver failure.

Bleeding time is prolonged in conditions in which platelets are defective or less in number, and the vascular response to injury is impaired. Clotting time is prolonged in conditions in which clotting factors are defective or deficient.

Conditions in which BT is prolonged, but CT is normal
- Thrombocytopenia due to any cause
- Thrombasthenia
- Idiopathic thrombocytopenic purpura

Conditions in which CT is prolonged, but BT is normal
- Hemophilia
- Christmas disease
- Any bleeding disorder in which clotting factors are deficient.

Hemophilia

Hemophilia occurs due to the deficiency of factor VIII. It is an X-linked recessive bleeding disorder. The abnormality is located on the X chromosome. Women are carriers and usually do not suffer from the disease because they are protected by the second X chromosome, which is usually normal. The disease manifests with a bleeding tendency that usually appears in infancy, but, which in mild cases may appear in adult life. Bleeding from wounds is a characteristic symptom, which is usually slow and persists from days to weeks in spite of the presence of large clots. Bleeding may also occur spontaneously into the tissues, joints and cavities of the body. The patient is treated with fresh blood transfusions because factor VIII is lost rapidly on storage. The better alternative is to administer a factor VIII concentrate.

Christmas Disease

Christmas disease occurs due to deficiency of factor IX. It is clinically indistinguishable from hemophilia. Therefore, it is also called hemophilia B.

Purpura

Purpura is a group of diseases that occur due to thrombocytopenia. The two commonest forms of purpura are idiopathic thrombocytopenic purpura (ITP) and drug-induced purpura (which is also commonly seen in von Willebrand disease). Purpura induced by a vascular defect may be seen in vitamin C deficiency.

VIVA

1. What are the methods of determination of BT, and what are their normal values?
2. What are the precautions taken for determining BT by the Duke and Ivy methods?
3. Which method is more reliable for determining BT, and why?
4. What is the clinical significance of determining BT by the Duke and Ivy methods?
5. What are the methods of determination of CT, and what are their normal values?
6. What are the precautions to be taken while determining CT by the capillary tube and Lee–White methods? Which method is more reliable, and why?
7. What is the clinical significance of determination of CT by the capillary tube and Lee–White methods?
8. Why is CT normally more than BT?

   Ans: BT is the time from onset of bleeding to stoppage of bleeding. Bleeding stops due to the formation of a temporary hemostatic plug. CT is the time taken from onset of bleeding to formation of the definitive hemostatic plug (clot). Temporary hemostatic plug formation occurs earlier than the definitive hemostatic plug. Therefore, normally, CT is more than BT.

9. What are hemostasis and homeostasis?

   Ans: Hemostasis means arrest of bleeding. Homeostasis is defined as maintenance of constancy of the internal environment of the body, that is, milieu interior. As hemostasis tries to maintain constancy of blood volume, it is part of the total homeostatic mechanism.

10. What are the mechanisms of hemostasis?
11. What are the steps of blood coagulation, and how do you detect the defects in these steps?
12. What are the tests to detect defects in the vascular response of hemostasis?
13. What are the tests to detect defects in platelets?

    Ans: Defects in platelets can be detected by:
    - bleeding time
    - platelet count
    - platelet aggregation studies
    - platelet adhesiveness test
    - clot retraction test
    - prothrombin consumption test

14. What is normal prothrombin time and what is its clinical significance?
15. What is the normal partial thromboplastin time and what is its clinical significance?
16. What is the normal value of activated partial thromboplastin time (APTT), and what is its clinical significance?
17. What is normal thrombin time (TT), and what is its clinical significance?
18. What is plasma recalcification time (PRT), and what is its clinical significance?
19. What is hemophilia?
20. What is 'Simplate Method' of BT determination, and what is its advantage?

    Ans: In Duke and Ivy bleeding time methods, there is no full control on the depth of the wound made by a lancet or a needle. The widely practised technique is to use an automated scalpel to control the depth and length of the wound, which is usually

1 mm deep and 9 mm long. The blood pressure cuff is inflated to 40 mm of Hg to distend the capillary bed of the forearm. The normal bleeding time in this method is < 7 minutes.

21. *What are the factors that influence BT and CT?*

Ans:

Factors influencing BT
– Size (breadth and depth) of the wound
– Degree of hyperemia of skin puncture site
– Number of platelets and their functional status
– Functional status of the blood vessels
– Body temperature or temperature of the part to be pricked: If the part is cold, bleeding is less due to vasoconstrictions. Rubbing the part (hyperemia) promotes bleeding.
– Environmental temperature: In cold weather, due to low temperature, BT becomes less (due to vasoconstriction)

Factors influencing CT
– Nature of contact surface. Siliconised surface may prolong the CT.
– Blood level of clotting factors.
– Skin temperature: Low temperature may prolong the CT.

22. *Name the conditions in which bleeding time is prolonged, but CT is normal.*

Ans: Prolongation of BT with normal CT is seen in:
i)   Thrombocytopenia (decreased production of platelets or increased destruction of platelets).
ii) Thrombasthenia (functional platelet defects).
iii) Drugs—aspirin, large doses of penicillin, corticosteroids, sulfa drugs.
iv) von Willebrand disease
v)   Other diseases—uremia, cirrhosis, leukemia, etc.
vi) Vessel wall defects (acquired, but may be inherited).
vii) Allergic purpura—there is damage to capillary wall by antibodies.
viii) Infections—typhus, bacterial endocarditis, hemolytic streptococci, etc.
ix) Vitamin C deficiency—Petechia, and bleeding from gums occur due to decreased intracellular substance and less stable capillary basement membrane.
x)   Senile purpura—in the elderly, small vessels rupture due to increased mobility of skin resulting from loss of elastic and connective tissues around blood vessels.
xi) Connective tissue diseases

23. *How is the severity of bleeding linked to the level of platelet count?*

Ans: The level of platelet deficiency is the main factor that contributes to severity of bleeding.
Above $100,000/mm^3$—No clinical symptoms, bleeding is rare.
$50,000–100,000/mm^3$—Bleeding may occur after major surgeries
$20,000–50,000/mm^3$—Bleeding occurs with minor trauma
Below $20,000/mm^3$—Spontaneous hemorrhages in urinary and GI tract, nose bleeds, etc.
At $< 20,000/mm^3$—Cerebral hemorrhages may occur

24. *Give the causes of thrombocytopenia.*

Ans:

A. Decreased production
  – Bone marrow suppression: Drugs (sulphas, chloramphenicol, cytotoxic drugs); irradiation, toxemic conditions, and aplastic anemia.
  – Bone marrow infiltration: Leukemias and secondary deposits of malignant disease.
  – Periodic thrombocytopenic purpura (purpura hemorrhagica)

B. Increased destruction
  – Drugs: Thiazides, quinine, ethanol, estrogens, methyldopa, quinidine
  – Idiopathic thrombocytopenic purpura
  – Hypersplenism (Sequestration and destruction in spleen)
  – Disseminated intravascular coagulation
  – Hemorrhage with severe transfusion

25. *Give the causes of thrombocytosis.*

Ans:

A. Primary thrombocytosis (thrombocythemia): It is a myeloproliferative disease involving megakaryocytes.

B.   Secondary (or reactive) thrombocytosis: Often occurs after removal of spleen or after severe hemorrhage.

26. *What is the mechanism of clotting in the glass capillary tube in your experiment?*

   Ans: When blood comes in contact with the glass surface of the capillary tube (similar to the injury of blood vessel), it initiates intrinsic blood coagulation. Activation of platelets causes release of phospholipids (PPL). The PPL, along with high-molecular-weight kininogens and kallikrein, converts factor XII to XIIa that facilitates the intrinsic mechanism of clotting.

27. *Give the causes of prolongation of clotting time*

   Ans:

   A. Hereditary coagulation disorders
   - Hemophilias A, B, C, D
   - von Willebrand disease
   - Afibrinogenemia and dysfibrinogenemia
   - Deficiency of factor XIII

   B. Acquired coagulation disorders
   - Vitamin K deficiency
   - Liver diseases: There is a decrease of all clotting factors except VIII. There is also a reduced uptake of vitamin K, and abnormalities of platelet function.
   - Intravascular clotting: Clotting factors are used up and bleeding may occur.
   - Anticoagulant therapy: Patients receiving heparin or wafarin show an increased CT.
   - Newborns: Premature babies have a tendency to bleed due to low levels of certain clotting factors in the plasma, especially prothrombin. Usually, normal levels of the clotting factors are reached by the 2nd or 3rd week after birth.

28. *How is the fluid state of blood maintained in the body?*

   Ans: A balance between clotting and anticlotting mechanisms prevents intravascular clotting. In addition, continuous nature of blood flow and endothelial factors contribute to fluidity of blood.

   1. Continuous flow of blood (dynamic circulation)
   2. Endothelial factors:
   - Smoothness of endothelial surface (damage to endothelium causes this activation).
   - The glycocalyx layer on the endothelium repels clotting factors and platelets.
   - Thrombomodulin removes thrombin as soon as it is formed.
   - Prostacyclin secreted by endothelium counteracts platelet aggregation.
   3. Antithrombin action of antithrombin III—Heparin complex and fibrin.
   4. Fibrinolytic (Plasmin System).

29. *Define thrombosis and embolism and give the causes for each.*

   Ans: Thrombosis is an intravascular clot. Generally, thrombosis develops due to two mechanisms:
   - Local damage or roughness of endothelial surface of blood vessel: This usually occurs at the site of atheromatous plaques (sites more prone are coronaries, carotid arteries, cerebral arteries), on damaged cardiac valves, or in veins of the lower limbs. At the site of atheromatous plaque, platelets aggregate, adhere and are activated, and slowly initiate the intrinsic system of clotting.
   - Slowing of blood flow (stasis): Decreased flow of blood in the pelvic and leg veins causes accumulation of clotting factors. This usually occurs in prolonged confinement to bed (fractures, major surgery, severe burns), during long flights in aeroplanes, as a complication of pregnancy, etc.

      Emboli are small fragments of a thrombus that after getting dislodged from thrombus enter the downstream blood and block smaller vessels. This process is called embolism. Also, an embolus can be a blood clot, an air bubble, fat globules from broken bones, and a piece of tissue debris. Lodgment of emboli (embolism) in smaller arteries of any vital organ such as heart, lung or brain could be life-threatening and should be treated with fibrinolytics and anticoagulant agents.

Chapter 18

Platelet Count

Learning Objectives

After completing this practical, you will be able to (MUST KNOW):

1. Describe the importance of performing platelet count in practical physiology.
2. List the methods of performing platelet count.
3. Perform platelet count by the Rees–Ecker method and peripheral blood smear method.
4. List the precautions and possible sources of error in the Rees–Ecker method.
5. State the normal value of platelet count.
6. List the functions of platelets.
7. Name the conditions that alter platelet count.

You may also be able to (DESIRABLE TO KNOW):

1. Explain the role of platelets in hemostasis (temporary hemostatic plug formation and blood coagulation).
2. Name the granules of platelets and list the chemicals present in these granules.
3. Describe the regulation of thrombopoiesis.
4. List the principle and advantages of platelet count by the Brecher-Cronkite method.
5. Explain the causes of thrombocytopenia and thrombocytosis.

INTRODUCTION

Platelets are anuclear cytoplasmic fragments of megakaryocytes. They play an important role in hemostasis (the control of bleeding) and the formation of clots within the blood vessels.

Development

Platelets are developed from megakaryocytes, the giant cells in the bone marrow. The development of platelets is known as thrombopoiesis. The steps of thrombopoiesis are shown in Fig. 18.1.

Megakaryocytes form platelets by pinching off bits of cytoplasm and extruding them into the circulation. The production and release of platelets from the bone marrow normally remains constant. Production is depressed by transfusion of platelets, and is enhanced by removal of platelets from the blood (thrombocytopheresis). This indicates that there is a feedback regulatory mechanism for platelet production. Thrombopoietin, a hormone, is probably involved in this process. Platelet production is also regulated by the colony stimulating factors (GM-CSF), IL1, IL3 and IL6.

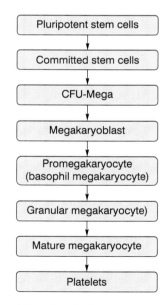

Fig. 18.1   Steps of thrombopoiesis.

Life History

Platelets normally have a half-life of about 4 days. Their survival time in circulation is about 8–12 days. Aged platelets are removed from the circulation by the reticuloendothelial system. The spleen is an important site of destruction of platelets. Therefore, platelet count increases after splenectomy and decreases in hypersplenism.

Normal Count

In adults: 1.5–4 lakhs/mm^3 of blood

Structure

Platelets are small, anucleated, granulated, spherical or oval bodies, 2–4 μm in diameter. They contain microtubules and microfilaments. The cytoplasm contains two types of granules: alpha and dense. The alpha granules contain PDGF (platelet-derived growth factor), platelet factor 3 (a phospholipid), fibronectin, plasminogen, platelet fibrinogen, proaccelerin (factor 5), thrombospondin, alpha-2 plasmin inhibitor and hydrolases. The dense granules contain serotonin, ADP and calcium ions.

Functions

Platelets perform four main functions in the body: (1) temporary hemostasis (arrest of bleeding), (2) clotting of blood, (3) phagocytosis of small particles and organisms and (4) storage and transport of chemicals.

Temporary Hemostasis

The most important function of platelets is the arrest of bleeding. The initial events following damage to the blood vessels are vasoconstriction and temporary hemostatic plug formation. This is followed by conversion of the temporary plug into the definitive clot. The formation of a hemostatic plug at the site of injury immediately stops bleeding. This hemostatic plug is formed by platelets and is their primary function. The hemostatic plug is known as the platelet plug. The temporary hemostatic plug is formed by three properties of platelets: adhesion, aggregation and release reaction.

Platelet adhesion   Platelets adhere to the exposed collagen of the lining of the damaged blood vessels. The von Willebrand factor facilitates platelet adhesion.

Platelet aggregation   Platelets have the tendency to stick to each other and to the damaged vessel wall. This phenomenon is called platelet aggregation. Fibrinogen, thrombin and PAF (platelet activating factors) foster platelet aggregation.

Platelet activation and release reaction   The binding of platelets to collagen initiates platelet activation. Activation is also produced by ADP and thrombin. The activated platelets change their shape, put out pseudopodia, and discharge the contents of their granules. This is known as **release reaction of platelets**. When platelets adhere to the collagen in the damaged vessel wall, ATP in the adhered platelets is converted to ADP. **ADP and collagen** activate phospholipase A2, which causes hydrolysis of membrane phospholipids to form arachidonic acid. Arachidonic acid is then converted to endoperoxides by cyclo-oxygenase. Endoperoxides, when acted upon by thromboxane synthase, form thromboxane A$_2$. **Thromboxane A$_2$** causes vasoconstriction and platelet aggregation, and also increases calcium influx into the platelets. Increased intracellular calcium brings about contraction of microfilaments that cause movement of granules to the canaliculi of the cells. Granules fuse with the canalicular membrane and finally discharge their contents to the exterior through the open canaliculi (release reaction).

Blood Clotting

Platelets participate in the clotting process because platelet factor 3 (platelet phospholipids) is needed for formation of Xa (activation of the Stuart–Prower factor) and for the conversion of prothrombin to thrombin by factor Xa and Va. Another important function of platelets is to promote clot retraction. This is the shrinkage of the clot, which depends on metabolically active platelets. This is produced by contraction of attached platelet pseudopodia in the polymerised fibrin, which contains actin–myosin-like proteins. If the clot does not retract, it may not be stable and may disintegrate.

Phagocytosis

Carbon particles, immune complexes and viruses undergo phagocytosis by platelets in the circulation.

Storage and Transport

Platelets take up 5-HT and synthesise, store and transport serotonin. They also store and transport heparin.

METHODS OF COUNTING

Several problems are encountered in the counting of platelets because:

1. They are small and difficult to discern.
2. They have an adhesive character and attach readily to glassware, particles or debris in the diluting fluid.
3. They clump easily.
4. They are not evenly distributed in the mixture of blood and diluting fluid.
5. They readily disintegrate in blood diluted with fluid making it difficult to distinguish them from debris.

Therefore, unless carefully done, accurate counting of platelets becomes impossible.

Three methods are frequently used for platelet count. These are:

1. Hemocytometry (direct count)
2. Study of blood smear (indirect count)
3. Automated counting

Platelet Count by Hemocytometry

Two methods of platelet count by hemocytometry are frequently used: (1) the Rees–Ecker method and (2) the Brecher–Cronkite method. The details of the Rees–Ecker method will be discussed, as this is the method usually followed in our laboratories.

The Rees–Ecker Method for Manual Platelet Count

Principle

Whole blood is diluted with a solution of brilliant cresyl blue which stains the platelets light blue. The diluent also prevents coagulation. No attempt is made to lyse the red cells. Platelets are then counted by hemocytometry.

Requirements

I. Equipment

1. Microscope
2. Hemocytometer (RBC pipette and counting chamber)
3. Materials for sterile finger prick
4. Petri dish
5. Filter papers

Instead of Neubauer's hemocytometer, a specially designed Spencer–Brightline hemocytometer is used for platelet counts. This uses the Spencer–Brightline counting chamber. The metallic surface of this chamber makes it easier to see the platelets. The cell distribution also appears better, since the chamber's surface is smoother. If the Spencer–Brightline hemocytometer is not available, Neubauer's hemocytometer may be used.

II. Reagent   The diluent used for counting platelets must meet certain requirements. It must:

1. Provide fixation to reduce the adhesiveness of the platelets
2. Prevent coagulation
3. Prevent hemolysis
4. Provide a low specific gravity so that the platelets settle in one plane.

The **Rees–Ecker fluid** meets all these requirements. 1% ammonium oxalate can be used, but it is not as good as the Rees–Ecker fluid.

Composition of the Rees–Ecker fluid

1. Sodium citrate—prevents coagulation, preserves RBC and provides the necessary low specific gravity.
2. Formalin—acts as a fixative.
3. Brilliant cresyl blue—identifies the diluent.

Note: Brilliant cresyl blue does not stain the platelets, as it is not essential for counting. Dye is used only for identification of the diluent.

4. Deionised water—acts as a solvent.

Note: The Rees–Ecker fluid must be stored in the refrigerator and filtered before each use.

III. Specimen   Capillary blood (from a finger puncture) can be used. Generally, venous blood gives more satisfactory results, as platelet count in capillary blood is usually less than that of venous blood. This difference is due to clumping of platelets at the site of puncture in finger prick blood collection. The venous blood that is collected should be anticoagulated with EDTA because EDTA reduces the tendency of platelet clumping. If venous blood is used, the test should be performed within 2 hours of collecting blood.

Procedure

1. Clean the RBC pipette and Neubauer's chamber thoroughly.

Note: All glassware must be scrupulously cleaned. This is to prevent adhesion and aggregation of platelets. Anything in the pipette to which the platelets could adhere must be removed. 95 per cent ethanol is used to clean the hemocytometer. A lint-free cloth should be used.

2. Puncture the fingertip and suck the blood exactly up to the 0.5 mark of the RBC pipette.

3. Rapidly dilute the blood with the Rees–Ecker fluid to the 101 mark of the pipette.

4. Shake the pipette immediately after dilution for at least 1 minute.

5. Discard 3–5 drops of the solution from the pipette.

6. Charge the Neubauer's chamber.

7. Cover the charged chamber with a petri dish lined with moist filter paper and allow 15 minutes for the platelets to settle in the chamber.

Note: The chamber is covered to prevent evaporation.

8. After 15 minutes, count the platelets under a high-power objective.

Note: The platelets are bluish and must be distinguished from debris. Platelets are oval or round bodies, normally 2–4 mm in diameter and refractile in nature.

9. Count the platelets in all the 25 medium squares of the RBC square, that is, in 1 mm^2 area or 1/10 mm^3 volume.

10. Enter the results in the squares drawn on paper.

Calculations

The cells are counted in 25 medium squares, and each of these squares has 16 smaller squares.

The area covered by the 25 medium squares is 1 mm^2.

Platelet count/ml or mm^3 of blood

$$= \frac{\text{Number of platelets counted}}{\text{Volume of fluid}} \times \text{dilution}$$

Dilution is 200.

Volume of fluid in 1 mm^2 = 1 × 1/10

= 1 × 0.1 = 0.1 ml or mm^3

Platelet count/ml or mm^3 of blood = Number of platelets counted × 200/0.1

= Number of platelets counted × 2000

Precautions and Sources of Error

1. The glassware must be scrupulously cleaned. Debris and dust are the main sources of error as they are easily mistaken for platelets.

2. The diluting fluid must be filtered just before use (to remove stained particles from the stain).

3. If venous blood is used, the platelets must be counted within 2 hours. Delay causes disintegration and clumping of platelets.

4. Blood should be rapidly diluted. This is essential because the platelets may form clumps.

5. Blood must be thoroughly mixed with the diluent by shaking the contents of the pipette for at least one minute. Inadequate mixing results in clumping of platelets.

6. The charged chamber should be kept for 15 minutes under a petri dish to prevent evaporation and for the cells to settle down.

7. Other precautions of hemocytometry (as described in Chapter 6) should also be followed.

Important Notes

1. It is ideal to make a duplicate count to minimise errors. This is done by charging both sides of the counting chamber simultaneously, and counting both the sides separately.

2. A blood smear should be made and stained simultaneously to check and compare the value observed in the direct method.

3. If the count is low, the WBC pipette can be used for dilution for recounting. The calculation can be done by using the correct dilution factor.

4. If other hematologic tests are to be performed with platelet count, and blood is used from the same puncture, it is necessary to draw the blood for platelet count first before drawing blood for other tests.

5. The finger should not be squeezed excessively to collect blood.

6. In spite of all precautions, the error of platelet count in this method is 15–30 per cent.

The Brecher–Cronkite Method

Principle

This method uses phase-contrast microscopy. Ammonium oxalate is one of the constituents of the diluent that completely lyses the red cells. Platelets are then counted with a phase-hemocytometer and phase-contrast microscope to enhance the refractileness of the platelets.

Advantages

1. Identification of platelets is easier.
2. The error involved is low (5–10 per cent).

Platelet Count by Study of Blood Smear

Principle

The principle is the same as that of making a blood smear.

Procedure

1. Place a drop of 14% magnesium sulphate solution on the tip of a finger and prick through this drop of solution.

   Note: Magnesium sulphate prevents clumping of blood.

2. Make a blood smear and stain with Leishman stain.
3. Count platelets per 1000 red cells.

Normal Count

The normal ratio of platelets to RBCs is 1 : 20.

Note: Total red cell count can be done separately. If the red cell count is $5,000,000/mm^3$, and platelet count in the indirect method is 1 : 20, the indirect absolute count of platelets will be $250,000/mm^3$ of blood.

Platelet Count by Automated Method

Automated platelet counting is done with an S Plus Coulter counter. In the S Plus model, platelets and red cells pass through the apertures. The particles that are between 2 and 10 fL are counted as platelets. A platelet graph is also plotted according to the size distribution of the platelets counted.

DISCUSSION

Platelets participate in the coagulation of blood and are, therefore, associated with the hemostatic mechanisms of the body.

Clinical Significance

Platelet count is usually ordered as a part of the laboratory diagnosis of a bleeding disorder. When platelet count increases in the blood, the condition is known as thrombocytosis, and when the count decreases, the condition is called thrombocytopenia. Thrombocytopenia can be caused by impaired production or increased destruction of the platelets. Prolonged bleeding time is the hallmark of thrombocytopenia. When platelet count is less than $50,000$ per mm^3 of blood, the count is called critical count, as bleeding may occur spontaneously, as below this count hemorrhagic tendency appears. However, count below $20,000$ leads to spontaneous hemorrhage.

The hemorrhagic tendency is proportional to the degree of thrombocytopenia and is characterised by petechiae, ecchymoses, menorrhagia and bleeding from mucous membranes into the central nervous system. To differentiate the causes of thrombocytopenia, the bone marrow should be carefully examined. If megakaryocytes are absent in the bone marrow, this implies failure of platelet production.

Conditions That Alter Thrombocyte Count

Thrombocytosis

1. Polycythemia vera
2. Chronic myeloid leukemia
3. Iron deficiency anemia
4. Splenectomy
5. Inflammatory disorders: Rheumatoid arthritis, inflammatory bowel disease
6. Following major surgery
7. Acute or chronic hemorrhage
8. Essential thrombocytosis

Thrombocytopenia

A. Increased platelet destruction
   I. Immune-mediated
      1. Primary: Idiopathic thrombocytopenic purpura
      2. Secondary:
         a) Autoimmune: SLE
         b) Allo-immune: Post-transfusion
         c) Drug-induced
            • Quinidine
            • Sulfa compounds
            • Heparin
         d) Infection: HIV, cytomegalovirus

II. Non-immune-mediated
    1. DIC
    2. Hemolytic-uremic syndrome
    3. Thrombotic thrombocytopenic purpura
B. Decreased production
   I. Diseases of bone marrow
     1. Aplastic anemia
     2. Marrow infiltration
       • Leukemia
       • Disseminated cancer
     3. Drug-induced
       • Thiazides

     • Cytotoxic drugs
     • Alcohol
    4. Infections: Measles, HIV
  II. Ineffective megakaryopoiesis
    1. Megalobastic anemia
    2. Myelodysplastic syndrome
C. Sequestration of platelets
   I. Hypersplenism
     • Portal hypertension
     • Lymphomas
     • Myeloproliferative disorders
  II. Hemodilutional

VIVA

1. Why does the platelet count produce inaccurate results unless performed very carefully?
2. What are the different methods of platelet count?
3. What is the principle of the Rees–Ecker method?
4. What are the advantages of using the Spencer–Brightline counting chamber for platelet count?
5. Why is the Rees–Ecker fluid an ideal diluent for platelet count?
6. What is the composition of the Rees–Ecker fluid and what are the functions of each constituent?
7. Why is the Rees–Ecker fluid filtered before every use?
8. Why is venous blood preferred to capillary blood for platelet count?
9. Why is glassware cleaned thoroughly for platelet count?
10. Why is the blood rapidly diluted and thoroughly mixed with the diluting fluid?
11. Why is the charged chamber covered by a petri dish for 15 minutes?
12. How do you identify platelets under the high-power objective?
13. What are the sources of error in the manual method of platelet count?
14. What is the other method of platelet count using the principle of hemocytometry and what are its advantages?
15. How is the indirect count of platelets performed?
16. What are the precursor cells for platelets?
17. What are the factors that regulate the development of platelets?
18. What is the lifespan of platelets and how are they removed from circulation?
19. What is the normal platelet count?
20. What are the properties of platelets? What are its functions?
21. What are the causes of thrombocytosis and thrombocytopenia (Refer 'Viva' of previous chapter)?
   In addition, all the questions of previous chapters, especially questions related to bleeding time, may be asked here.

CHAPTER 19

Reticulocyte Count

Learning Objectives

After completing this practical, you will be able to (MUST KNOW):

1. Describe the importance of performing reticulocyte count in practical physiology.
2. State the value of normal reticulocyte count in newborns and adults.
3. Identify reticulocytes in the smear prepared by using supravital staining.
4. Perform reticulocyte count by the manual method.
5. List the precautions and sources of error for reticulocyte count.
6. Explain the meaning of supravital staining, and name the supravital stains.
7. List the common causes of reticulocytosis and reticulocytopenia.

You may also be able to (DESIRABLE TO KNOW):

1. Explain the structure, function and fate of reticulocytes.
2. Explain the reticulocyte response.
3. Explain the physiological and clinical significance of reticulocyte count.
4. Explain the physiological basis of reticulocytosis in different conditions.
5. Describe the method of absolute reticulocyte count.
6. State the principle and advantages of reticulocyte count by the automated method.
7. Explain the phenomenon of punctate basophilia.

INTRODUCTION

Reticulocytes are juvenile red cells that pass into the bloodstream from the bone marrow. During the process of development, the nuclei are lost but not the cytoplasmic RNA. Therefore, reticulocytes do not possess nuclei, but contain a network of reticulum in the cytoplasm, which represents the remnants of basophilic cytoplasm (the RNA) of the precursor cells. On **vital staining** with cresyl blue, the reticular network appears in the form of a heavy wreath, or clumps of small dots, or as a faint thread connecting two small nodes (Fig. 19.1). The ribosomal and cytoplasmic remnants of reticulocytes pick up a supravital stain when the stain is allowed to penetrate the cells while in the living condition. **Supravital stains** may also reveal basophilic stippling. In pathological conditions, the stained basophilic materials present in the form of clumps in the cytoplasm appear as discrete blue particles (punctate basophilia). The basophilic stippling represents precipitation of RNA in the cytoplasm. Such stippling is seen in red cells in toxic conditions such as heavy metal poisoning, especially lead poisoning.

Reticulocyte Production

Reticulocytes are produced in the bone marrow from late (orthochromatic) normoblasts. The nucleus is extruded from the late normoblast to form reticulocytes. Reticulocytes lose their mitochondria, ribosomes and basophilic tint to form mature erythrocytes. One per cent of the circulating red cells is replaced every day by newly formed red cells. With the release of young red cells into the circulation, a few reticulocytes are also released. When the bone marrow sends out red cells at an increased rate, more reticulocytes are released. Thus, the number of reticulocytes in peripheral blood is an **index of erythropoiesis** (production of red cells). Reticulocytes are the immediate precursors of red cells. Therefore, whenever the demand for red cells in the circulation increases, reticulocyte formation and release is also accentuated. Sometimes the demand may be so high that nucleated red cells are also released from the bone marrow.

Lifespan

Reticulocytes stay in circulation for about 24 hours before they mature into erythrocytes. Most of the reticulocytes are present in the bone marrow where they actually mature into red cells.

Normal Count

In adults, the count is 0.5–1 per cent of the red cells. In newborns, the count is 2–6 per cent. The number falls during the first year to less than 1 per cent and the level is maintained throughout life.

METHODS OF COUNTING

Reticulocyte count can be done by manual methods and automated methods. The manual method includes the relative count and absolute count. A relative count is taken against the number of red cells and then expressed as a percentage of red cells. An absolute count is taken against the relative count and the total RBC count.

Manual Method (Relative Count) of Reticulocyte Count

Principle

The RNA content of the reticulocytes can be detected by exposing the living cells to a supravital stain. In supravital staining, the living blood cells are mixed with the stain as opposed to differential leucocyte count, where the smear is made before staining. In one method, the stain is sprayed on the slide and blood is added to the stain. In the other method, the stain is mixed with a drop of blood and covered with a coverslip. The mixture is sealed on the slide and viewed in liquid form under the microscope.

Requirements

1. Supravital stains
2. Glass slides
3. Watch glass
4. Filter paper
5. Microscope
6. Equipment for sterile finger puncture

Supravital stains

These are dyes that are used for staining the living cells in vitro (outside the body). Usually in practice, living cells are stained (for diagnostic purposes) outside the body. Vital stains are used for staining living cells in vivo (rarely used nowadays). Therefore, supravital stains (not vital stains) are commonly used.

i)   Brilliant cresyl blue stain

Function of each constituent

- Brilliant cresyl blue—stains the RNA of reticulocytes.
- Sodium citrate—prevents coagulation.
- Sodium chloride—provides isotonicity.

Brilliant cresyl blue is prepared as a 1% solution in isotonic saline or methyl alcohol.

ii)   New methylene blue stain

Composition

New methylene blue is prepared as a 1% solution in isotonic saline and then diluted to 100 ml with 3.8% sodium citrate. New methylene blue is chemically different from methylene blue, which is a poor reticulocyte stain. It is preferred to brilliant cresyl blue as it deeply stains the filamentous net-like structures (reticulum) present in the cytoplasm of reticulocytes so that they are easily identified.

Function of each constituent

- New methylene blue—stains the RNA of reticulocytes.
- Sodium oxalate—prevents coagulation.
- Sodium chloride—provides isotonicity.

Procedure

1. Clean the glass slides thoroughly.
2. Take a drop of stain on a clean slide.
3. Make a sterile finger prick to get a drop of blood.
4. Add the drop of blood to the stain.
5. Mix the blood gently with the help of the blunt edge of a slide without touching the specimen slide.
6. Cover the slide with a watch glass lined with moist filter paper for 15 minutes to prevent evaporation.
7. Select a spreader.
8. After 15 minutes, place the edge of a spreader on the mixture, transfer the portion of mixture sticking to the spreader to another slide, and immediately make a thin smear.
9. Make a minimum of 2–3 such smears.
10. Allow the smear to dry.
11. Examine the smear first under a low-power objective and locate a thin portion of the smear where the red cells are evenly distributed.
12. Carefully change to the oil-immersion objective. Focus sharply and try to locate an area in which there are approximately 100–150 red cells visible in the oil-immersion field.

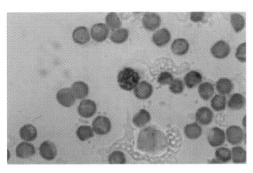

Fig. 19.1 Reticulocyte (supravital staining). Note the only one reticulocyte in the field and appreciate the reticulin network in that cell.

13. Identify reticulocytes and red cells.

> **Note:** Reticulocytes are identified by the fine, deep, violet filaments and granules arranged in a network. Red cells stain pale blue. Red cells are slightly smaller in size than reticulocytes (see Fig. 19.1).

14. Enumerate the reticulocytes and red cells in each field. Count a minimum of 1000 cells (minimum of 10 fields).

> **Note:** Counting is easier if the size of the microscopic field is reduced. This can be done by placing in the eyepiece of the microscope a small circular piece of black paper in which a hole of 5 mm diameter has been made with a puncher.

15. Enter your observation in a tabular form, as given in Table 19.1.

Calculation

$$RC = \frac{\text{Number of reticulocytes counted}}{\text{Total number of cells counted}} \times 100$$

where, RC is the reticulocyte count (per cent).

For example, let us assume the total number of cells counted (reticulocytes + RBCs) to be = 1500. Number of reticulocytes seen (in 15 fields) = 15.

Table 19.1 Observation for reticulocyte count.

Field no.	Number of reticulocytes	Number of RBCs	Total number of cells
	(1)	(2)	(1 + 2)
1.			
2.			
3.			
4.			
. . .			
. . .			
15.			

$$\text{Reticulocyte count (\%)} = \frac{15 \times 100}{1500} = 1 \text{ per cent}$$

Precautions and Sources of Error

1. Staining time should not be less than 10 minutes.
2. Mixing of the blood with the stain should be done gently but thoroughly prior to making the smear. This is important because the reticulocytes have a lower specific gravity than mature red cells, and therefore, settle on top of the red cells in the mixture. Thus an unmixed or poorly mixed blood specimen will not give the correct result.
3. Reticulocytes should be properly identified. The red cells showing highly refractile areas may be confused with reticulocytes. These artifacts in the red cells are probably due to moisture in the air and poor drying of the smear. Use a fresh specimen.
4. Careful focusing of the microscope is essential in the reticulocyte count. Stained platelet granules and leucocyte granules must not be mistaken for a reticulocyte. Precipitated stain might also be mistaken for reticulum within the erythrocytes. To minimise this possibility, the dye must be filtered immediately before use. Immediate drying of the smear also prevents formation of the crystalline objects that sometimes appear in the red cells.
5. Supravital stains also stain other **red cell inclusions** in addition to staining the RNA in the reticulocytes. These include Howell–Jolly bodies, Heinz bodies and Pappenheimer bodies. These bodies are present in different pathological conditions. In a reticulocyte count, if these bodies are present, they should be counted separately.
6. Equal volumes of staining fluid and blood specimen should be used. In case of low hematocrit value (anemia), use a large proportion of blood, and when the hematocrit is high (polycythemia), use a smaller volume of blood. This variation in dilution helps in the spreading out of 100–150 red cells per microscopic field making it easier to count. Therefore, hematocrit or hemoglobin content of the blood should be determined prior to reticulocyte count. At least the lower palpebral conjunctiva should be examined to clinically assess the hemoglobin status of the subject.

Manual Method (Absolute Count) of Reticulocyte Count

A direct absolute count of reticulocytes by hemocytometry is not possible. An indirect count is taken against the number of red cells and expressed as a percentage of red cells. This relative value can be converted to an absolute value by performing the total RBC count of the same sample of blood.

Absolute count of reticulocytes/ml of blood

$$= \frac{RC\ (\%) \times RBC\ count/ml\ of\ blood}{100}$$

where RC is reticulocyte count (per cent).

Normal value   20,000–50,000/mm^3 of blood

Automated Method of Reticulocyte Count

With the use of automated techniques, the process of counting reticulocytes has become easier. This is done by the principle of flow cytometry.

Principle

Cells are stained with a fluorochrome dye that preferentially stains RNA. The cells are counted by a fluorescent technique. The RNA containing reticulocytes will fluoresce when exposed to ultraviolet light. This instrument can count thousands of reticulocytes in just a few seconds.

Advantages

1. The process of counting is made easy.
2. It takes very little time.
3. It is an accurate method.

DISCUSSION

Physiological Significance

The number of reticulocytes in circulation indicates the degree of activity of the bone marrow. When the marrow is very active, the reticulocyte count increases; and when the marrow is suppressed, the reticulocyte count decreases. Therefore, the number of reticulocytes in the peripheral blood is a good index of bone marrow activity, especially of erythropoiesis. Reticulocyte count is proportionate to the red cell production.

Clinical Significance

Reticulocyte Response

The reticulocyte count is performed to follow-up therapeutic response for anemias in which the patient is deficient in one of the substances essential for the synthesis of red cells. When therapy begins, new red cells will be formed and released rapidly into the circulation before the cells are fully matured. Many reticulocytes are released with the release of young red cells. The corresponding increase in reticulocyte count is called reticulocyte response. Reticulocyte response indicates a **favourable response to treatment**. This is typically observed in the **treatment of pernicious anemia and iron deficiency anemia**. When vitamin B12 is administered as part of the treatment of pernicious anemia, the number of reticulocytes increases in the blood in the initial phase of the treatment. This indicates that the patient is responding well to the treatment. Similarly, the reticulocyte count increases in the blood when iron is given in the treatment of iron deficiency anemia. Thus, the reticulocyte count is performed to assess the response of the patient to the treatment in pernicious and iron deficiency anemia.

Detection of Types of Anemia

The reticulocyte count may provide useful information about the type of anemia, as it is elevated in conditions in which the erythroid precursors can increase the production of red cells in response to an increase in the demand for them. This is commonly seen in hemolytic anemia in which erythropoietic activity remains unimpaired. This is also seen in blood-loss anemia.

Conditions That Alter Reticulocyte Count

An increase in reticulocyte count is known as reticulocytosis, and a decrease in reticulocyte count is known as reticulocytopenia.

Reticulocytosis

Physiological
1. Newborns and infants
2. High altitude

Pathological

1. Hemolytic anemia
2. Acute hemorrhage
3. During treatment of deficiency anemias (reticulocyte response)
4. Any condition that stimulates the bone marrow to produce red cells

Reticulocytopenia

1. Aplastic anemia
2. Myxedema
3. Hypopituitarism

4. Leuco-erythroblastic anemia

The **leuco-erythroblastic blood picture** is used to describe the presence of immature myeloid and nucleated red cells in the peripheral blood often as a consequence of a disturbance of the bone marrow architecture by abnormal tissues (infiltration). It is seen in:

◈ secondary carcinoma of bone
◈ myelofibrosis
◈ after splenectomy in thalassemia major
◈ multiple myeloma

There is no physiological reticulocytopenia.

VIVA

1. What is the normal reticulocyte count in adults?
2. What is the normal reticulocyte count in newborns and at what age does it reach the adult value?
3. What are the methods of reticulocyte count?
4. What is a supravital stain? Give examples. How does it differ from the vital stain?
5. What is the composition and function of each constituent of brilliant cresyl blue stain?
6. What are the sources of error in the manual method of reticulocyte count?
7. What happens when blood is not properly mixed with the stain?
8. How do you identify reticulocytes in the smear?
9. Why should equal volumes of staining fluid and blood be used for the reticulocyte count?
10. How do you perform absolute reticulocyte count?
11. What is the principle and what are the advantages of the automated method of reticulocyte count?
12. What is the lifespan and fate of reticulocytes?
13. How do reticulocytes develop in the bone marrow?
14. What is the physiological significance of reticulocyte count?
15. What is the clinical significance of reticulocyte count?
16. What is reticulocyte response and what is its significance?
17. What are the conditions of reticulocytosis and reticulocytopenia?
18. What is the cause of reticulocytosis at high altitudes?
19. What is punctate basophilia? In what conditions is it seen?

CHAPTER 20

Determination of Specific Gravity of Blood

Learning Objectives

After completing this practical, you will be able to (MUST KNOW):
1. List the methods of determination of specific gravity of blood.
2. Learn the principle of determination of specific gravity of blood by Philips and Vanslyke's copper sulphate method.
3. List the factors that affect specific gravity of blood.
4. Give the conditions that alter specific gravity of blood.

INTRODUCTION

The specific gravity of blood is the ratio of the weight of blood to the weight of an equal volume of water at 4°C. It depends on hematocrit, plasma proteins and water content of blood. The specific gravity of blood gives an idea of the solute and water content of blood. Under normal conditions, specific gravity is a good index of the hemoglobin content of blood. It has proved to be useful in screening blood donors and in emergency cases of burns that need repeated transfusion. This method was extensively used during World War II in assessing battle casualties requiring blood transfusion.

METHODS

Specific gravity of blood can be determined by (1) direct and (2) indirect methods. Indirect methods are of two types: Hammar Schlag's method, and Philips–Vanslyke's copper sulphate method.

Direct Method

Equal volume of blood and water are taken in two capillary tubes called pyconometers and the liquids are weighed. The ratio of the weights of the liquids gives the specific gravity of blood.

Indirect Method

Hammar Schlag's Method

In this method, the specific gravity of blood is determined by equalising the density of two miscible liquids like chloroform (specific gravity 1.470) and benzene (specific gravity 0.880) to that of blood.

Philips–Vanslyke's Copper Sulphate Method

Principle

Two miscible liquids of known but different specific gravities are mixed in varying proportions to give a number of solutions covering the expected range of specific gravity. A drop of blood is then allowed to fall in each of the solutions and the behaviour is studied. The specific gravity of blood is compared with solutions of copper sulphate of known specific gravities.

Requirements

1. Stock solution of copper sulphate of specific gravity 1.100.
2. Distilled water
3. Test tubes
4. Dropper

Procedure

1. Prepare copper sulphate solution (10 ml) of specific gravities ranging from 1.050 to 1.068 by mixing distilled water with stock solution of copper sulphate in different test tubes as given in the Table 20.1.
2. Mix solution in each tube properly.
3. Pour a drop of blood into each tube from a height of about 1 cm above the solution with the help of a pipette.

Table 20.1   Copper sulphate solutions in a range of specific gravities.

Test tube	1	2	3	4	5	6	7	8	9	10
Copper sulphate solution (ml)	4.9	5.1	5.3	5.5	5.7	5.9	6.1	6.3	6.5	6.7
Distilled water (ml)	5.1	4.9	4.7	4.5	4.3	4.1	3.9	3.7	3.5	3.3
Specific gravity of solution	1.050	1.052	1.054	1.056	1.058	1.060	1.062	1.064	1.066	1.068

4. Observe the behaviour of the blood-drop in the solution of the tubes.

Note: The blood-drop will travel for some distance because of the momentum and will sink if it is heavier than the solution, or will float on the surface of the solution if it is lighter.

5. Note the tubes (specific gravity of the solution) in which the blood-drop remains suspended at the centre of the solution for 15–20 seconds. This gives the specific gravity of the blood sample.

Note: The blood-drop floats in copper sulphate solution due to the covering of copper proteinate layer, which is stable for about 15–20 seconds.

Normal Values

The normal range of specific gravity of blood varies from 1.048 to 1.066.

Average value in males   : 1.057
Average value in females : 1.053

Precautions

1. While preparing the solution, the ratio of water in copper sulphate must be measured accurately.
2. The blood should be dropped into the copper sulphate solution from a height of about 1 cm from the upper level of the solution.
3. The reading should be taken within 10–15 seconds.

DISCUSSION

Physiological Significance

The specific gravity of blood may alter due to alteration in the solute content, water content, or cell content of the blood. Any condition that leads to hemoconcentration, like diarrhea, vomiting and excessive sweating, increases the specific gravity of the blood, and conversely any condition that causes hemodilution, like excessive saline infusion, pregnancy and so on, decreases the specific gravity. Specific gravity gives the indication about the solid and water content of the blood.

Factors That Affect Specific Gravity of Blood

1. The number of RBCs in the blood.
2. Hemoglobin content of the blood.
3. Plasma protein concentration.
4. Water content of the blood.

Clinical Significance

Conditions That Affect Specific Gravity of Blood

Conditions that increase specific gravity

Physiological
1. High altitude
2. Newborns and infants
3. Excess sweating

Pathological
1. Diarrhea
2. Vomiting
3. Dehydration
4. Polycythemia

Conditions that decrease specific gravity

Physiological
1. Pregnancy
2. Excess water intake

Pathological
1. Different conditions in which there occur overhydration (increased water content of blood) for example nephritic syndrome.

VIVA

1. *What is the importance of the determination of specific gravity of blood?*
2. *What are the methods of determination of specific gravity of blood?*
3. *What is the principle of Philips–Vanslyke's copper sulphate method?*
4. *What are the precautions of Philips–Vanslyke's copper sulphate method?*
5. *What is the clinical significance of estimation of specific gravity of blood?*
6. *What are the factors that affect specific gravity of blood?*
7. *Name the conditions that alter the specific gravity of blood.*

CHAPTER 21

Stethography

Learning Objectives

After completing this practical, you will be able to (MUST KNOW):

1. Define stethography.
2. Tie the stethograph at the proper position around the chest of the subject.
3. Record respiratory movements (normal and following different maneuvers).
4. List the precautions taken during stethographic recordings.

5. Define breaking point.
6. List the factors that affect the breaking point.
7. Define and give examples of periodic breathing.

You may also be able to (DESIRABLE TO KNOW):

1. Explain the effects of exercise and hyperventilation on respiration.
2. Explain the differences in breath-holding time following inspiration and expiration.

INTRODUCTION

Stethography is the method by which respiratory movements are recorded. Stethography is useful in assessing the breath holding time (BHT) following inspiration and expiration, and in response to different stimuli. Physiologically, BHT is a determinant of the respiratory capacity of the individual. This can be used as a tool in the assessment of respiratory fitness.

METHODS

Method of Using a Stethograph

Principle

The stethograph is tied around the chest of the subject. The movement of the chest causes a change in the air pressure in the stethograph, which is recorded on a moving drum.

Requirements

1. **Stethograph**   The stethograph (Fig. 21.1) consists of a corrugated rubber tube with a stopper at each end and an air outlet pipe connected to the tambour.

2. **Marey's tambour**   It is a metallic cup with a side tube and a rubber diaphragm mounted at the top

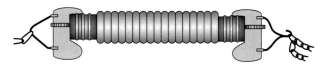

Fig. 21.1   Stethograph.

(Fig. 21.2). A writing lever is attached to a small metal disc, which rests on the rubber diaphragm. The side tube of the metal cup is connected to the stethograph by a rubber tube.

3. Kymograph
4. Drinking water

Procedure

1. Ask the subject to sit comfortably on a stool with his/her back towards the recording apparatus.
2. Tie the stethograph around the chest of the subject at the level of the fourth intercostal space and connect it to the tambour.

Note: Check that when the stethograph is connected to the tambour, the pressure change in the stethograph is transmitted to it. It is confirmed by movement of the lever with movement of the chest.

3. Bring the writing lever in contact with the paper of the kymograph and set the drum to move at a slow speed (2.5 mm/s).
4. Record normal respiration for about 5 cm.
5. Ask the subject to drink water and record the effect

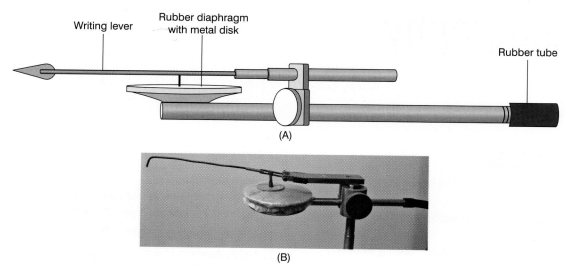

Fig. 21.2   Marey's tambour. (A) Diagrammatic representation; (B) A photograph.

of deglutition on respiratory movement. Then take a normal tracing.

6. Take a normal tracing and ask the subject to hold his breath as long as possible after quiet inspiration and expiration and following deep inspiration and deep expiration, and record the effects.

> **Note:** The effects of all these respiratory maneuvres should be recorded separately. Normal tracings should be recorded before and after each recording.

7. Record normal respiration and stop the drum. Ask the subject to take deep breaths as rapidly as possible for one and a half minutes. Immediately after hyperventilation, start the drum and record the effect on respiratory movement.

8. Record normal respiration. Disconnect the stethograph from Marey's tambour and ask the subject to exercise (spot jogging) for one minute. Immediately after exercise, connect the stethograph to the kymograph and record the effect of exercise on respiratory movement.

Precautions

1. The subject should sit comfortably and in an erect posture.

2. The tambour should be tied at the level of the fourth intercostal space because expansion of the chest is maximum at this level.

3. Before and after the recordings for each maneuver (for example, swallowing water), normal tracings should be taken.

4. The recording should not be made during the act of hyperventilation but immediately after.

5. The stethograph must be disconnected from the tambour during exercise, and recording should be made immediately after exercise.

6. For BHT, the recording should be made after quiet inspiration and quiet expiration, and forceful inspiration and forceful expiration.

Observation

Note that downstroke is inspiration and upstroke is expiration. Note that apnea occurs during the act of deglutition. Study the duration of BHT following normal and deep inspiration and expiration. Observe the breathing pattern following hyperventilation and exercise (Fig. 21.3).

DISCUSSION

Deglutition Apnea

During deglutition (drinking of water), respiration stops temporarily. This is called deglutition apnea. It is due to closure of the glottis, which helps in passage of food or water in the esophagus and prevents entry of food materials into the respiratory tract.

Breath-Holding Time (BHT)

BHT is the maximum time for which the subject can hold his breath. BHT is greater following inspiration

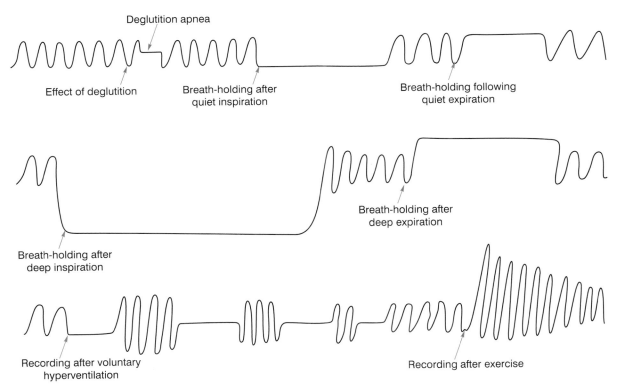

Fig. 21.3 Recording of respiratory movements to study the effect of deglutition, voluntary hyperventilation and exercise, and to determine breath-holding time (BHT).

than expiration. Respiration can be voluntarily held for some time, but eventually, the voluntary control is overridden. The point at which breathing can no longer be voluntarily inhibited is called the **breaking point**. The breaking is due to **rise in arterial pCO_2 and the *fall in pO_2***, as body tissues continue to utilise oxygen and produce carbon dioxide. The rise in arterial pCO_2 and fall in pO_2 stimulate central and peripheral chemoreceptors, which stimulate respiration. **Generally, breaking point is reached at alveolar pO_2 of 56 mm Hg and alveolar pCO_2 of 49 mm Hg.** It has been suggested that proprioceptive impulses from respiratory muscles and joints may be involved in the breaking point.

Factors Affecting Breaking Point

1. **Breathing 100 per cent oxygen** increases BHT. Breathing 100 per cent oxygen before holding breath increases alveolar pO_2, so the breaking point is delayed.
2. **Hyperventilation** at room air increases BHT. This is because hyperventilation removes CO_2 from the blood and therefore delays breaking point.

3. **Psychological factors** play a role. Encouragement delays breaking point.

Hyperventilation

Periodic breathing occurs following voluntary hyperventilation. There occurs apnea followed by a brief period of hyperpnea. The apnea occurs due to removal of carbon dioxide during hyperventilation, so respiration stops temporarily. This causes accumulation of carbon dioxide, which stimulates respiration; as a result, there is hyperventilation.

Periodic breathing (Cheyne–Stokes breathing) is characterised by alternating apnea and hyperventilation. It is seen **physiologically** in sleep (especially in infants), at high altitude and following voluntary hyperventilation, and **pathologically** in left ventricular failure and brain damage.

Exercise

During exercise, hyperventilation occurs due to stimulation of respiratory centres by increased discharge from the proprioceptors in the joints, ligaments and muscles. Though the increase in respiration is proportionate to the increase in oxygen consumption, the role of oxygen in the stimulation of hyperventilation is still not clear. **Increased body temperature, increased K$^+$ level and lactic acid concentration** play a role in hyperventilation. But, as the exercise is mild to moderate here, hyperventilation is mainly due to increased proprioceptive information from the exercising muscles and joints.

Hyperventilation persists after intense exercise due to increased arterial H$^+$ concentration, which occurs due to lactic acidemia. Sometimes, a pattern of periodic breathing is also observed following exercise.

VIVA

1. What is stethography?
2. Why is the stethograph tied at the fourth intercostal space around the chest?
3. What are the precautions taken for stethography?
4. What is deglutition apnea? What is its cause?
5. What is breaking point? What are its causes?
6. What are the factors that affect breaking point?
7. What are the causes of periodic breathing that occurs following voluntary hyperventilation?
8. What are the effects of exercise on respiratory movement?
9. What is periodic breathing? Give examples.
10. Briefly explain the effects of pO_2 and pCO_2 on respiration.

CHAPTER 22

Vitalography and Effect of Posture on Vital Capacity

Learning Objectives

After completing this practical, you will be able to (MUST KNOW):
1. Define vital capacity.
2. Record the effect of posture on vital capacity.
3. List the precautions taken during the recording.
4. State the normal value of vital capacity.
5. List the factors that affect vital capacity.

You may also be able to (DESIRABLE TO KNOW):
1. Explain the variation in vital capacity in different conditions.
2. List the reasons for alteration in vital capacity with change in posture.
3. Explain the physiological significance of vital capacity.

INTRODUCTION

Vital capacity (VC) is the maximum volume of air that can be expired from the lungs by forceful effort following a maximal inspiration. VC is computed as the sum of tidal volume, inspiratory reserve volume and expiratory reserve volume. The average value of VC is 4.5 litres in males and 3.3 litres in females. VC depends on the growth and development of the subject and the physical training he/she has received. Change of posture also affects vital capacity.

Factors Affecting Vital Capacity

Physiological Factors

1. **Posture**   VC is greater in an erect posture than in the sitting and lying postures (for explanation, see Discussion).
2. **Age**   VC is high in young adults, and low in children and old people. As age advances, compliance of the lungs and chest wall decreases, and therefore vital capacity decreases.
3. **Gender**   VC is greater in males because the size of the chest is larger and muscle power is more in males.
4. **Physical build**   VC is low in obese and very thin persons. It is high in well-built persons. Vital capacity depends on chest size, muscle power and body surface area of the individual.

5. **Pregnancy**   VC is low during pregnancy because chest expansion decreases as abdominal size increases.
6. **Physical training**   VC is higher in trained athletes than in untrained individuals. It is even higher in swimmers and divers.

Pathological Factors

1. VC decreases in the **diseases of the chest wall** (for example, kyphoscoliosis), **lungs** (for example, emphysema, fibrosis, pulmonary edema) and **pleura** (for example, pleural effusion, pneumothorax).
2. VC decreases in **diseases of the abdomen** in which lung expansion is restricted as seen in abdominal tumours and ascites.

METHODS

Method to Demonstrate the Effect of Posture on VC

Principle

Change in posture changes the ability to carry out physical effort and the ventilatory capacity of the lungs. Therefore, posture affects the vital capacity.

Requirements

1. Student's spirometer (vitalometer) (Fig. 22.1).
2. Mouthpiece

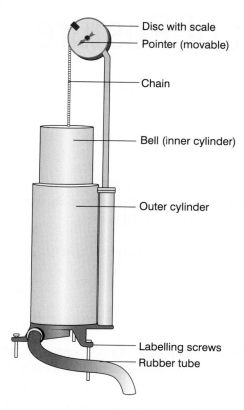

Fig. 22.1   Student's spirometer.

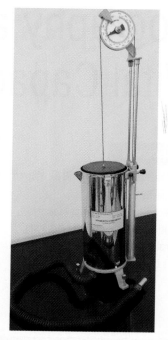

Fig. 22.2   Recording of vital capacity using student's spirometer. Note the change in the position of the pointer (red arrow) from the zero mark after the maneuver.

Procedure

1. Adjust the reading of the vitalometer to the zero mark.
2. Ask the subject to lie down comfortably on a couch.
3. Connect the mouthpiece of the vitalometer to the subject's mouth.
4. Ask the subject to exhale forcefully to the maximum after taking a deep inspiration.
5. Record the vital capacity from the scale of the vitalometer (Fig. 22.2).
6. Change the position of the arrow to zero and ask the subject to repeat the maneuvre.
7. Record vital capacity three times, with a gap of at least two minutes between each, and record the best one.
8. Ask the subject to sit on a stool with his/her spine erect.
9. Record vital capacity (as described above) three times and record the best reading.
10. Ask the subject to stand up.
11. Record the vital capacity three times and record the best reading.
12. Compare the vital capacities recorded in the three positions.

Observation

Note that the vital capacity is maximum in the erect posture, and minimum in the supine posture.

Precautions

1. Each time, before recording vital capacity, the arrow mark of the scale should be adjusted to zero.
2. In the sitting and standing postures, the spine of the subject should be erect.
3. The subject should be trained and encouraged to put his/her maximum effort possible.
4. A minimum of three attempts should be made in all the postures and the best of the three should be taken.
5. The gap between each attempt should be a minimum of one to two minutes.
6. The test should not be performed on a full stomach.

DISCUSSION

Vital capacity (VC) ranges between 3.2 to 4.8 l. It is more in males and about 20% lower in females.

VC is **more in the erect posture** than in supine and sitting postures because of the following reasons:

1. **More physical (muscular) effort** is applied in the erect posture.
2. In the **erect posture**, the diaphragm descends; therefore, the **capacity of the thoracic cage increases**. In the **supine position**, the diaphragm is pulled upward because the abdominal viscera push the diaphragm. Therefore, the **capacity of the thoracic cage decreases**. Hence, vital capacity is greater in the erect posture than in the supine position.
3. In the **supine position**, due to elimination of the effect of gravity, the **blood flow to the lungs increases**. This decreases vital capacity. In the **standing posture**, blood is pooled in the lower extremities, therefore venous return decreases. This **decreases pulmonary blood flow**. Thus vital capacity increases on standing.

Two-Stage Vital Capacity

Two-stage vital capacity is defined as the sum of the inspiratory capacity (IC) and expiratory reserve volume (ERV) measured separately with the help of a spirometer.

Physiological Significance

Vital capacity indicates **the strength of the respiratory muscles**. Therefore, the maximum inspiratory and expiratory effort of the person can be assessed by determining vital capacity. VC is more in trained individuals such as athletes, swimmers, runners and divers.

Prediction of Vital Capacity

Various formulas have been introduced to predict VC in individuals based on their race, ethnicity, age and gender. Various respiratory disorders are diagnosed by comparing the actual value (recorded value) with the **predicted value**.

OSPE

I.   Determine the vital capacity of the given subject in the sitting posture by using the student's spirometer.

Steps
1. Adjust the zero reading of the vitalometer.
2. Ask the subject to sit comfortably on a stool.
3. Instruct him to put in the maximum effort during recording.
4. Connect the mouthpiece of the vitalometer to the mouth of the subject.
5. Ask the subject to exhale forcefully to the maximum after taking a deep inspiration and note the reading.
6. Ask the subject to repeat the procedure three times, and record the best one.

II. Record the effect of standing (from lying-down posture) on the vital capacity of the given subject.

Steps
1. Adjust the zero reading of the vitalometer.
2. Ask the subject to lie down comfortably in the supine posture on a couch.
3. Instruct the subject to put in the maximum effort during recording.
4. Connect the mouthpiece of the vitalometer to the mouth of the subject.
5. Ask him/her to exhale forcefully and maximally following a deep inspiration and record the reading from the vitalometer scale.
6. Ask the subject to stand up erect.
7. Adjust the zero reading of the vitalometer.
8. Ask him/her to exhale forcefully and maximally following a deep inspiration and record the reading from the vitalometer scale.
9. Compare both the readings and report.

VIVA

1. Define vital capacity.
2. What is the normal value of VC in males and females?
3. What are the factors that affect vital capacity?
4. What are the precautions for recording vital capacity?
5. Why is the vital capacity greater in the standing posture than in the sitting and supine postures?
6. What is the physiological significance of VC?
7. What is two-stage vital capacity?
8. What is the importance of prediction of VC?

CHAPTER 23

Pulmonary Function Tests and Spirometry

Learning Objectives

After completing this practical, you will be able to (MUST KNOW):

1. Describe the importance of performing this practical in clinical physiology.
2. Classify the pulmonary function tests (PFTs).
3. Record the lung volumes and capacities and FEV_1 by spirometry.
4. Define lung volumes and capacities.
5. State the normal values of all PFTs.
6. Explain the differences between patterns of FEV_1 in obstructive and restrictive lung diseases.

7. State the importance of FVC and FEV_1 in the diagnosis of respiratory diseases.
8. Name the common conditions that alter the result of PFTs.

You may also be able to (DESIRABLE TO KNOW):

1. Explain the significance of all PFTs.
2. Explain the disturbances in pulmonary circulation, diffusion, and ventilation–perfusion ratio in the pathophysiology and diagnosis of respiratory diseases.

INTRODUCTION

The most important function of the lung is to maintain tension of oxygen and carbon dioxide of the arterial blood within the normal range. This is achieved by uptake of oxygen from the inspired air and giving up of carbon dioxide in the expired air. Thus, tissue oxygenation is adequately maintained and accumulation of carbon dioxide in excess in the body is prevented by the lung. The fundamental mechanisms involved in attaining this goal are ventilation, diffusion and perfusion. Therefore, pulmonary function tests (PFTs) should be aimed at assessing different aspects of ventilation, diffusion and perfusion.

The assessment of the type and degree of functional impairment caused by various diseases affecting the respiratory systems requires an understanding of the basic principles of respiratory physiology. Some of the pulmonary function tests may require elaborate equipment and procedures, but most of the tests are simple, non-invasive and inexpensive.

Classification of PFTs Based on Lung Function

From the physiological point of view, PFTs are best classified by categorising different tests to assess ventilation, ventilation–perfusion relationship and diffusion, and to measure dead space, compliance,

airway resistance and pulmonary blood flow and pressure.

Parameters That Assess Ventilation

A. Static lung volumes and capacities

1. Lung volumes
   - Tidal volume
   - Inspiratory reserve volume
   - Expiratory reserve volume
   - Residual volume
2. Lung capacities
   - Vital capacity
   - Inspiratory capacity
   - Functional residual capacity
   - Total lung capacity

B. Mechanics of breathing (Dynamic lung volumes and capacities)

1. Timed vital capacity
2. Maximum mid-expiratory flow rate
3. Maximum voluntary ventilation
4. Peak expiratory flow rate
5. Maximum expiratory flow–volume curve
6. Closing volume

Study of Ventilation–Perfusion Relationship

Uniformity of ventilation is assessed by:

1.   Nitrogen washout method (Breath nitrogen test)
2.   Radioactive xenon method

Assessment of Diffusion

1.   Measurement of pO_2 and pCO_2 in arterial blood
2.   Measurement of diffusing capacity of O_2 and CO_2

Determination of Pulmonary Blood Flow and Pressures

Measurement of mean pulmonary artery pressure, pulmonary capillary wedge pressure, pulmonary blood flow and pulmonary vascular resistance.

Assessment of Ventilation

Ventilation is the process of movement of air in and out of the gas exchanging units of the lung, that is, the alveoli. Its adequacy depends on the lung volumes and capacities and the mechanics of breathing. The various **lung volumes and capacities are indices of static dimensions** of the lung at various stages of inflation (Fig. 23.1). The mechanics of breathing deal with static as well as dynamic mechanical properties of the respiratory apparatus.

Lung Volumes

1. Tidal volume   Tidal volume (TV) is the volume of air inspired or expired during quiet breathing. This

is 500 ml in adults. About 150 ml of this volume occupies the upper airways up to the respiratory bronchioles, and this amount does not take part in gas exchange. This is called **anatomical dead space**. The remaining volume, that is, 350 ml, is available for alveolar ventilation.

Minute ventilation (MV)   This is the volume of air that can be breathed in or out of the lung in one minute.

$$MV = TV \times \text{respiratory rate per min.}$$

This is also called **resting minute volume (RMV)** or **pulmonary ventilation (PV)**. Normal value of MV is 6 litres/min.

2. Inspiratory reserve volume   The volume of air inspired with a maximal inspiratory effort in excess of the tidal volume is called the **inspiratory reserve volume (IRV)**. The **normal value of IRV** is 3 litres in men and 2 litres in women. Inspiratory muscles should be used to the maximum when measuring IRV.

3. Expiratory reserve volume   The volume of air that can be expired with a maximum expiratory effort after passive expiration is called **expiratory reserve volume (ERV)**. The **normal value of ERV** is 1 litre in men and 0.7 litres in women. Expiratory muscles should be used to the maximum when measuring ERV.

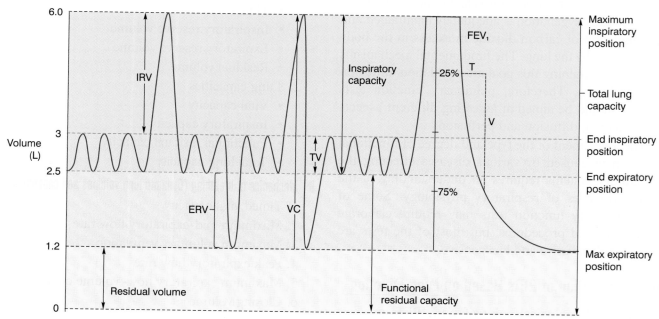

Fig. 23.1   Lung volumes and capacities (TV: Tidal volume; IRV: Inspiratory reserve volume; ERV: Expiratory reserve volume; VC: Vital capacity; VC = IRV + ERV + TV; FEV_1: Forced expiratory volume in first second). For calculation of $FEF_{25-75\%}$, note T as time and V as volume as drawn from FEV_1 curve.

4. Residual volume The volume of air left in the lung at the end of a maximal expiratory effort is the **residual volume (RV)**. The **normal value of RV** is 1.2 litres in men and 1.1 litres in women.

Lung Capacities

1. Vital capacity (VC) The maximum amount of air that can be expired forcefully after a maximal inspiratory effort is called the vital capacity (VC). The **normal value** of VC is about 4.5 litres in men and about 3 litres in women.

Forced vital capacity (FVC) The total volume expired forcefully with greatest force and speed after a maximal inspiration is the FVC. FVC differs very little from VC in the normal subject, but it is proportionately more reduced when there is airway obstruction with air trapping.

2. Inspiratory capacity This is the maximum amount of air that can be inspired from the resting expiratory level. This is the IRV + TV. It is about 3.5 litres.

3. Functional residual capacity (FRC) This is the amount of air remaining in the lungs at the end of a normal expiration at rest.

$$FRC = ERV + RV$$

4. Total lung capacity The volume of air present in the lungs at the end of maximal inspiration is the total lung capacity (TLC). The **normal value** is 6 litres in men and 4.2 litres in women.

> **Note:**
> 1. All static volumes are measured by spirometer, except RV, FRC and TLC.
> 2. Values of lung volume and capacities should be uniform and converted with standard temperature and pressure, dry (STPD) for comparison using gas equation.
> 3. RV and TLC are calculated after measuring FRC, which is done by nitrogen-washout method or helium dilution technique.

Assessment of Mechanics of Breathing

In carrying out the process of ventilation, certain forces are required to overcome the elastic recoil of the lung and thorax, the non-elastic resistance caused by the movement of tissues during breathing, and the airway resistance. Thus, assessment of mechanics of breathing is aimed at assessing compliance and airway resistance.

Compliance

Compliance measures the relative stiffness and distensibility of the lungs and thorax. The elastic recoil of the lung, which is measured under static condition, is called compliance. Compliance is defined as the **volume change per unit transpulmonary pressure difference** between the esophageal or intrapleural pressure and the mouth pressure. If the volume change per unit pressure change is higher than normal, the tissues are more distensible, and if it is less, the tissues are stiffer than normal. Patients with decreased compliance put more respiratory effort to achieve adequate alveolar ventilation and therefore they are dyspneic.

Airway Resistance

This represents the frictional resistance to airflow through the conducting air passages. Patients with increased **airway resistance** often present serious mechanical problems and develop **dyspnea**. The degree of dyspnea depends on the severity of the increased airway resistance.

Dynamic Lung Volumes and Capacities

Dynamic lung volumes and capacities give a fair idea of the mechanics of breathing.

1. Timed vital capacity This is also called forced expiratory volume in the first second (FEV_1). This is defined as the fraction of the vital capacity expired in the specified time, for example, FEV_1, that is, the fraction of vital capacity expired in the first second. This test measures the vital capacity in relation to time and gives the portion of the vital capacity expired in a specified time. This is an index of airflow rate. In normal conditions, **80–85 per cent of the forced vital capacity is expired in the first second**, 95 per cent in two seconds (FEV_2) and 97–100 per cent in three seconds (FEV_3). It is one of the most useful tests to detect generalised airway obstruction. It is a relatively insensitive indicator of small airway obstruction.

2. Maximum mid-expiratory flow rate (MMEFR) This is the maximum flow achieved during the middle third of the total expired volume. This is expressed as forced expiratory flow at 25–75 per cent of the lung volume ($FEF_{25-75\%}$). $FEF_{25-75\%}$ indicates the patency of small airways. The measurement of flow rate between 200 and 1200 ml ($FEF_{200-1200ml}$) in litres per second indicates the patency of larger airways.

3. Maximum voluntary ventilation (MVV) This is also called maximum breathing capacity (MBC). MVV is the maximum volume of air that can be breathed out per minute by maximal voluntary effort. The normal value of MVV is 150 l/min in adult males and 125 l/min in adult females.

Breathing reserve (BR) This is the maximum amount of air that can be breathed in and out of the lung above the minute ventilation (MV). BR = MVV − MV. Normal value of BR ranges from 115 l to 160 l.

Dyspneic index (DI)

$$DI = \frac{BR}{MVV} \times 100.$$

Normally it is 90%. When DI is <60%, dyspnea occurs at rest. DI is also known as **breathing reserve ratio (BRR)**.

4. Peak expiratory flow rate (PEFR) It is the maximum velocity in litres per minute with which air is forced out of the lungs. PEFR can be read directly from the dial of the peak flow meter. The normal value of PEFR is 400–600 l/min or 6–10 l/sec.

5. Maximum expiratory flow volume curve (MEFVC) Because of the limitation of FEV_1, certain other tests are performed to detect airway obstruction in its early phase. These include V_{max} 75 per cent, response of maximum expiratory flow volume curve (MEFVC) to inhalation of helium, and closing volume. In MEFVC, flow is plotted against volume exhaled. V_{max} 75 per cent is the volume achieved after exhaling 75 per cent of the total FVC.

Flow–Volume curve The flow rate is plotted against the lung volume to obtain a flow–volume curve (Fig. 23.2A) and a flow-volume loop (Fig. 23.2B). The subject expires maximally and forcefully to residual volume following a deep inspiration (TLC). The flow rate quickly reaches a maximum and then falls slowly. In obstructive diseases, the volume is greater because of air trapping, and the flow rate is less in airway obstruction.

6. Closing volume (CV) This test detects small airway obstruction by measuring the volume of gas remaining in the lung after closure of small airways in the gravity-dependent lung areas.

Ventilation–Perfusion Relationship

The inspired air is not distributed evenly even in normal conditions. In an erect posture, resting ventilation per unit volume of lung is greater at the

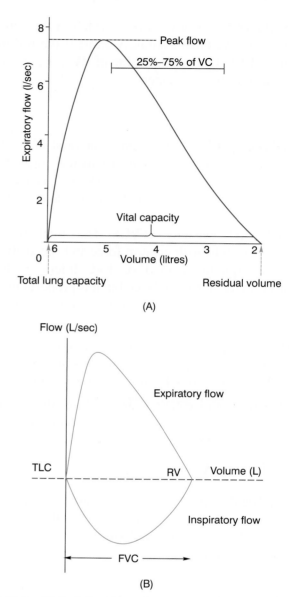

Fig. 23.2 (A) Expiratory flow–volume curve; (B) Normal flow–volume loop.

bases than at the apices. The difference in values is less pronounced when lying down and during exercise. In disease states, the distribution becomes more uneven resulting in hypo- and hyperventilated areas. Such non-uniform distribution of inspired gas leads to decreased oxygen tension in the arterial blood. The uniformity of distribution of inspired air is measured by the **nitrogen washout method**. An alveolar gas sample after 7 minutes of breathing oxygen normally contains less than 2.5 per cent of nitrogen. The higher the percentage of nitrogen in the alveolar sample, the greater the degree of non-uniformity of distribution of inspired gas.

Diffusion

Diffusion is the physical process by which gas moves across a membrane from the region of higher partial pressure to the region of lower partial pressure. In the lungs, oxygen moves from the alveoli to the pulmonary capillaries and carbon dioxide moves in the opposite direction. The **diffusion capacity of carbon dioxide is twenty times that of oxygen**. Therefore, diffusion problems usually do not produce carbon dioxide retention.

PaO$_2$ and PaCO$_2$ depend on diffusion of the gases through the alveolocapillary membrane. It is difficult to measure the diffusing capacity of the gases. Therefore, measurement of the arterial blood gas tension is essential in the evaluation of pulmonary functions. The **normal value** of PaO$_2$ is 90–95 mm Hg, and that of PaCO$_2$ is 36–44 mm Hg.

Pulmonary Blood Flow and Pressure

Pulmonary function test is incomplete without the study of pulmonary circulation. Measurement of pressures, vascular resistance, blood volume and distribution of blood flow in the pulmonary circulation help in detecting vascular occlusion and decreased pulmonary capillary volume.

The pulmonary vasculature accommodates 5 l/min of right ventricular output. The vessels are comparatively thin-walled and provide less resistance to flow in comparison to systemic vessels. The **normal mean pulmonary artery pressure is 15 mm Hg**. In an erect posture the arterial pressure is lowest at the apex and highest at the lung bases.

METHODS

Method to Study Various Lung Functions

Principle

Subject exhales forcefully into the instrument, and this is used to detect different parameters which reflect various lung functions.

Requirements

1. Recording spirometer A recording spirometer (Fig. 23.3A) is a spirometer with a recording kymograph.

The spirometer consists of a hollow double-walled vessel. The space between the two walls contains water; making it airtight. In the space between the two walls, an inverted hollow cylindrical bell of 9 l capacity is placed. The bell is attached to a counterbalance with a chain which passes over a pulley. The counterbalance carries a pen for writing on the kymograph paper. The kymograph operates at speeds of 60 and 1200 mm/min. The spirometer records the volume and capacities of the lung.

Computerised spirometer Nowadays, lung functions are assessed by using a computerised spirometer (Fig. 23.3B) rather than the recording spirometer.

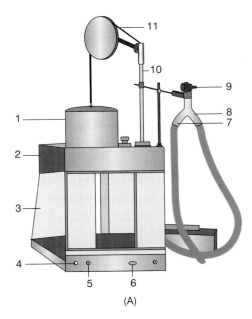

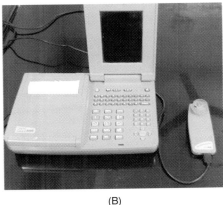

Fig. 23.3A (A) Spirometer (Expirograph) (1: Bell of the spirometer; 2: Paper speed selector; 3: Paper; 4: Pilot lamp; 5: On–off (power) switch; 6: Writing pen-holder; 7: Expiratory valve; 8: Inspiratory valve; 9: Bidirectional valve tap; 10: Bell supporter; 11: Pulley); (B) Computerised spirometer.

2. Wright's peak flow meter This is a simple portable device for measuring ventilatory functions (Fig. 23.4). It has a mouthpiece which is connected to a body piece that contains a calibrated scale with marker. The calibrations are from 60–800 litres per minute.

3. Douglas bag This is a bag to collect air when a person breathes into it. This is used for determining MVV.

4. Gas volume meter

Procedure

Lung volumes and capacities

1. Fill three-fourths of the bell of the spirometer with air or 100 per cent oxygen.
2. Ask the subject to sit comfortably and relax.
3. Adjust the speed of the spirometer at 60 mm/min.
4. Place a sterilised mouthpiece in the subject's mouth in such a way that the mouthpiece remains fitted between the teeth and the lips.
5. Connect the mouthpiece to the spirometer.
6. Close the nostrils with the help of a nose clip.
7. Ask the subject to breathe in and out normally through the mouth; this is the tidal volume.
8. Ask the subject to breathe in as much as possible after a normal expiration, this is the IRV; then also record a few normal breaths.
9. Ask the subject to exhale as much as he can after a normal inspiration to record ERV and record a few normal breaths after that.
10. Ask the subject to breathe out forcefully with maximum effort after taking a deep inspiration. This records VC.

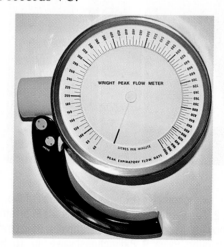

Fig. 23.4 Wright's peak flow meter.

11. Calculate TV, IRV, ERV, VC, and IC from these recordings (height 1 mm = 30 mL) as depicted in Fig. 23.1.

Timed vital capacity (FEV₁)

1. Ask the subject to sit comfortably and place the mouthpiece and nose clip as described above.
2. Record few normal tidal respiration by asking the subject to take quiet breaths, at 60 mm/min speed of spirometer.
3. Ask the subject to **take maximum inspiration** and hold his breath. Immediately change the speed of the spirometer to 1200 mm/min and ask him to exhale as rapidly and as forcefully as he can, to record timed vital capacity.
4. Repeat the procedure three times and note the best one.
5. Calculate FEV₁ from the obtained recording.

Calculation of FEV₁ To calculate FEV_1, draw a vertical line from the top of the beginning of the curve, and take 20 mm (=1 sec) from its base to the right to check at what percentage it intersects the curve (Fig. 23.6). Likewise, FEV_2, FEV_3 and FEV_4 are calculated by intersecting the curve with vertical lines at every 20 mm.

Calculation of FEF₂₅₋₇₅% Divide the FEV_1 curve (Fig. 23.1) equally into four parts. Draw a horizontal line from the 25% mark and a vertical line from the 75% mark, and mark the point of intersection. The horizontal limb denotes time (T) and the vertical limb denotes volume (V).

Maximum voluntary ventilation

1. Ask the subject to sit comfortably.
2. Connect the mouthpiece of the Douglas bag to the subject's mouth.
3. Ask the subject to breathe as deeply (inhale to maximum) and as rapidly **as he can for 15 seconds into the Douglas bag**.
4. Measure the air collected in the Douglas bag with the help of a gas volume meter and multiply the volume by 4 to derive MVV.

Alternative method MVV can also be recorded by recording FEV_1 in a spirometer and multiplying the value by 38. This gives an approximate value of MVV.

Peak expiratory flow rate

1. Ask the subject to sit comfortably.
2. Connect a Wright's peak flow meter to the subject's mouth.

3. Ask the subject to inhale maximally and then blow out as fast as he can into the flow meter.

4. Note the reading from the dial of the flow meter.

5. Repeat the procedure minimum three times at a gap of two minutes each and take the value of the best performance.

Using computerised spirometer Entire lung functions are assessed by using a computerised spirometer (Fig. 23.3B). Ask the subject to exhale as much as he can after a normal inhalation. He is instructed to breathe out forcefully with maximum effort after a deep inhalation. This records all lung volumes and capacities with the predicted values (Fig. 23.5).

Gas sampling and analysis

Respiratory gas analysis Samples of inspired (atmospheric) air, mixed expired (from the Douglas bag) air and alveolar (collected by the Haldane–Priestley method) air are taken for analysis of partial pressure of oxygen, carbon dioxide and nitrogen. Gas analysers show the partial pressure of different gases.

Blood gas analysis The oxygen content of the blood is determined by Haldane's gas analysis apparatus. Arterial and venous blood are collected and sent for analysis. The oxygen-carrying capacity of blood is estimated by the Van Slyke gasometry method. The partial pressure of carbon dioxide is also determined with the help of gasometers.

Pulmonary blood flow Assessment of pulmonary circulation depends upon measuring pulmonary vascular pressures and cardiac output. These are usually measured in intensive care units with the facilities of invasive monitoring. With a flow-directed pulmonary arterial (Swan–Ganz) catheter, the pulmonary arterial and pulmonary capillary wedge pressures are measured directly. The cardiac output is obtained by the thermodilution method. **Pulmonary vascular resistance (PVR)** is calculated as:

$$PVR = \frac{80 \ (PAP - PCW)}{CO}$$

where PAP = Mean pulmonary arterial pressure in mm Hg, PCW = Pulmonary capillary wedge pressure in mm Hg, and CO = Cardiac output in l/min.

Precautions

1. The subject should be comfortable and relaxed.

2. The apparatus should be sterilised and cleaned properly.

3. The subject should be trained adequately to perform different maneuvers like inhaling and exhaling maximally, and so on.

4. The subject should sit with his/her spine erect.

5. A minimum of three recordings should be taken for FEV_1, MVV, and PEFR at a gap of two minutes each and the best of the three should be taken for the final reading.

6. For recording of FVC and FEV_1, the subject should be encouraged to put his maximum effort to exhale fast and to the maximum extent possible.

Observation

Nowadays, all PFT parameters such as all lung volumes and capacities and FEV_1 including flow-volume curve are reorded in the computerised sprometer. Also, predicted values are displayed in the screen for comparison of the recorded values with the standard one matched for age and gender (Fig. 23.5).

DISCUSSION

Normal Values of PFT

The normal values of PFT in an adult male are as follows:

TV	: 500 ml
IRV	: 3000 ml
ERV	: 1100 ml
FVC	: 4600 ml
FEV_1	: > 80 per cent of FVC
PEFR	: 400 to 600 l/min
RMV	: 6000 ml
MVV	: 125 to 170 l/min
Breathing reserve	: 115 to 160 l/min
Dyspneic index	: > 90 per cent

Dyspneic index is also known as breathing reserve ratio (BRR).

All lung volumes and capacities are about 15–25 per cent less in females. The values may be more in athletes and tall persons and may be less in non-athletes and asthenic persons.

Lung Volumes and Capacities

Lung volumes and capacities show a wide range of value in the normal population depending on the age,

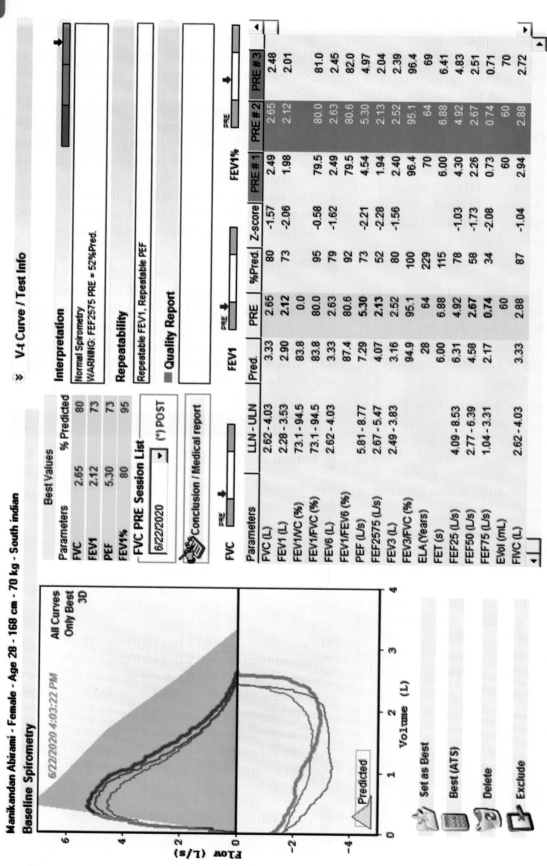

Manikandan Abirami - Female - Age 28 - 168 cm - 70 kg - South indian
Baseline Spirometry

6/22/2020 4:03:22 PM

All Curves
Only Best
3D

Best Values

Parameters		% Predicted
FVC	2.65	80
FEV1	2.12	73
PEF	5.30	73
FEV1%	80	95

FVC PRE Session List

6/22/2020 ▼ (*) POST

Conclusion / Medical report

V-t Curve / Test Info

Interpretation

Normal Spirometry
WARNING: FEF2575 PRE = 52%Pred.

Repeatability

Repeatable FEV1, Repeatable PEF

Quality Report

Parameters	Pred.	LLN - ULN	PRE	%Pred.	Z-score	PRE # 1	PRE # 2	PRE # 3
FVC (L)	3.33	2.62 - 4.03	2.65	80	-1.57	2.49	2.65	2.48
FEV1 (L)	2.90	2.28 - 3.53	2.12	73	-2.06	1.98	2.12	2.01
FEV1/VC (%)	83.8	73.1 - 94.5	0.0					
FEV1/FVC (%)	83.8	73.1 - 94.5	80.0	95	-0.58	79.5	80.0	81.0
FEV6 (L)	3.33	2.62 - 4.03	2.63	79	-1.62	2.49	2.63	2.45
FEV1/FEV6 (%)	87.4		80.6	92		79.5	80.6	82.0
PEF (L/s)	7.29	5.81 - 8.77	5.30	73	-2.21	4.54	5.30	4.97
FEF2575 (L/s)	4.07	2.67 - 5.47	2.13	52	-2.28	1.94	2.13	2.04
FEV3 (L)	3.16	2.49 - 3.83	2.52	80	-1.56	2.40	2.52	2.39
FEV3/FVC (%)	94.9		95.1	100		96.4	95.1	96.4
ELA(Years)	28		64	229		70	64	69
FET (s)	6.00		6.88	115		6.00	6.88	6.41
FEF25 (L/s)	6.31	4.09 - 8.53	4.92	78	-1.03	4.30	4.92	4.83
FEF50 (L/s)	4.58	2.77 - 6.39	2.67	58	-1.73	2.26	2.67	2.51
FEF75 (L/s)	2.17	1.04 - 3.31	0.74	34	-2.08	0.73	0.74	0.71
EVol (mL)			60			60	60	70
FIVC (L)	3.33	2.62 - 4.03	2.88	87	-1.04	2.94	2.88	2.72

Set as Best

Best (ATS)

Delete

Exclude

Fig. 23.5 PFT parameters recorded by computerised spirometer. Note that predicted and % of predicted values are displayed along with the recorded values.

sex and height of the subject. The Indian population shows significantly lower values compared to their western counterparts. Predicted normograms are available based on these variable factors. Deviations up to 20 per cent from the predicted value for a given age, sex and height are commonly seen in normal subjects. Serial measurements of these values are of great importance, because changes of even 5 per cent in a particular individual are likely to be of significance.

Vital Capacity

Conditions that decrease VC
1. Loss of functioning lung tissue
   - Interstitial pulmonary fibrosis
   - Chest deformity
   - Neuromuscular disease
   - Thickened pleura
2. Loss of distensibility of lung tissues or pleura
   - Atelectasis
   - Consolidation
   - Pulmonary edema
   - Pulmonary resection

Conditions that increase VC
1. VC is more in the western population compared to the Indian.
2. VC is higher in males.
3. VC is higher in athletes compared to non-athletes.
4. VC is higher in adults than in children and the elderly.
5. VC shows a higher increase in the standing posture than in the supine and sitting postures.

There is no pathological condition in which VC increases.

Mechanics of Breathing

Static Lung Compliance

Static lung compliance decreases in:
1. Pulmonary edema
2. Chronic pulmonary congestion
3. Kyphoscoliosis
4. Fibrothorax
5. Interstitial fibrosis
6. Atelectasis

Patients with decreased compliance have to put in more respiratory muscular effort to achieve adequate alveolar ventilation. Therefore, very often they are dyspneic.

Airway Resistance

Airway resistance increases in:
1. Bronchial asthma
2. Chronic bronchitis
3. Emphysema
4. Other diseases that are characterised by airway obstruction

Patients with increased airway resistance are often dyspneic, and dyspnea depends on the severity of airway obstruction.

Forced Vital Capacity (FVC)

FVC decreases in conditions in which there is obstruction to the airways resulting in air trapping, for example, bronchial asthma.

Timed Vital Capacity (FEV$_1$)

FEV$_1$ is the single most useful test to **detect generalised airway obstruction**. But this must be done properly to get the proper results, as it is effort-dependent. This is also relatively non-specific in the sense that it gives the idea of generalised obstruction (not specific for small airway obstruction).

FEV$_1$ decreases in obstructive diseases of the lung, for example, bronchial asthma.

Obstructive lung diseases

Obstructive lung diseases are characterised by reduction in airflow particularly FEV$_1$ and FEV$_1$/FVC less than 5th percentile of predicted.

FEV$_1$ decreases in asthma, emphysema, chronic bronchitis, bronchiectasis and cystic fibrosis.

Restrictive lung disease

Restrictive lung diseases are characterised by reduction in lung volume specifically TLC less than 5th percentile of predicted. Both FEV$_1$ and FVC are low. FEV$_1$/FVC is normal or increased. Restrictive lung diseases are due to the following:
1. **Extrapulmonary causes** of restrictive lung diseases are severe obesity, kyphoscoliosis and neuromuscular disorder.
2. **Interstitial lung diseases** causing restrictive lung disease include acute respiratory distress

syndrome (ARDS), pneumoconiosis, sarcoidosis and idiopathic pulmonary fibrosis.

Severity of spirometric abnormality based on FEV_1 (FEV_1 interpretation of % predicted) is shown in Table 23.1.

Table 23.1   Severity of spirometric abnormality based on FEV_1

FEV_1 % pred	Degree of severity
>70%	Mild obstruction
60–69%	Moderate obstruction
50–59%	Moderately severe obstruction
<35–49%	Severe obstruction
<35%	Very severe obstruction

FEV_1/FVC

The ratio of FEV_1/FVC is approximately 0.75–0.80. This is a more sensitive indicator of airway obstruction than FVC or FEV_1 alone.

FEV_1/FVC : Interpretation of absolute value:

◆ 80 or higher—Normal
◆ 79 or lower—Abnormal

MMEFR ($FEF_{25-75\%}$)

This is one of the **most sensitive indicators of patency of the small airways**. This is slowed in diseases that cause small airway obstruction.

$FEF_{200-1200ml}$

This is the flow rate between 200 and 1200 mL of FVC. It is one of the **sensitive indicators of patency of larger airways**. It is slower in diseases that cause large airway obstruction.

PEFR

As it measures peak expiratory flow rate during peak expiration, it decreases in airway obstruction. MMEFR and $FEF_{200-1200\ ml}$ are better indicators and more sensitive than PEFR.

MVV

The normal value is 150 l in adult males and 125 l in adult females. However, the value can be fallacious if the patient does not cooperate and fails to use maximum possible effort to perform the test.

MVV decreases in patients with subjective dyspnea.

Ventilation–Perfusion Relationship

In the erect position, ventilation per unit volume of lung is greater at the bases than at the apices. The perfusion is also not uniform in the erect posture due to the effect of gravity. But a greater degree of non-uniform perfusion occurs in diseases like pulmonary embolism and diseases with destruction of lung tissue. The arterial blood gas tension is primarily affected by the relationship of ventilation with perfusion. The normal ratio of ventilation to perfusion is 0.8. Alteration in this ratio affects PaO_2 more than $PaCO_2$.

Diffusion

The **pulmonary diffusing capacity decreases** during the following circumstances:

1. When the total surface area of the alveolar capillary membrane is reduced, as in:
    *   Emphysema
    *   Pulmonary embolism
    *   Thrombosis of pulmonary capillaries
    *   Following surgical removal of lung tissues
2. When there is a defect in the membrane (thickening of the membrane), as in:
    *   Asbestosis
    *   Sarcoidosis
    *   Progressive systemic sclerosis
    *   Collagen diseases
    *   Interstitial edema
    *   Interstitial fibrosis
    *   Diffuse metastatic lesions of the lung

The **pulmonary diffusing capacity increases** in exercise.

Disturbance in Pulmonary Circulation

Pulmonary vascular resistance (PVR) is increased by different mechanisms as given below:

1. Pulmonary arterial or arteriolar vasoconstriction in response to alveolar hypoxia increases PVR.
2. Intraluminal thrombi in pulmonary vessels decrease the luminal cross-sectional area and increase PVR.
3. Proliferation of smooth muscle within the vessel wall decreases luminal cross-sectional area and increases PVR.
4. Destruction of small pulmonary vessels either by scarring or by loss of alveolar wall, decreases total cross-sectional area of the pulmonary vascular bed and increases PVR.

When PVR increases, the pulmonary arterial pressure rises, this decreases right ventricular output.

PVR increases in:

1. Cardiac conditions that elevate left atrial pressure such as mitral stenosis.
2. Chronic pulmonary hypoxemia
   - COPD (chronic obstructive pulmonary diseases)
   - Interstitial lung disease
   - Chest wall diseases, for example, kyphoscoliosis
   - Obesity hypoventilation
   - Sleep apnea syndrome
3. Diseases affecting pulmonary vessels
   - Recurrent pulmonary embolism
   - Scleroderma (occludes small pulmonary arteries and arterioles)

Restrictive and Obstructive Lung Diseases

Commonly two major patterns of abnormal ventilatory function of the lung are encountered: restrictive, and obstructive lung disease. In the obstructive disease, the hallmark of dysfunction is the decrease in expiratory flow rates, particularly the MMEFR and FEV_1/FVC. The hallmark of restrictive disease is the reduction in FVC (Fig. 23.6).

In **obstructive diseases**, FEV_1 decreases as there is obstruction to the outflow of air from the lung, but TLC remains normal (TLC may increase due to air trapping). In **restrictive lung diseases**, TLC is decreased as there is a problem in lung expansion but

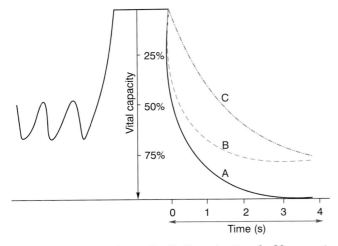

Fig. 23.6 Timed vital capacity (A: Normal pattern [>80 per cent expired in first second]; B: Restrictive pattern [total vital capacity is less, but FEV_1 as per cent of FVC is normal]; C: Obstructive pattern [FEV_1 is grossly reduced, even FEV_4 is less than 80 per cent]).

FEV_1 remains normal (as per cent of FVC) as there is no obstruction to the outflow of air from the lung.

Obstructive Diseases

1. TLC is normal or increased.
2. RV is elevated due to trapping of air during expiration.
3. Ratio of RV/TLC is increased.
4. VC is frequently decreased (not due to decreased lung volumes but due to increased RV).
5. FEV_1 is less than 80 per cent of TLC.
6. FEV_1/FVC decreases.
7. MMEFR decreases.

In the early phase of obstruction, which originates in the small airways, FEV_1/FVC may be normal, but decrease in MMEFR and an abnormal configuration in the terminal portion of forced expiratory flow–volume curve may indicate the presence of the disease.

Restrictive Diseases

The **hallmarks of a restrictive pattern** are:

1. Decreased TLC
2. Decreased VC
3. Decreased RV
4. Normal preservation of forced expiratory flow rates, especially FEV_1 expressed as percentage of FVC. The restrictive diseases can be broadly subdivided into parenchymal and extraparenchymal disease. Extraparenchymal dysfunction is again of two kinds, the extraparenchymal dysfunction in inspiration and the extraparenchymal dysfunction in inspiration plus expiration.

Restrictive parenchymal dysfunction

1. Decreased TLC
2. Decreased RV
3. Decreased VC
4. Normal or increased FEV_1/FVC

Restrictive extraparenchymal dysfunction

Inspiratory dysfunction In extraparenchymal inspiratory dysfunction, which usually occurs due to inspiratory muscle weakness or a stiff chest wall, the adequate distending forces are prevented from being exerted on an otherwise normal lung. Therefore, TLC is reduced but RV is not affected, and expiratory flow rates are preserved.

Inspiratory plus expiratory dysfunction This usually occurs in expiratory muscle weakness or due to deformed chest wall which is abnormally rigid at lung volumes below FRC. Therefore, RV is often significantly elevated. The ratio of FEV_1/FVC may be affected depending on the strength of the expiratory muscles.

Uses of PFTs

1. Assist in diagnosis of respiratory diseases.
2. Help in monitoring the efficiency of treatment.
3. Help in monitoring the progress of the disease.
4. Help in monitoring the efficacy of physical training.
5. Help in studying the prevalence of respiratory diseases in the community or respiratory industrial hazards.
6. Help in evaluating the respiratory fitness of the patients for general anaesthesia prior to surgery.
7. Assist in medico-legal cases to decide fitness or amount of compensation.
8. Used in evaluation of lung functions in research.

OSPE

I. Record vital capacity of the given subject by using recording spirometer.

Steps

1. Ask the subject to sit comfortably with an erect spine.
2. Check that the bell of the spirograph is filled up to three-fourths of its capacity with air.
3. Adjust the speed of the spirometer at 60 mm/min.
4. Place the mouthpiece into the mouth of the subject in such a way that mouthpiece remains between the teeth and the lips.
5. Connect the mouthpiece to the spirometer.
6. Instruct the subject to breathe in and out quietly through the mouth to record tidal volume.
7. Ask the subject to exhale as much as she can immediately following a deep inspiration.

II. Record FEV1 of the given subject and report your findings.

Steps

1. Ask the subject to sit comfortably with an erect spine.
2. Check that the bell of the spirograph is filled up to three-fourths of its capacity with air.
3. Adjust the speed of the spirometer at 60 mm/min.
4. Place the mouthpiece into the mouth of the subject in such a way that the mouthpiece remains between the teeth and the lips.
5. Connect the mouthpiece to the spirometer.
6. Instruct the subject to breathe in and out quietly through the mouth to record a few tracings of tidal volume.
7. Ask the subject to take a deep breath and hold it.
8. Immediately change the speed of the spirometer to 1200 mm/min and ask the subject to exhale to the maximum and as rapidly as possible.
9. Switch off the spirometer as soon as FEV_1 is recorded.

VIVA

1. What are the uses of pulmonary function tests?
2. Name different PFTs.
3. What are lung volumes and capacities?
4. Define vital capacity. What is the normal value of vital capacity in males and females and why is there a difference?
5. Define residual volume. What is its normal value?
6. What is the significance of functional residual capacity and how is it determined? In which condition is it altered?

Ans: FRC maintains a constant RV and at the same time it allows continuous exchange of gases in both phases of respiration. It checks sudden fall in partial pressure of gases in blood. It is measured by the helium dilution and nitrogen washout methods. FRC increases in conditions in which air trapping occurs, like asthma, emphysema and so on.

7. What are the tests that determine the mechanics of breathing (compliance and airway resistance)?

8. What is timed vital capacity and what is its significance?

9. What is MMEFR and what is its significance?

10. What is MVV and what is its normal value?

11. What are the precautions for PFT?

12. Why are most of the parameters of PFT recorded at least three times, and the best of three taken for consideration?

13. Name the conditions in which vital capacity decreases.

14. Name the conditions in which FEV_1 decreases.

15. Why is the ratio of FEV_1/FVC a better indicator of obstruction than the FEV_1 and FVC alone?

16. What are the differences between restrictive and obstructive lung diseases and how do you differentiate between these two patterns?

17. What are the diagnostic hallmarks of obstructive lung disease?

18. What are the two subcategories of restrictive extraparenchymal dysfunction? Name one test to differentiate these two dysfunctions.

19. Name the tests to detect the abnormalities of pulmonary circulation.

20. What are the mechanisms of increased pulmonary vascular resistance?

21. Name the diseases in which pulmonary vascular resistance increases.

22. What are the lung volumes and capacities that cannot be recorded by a simple spirometer?

Ans: RV, FRC and TLC cannot be recorded by a simple spirometer.

23. What is the breathing reserve ratio? What is its clinical significance?

24. What is minute ventilation? What is its normal value?

25. What is $FEF_{200-1200ml}$? What is its significance?

CHAPTER 24

Cardiopulmonary Resuscitation

Learning Objectives

After completing this practical, you will be able to:
1. Give the meaning of cardiopulmonary resuscitation (CPR).
2. Give the indications for CPR.
3. Give the objectives of CPR.
4. List the measures for basic life supports.
5. Describe the procedure for mouth-to-mouth breathing and external cardiac massage.
6. List the measures for advanced life supports.

INTRODUCTION

The supportive and specific treatment given immediately to patients, in whom for some reasons the cardiac and the ventilatory activities have stopped, is called cardiopulmonary resuscitation (CPR). CPR is given in an acute medical emergency that requires adequate life-saving procedures. Therefore, it should be carried out by a well-trained and experienced team.

Indications for CPR

CPR is indicated in conditions of cardiorespiratory arrest. The common situations that can lead to cardiorespiratory arrest include:
1. Primary cardiac arrhythmias
2. Arrhythmias associated with acute myocardial infarction
3. Electric shock
4. Poisoning
5. Trauma
6. Drowning
7. Pulmonary embolism
8. Muscular relaxation during surgery
9. Anaphylactic shock
10. Head injury
11. Cardiac surgery
12. Cardiac tamponade
13. Acute pulmonary edema
14. Chronic lung disease (rare)

The main mechanisms responsible for **cardiac arrest** or cessation of heart action are cardiac asystole, and ventricular fibrillation.

Diagnosis of Cardiac Arrest

Features of cardiac arrest are:
1. Absence of pulsation of large arteries.
2. Absence of heart beats
3. Gasping movements followed by total arrest of respiration
4. Blood pressure not recordable
5. Dilated pupils, not responding to light.
6. Pallor (pale and cold skin) and cyanosis.
7. Unconsciousness.

Objectives of CPR

1. To provide adequate pulmonary ventilation so that partial pressure of oxygen in the arterial blood is maintained.
2. To facilitate pumping of the heart so that effective circulation in maintained.

METHODS

General Plan for CPR

CPR can be divided into two broad supportive measures: Emergency measures and definitive treatments.

Classically, they are described as **A B C D E F G H I**, administered in two phases (Phase I and Phase II).

A : Airways
B : Breathing
C : Circulation
D : Drugs
E : ECG monitoring
F : Fibrillation treatment (with defibrillator)
G : Gauging for restoration of breathing and circulation
H : Hypothermia
I : ICU Management

The two phases of management are:

1. **Phase I** Emergency Measures (Basic life support): This consists of A, B, and C.
2. **Phase II** Definitive Treatment (Advanced life support): This consists of D, E, F, G, H and I.

Phase I: Basic Life Support

Basic life support should be started immediately. A clear airway and presence of breathing are essential parts of successful resuscitative measures. Unless adequate ventilation is achieved, attempts to restore circulation become futile. The steps are:

1. Assess the responsiveness of the patient by gently shaking the subject.
2. Position the patient on a firm, flat surface.
3. Open the mouth and remove vomitus, mucus or debris if visible.
4. To extend the neck, place the palm of one hand on the patient's forehead and apply firm pressure to tilt the head backward. At the same time, place the palm of the other hand under the chin to support it (**head tilt – chin lift maneuver**). This raises the tongue away from the spine and opens the airway.

   To ventilate the lungs of the patient, perform any of the following three maneuvers. Mouth-to-mouth breathing is performed in adults and mouth-to-nose breathing is preferred in infants and children. Holger Nielson method is usually not performed unless there are respiratory problems as seen in drowning.

5. Mouth-to-mouth respiration (Fig. 24.1)
   - Clear the airway.
   - Extend the neck.
   - Close the nostrils (of the patient) by pinching with the thumb and the index finger of the right hand.
   - Take a deep breath.
   - Apply your mouth close to the patient's mouth and exhale forcefully into the subject's mouth.
   - Look for chest expansion and abdominal distension.
   - Repeat and maintain the breathing at a rate of 10–15 per minute.

Mouth-to-nose respiration Ideally, it is suitable for children. The steps are same as those of mouth-to-mouth respiration except that the mouth of the patient is closed and the rescuer breathes into the nostrils of the subject.

Manual manipulation of the thorax (**Holger–Nielson method or back pressure – armlift method**)
- Lay down the patient in prone position.
- Abduct the arms at the shoulder and flex the elbows.
- Turn the head to one side resting on the hands.
- Kneel down with one knee near the patient's head.
- Hold the patient's arm and straighten yourself to raise the subject's arm until resistance is felt. The details are demonstrated in Fig. 24.2A–C.

> **Note:** During this maneuver, the thorax of the patient expands and the intrathoracic pressure drops and inspiration takes place.

- Then gently drop the patient's arm.
- Place your hands with fingers spread apart on the back of the subject in the midaxillary space, and slightly compress to produce expiration (Fig. 24.2D and E).

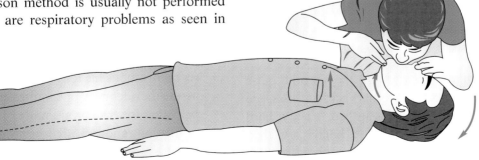

Fig. 24.1 Proper method for opening the airway with the head tilted and chin lifted to administer mouth-to-mouth respiration.

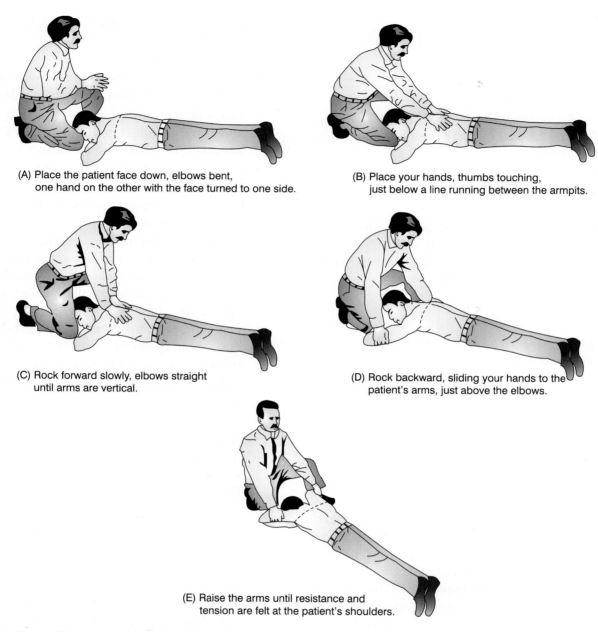

(A) Place the patient face down, elbows bent, one hand on the other with the face turned to one side.

(B) Place your hands, thumbs touching, just below a line running between the armpits.

(C) Rock forward slowly, elbows straight until arms are vertical.

(D) Rock backward, sliding your hands to the patient's arms, just above the elbows.

(E) Raise the arms until resistance and tension are felt at the patient's shoulders.

Fig. 24.2   Holger–Nielson method for artificial respiration.

- Repeat the whole cycle 10–12 times per minute.
6. Palpate the carotid pulse.

Note: Palpation for at least 10 seconds is recommended to ensure that slow, irregular, or very weak pulses are not missed.

7. *External cardiac massage* If the carotid pulse is not felt, perform external cardiac massage (Fig. 24.3). If the patient is in bed, place a hard board under the patient. The hands are then positioned about 3 cm above the xiphoid process and to the left with the shoulders of the rescuer vertically above the chest of the subject. With the heel of the hand and the fingers off the chest, the sternum is compressed 4–5 cm thrusting straight down towards the spine. The recommended compression rate is 80–100 per minute. The rescuer responsible for airway management should assess the adequacy of compression by periodically palpating for the carotid pulse. The compression–ventilation ratio is 5 : 1.

8. If pulse returns, ventilation should be continued as required.

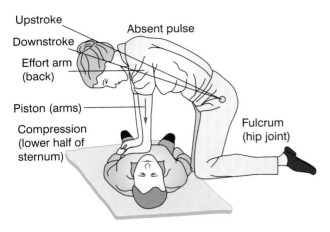

Fig. 24.3 Proper technique for chest compressions (uses principles of lever). Note that the forearm and arm are straight (elbows extended). The recommended compression is 80–100 per minute. Fifteen chest compressions are performed before ventilating twice when there is a single rescuer. Palpate the carotids for detecting a pulse every two minutes.

Phase II : Advanced Life Support

Advanced life support comprises primary and adjunctive therapies.

Primary therapies

Primary therapies for advanced life support include:

1. Defibrillation
2. Airway management and oxygen therapy

Defibrillation This is one of the most important modalities of treatment of CPR. It should be started as early as possible. The time between the onset of the arrest to the successful defibrillation is the major determinant of survival in cardiac arrest due to ventricular fibrillation. A fibrillating heart cannot pump blood, as effective contractions do not occur. Defibrillation converts fibrillation into flutter or normal rhythm so that effective ventricular contractions occur and heart pumps blood.

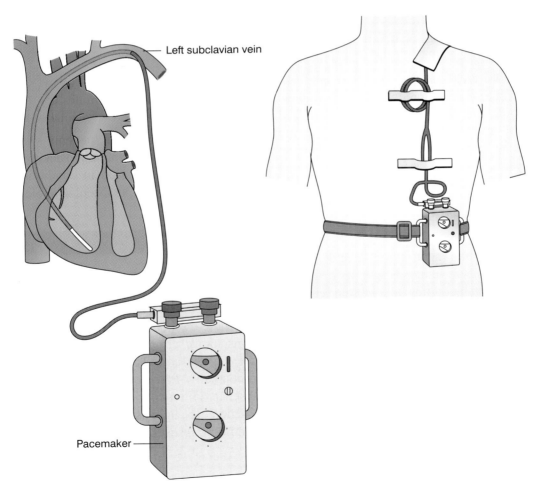

Fig. 24.4 Temporary pacemaker. The transvenous catheter electrode is attached to a battery-powered external pacemaker. The catheter is wedged in the apex of the right ventricle.

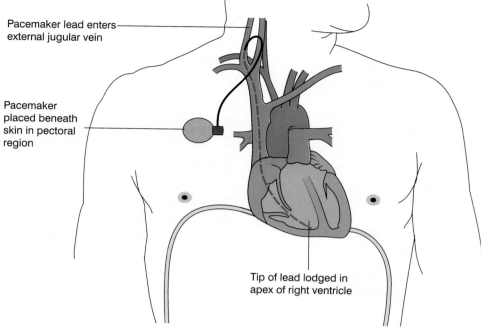

Fig. 24.5   Permanent pacemaker.

Adrenaline and sodium bicarbonate are administered intravenously.

Airway management and oxygen therapy   Hundred per cent oxygen should be administered and endotracheal intubation should be carried out by a qualified individual as soon as possible. But, the basic life support should be carried out by a qualified individual as soon as possible. But, the basic life support should not be delayed or interrupted for more than 30 seconds for intubation.

Adjunctive therapies

1. Self-induced cough   When the arrest is detected before loss of consciousness, self-induced vigorous coughing can produce minimum blood flow to the brain required to maintain consciousness temporarily until definitive treatment is initiated.

2. Precordial thump   A quickly applied solitary precordial thump may convert ventricular fibrillation or asystole to a normal rhythm.

3. Atropine sulphate   Atropine sulphate (0.5 mg) is injected intravenously every 5 minutes for the treatment

of bradycardia. It may also help in the treatment of cardiac asystole.

4. Sodium bicarbonate   It is given as 1 mEq/kg intravenously every 10 minutes for the treatment of cardiac arrest due to hyperkalemia or acidosis.

5. Pacemakers   It helps in patients with problems of abnormal impulse formation. Packing is carried out early during resuscitation in conditions of refractory bradyarrhythmias or persistent asystole (Figs. 24.4 and 24.5).

DISCUSSION

There are different methods to assist ventilation in CPR like Sylvester-Brosche method, Drinker's method, Paul-Bunnel method and Rocking method. But these methods are not routinely followed. Despite resuscitative efforts, a patient in cardiac arrest may not recover and regain spontaneous ventilation and circulation. Persistent deep unconsciousness and absence of respiration, reflex response or pupillary reaction to light suggest cerebral death. In this condition, resuscitative efforts are unproductive.

VIVA

1. *What do you mean by cardiopulmonary resuscitation?*
2. *What are the causes of cardiorespiratory arrest?*
3. *What are the indications for CPR?*
4. *What are the signs of cardiac arrest?*
5. *What are the objectives of CPR?*
6. *What are the basic life supports?*
7. *How is mouth-to-mouth respiration carried out?*
8. *How is mouth-to-nose respiration carried out?*
9. *What is the Holger–Nielson method of CPR?*
10. *How is external cardiac massage carried out?*
11. *What are the advanced life supports?*
12. *What is the physiological basis of use of defibrillation in cardiac arrest due to ventricular fibrillation?*
13. *What is internal cardiac massage?*

     Ans: It is performed if cardiac arrest occurs during cardiac surgery. The heart is directly compressed rhythmically at a rate of 80/min.

14. *What is the Paul–Bunnel method of CPR?*

     Ans: This is an alternative method to assist ventilation. Air tubes are wrapped around the chest. The thorax is rhythmically compressed by forcing air in and out of the tubes.

15. *What is the Rocking method of CPR?*

     Ans: The patient is laid on a stretcher and shoulder is strapped. Stretcher is rocked up and down 10 times per minute. The movements of the diaphragm stimulate respiration.

CHAPTER 25

Body Composition Analysis and Assessment of Basal Metabolic Rate

Learning Objectives

After completing this practical, you will be able to (MUST KNOW):

1. Understand the importance of assessment of body composition and metabolism.
2. Give the principle of BIA for assessment of body composition and metabolism.
3. Define BMR.
4. Give the normal value of BMR in males and females.

5. List the conditions necessary for the measurement of BMR.
6. Enumerate the factors that affect the BMR.

You may also be able to (DESIRABLE TO KNOW):

1. Say why measurement of BMR by BIA is a better one.
2. Explain the clinical importance of assessment of body composition and BMR.

BODY COMPOSITION ANALYSIS

INTRODUCTION

Body mass index (BMI), waist circumference (WC), waist-to-hip ratio (WHR), waist-to-height (WhtR) and skin fold thickness have been reported as the predictors of cardiovascular (CV) risk. However, body fat (BF) mass, body lean mass and body fat mass index (BFMI) are better predictors of CV risks.

Body composition is determined by **bioelectrical impedance analysis (BIA)**, a method which involves the measurement of bioelectrical resistive impedance (R). This method is regarded as safe and reliable, and based upon the principle that the electrical conductivity of the fat free tissue mass is far greater than that of fat. Measurements at 5/50/100/200 kHz were obtained using the multiple frequency BIA instrument Bodystat. BIA included BF, lean body mass, body cell mass (BCM), total body water (TBW), intracellular water (ICW) and extracellular water (ECW). The current range of 50–100 kHz displays BF, BF %, BF mass index (BFMI), lean body mass, basal metabolism (BM), and activity metabolism (AM).

METHODS

Method to Assess Body Mass Composition

▌ Principle

Bioimpedance analysis is based on the principle that the volume of a conductor (in the human body, this is the highly conductive body water) is proportional to its length and inversely proportional to its electrical resistance as defined by

$$\text{Volume} = \frac{\rho\, L^2}{R}$$

where ρ is the resistivity (ohm cm) of the conductor, L is the conductor length (cm, for whole body measurements in humans; stature is used as a surrogate for the unknown true conductive length), and R is the electrical resistance of the conductor (ohm).

BIA devices determine the body composition by measuring the electrical impedance of an imperceptible electric current passing through the body. Impedance is a vector composed of two frequency-dependent parameters, resistance and reactance. Reactance is a measure of body cell mass and resistance reflects total body water.

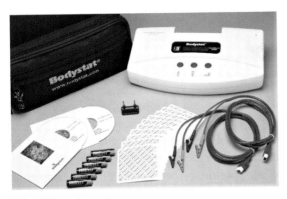

Fig. 25.1   BIA equipment

Requirements

Equipment   Bodystat Quad Scan 4000, with its accessories (Fig. 25.1)

Accessories used   Body stat electrodes

Software   Quad scan 4000 software

Preparation of the Subject

◈ The subject is instructed to avoid eating or drinking for 4 h prior to the test, and to avoid exercise and alcohol for 24 h prior to the test.

◈ Assess the hydration status by clinical examination and ensure that no metals have be worn by the subject

◈ The subject is placed in the supine position with no parts of the body touching another for at least 10 min in standardised conditions (quiet environment and ambient temperature).

◈ The electrodes are placed on the dorsal surfaces of the hand and foot proximal to metacarpal–phalangeal and metatarsal–phalangeal joints respectively.

Laboratory temperature   Thermo-neutral temperature has to be maintained in the lab throughout the procedure.

Procedure

1. Obtain consent of the subject.
2. Record participant's height, weight, waist and hip circumference as per standard methods (data to be fed to the machine for analysis).
3. Check that there is sufficient battery power in the machine prior to commencing by switching on the machine and checking the battery indicator (series of bars on the left of the display)
4. Assess the physical activity of the participant using the International Physical Activity Questionnaire (IPAQ).

5. Clean the area with spirit and cotton before electrode placement.
6. Let the subject lie down in supine position for 10 minutes. The arms should be abducted from the trunk and both legs should be abducted by placing rolled blanket or towel (separate the legs 30° to 40°).
7. Place two signal-introducing electrodes on the right side on the dorsum of the hand and foot close to the metacarpal-phalangeal and metatarsal-phalangeal joints respectively (Fig. 25.2).
8. Apply two voltage-sensing electrodes in the pisiform prominence of the wrist and between the medial and lateral malleolus of the ankle (the distance between the electrodes should be 5 cm (Fig. 25.2).
9. Feed all the anthropometric details measured from the subject into the machine. The current of 500 to 800 micro amperes with 50 KHz frequency is applied to the body via the cables of BIA equipment.
10. By measuring the impedance and by applying predictive equations used in the hardware unit, the machine estimates the body composition, and the

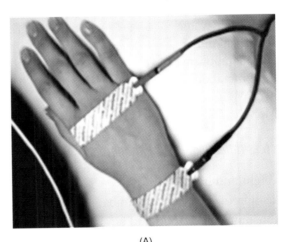

(A)

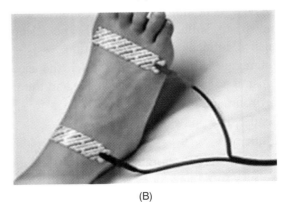

(B)

Fig. 25.2   Electrode placements. (A) In the arm; (B) In the leg.

results are displayed on the LCD screen and also stored in the apparatus.

Results

Results (various parameters) are noted from the LCD screen of the equipment. BIA is a simple, inexpensive, quick and non-invasive technique for measuring many body composition parameters. Following parameters are recorded:

- Body weight (kg)
- Body cell mass (kg)
- Body cell mass (%)
- Extracellular mass (kg)
- Fat-free mass (%)
- Body fat (kg)
- Body mass index (BMI)
- Body fat mass index (BFMI)
- Fat-free mass index (FFMI)
- Phase angle
- Total body water
- Extracellular water
- Intracellular water
- Third space water
- Nutritional index
- Basal metabolism (BM)
- Active metabolism (AM)
- BM/BW
- BM/BF

Factors Influencing BIA Parameters

1. Weight and height
2. Position of the body and limbs
3. Consumption of food and beverages
4. Level of physical activity before BIA measurements
5. Medical conditions and medication which are known to influence the fluid and electrolyte balance, influence body composition.
6. Cutaneous disease that may alter the electrical transmission between the electrode and the skin
7. Environmental conditions
8. Gender, age and skin temperature
9. Ethnicity
10. Technical fault: non-adherence of electrodes, use of wrong electrodes, loosening of cable clip, interchanging of electrodes

BASAL METABOLIC RATE (BMR)

INTRODUCTION

The total energy expenditure of the body is the sum of the energy required to carry out various body activities. Basal metabolism is the lowest level of energy production. The body metabolism is directly linked to the production of body heat. The measurement of heat production under basal conditions is called basal metabolic rate (BMR). It is measured as $kcal/h/m^2$ body surface area (BSA).

For measurement of BMR, the following basal conditions are required:

1. Minimum 12 hours of fasting
2. Complete physical and mental rest
3. Comfortable ambient temperature (about 25°C).

BMR is estimated by measuring the oxygen consumption of the subject for 6 minutes under basal conditions. Normal values of BMR (in adults):

- Males: 40 $kcal/h/m^2$ BSA
- Females: 37 $kcal/h/m^2$ BSA.

A ± 10% is considered to be normal.

MEASUREMENT OF BMR

BMR is measured by measuring oxygen consumption in the basal state. Oxygen consumption can be measured by three methods:

Open Circuit Method

Expired air is collected in a Douglas bag and then analysed for carbon dioxide and oxygen content. The difference in the composition of the atmospheric air and the expired air when computed for the total expired indicates total oxygen consumption.

Closed Circuit Breathing

This is the most commonly used method for measuring BMR. The indirect principle is employed whereby oxygen consumption of the subject is measured and is then translated into forms of heat production.

Calculations

Calculation of O_2 consumption per minute

$$= \frac{\text{Initial level of O}_2 - \text{Final level of O}_2 \text{ (after 6 minutes)}}{6}$$

Oxygen utilisation per hour (60 min), i.e., A = Oxygen utilisation in 6 min × 10 at BTPS (body temperature, ambient pressure, saturated with water vapour)

Oxygen utilisation at STPD (B) = A × Correction factor (C) = B × 4.82*

Hence, BMR of the subject = (B × 4.82)/BSA in kcal/h/m² Refer appendix for BSA nomogram and Du Bois nomogram.

BIA Method

The bioelectrical impedance analysis (BIA) for body composition measures basal metabolism and active metabolism and provides the ratio of metabolism to body weight and body fat (BM/BW, BM/BF), which are more accurate methods of estimation of body metabolism. Presently, BMR is assessed by the BIA method, as described in detail under the heading "Assessment of Body Composition."

DISCUSSION

Physiological and Clinical Significance

1. Body composition is required for assessing the cardiovascular risk of the individual, in many clinical and research settings.

2. Body metabolism and composition are needed for diagnosing various pathological conditions, e.g., hypothyroidism and hyperthyroidism.

3. It helps in understanding the effects of nutrition on the BMR, which in turn may help in preparing a dietary plan for a patient.

Factors That Affect the BMR

Factors That increase BMR

- Obesity
- More muscle mass
- Greater height (more surface area)
- Children and young adults
- Elevated levels of thyroid hormone
- Stress
- Fever, illness
- Male gender
- Pregnancy and lactation
- Certain stimulants such as caffeine and tobacco

Factors That Decrease BMR

- Older age
- Lower lean body mass
- Lower height
- Depressed levels of thyroid hormone
- Fasting and starvation
- Female gender

VIVA

1. What is the importance of assessment of body composition?
2. What is the principle of BIA?
3. What is BMR?
4. What is the normal value of BMR?
5. What are the conditions necessary for the measurement of BMR?
6. What are the factors that affect the BMR?
7. Why is the measurement of BMR by BIA a better method?

CHAPTER 26

Electrocardiography

Learning Objectives

After completing this practical, you will be able to (MUST KNOW):

1. Define ECG.
2. Classify ECG leads.
3. Handle the ECG machine properly.
4. Record ECG.
5. List the precautions taken while recording ECG.
6. List the uses of ECG.
7. Identify the different waves and complexes of ECG.
8. State the cause of production of the P wave, QRS complex and T wave.
9. Calculate the heart rate and mean QRS axis.
10. Define and state the normal duration and significance of PR interval, QRS complex and QT interval.

You may also be able to (DESIRABLE TO KNOW):

1. Explain the physiological significance of different waves, complexes and intervals.
2. List the conditions that cause alteration in different waves, complexes and intervals.
3. Explain the physiological basis of such alterations.

INTRODUCTION

Electrocardiography is the method of recording an electrocardiogram (ECG). ECG is the recording, and electrocardiograph is the machine that records the ECG. It is one of the most important and commonly ordered diagnostic tests in clinical practice.

ECG is the graphic recording of the electrical activities of the heart. The body is a volume conductor, that is, body fluids are good conductors of electricity. Therefore, electrical changes occurring in the heart with each heart beat are conducted all over the body and can be picked up from the body surface. The record of these electrical fluctuations during the cardiac cycle is called an electrocardiogram. Thus, the ECG recorded at the body surface represents the **algebraic sum of the action potential of the individual cardiac muscle fibres.**

Uses of ECG

An ECG is useful in the diagnosis of many heart diseases. It is regularly recorded before any surgical intervention to assess the cardiac status of the patient. However, it does not give direct information concerning the mechanical performance of the heart. It may be completely normal in a patient with organic heart disease or may show some non-specific abnormalities in a normal subject. Therefore, the ECG must be interpreted with the clinical features of the patient and with the findings of other investigations.

ECG investigation is done in the following conditions:

1. Anatomical orientation of the heart
2. Relative size of the chambers of the heart
3. A variety of disturbances of rhythm and conduction
4. To detect ischemia of the myocardium, if present
5. The location, extent and progress of myocardial infarction
6. The effects of altered electrolyte concentration
7. The influence of certain drugs like digitalis
8. Evaluation of electronic pacemaker function

METHODS

Electrocardiography

Principle

Electrical activities generated with each beat are conducted from the heart to the body surface, which are picked up and recorded by the electrocardiograph.

Requirements

1. ECG machine

In modern electrocardiography, two types of ECG apparatus are used: the string galvanometer and the radio-amplifier. The apparatus should be sensitive to potential changes of the order of microvolts and have a frequency response of 50–100 Hz. The use of the string galvanometer needs experience. This apparatus is not used in routine practice because the photographic paper used for recording needs to be developed. At present, the transistor amplifier and cathode ray tubes are used for this purpose. It has a main switch which regulates the power supply; a lead selection switch which selects various leads;

a calibration switch, used for calibration; and a start–stop switch to regulate paper speed (Fig. 26.1A).

2. Electrodes and electrode jelly

Limb electrodes are flat metal plates that are kept in position by plastic flat-clip type of clamps, usually red, yellow, green and black in colour and chest electrodes are metal cups that are kept in position by suction produced by rubber bulbs, usually blue in colour (Fig. 26.1B). Electrode jelly (also known as cardiac jelly) is a specially made paste that contains fine sand or glass particles used for placing electrodes on the body surface. It helps in establishing proper contact of the electrode plates to the body.

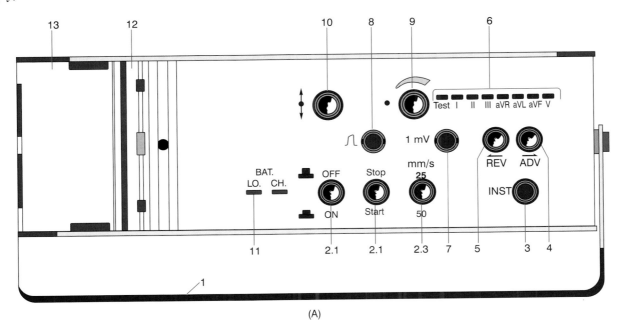

(A)

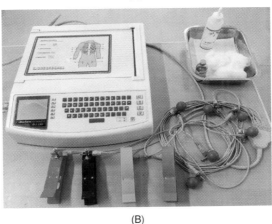

(B)

Fig. 26.1 (A) Schematic diagram of the front view of an ECG machine (1: Handle; 2.1, 2.2 and 2.3: Control switches; 3: Stylus adjuster; 4 and 5: Lead positioners; 6: Lead selection button; 7: Voltage selection; 8: Filter A/C; 9: Gain; 10: Stylus deflector; 11: Battery strength indicator; 12 Stylus protector; 13: Table for guiding paper movement (*Source:* Cardidat 108T/MK-VI; BPL Ltd.); (B) ECG machine, electrodes and jelly.

3. ECG paper

This is the strip of graph paper which has vertical and horizontal lines 1 mm apart. The horizontal axis represents time whereas the vertical axis denotes amplitude. There is a heavy line every 5 mm in both the planes. Thus, there are small squares of 1 mm × 1 mm, and big squares of 5 mm × 5 mm. The ECG paper is a heat-sensitive, plastic-coated paper. The ECG is inscribed on this paper by a hot stylus.

Paper speed   Conventional ECG is taken at a speed of 25 mm/s. One small square (1 mm) corresponds to 0.04 seconds, while the big square (5 mm) is equivalent to 0.20 seconds (Fig. 26.2). When the ECG paper runs through 5 big squares, one second recording has been taken.

Sensitivity   Voltage is measured along the vertical axis. Usually, a 10 mm deflection is equivalent to 1 mV. There is provision to change the sensitivity in special circumstances, for example, when ECG complexes are too small, the sensitivity can be doubled so that a 1 mV deflection is equivalent to 20 mm. When ECG complexes are too large, sensitivity may be reduced to half from the original so that 1 mV is equivalent to 5 mm. The process of determination of sensitivity is called standardisation. It is displayed by pressing the calibration button before and after an ECG is recorded.

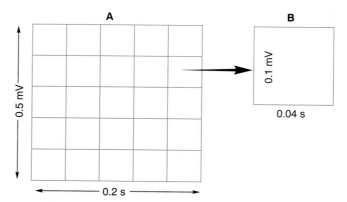

Fig. 26.2   Squares of the ECG paper. (A) Large square; (B) Small square. Time depicted in figures represents the time of the paper speed of 25 mm/s.

4. ECG leads

The ECG leads are broadly classified into two categories, the direct and the indirect (Fig. 26.3). A lead or an electrode is a metal plate (flat discs of dimension 7.5 × 5 cm, non-corrosive) applied snugly over an appropriate body part. For better contact of the leads, ECG jelly is applied after the skin surface is cleaned thoroughly.

Direct leads   Leads applied directly to the surface of the heart to record ECG are called direct leads. These leads are used to record cardiac activities during cardiac surgery or during an experiment.

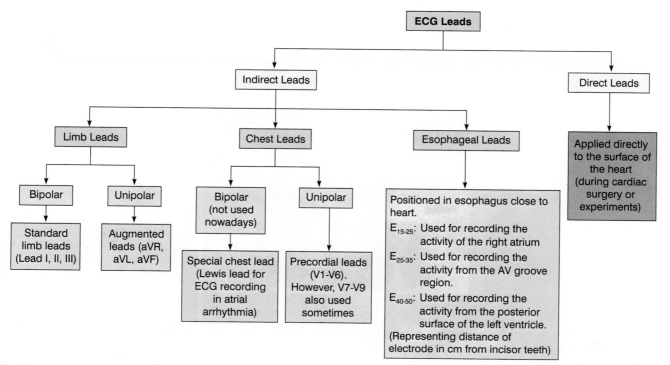

Fig. 26.3   Classification of ECG leads.

Indirect leads   Leads applied away from the heart to record the cardiac activities are called indirect leads. The different indirect leads are limb leads, chest leads and esophageal leads.

Limb leads   Limb leads are of two types, bipolar and unipolar.

Bipolar limb leads   Bipolar standard limb leads (I, II and III) are the original leads selected by Einthoven to record electrical potential on the frontal plane. In the method of bipolar leads, two similar electrodes are placed on the body surface and the potential difference between these two electrodes is recorded. The electrodes are attached to the right arm, left arm and left foot as depicted in the Einthoven triangle (Fig. 26.4). Another electrode is applied to the right leg, which acts as a ground wire to prevent external disturbances during recording.

Lead I   Between the right arm (negative electrode) and the left arm (positive electrode).

Lead II   Between the right arm (negative electrode) and the left leg (positive electrode).

Lead III   Between the left arm (negative electrode) and the left leg (positive electrode).

Unipolar limb leads   In this method, one electrode is active while the other is indifferent. There are three unipolar limb leads: aVR, aVL and aVF. Here 'a' stands for augmented leads. The potential recorded in aVL is one-and-a-half times that recorded in VL, and similarly for aVR and aVF. Therefore, these leads are called augmented leads. 'V' stands for voltage, and R, L and F indicate that the exploring (active) electrode is on the right arm, left arm and left foot respectively. The other (indifferent) electrode is connected to the remaining two leads through a high-resistance coil. For example, while recording from lead aVL the active electrode is placed on the left arm, the indifferent electrode is connected through a high resistance to the other two electrodes placed on the left foot and right arm.

aVR   Between the right arm (positive electrode) and left arm + left leg (negative electrode).

aVL   Between the left arm (positive electrode) and right arm + left leg (negative electrode).

aVF   Between the left foot (positive electrode) and right arm + left arm (negative electrode).

Vector of augmented limb lead = 3/2 vector of unaugmented limb lead.

$$aVR = VR - \frac{VL + VF}{2}$$

$$2aVR = 2VR - (VL + VF)$$

Since VR + VL + VF = 0 (Einthoven triangle),

$$VR = -(VL + VF)$$

$$2aVR = 2VR + VR$$

$$aVR = \frac{3}{2} VR$$

Chest leads   Chest leads are of two types, bipolar and unipolar.

Bipolar chest leads   These leads were used before the discovery of unipolar chest leads. These leads record differences of potential between any given position on the chest and on one extremity. They are not used now because the potential in the extremity appreciably alters the pattern of the chest leads.

Lewis lead   This is a special bipolar chest lead used for recording ECG in atrial arrhythmias. This lead amplifies the waves of atrial activity.

Unipolar chest leads   There are six chest leads that are used routinely: V_1 to V_6. There are three other chest leads ($V_7–V_9$). The chest leads employ an exploring electrode on the chest surface. The reference electrode is connected to the right arm, left arm and left leg through a high resistance, called **Wilson's terminal**, which is maintained at zero potential. The right leg is connected with a grounding electrode to

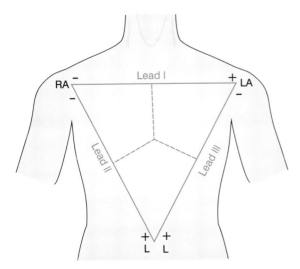

Fig. 26.4   Einthoven's triangle (RA: right arm; LA: Left arm; LL: Left leg). Note that perpendiculars drawn from the midpoint of each limb of the triangle intersect at the centre of the electrical activity.

avoid electrical interference. The position of the chest electrodes (positive electrodes) on the chest surface in different leads are as follows:

V_1 In the right fourth intercostal space at the right border of the sternum.

V_2 In the left fourth intercostal space at the left border of the sternum.

V_3 At the midpoint between V_2 and V_4.

V_4 In the left fifth intercostal space on the midclavicular line.

V_5 In the left fifth intercostal space on the anterior axillary line.

V_6 In the left fifth intercostal space on the midaxillary line.

V_7 In the left fifth intercostal space on the posterior axillary line.

V_8 In the left fifth intercostal space on the posterior scapular line.

V_9 In the left fifth intercostal space on the back just left to the spine.

Esophageal leads   In these leads, an electrode is fixed on the tip of the esophageal catheter, which is positioned in the esophagus close to the heart chambers. The leads are designated as E_{18}, E_{20} and so on. In this, E stands for 'esophageal', and the number indicates the distance of the electrode from the incisor teeth expressed in centimetres.

E_{15-25} Used for recording the activity of the right atrium.

E_{25-35} Used for recording the activity from the AV groove region.

E_{40-50} Used for recording the activity from the posterior surface of the left ventricle.

Procedure

1. Ask the subject to lie down on a couch comfortably.
2. Clean the skin thoroughly with alcohol around the left and right wrists and left and right leg just above the ankle joint and apply jelly.
3. Connect the electrodes in these positions.
4. Switch on the machine and keep the stylus at the centre of the paper.
5. Adjust the sensitivity to get a standard calibration of 1 cm / 1 mV by pressing the 'CAL' button 3 to 4 times.
6. Adjust the lead selector knob to record ECG of the 12 leads in the following order: I, II, III, aVR, aVL and aVF.

7. Place the chest electrodes in an appropriate position on the chest after thorough cleaning and application of jelly, and record the ECG from V_1 to V_6.
8. Again take the standard calibration.
9. Tear out the paper from the machine and label the record.
10. Write the name and age of the subject and the date of the recording.
11. Calculate heart rate and QRS axis as described in the 'Discussion'.
12. Study and interpret the ECG as described under 'Discussion' (Systematic Interpretation of ECG).

Precautions

1. The subject should be totally relaxed.
2. The skin in the area where the electrodes are connected should be thoroughly cleaned and jelly should be applied to decrease skin resistance.
3. The right foot should be connected for grounding.
4. Ensure that the leads are properly applied at the appropriate places and are in good contact with the body surface.
5. Before starting the recording, ensure that the required voltage is available at the mains and that the instrument is properly earthed.
6. Standardisation should be done before and after the recording, to ensure that proper standard was maintained throughout the recording.
7. A minimum of three ECG complexes should be recorded for each lead.
8. The stylus should be adjusted so that it records at the centre of the paper.
9. Recording of 12 leads should be done in proper sequence as I, II, III, aVR, aVL, aVF and V1 to V6.

DISCUSSION

Features of a Good ECG

1. Optimal standardisation of the calibration signal forms rectangles. The corners of the signal form a right angle.
2. The base line is stable.
3. It contains a minimum of three complexes of each lead.
4. It contains a long strip of II and V1 if arrhythmia is suspected or present.

5. There is no interference by alternating current.

6. ECG complexes are recorded at the centre of the paper and do not overshoot the margins.

Normal ECG

The ECG tracing shows different waves, intervals and segments (Fig. 26.5).

Waves

P wave   This is the deflection produced by atrial depolarisation.

QRS complex   This consists of Q, R and S waves. The QRS complex is the deflection produced by ventricular depolarisation.

Q wave   This is the initial negative deflection in the QRS complex.

R wave   This is the positive deflection in the QRS complex.

S wave   This is the second negative deflection in the QRS complex.

QS complex is the term used when the entire QRS complex is negative, without any positive deflection.

T wave   This is the positive deflection produced by ventricular repolarisation.

U wave   This is the final positive deflection in the ECG. This wave is not always present normally. It occurs due to slow repolarisation of the papillary muscle.

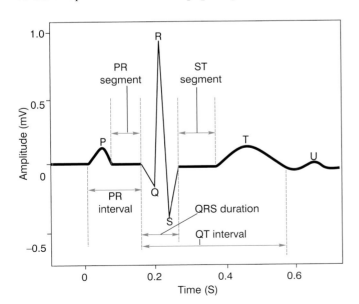

Fig. 26.5   Normal ECG showing different waves, segments and intervals.

Segments

PR segment   This lies between the end of the P wave and the beginning of the QRS complex.

ST segment   This lies between the end of the QRS complex and the beginning of the T wave. The point where the QRS complex ends and the ST segment begins is called **the J point**. There is no electrical activity at the J point. Elevation of the J point (even 1 mm from the base) suggests myocardial ischemia.

Intervals

PR interval

Definition   This is the interval between the beginning of the P wave to the beginning of the QRS complex.

Normal duration   The range of PR interval is 0.12–0.20 seconds (average 0.18 s). PR interval shortens as the heart rate increases, from the average of 0.18 s at the rate of 70 to 0.14 s at the rate of 130.

Significance   This represents atrial depolarisation and conduction through the AV node.

QRS interval (QRS duration)

Definition   This is the interval of the QRS complex. It is measured from the beginning of the Q wave (or R wave if the Q wave is absent) to the J point.

Normal duration   The normal range is 0.08–0.10 seconds.

Significance   This represents ventricular depolarisation. Atrial repolarisation also occurs in this period.

QT interval

Definition   This is the interval of the QRS complex and T wave. It is measured from the beginning of the QRS complex to the end of the T wave.

Normal duration   The normal range is 0.40–0.43 seconds.

Significance   This represents ventricular depolarisation and ventricular repolarisation. It corresponds to the duration of electrical systole.

ST interval

Definition   This is the interval between the J point and the end of the T wave. It is calculated by deducting QRS interval from the QT interval.

Normal duration   The average duration is 0.32 seconds.

Significance   This represents ventricular repolarisation.

PP interval

Definition This is the interval measured between either the peaks or the beginnings of two successive P waves.

Significance The PP interval is measured for calculating the atrial rate.

RR interval

Definition This is the interval between two successive R waves. It is measured between the peaks of two successive R waves.

Significance The RR interval is measured for calculating the heart rate (the ventricular rate).

The duration, amplitude, causes and significance of ECG components are summarised in Table 26.1.

▋ Normal 12-Lead ECG

The deflection of waves in a particular lead is governed by a basic law; that is, a positive (upward) deflection is seen in any lead if electrical depolarisation spreads towards the positive pole of that lead, and a negative (downward) deflection is seen if depolarisation spreads towards the negative pole of the lead. An isoelectric or biphasic deflection is seen when the depolarisaton starts in the SA node and spreads downwards to the subject's left (towards the positive pole of lead II and away from the positive pole of lead aVR). The P wave is always positive in lead II and negative in lead aVR (Fig. 26.6). Ventricular septum depolarises from left to right (towards lead V1 and away from lead V_6). This produces a small q wave (septal q wave) in V_6

Table 26.1 Waves, intervals and segments of ECG.

Waves, intervals and segments	Duration and amplitude	Cause	Significance
P wave	Duration: 0.08–0.10 sec Amplitude: Usually < 2.5 mm in lead II	Due to atrial depolarisation	If duration >0.10 sec, indicates left atrial enlargement If amplitude >2.5 mm, represents right atrial enlargement
QRS complex	Duration: 0.08–0.10 sec Amplitude is quite variable from lead to lead.	Due to ventricular depolarisation	If duration >0.10 sec, may indicate bundle branch block
T wave		Represents ventricular repolarisation	Normal T wave is usually in the same direction as the QRS complex in right precordial leads. T wave is always upright in lead I, II, V3-6, and always inverted in lead aVR.
U wave		Slow repolarisation of papillary muscles	
PR segment	Isoelectric	Extends from the end of P wave to the start of QRS complex	
PR interval	Isoelectric Duration: 0.12-0.20 sec Average: 0.18 sec	Beginning of P wave to the start of QRS complex It includes the conduction delay in the AV node	PR Interval is measured for calculating atrial rate. PR Interval shortens as the heart rate increases
QT interval	QT interval: 0.39 sec at a heart rate of 60/min Duration of QTc: 0.35-0.43 sec	Onset of Q wave to the end of the T wave Represents ventricular depolarisation + repolarisation and corresponds to the duration of electrical systole	Shortens with tachycardia and lengthens with bradycardia so it must be corrected for the effect of the associated heart rate (QTc)
ST segment	Isoelectric	Extends from the J point to the onset of T wave	Convex or straight upward ST segment elevation (e.g., in lead II, III and aVF) is abnormal and suggests transmural injury or infarction. ST segment depression is always abnormal, though often non-specific.
ST interval		End of S wave to the end of T wave	
RR interval	Duration of the cardiac cycle		RR interval is measured for calculating heart rate (ventricular rate).

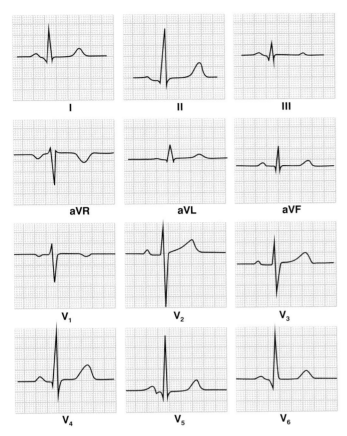

Fig. 26.6   Normal 12-lead ECG.

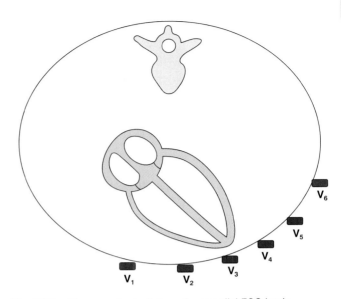

Fig. 26.7   Diagram of orientation of precordial ECG leads. Leads V₁ and V₂ overlie the right ventricle. Leads V₃ and V₄ are transitional leads between the right and left ventricles, and leads V₅ and V₆ overlie the left ventricle.

and a small r wave (septal r wave) in lead V_1. During ventricular depolarisation, as left ventricular mass is more than right ventricular mass, the net direction of depolarisation is towards the left chest leads (Fig. 26.7). This produces tall 'R' wave in leads V_5 and V_6, and a deep s wave in leads V_1 and V_2. Chest leads between these two positions show a transitional pattern. In extremity leads, the QRS complex varies depending on whether the heart is more horizontal or vertical. When the heart is more vertical, leads II, III and aVF show a qR pattern and when the heart is more horizontal, leads I and aVL show a qR pattern. The T wave normally follows the direction of the QRS complex deflection. In chest leads, the T wave is positive in left-sided leads (and also in V_2). In V_1, the T wave may be positive or negative.

Systematic Interpretation of ECG

Routine screening of the ECG requires step-by-step examination of the ECG.

1. What is the heart rate? What is the atrial rate and what is the ventricular rate?

2. Is the rhythm regular or irregular?
3. What is the mean cardiac vector?
4. Are the P waves normal? Do the P waves have a fixed relation to the QRS complexes?
5. What is PR interval? What is the voltage duration and configuration of the QRS complex?
6. Is the ST segment isoelectric?
7. Are the T waves normal?
8. What is the QT interval? Is the QTc appropriate for the heart rate? (QTc is the QT interval corrected for the rate.)

Rate

The heart rate should be calculated first. The comment should be made on both atrial and ventricular rates. Usually, the heart rate means the ventricular rate.

At a paper speed of 25 mm/s:

$$\text{Atrial rate/min} = \frac{1500}{\text{PP interval in mm}}$$

$$\text{Ventricular rate/min} = \frac{1500}{\text{RR interval in mm}}$$

Normally the RR interval is equal to the PP interval but sometimes, the ventricular rate may be different from the atrial rate.

When the RR interval is irregular, as in atrial fibrillation, the number of QRS complexes are counted over 5 seconds in the rhythm strip and this number is multiplied by 12 to provide the number of QRS complexes in 60 seconds (1 minute). This enables the measurement of the average ventricular rate.

The normal heart rate is 60–100 per minute.

Rhythm

Normally the rhythm is regular. It is seen by calculating successive cycle lengths (RR intervals). However, there may be minor variations of rhythm. A variation up to 10 per cent in the adjacent cycle length is considered normal.

Mean QRS Axis (Cardiac Vector)

Cardiac vector can be calculated roughly and accurately.

Rough estimation

Normal   For rough estimation of cardiac vector, QRS complexes are seen in lead I and aVF. When the QRS complexes are predominantly upright (that is, there is a dominant R in both leads), the axis is normal.

Right axis deviation   If the QRS complex in lead I is predominantly negative (that is, dominant S in lead I) while it is predominantly positive in aVF (that is, dominant R in aVF), there is right axis deviation.

Left axis deviation   If the QRS complex is predominantly positive in lead I but negative in aVF, left axis deviation is present. When the QRS complexes in both lead I and aVF are predominantly negative, the axis is intermediate.

Accurate estimation
The vector at any given moment in the two dimensions of the frontal plane can be calculated from any two standard limb leads. The height of QRS complexes in mm in lead I, II, and III are measured and an Einthoven's triangle is drawn (Fig. 26.8A). In each lead, distances equal to the height of the R wave minus the height of the largest negative deflection in the QRS complex are measured. These distances are drawn from the midpoint to the side of the triangle representing that lead. Perpendicular lines are drawn from the midpoint of the arms of the triangle to the centre and from the end of the QRS complexes drawn on the triangle. An arrow is drawn from the centre of the triangle to the point of intersection of the perpendiculars extended from the distances measured on the sides. This arrow represents the magnitude and direction of the mean QRS vector. The normal direction of the mean QRS vector is generally said to be −30 to +110 degrees (Fig. 26.8B). If the axis falls to the left of −30°, left axis deviation is

present and if the axis falls to the right of +110°, right axis deviation is present.

Waves and Intervals

P wave

Duration and amplitude   Normal P wave duration does not exceed 0.10 s and P waves are not more than 2.5 mm tall.

Configuration   Usually P waves are upright in lead I to aVF and V_3–V_6; inverted in aVR; and upright, inverted or biphasic in lead III, aVL, and V_1 and V_6. P wave morphology is best studied in lead II and V_1.

PR interval

Normal PR interval is 0.12–0.20 seconds, that is, 3–5 small squares. Normally, there should not be any variation in PR intervals.

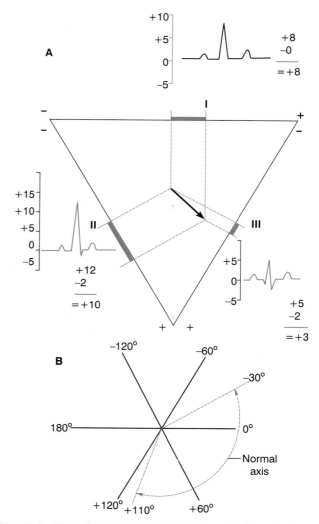

Fig. 26.8   Mean QRS axis. (A) Determination; (B) Normal value in a hexaxial system (Cabrera system).

QRS complex

Amplitude   In limb leads, that is, in lead I, II, III, aVR, aVL and aVF, the total amplitude of QRS should be 5 mm or more. In chest leads, the amplitude of QRS complex should be 10 mm or more.

Duration   The normal duration of the QRS complex does not exceed 0.11 seconds.

Configuration   Normally, the R wave is dominant in leads I, II, V_4–V_6 and the S wave is dominant in aVR, V_1 and V_2. Either R or S wave may be dominant in lead III, aVL, aVF and V_3 depending on the position of the heart.

Q wave

Normally, Q waves are small in leads I, aVL, V_5 and V_6. A QS complex is commonly found in aVR. There may be deep Q waves in lead III alone in normal individuals and may become less prominent on deep inspiration. Occasionally, a deep Q wave is found in V_1 and V_2. The depth of a Q wave is less than 25 per cent of the height of the ensuing R wave in most leads and may be up to 50 per cent in aVL. Any Q wave with greater amplitude is considered pathological.

ST segment

The normal ST segment is isoelectric. ST depression less than 0.5 mm is not abnormal. ST elevation up to 1 mm in limb leads and in V_5 and V_6 and 2 mm in V_1–V_4 may be normal.

T wave

T waves are upright in leads I, II, V_4–V_6; inverted in aVR; and upright, inverted or biphasic in lead III, aVL, aVF and V_1–V_3.

QT interval

The upper limit of a normal QT interval is 0.42 s in males and 0.43 s in females. QT intervals should be measured in the lead where the end of the T wave is best discernible. QT interval varies with the heart rate. Therefore, **corrected QT interval (QTc)** is measured by using **Bazett's formula**.

$$QTc = \frac{QT}{\sqrt{RR}}$$

(where, QT is the QT interval and RR is the RR interval in seconds).

Abnormal ECG

Abnormalities of Heart Rate

The physiological basis for alteration in heart rate has been described in Chapter 27.

Bradycardia
1. Sinus bradycardia
   - Athletes
   - Sick sinus syndrome
   - Drugs (e.g., beta blockers)
   - Obstructive jaundice
   - Raised intracranial pressure
   - Myxedema
2. Junctional (nodal) rhythm
3. Complete heart block

Tachycardia
1. Sinus tachycardia
   - Anxiety
   - Fever
   - Hypoxemia
   - Thyrotoxicosis
   - Cardiac failure
   - Acute carditis
2. Ectopic (re-entrant) tachycardia
3. Atrial premature beats
   - Anxiety
   - Excess tea or coffee intake
   - Viral infections
   - Rheumatic heart disease
   - Digitalis toxicity
   - Cardiomyopathies
4. Paroxysmal supraventricular tachycardia
5. Atrial fibrillation
   - Rheumatic heart disease with mitral stenosis
   - Coronary artery disease
   - Cardiomyopathies
   - Thyrotoxicosis
6. Atrial flutter
   - Rheumatic heart disease
   - Coronary artery disease
7. Ventricular premature beats
8. Ventricular tachycardia

Abnormal Axis Deviation

Right axis deviation
1. Right ventricular hypertrophy
2. Left posterior hemiblock

3. WPW syndrome
4. Dextrocardia

Left axis deviation

1. Left ventricular hypertrophy
2. Left anterior hemiblock
3. WPW syndrome
4. Inferior myocardial infarction
5. Obstructive airway disease

P Wave Abnormalities

P wave may be abnormal due to atrial enlargement and intra-atrial conduction abnormalities. Atrial enlargement results in tall and peaked P waves.

Abnormal PR Interval

Short PR interval

1. WPW syndrome
2. Nodal rhythm
3. Atrial premature beats

Long PR interval (first degree AV block)

1. Rheumatic carditis
2. Digitalis effect
3. Coronary artery disease

Abnormalities of QRS Complex

Amplitude

1. Low amplitude
   - Marked emphysema
   - Myxedema
   - Pericardial effusion
   - Cardiomyopathy
2. High amplitude
   - Ventricular hypertrophy

Pathological Q waves

Depth of Q wave more than 25 per cent of the height of the ensuing R wave, or more than 0.04 s in duration, is considered pathological. Common causes are:

- Acute or old myocardial infarction
- Unstable angina
- Dilated cardiomyopathy
- Hypertrophic cardiomyopathy

Abnormalities of ST Segment

ST elevation

1. Acute myocardial infarction
2. Acute pericarditis

ST depression

Commonly seen in myocardial ischemia.

Abnormalities of T Wave

Tall T wave

1. Hyperkalemia
2. Acute myocardial infarction

Inverted T wave

I. Physiological
   - Young children
   - Deep inspiration (occasionally)
   - After a heavy meal (occasionally)
II. Pathological
   - Ventricular hypertrophy (due to strain)
   - Bundle branch block
   - Digitalis effect
   - Myocardial ischemia

Abnormal QT Interval

Prolonged QT interval

1. Hereditary
2. Antiarrhythmic drugs, like quinidine
3. Hypokalemia
4. Acute myocardial infarction

Shortened QT interval

This is of less clinical significance and may be seen in hypercalcemia.

VIVA

1. Define ECG.
2. What are the uses of ECG?
3. What are the types of ECG machines used to record ECG in the laboratories?
4. How does the stylus write on the ECG paper?
5. What is the need for standardisation before and after the recording of ECG?
6. What are the types of ECG leads?
7. What is Einthoven's triangle?
8. Where should the different chest leads be placed?
9. What is the use of esophageal leads?
10. What are the precautions taken during recording of ECG?
11. Why is the right leg connected during ECG recording?
12. How is the main line frequency interference kept free from the ECG recording?

   Ans: Main line frequency disturbance is kept free by keeping electrode resistance below 10,000 ohms, using a single grounding electrode from the subject, and keeping all AC cords away from the subject.

13. What does a QRS complex represent?
14. What do the P, QRS, T and U waves represent?
15. What is ST segment and what is its significance?
16. What is the 'J' point? What is its significance?
17. How do you calculate the PR interval? What is its normal duration? What is its significance?
18. How do you calculate the QRS interval? What is its normal duration? What is its significance?
19. How do you calculate the QT interval? What is its normal duration? What is its significance?
20. How do you calculate the ST interval? What is its normal duration?
21. How do you calculate the PP interval? What is its significance?
22. How do you calculate the RR interval? What is its significance?
23. How do you calculate the heart rate?
24. How do you calculate ventricular rate when the RR interval is irregular?
25. How do you determine the QRS axis (cardiac vector)?
26. What do you mean by right and left axis deviation? Give examples.
27. What are the causes of tachycardia?
28. What are the causes of bradycardia?
29. What are the causes of short and long RR interval?
30. What are the causes of high and low amplitudes of QRS complex?
31. When does a Q wave become pathological? What are the conditions of pathological Q wave?
32. What are the conditions of ST depression and ST elevation?
33. What are the causes of tall T wave?
34. What are the causes of inverted T wave?
35. What are the causes of prolonged QT interval?

CHAPTER 27

Examination of the Radial Pulse

Learning Objectives

After completing this practical, you will be able to (MUST KNOW):

1. Outline the importance of examination of radial pulse in clinical physiology.
2. Define arterial pulse.
3. List the parameters to be considered for the clinical examination of radial pulse.
4. Examine the radial pulse properly (with proper sequence and procedure).
5. List the common causes of tachycardia, bradycardia, irregular pulse, high and low volume pulses, water hammer pulse, pulsus paradoxus and pulsus alternans.

You may also be able to (DESIRABLE TO KNOW):

1. Define and describe different abnormal pulses.
2. Explain the causes of variation of different parameters of the arterial pulse.
3. State the physiological basis of the changes in the different parameters of the arterial pulse in different conditions.
4. Explain the mechanism of genesis of tachycardia, bradycardia, irregular pulse, high and low volume pulse, water hammer pulse, pulsus paradoxus and pulsus alternans in different conditions.

INTRODUCTION

Examination of the radial pulse is an important and essential part of the clinical examination of a patient. It is not only important for examination of the cardiovascular system but also for any systemic examination of the patient, because arterial pulse is one of the vital signs that must be checked along with the general examination.

Definition

Arterial pulse is defined as the rhythmic expansion of the arterial wall due to transmission of pressure waves along the walls of the arteries, which are produced during each systole of the heart.

Importance

Examination of the arterial pulse provides physiological information regarding:

1. The working of the heart
2. The circulatory state and hemodynamics (blood volume, blood pressure and so on)
3. The condition of the blood vessels
4. The state of autonomic activity in the body at that moment
5. The mental state of the subject
6. The state of body metabolism and temperature

The Radial Pulse

Clinically, the radial pulse is preferred for the examination of arterial pulse for the following reasons:

1. It is clinically easily accessible for its peripheral location in the upper limb.
2. It is easy for palpation as it lies over the radial bone.
3. It is easy for assessing the condition of the arterial wall (to roll the artery against the bone).

Arterial pulse tracing   The pulse tracing recorded by sphygmograph or Student's physiograph from the radial artery shows the following waves (Fig. 27.1). The pulse wave has an upstroke and a downstroke. The 'p' wave (**percussion wave** or tidal wave) occurs due to ejection of blood from the ventricle during systole. The 'd' wave (**dicrotic wave**) occurs due to rebound of blood against the closed aortic valve during diastole. The 'n' (**dicrotic notch**) represents the closure of the aortic valve. Sometimes, in the upstroke of the pulse wave, a small 'a' or anacrotic wave is seen, which occurs due to change in the velocity of ejection of blood from the ventricle towards late systole.

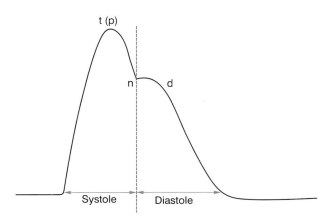

Fig. 27.1   The radial pulse tracing (t: tidal [percussion: p] wave; n: dicrotic notch; d: dicrotic wave).

METHODS

Method of Examination of Radial Pulse

Principle

With each ventricular contraction, not only is the blood pumped into the aorta but also pressure waves that are transmitted along the walls of the vessels are generated. These pressure waves expand the arterial wall, and the expansion is palpated as a pulse.

Procedure

The arterial pulses are detected by gently compressing the vessel against the bone. The radial pulse is examined by compressing the radial artery against the head of the radius. For better elicitation of the pulse, the forearm of the subject should be semipronated and the wrist slightly flexed (Fig. 27.2A).

The following aspects (parameters) of the pulse are examined.
1. Rate
2. Rhythm
3. Volume (amplitude)
4. Character
5. Condition of the arterial wall
6. Radiofemoral delay (presence or absence of delay of the femoral pulses compared with the radials)
7. Other peripheral pulses

Rate

Count the rate of the pulse, not immediately after placing the finger on the artery, but when the nervousness of the patient subsides. Count the pulse completely for one minute.

> **Note:** Pulse rate should be counted only when the pulse resumes its normal rate. Therefore, it is advised to feel the radial pulse gently while eliciting the history of the patient. The pulse should be counted for a minimum of one minute. The counting of pulse for 5 or 10 seconds and multiplying it by 12 or 6 to get the rate per minute is not correct, at least for beginners. The ideal time is 2 minutes and the average of the two may be taken.

In conditions of irregularities of the heart, the counting of radial pulse may not reflect the true ventricular contractions. In these conditions, the heart beat should be counted by auscultating the apex. The difference between the pulse rate and the heart rate is called **pulse deficit**. It should also be noted that the pulse rate can never be more than the heart rate.

Rhythm

Rhythm is the spacing order at which successive pulse waves are felt. When spacing between all the waves is constant, the pulse is said to be regular. When spacing is not constant, the pulse is said to be irregular. The irregular pulse may have a fixed pattern of irregularity (irregular at regular intervals) or the irregularity may not have any pattern (irregularly irregular).

Volume

It is the degree of expansion of the arterial walls during each pulse wave. Usually in physiological conditions, the volume is normal and equal on both the sides. Normal volume cannot be described but can only be appreciated by palpating the artery of a normal individual. The pulse volume gives an indication of the stroke volume of the left ventricle.

Character

Study the character of the arterial pulse waves. The character of a normal pulse is described as 'normal' when no abnormalities are detected. The abnormalities may be seen in rate, rhythm or amplitude of the pulse. Depending on these changes, various types of abnormal pulses are described. It should be noted that the character of the pulse is best appreciated by palpating the carotid artery in the neck.

Condition of the arterial wall

Place three middle fingers on the artery to assess the condition of the arterial wall. Obliterate the flow of blood into the artery by pressing the index finger, and

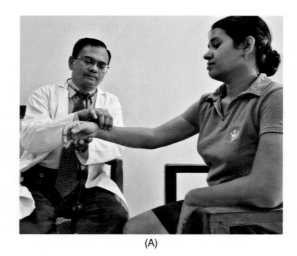

(A)

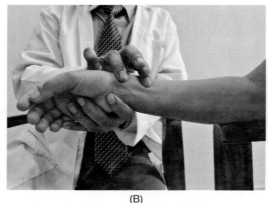

(B)

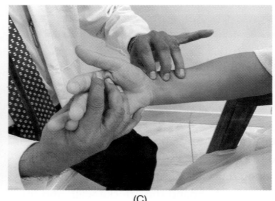

(C)

Fig. 27.2   (A) Examination of the radial pulse. Note that the subject's hand is supported by the examiner's left hand, subject's forearm is semiflexed and semipronated, and the wrist is slightly flexed; (B) Procedure of assessment of the condition of arterial wall. First, the artery is fixed and emptied by index finger and ring finger; (C) Then with the help of middle finger, the artery is rolled against the bone to feel the wall thickness.

empty the vessel by the ring finger (Fig. 27.2B). Then palpate the artery with the middle finger. Roll the artery against the bone to assess the thickness of the arterial wall (Fig. 27.2C).

Normally, the arterial wall is not palpable or is just palpable. But, in old age, it is well palpable (thickened) and may be tortuous.

Delay

Compare the appearance of the femoral pulse with the appearance of the radial pulse and mark if any delay is present between them. Normally there is no radiofemoral delay. Also compare with the radial pulse of the opposite side.

Other peripheral pulses

Palpate the femoral, popliteal (Fig. 27.3A), posterior tibial (Fig. 27.3B) dorsalis pedis (Fig. 27.3C), brachial (Fig. 27.3D), superficial temporal (Fig. 27.3E), frontal

branch of superficial temporal (Fig. 27.3 F) and carotid (Fig. 27.3G) arteries of both the sides as detailed in the caption of Fig. 27.3 and appreciate if the pulses are well felt and appear simultaneously on both sides.

Precautions

1. The subject should relax and rest for a minimum of five minutes.
2. The subject's forearm should be semipronated and the wrist should be semiflexed.
3. Pulse rate should be counted for a minimum of one minute. If irregularity is detected, the pulse should be counted for a minimum of three minutes and the average of the three should be taken as the pulse rate.
4. If the pulse is irregularly irregular, heart beats must be auscultated to detect pulse deficit, if present.
5. Pulses of both the sides should be examined and compared.

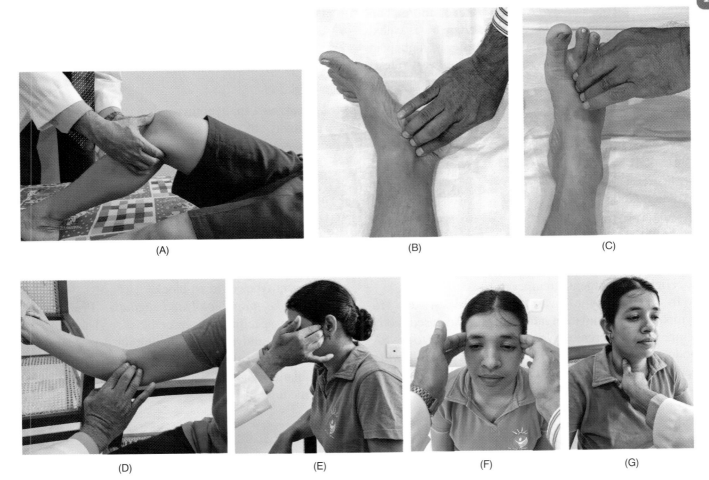

Fig. 27.3   Procedure of examination of other peripheral pulses and carotid pulse. (A) Popliteal artery is palpated in the popliteal fossa by flexing the knee joint to relax the popliteal fascia and hamstrings and by keeping the fingers of both hands from the two sides on the inferior part of the fossa; (B) Posterior tibial artery is palpated by placing the fingers just below the medial malleolus; (C) Dorsal pedis artery is palpated by keeping the fingers on the dorsum of the foot in the upper part of the groove between the big toe and the 2nd toe; (D) Brachial artery is palpated in the antecubital fossa by partially flexing the elbow joint and by placing the fingers just medial to the insertion of the biceps tendon; (E) Superficial temporal artery is palpated by placing the fingers above the zygomatic arch in front of the tragus of the ear; (F) Frontal branch of the superficial temporal artery is palpated by placing the fingers on both sides of the face above the outer part of the orbit; (G) Carotid artery is palpated by firmly placing the tip of the thumb or index finger between the sternomastoid and trachea roughly at the level of the cricoid cartilage.

6. Femoral artery must be examined simultaneously with radial artery to detect radiofemoral delay, if present.
7. The radial pulse should be examined with the middle three fingers to check the condition of the arterial wall. The index finger should be used to obliterate the flow of blood, the ring finger should be used to empty the vessel and the middle finger should be used to palpate and roll the artery against the bone.
8. If the artery is thickened and tortuous, the brachial artery should be examined for locomotor brachii.
9. The condition of the other peripheral pulses should be assessed.

10. If alternating pulses appear to be strong and weak, sphygmomanometry should be done to confirm the presence of pulsus alternans.

DISCUSSION

Pulse Rate

The normal pulse rate is 60–100 per minute. The heart rate is primarily under the control of the autonomic nervous system. The heart rate increases with increased sympathetic activity and decreases with increased parasympathetic activity. A heart rate of more than 100 is called **tachycardia**, and less than 60 is called **bradycardia**. Normally, the heart rate is higher in children and low in elderly persons. The heart rate is higher in inspiration and lower in expiration.

Conditions That Alter Heart Rate

Tachycardia

Physiological

- Exercise
- After eating
- Anger
- Emotion and excitement
- Infants and children
- Pregnancy
- High environmental temperature

In exercise, the heart rate increases due to sympathetic stimulation and due to increased body temperature. Increased sympathetic discharge to the SA node causes tachycardia. Tachycardia occurs following eating due to increased body metabolism that increases body temperature. The heart rate increases in anger, emotion and excitement due to increased sympathetic activity. The exact cause of tachycardia in pregnancy is not known, but it may be due to the direct action of progesterone on the SA node.

Pathological

- *Fever* Increased body temperature causes tachycardia by directly stimulating the SA node.
- *Anemia* Tachycardia occurs in anemia as a compensatory mechanism to improve blood (oxygen) supply to the tissues.
- *Thyrotoxicosis* Thyroxine increases the number of beta receptors in the heart and also increases the sensitivity of the beta receptors to catecholamines.
- Beriberi
- Paget's disease
- Arteriovenous fistula
- Heart failure
- Paroxysmal atrial tachycardia
- Ventricular or supraventricular tachycardia
- Other tachyarrhythmias
- Shock as seen in hemorrhage

Bradycardia

Physiological

- *Athletes* Heart rate is lower in athletes because of their increased vagal tone

- Fear
- Grief
- Very old age
- Meditation and pranayama

Pathological

- *Myxedema* In hypothyroidism, the number and sensitivity of beta receptors to catecholamines decreases.
- *Increased intracranial pressure, as in brain tumours* Increased intracranial pressure decreases heart rate by activating Cushing's reflex.
- *Obstructive jaundice* In obstructive jaundice, the concentration of bile salt increases in the blood. The toxic effect of bile salt inhibits the SA node, and therefore produces bradycardia.
- Different types of heart block.
- *Drugs like propranolol and digitalis* Propranolol is a non-specific β-receptor blocker. Therefore, it produces bradycardia by inhibiting β-receptors of the SA node. Digitalis produces bradycardia by stimulating vagal nuclei (increases vagal activity) in the medulla.

Rhythm

The normal rhythm is regular. Irregular rhythms may be regularly irregular or irregularly irregular. Irregular rhythm may be due to sinus irregularity or premature contraction.

Sinus Irregularity

This is called **sinus arrhythmia**. In this type of irregularity, the pulse rate constantly changes with respiration. Normally, the pulse rate is greater in inspiration than in expiration. In sinus arrhythmia the variation of heart rate in expiration and inspiration is more marked.

Premature Contraction

This is called extrasystole. It occurs due to generation of impulse from an ectopic focus present in the ventricle. Therefore, this is also called **ectopic beat**.

Irregularly Irregular Pulse

This is commonly seen in atrial fibrillation. In this condition, irregularity occurs not only in the interval between the beats, but also in the volume of the beats.

Irregularity associated with heart blocks

1. Partial heart block with dropped beat
2. Atrial flutter with irregular block

In these conditions, irregularity occurs due to block in conduction, which occurs irregularly.

Pulse Deficit

This is the difference between the pulse rate and the heart rate. Normally, there is no pulse deficit. However, in conditions of irregular rhythm, some of the heart beats may be weak. The heart may beat but the contraction may not be sufficient enough to generate pressure waves in the walls of the arteries. Therefore, the pulse rate may be less than that of the rate of heart contraction. Pulse deficit is usually seen in atrial fibrillation in which the deficit is more than ten. Pulse deficit seen in other types of heart blocks is usually less than ten.

Volume

The volume of the pulse is a rough guide to the pulse pressure. Pulse pressure is the difference between the systolic and diastolic pressure. The systolic pressure mainly depends on the stroke volume and the diastolic pressure on the compliance of the arteries. Therefore, the volume of the pulse gives an indication of the stroke volume and the compliance of the vessels. In normal conditions, where the compliance of the vessels is normal, the volume of the pulse mainly reflects the stroke volume.

When the volume of the pulse decreases, the pulse is called low volume pulse and when the volume increases, the pulse is called high volume pulse.

Conditions That Alter the Volume of the Pulse

Low volume pulse

A low volume pulse is also known as **pulsus parvus** (Fig. 27.4D). It occurs when the stroke volume of the heart decreases or when the pulse pressure decreases. Pulsus parvus is seen in:

◆ Aortic stenosis
◆ Obstructive cardiomyopathy
◆ Pericardial effusion
◆ Constrictive pericarditis
◆ Pulmonary stenosis
◆ Tight mitral stenosis

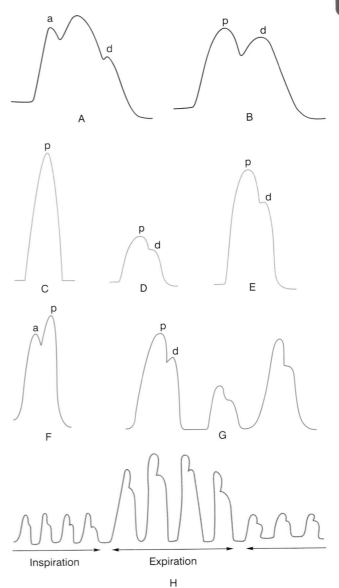

Fig. 27.4 Abnormal pulses. (A) Anacrotic pulse (note that the anacrotic wave is prominent); (B) Dicrotic pulse (note that the dicrotic wave is abnormally large); (C) Collapsing pulse (dicrotic notch absent); (D) Pulsus parvus; (E) Pulsus magnus; (F) Pulsus bisferiens; (G) Pulsus alternans; (H) Pulsus paradoxus.

Shock due to any cause. In shock, it becomes thready pulse (low volume and increased rate)

High volume pulse

The high volume pulse is called **pulsus magnus** (Fig. 27.4E). It is seen in conditions in which the stroke volume is greater and there is widening of the pulse pressure. Pulsus magnus is seen in:

◆ Aortic incompetence
◆ Thyrotoxicosis

- ❖ Patent ductus arteriosus
- ❖ Beriberi
- ❖ Anemia
- ❖ Fever
- ❖ Old age (due to increased pulse pressure)
- ❖ Exercise

Character

The character of a pulse is described as normal when no abnormalities are detected. Different types of abnormal pulses are described in clinical medicine. Common among these are anacrotic pulse, dicrotic pulse, water hammer pulse, pulsus bisferiens, pulsus paradoxus and pulsus alternans.

Anacrotic Pulse

This is also called anadicrotic pulse, which means two upbeats. A secondary wave occurs in the upstroke of the pulse. It is commonly found in aortic stenosis. The upstroke is slow and sloping (Fig. 27.4A). The anacrotic wave is exaggerated and has 2 upbeats. Therefore, this pulse is called anacrotic pulse.

Dicrotic Pulse

A better name for this is 'twice-beating pulse'. The dicrotic wave is prominent in this pulse and gives the impression of two beats. Therefore, this is called dicrotic pulse (Fig. 27.4B). It is commonly seen in febrile states, especially in typhoid fever.

Water Hammer Pulse

This is also called collapsing pulse or **Corrigan's pulse**. This is typically seen in aortic regurgitation. The collapsing pulse is characterised by a **rapid upstroke and a rapid downstroke** (descent) of the pulse wave. A dicrotic notch is usually absent (Fig. 27.4C). The rapid upstroke is due to greatly increased stroke volume and the rapid descent is due to the collapse of the pulse. The pulse pressure is therefore very high, sometimes as high as 100 mm Hg.

Causes

1. Common causes
   - Aortic incompetence
   - Patent ductus arteriosus
2. Less common causes
   - Arteriovenous fistula

- Ventricular septal defect (VSD)
- Hyperkinetic circulatory states, for example, thyrotoxicosis, severe anemia and beriberi.

Note: The **collapsing pulse** is better appreciated when the patient's arm is elevated and the wrist is grasped with the palm (of the examiner's hand) against the palmar surface of the wrist of the subject (Fig. 27.5).

Physiological basis   The collapsing pulse occurs due to rapid upstroke and rapid downstroke of the pulse wave. The **rapid upstroke** is due to a forceful, high-amplitude and steep-rising percussion wave which gives a sharp tap to the palpating hand and the **rapid downstroke** is due to a rapid fall of the descending limb of the pulse wave, which results in sudden disappearance of the pulse from the palpating hand.

The steep rise of the ascending limb of the pulse wave is due to increased end diastolic volume (EDV) of the left ventricle, which causes forceful ejection of blood during systole. This is because during diastole, in addition to the ventricular filling from the left atrium, the filling also occurs from the aorta through the incompetent aortic valve. The aortic valve does not close completely, so blood from the aorta enters into the left ventricle during diastole. This increases the total EDV of the left ventricle. So, during systole, the force of contraction of the left ventricle increases

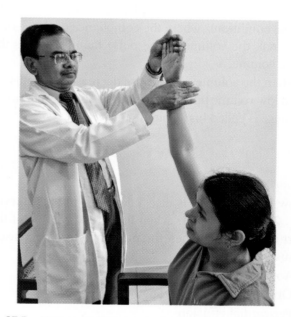

Fig. 27.5   Method of eliciting water-hammer pulse. Note that the collapsing pulse is better appreciated with the patient arm elevated and the examiner palm is placed firmly against the surface location of the radial artery in the wrist.

due to the **Frank–Starling mechanism**. Therefore, there is a steep rise in the percussion wave during systole.

The steep fall of the descending limb of the pulse wave is due to the collapse (sudden disappearance) of the pulse wave from the palpating hand. This occurs due to two factors:
1. the diastolic run-off of blood into the left ventricle and
2. rapid run-off of blood into the periphery because of decreased systemic vascular resistance.

Pulsus Bisferiens

Pulsus bisferiens is a combination of the low-rising pulse (anacrotic pulse) and the collapsing pulse (Fig. 27.4F). This is typically seen in aortic stenosis associated with aortic incompetence.

Pulsus Paradoxus

This is a misnomer since there is nothing paradoxical in this type of pulse. Actually, this is an accentuation of the normal phenomenon where the volume of the pulse decreases during inspiration and increases during expiration. In pulsus paradoxus, **during inspiration, the volume of the pulse is grossly decreased**, or may be absent in severe cases (Fig. 27.4H).

Causes
1. Common causes
   - Constrictive pericarditis
   - Pericardial effusion
2. Less common causes
   - Emphysema
   - Asthma (in the acute phase of severe asthma)
   - Massive pleural effusion
   - A mass in the thorax
   - Advanced right ventricular failure

Mechanisms (physiological basis)
1. During inspiration, the intrathoracic pressure becomes more negative. Blood pools in the pulmonary vascular bed. This decreases venous return to the left atrium. So, left atrial filling decreases, which results in decreased left ventricular stroke volume. Therefore, the volume of the pulse decreases in inspiration. This is more accentuated in the above conditions.
2. During inspiration, the intrapericardial pressure increases due to the traction from the attachments referred to the pericardium. This decreases venous return to the heart and results in low stroke volume. This is accentuated in pericardial effusion and constrictive pericarditis.
3. In constrictive pericarditis and pericardial effusion, the filling of the atria and ventricles decreases due to restriction to the expansion of the heart chambers. The limitation in the diastolic filling of the atria and the ventricles during inspiration results in lowering of left ventricular stroke volume.
4. In advanced stages of right ventricular failure, increase in lung volume in inspiration accommodates more blood than normal due to much decreased pulmonary vascular resistance. There is as such decreased right ventricular output. Therefore, these two factors result in decreased left ventricular stroke volume (due to decreased venous return to left atrium).
5. In acute and severe bronchial asthma, the increased respiratory effort makes intrathoracic pressure more negative during inspiration. So, there is more pooling of blood in the pulmonary veins, which results in decreased left ventricular stroke volume.

Pulsus Alternans

The pulse is regular, but alternate beats are strong and weak (Fig. 27.4G). It is difficult to appreciate pulsus alternans by palpating the artery. Diagnosis is confirmed while measuring blood pressure. There will be a difference of 5–20 mm Hg in the systolic pressure between two alternate beats. When the mercury is being lowered, the stronger beats are heard first, and on further lowering, the weaker beats also become audible, thus suddenly doubling the number of audible beats.

Causes
1. *Left ventricular failure*—this is the commonest cause of pulsus alternans.
2. Toxic carditis

Physiological basis In left ventricular failure, because of the decreased myocardial contractility, the left ventricular stroke volume decreases. This results in low pulse volume. So, the amount of blood left in the ventricle at the end of systole (end systolic volume of the left ventricle) increases. Therefore, prior to the next ventricular contraction, the ventricular volume (EDV) is also increased. This increases the force of contraction of the left ventricle in the next beat due to the Frank–Starling mechanism. Hence, the second beat becomes stronger. Likewise, the strong beats alternate with the weak beats.

Condition of the Arterial Wall

Normally, in young individuals, the arterial wall is soft and elastic or may not be palpable. In the elderly, it is palpable, hard and may be tortuous. This is due to thickening of the arterial wall by atherosclerosis. In such a condition, the brachial and temporal arteries may be quite prominent and tortuous. The brachial artery may exhibit a typical dancing movement with each beat, called locomotor brachii.

Radiofemoral Delay

Normally, there is no delay between the appearance of pulse in the radial and femoral arteries. Radiofemoral delay is typically seen in coarctation of the aorta (especially when the constriction is present distal to the origin of the left subclavian artery).

Other Peripheral Pulses

In the absence of any pathology, all the peripheral pulses are well felt and appear simultaneously on both sides. Peripheral pulses may not be felt properly in peripheral vascular diseases.

Arterial Pulse Tracing

Arterial pulse tracing is done mainly to study the difference in central and peripheral pulses. The recording of the **arterial pulse from a central artery** like the aorta is characterised by a fairly rapid rise to a somewhat rounded peak. The anacrotic shoulder present on the ascending limb occurs at the time of peak rate of aortic flow just before the maximum pressure is reached. The less steep descending limb is interrupted by a sharp downward deflection synchronous with aortic valve closure, called incisura. **Recording from the peripheral artery** shows a steep upstroke, less apparent anacrotic shoulder and replacement of incisura by a smoother dicrotic notch (Fig. 27.6). Arterial pulse tracing is usually not done in clinical practice as physicians can diagnose cardiovascular problems by clinical examination of the arterial pulses. The pulse tracing is used more for physiological and research purposes.

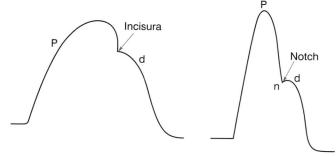

Fig. 27.6   Arterial pulse recorded from: (A) A central artery; (B) A peripheral artery (P: Percussion wave; d: Dicrotic wave; n: Dicrotic notch).

OSPE

Examine the radial pulse of the given subject and report your findings.

Steps

1. Stand on the right side of the subject and hold the right hand of the subject in a semipronated and slightly flexed position and support the limb.
2. Place your three middle fingers on the radial artery just above the wrist.
3. Count the pulse for 1 minute and check for volume and character of the pulse.
4. Check the condition of the arterial wall by obliterating the blood flow with one index finger, by emptying the vessel peripherally by ring finger and palpating and rolling the artery on the bone by the middle finger.
5. Ompare with the pulses of the opposite side.
6. Examine the femoral artery to check for radiofemoral delay.
7. Report your findings.

VIVA

1. Define arterial pulse.
2. What is the importance of examination of the radial pulse in clinical medicine?
3. What are the precautions to be taken during examination of the radial pulse?
4. What are the different aspects of the pulse, which are examined during clinical examination of the radial pulse?
5. Why are the three middle fingers used for examining the radial pulse?
6. What is pulse deficit and what is its most common cause?
7. What is the normal pulse rate and what is the main factor that regulates it?
8. What are the physiological conditions that cause tachycardia?
9. What is the cause of tachycardia in exercise?
10. Why does tachycardia occur after eating?
11. What are the causes of tachycardia in pregnancy?
12. Name the pathological conditions in which tachycardia occurs.
13. What is the cause of tachycardia in thyrotoxicosis?
14. What is the cause of tachycardia in anemia?
15. What is the cause of bradycardia in trained athletes?
16. Why is the heart rate reduced during sleep?

   Ans. Sympathetic activity decreases and parasympathetic activity increases during sleep. Therefore, the heart rate is lower in sleep than in the awake state.

17. What is the cause of bradycardia in increased intracranial pressure?

   Ans: When intracranial pressure increases as seen in a brain tumour, the blood flow to the vasomotor centre (VMC) in the medulla decreases because of the compression of intracranial blood vessels. This causes local hypoxia and hypercapnia, and stimulates VMC, which results in intense vasoconstriction. This is called Cushing's reflex. Vasoconstriction increases blood pressure, which stimulates baroreceptors, and the activation of baroreceptor reflex results in bradycardia. Therefore, bradycardia rather than tachycardia is one of the important clinical features of raised intracranial pressure.

18. What is the relationship between pulse rate and blood pressure?

   Ans: Pulse rate is inversely proportional to the blood pressure but not vice versa. This is called Mary's law. When blood pressure increases, the baroreceptors present in the arterial side of the circulation are stimulated. This activates the baroreceptor reflex, which results in bradycardia and hypotension. Conversely, when blood pressure decreases, there is tachycardia. Therefore, heart rate is inversely proportional to the blood pressure. But, blood pressure may not change with change in heart rate.

19. What is sinus arrhythmia?
20. What are the causes of high volume and low volume pulses?
21. What is the physiological significance of examining the volume of the pulse?
22. What do you mean by the collapsing pulse and what is its physiological basis?
23. What is pulsus paradoxus and what are the conditions that produce it?
24. What is the physiological basis of pulsus paradoxus in constrictive pericarditis and pericardial effusion?

   Ans: In constrictive pericarditis and in pericardial effusion, the filling of the atria and ventricles decreases due to restriction to the expansion of the heart chambers. The limitation in the diastolic filling of the atria and the ventricles during inspiration results in lowering of left ventricular stroke volume.

25. What is pulsus alternans and what is the physiological basis of this pulse?
26. What is the significance of examining the femoral artery simultaneously with the radial artery?
27. What are the differences between central and peripheral pulses as recorded by arterial pulse tracing?

CHAPTER 28

Measurement of Blood Pressure

Learning Objectives

After completing this practical, you will be able to (MUST KNOW):

1. Define blood pressure; define systolic, diastolic, mean arterial and pulse pressure.
2. State the normal values of systolic, diastolic, mean arterial and pulse pressure.
3. Tie the BP cuff properly around the arm of the subject.
4. Raise the mercury column and decrease the mercury column of the sphygmomanometer at the required speed, during BP recording.
5. Detect the appearance and disappearance of sounds by placing a stethoscope on the brachial artery while measuring blood pressure.
6. Record bp by palpatory and auscultatory methods, and list the precautions of recording BP.
7. List the physiological variations of blood pressure.

8. Define hypertension and hypotension.
9. Name the reflexes involved in regulation of BP.
10. State the importance of baroreceptor reflex.

You may also be able to (DESIRABLE TO KNOW):

1. List the merits and demerits of different methods of measuring blood pressure.
2. Explain the mechanism of alteration in blood pressure in different physiological conditions.
3. Explain the physiological basis of different types of hypertension and hypotension.
4. Explain the mechanism of short-term and long-term regulation of blood pressure.
5. Correlate the change in BP in some common clinical conditions.

INTRODUCTION

Blood pressure (BP) is defined as the lateral pressure exerted by a column of blood on the walls of the arteries. Blood pressure usually means arterial pressure. The pressure in the arteries fluctuates during systole and diastole of the heart.

Systolic BP

Definition   Systolic blood pressure (SBP) is defined as the maximum pressure produced during the cardiac cycle. It is recorded during systole. Therefore, it is called systolic blood pressure.

Significance   SBP depends mainly on the cardiac output. Thus, SBP increases in conditions in which cardiac output is more.

Normal values   100–119 mm Hg (120 to 139 mm Hg is prehypertension)

Diastolic BP

Definition   Diastolic blood pressure (DBP) is defined as the minimum pressure recorded during the cardiac

cycle. It is recorded during diastole. Therefore, it is called diastolic pressure.

Significance   DBP depends mainly on peripheral resistance. Thus, DBP changes in conditions in which there is change in peripheral resistance. Peripheral resistance depends mainly on the diameter of the blood vessels and viscosity of the blood.

Normal values   60–79 mm Hg (80 to 89 mm Hg is prehypertension)

Pulse Pressure

Definition   Pulse pressure (PP) is the difference between the systolic and diastolic blood pressures.

Significance   This is the pressure that maintains the normal pulsatile nature of the flow of blood in the vascular compartment. The pulsatile nature of the flow is required for the perfusion of the tissues.

Normal values   20–50 mm Hg

Mean Arterial Pressure

Definition   Mean arterial pressure (MAP) is the average pressure produced during the cardiac cycle. It is calculated by adding one-third of the PP to the diastolic pressure.

$$MAP = DBP + 1/3\ PP$$

Because the duration of a systole is less than the duration of a diastole, MAP is slightly less than the value halfway between systolic and diastolic pressure. MAP also determines tissue perfusion.

Significance MAP is the pressure that helps in the forward movement of blood in the lumen of blood vessels. MAP also determines tissue perfusion.

Normal values   75–105 mm Hg

Casual Blood Pressure

Blood pressure measured at any time of the day is called casual blood pressure.

Basal Blood Pressure

Blood pressure recorded in the basal state is called basal blood pressure. It is recorded following complete physical and mental rest, for 15 to 20 min.

Classification of BP by Joint National Committee (JNC-7).

Category	Systolic BP (mmHg)	Diastolic BP (mmHg)
Normal	100–119	60–79
Prehypertension	120–139	80–89
Stage I Hypertension	140–159	90–99
Stage II Hypertension	160 or above	100 or above

Factors Affecting BP

Blood pressure = Cardiac output × Peripheral resistance

Thus, factors that affect cardiac output and peripheral resistance also affect blood pressure. Alteration in cardiac output mainly affects systolic pressure while alteration in peripheral resistance mainly affects diastolic pressure.

Factors Affecting Cardiac Output

Cardiac output = Stroke volume × Heart rate
Therefore, any factor that affects stroke volume or heart rate alters cardiac output. Stroke volume is affected by preload, afterload and myocardial contractility, and the heart rate is mainly affected by parasympathetic and sympathetic activities.

1. Preload

Preload is the end diastolic volume (EDV), that is, the amount of blood present in the ventricle at the end of the diastole. When the EDV increases, the cardiac output increases and when EDV decreases, the cardiac output decreases. This occurs due to the operation of the **Frank–Starling mechanism**. EDV depends on the venous return to the heart.

Factors that increase preload
- Increased total blood volume
- Increased venous tone
- Increased pumping action of skeletal muscle
- Increased negative intrathoracic pressure
- Increased atrial contraction

Factors that decrease preload
- Decreased blood volume
- Venodilation
- Increased intrapericardial pressure
- Decreased ventricular compliance

2. Afterload

Afterload is peripheral resistance. When peripheral resistance increases as in hypertension, the cardiac output decreases and when peripheral resistance decreases as in anemia, the cardiac output increases.

3. Myocardial contractility

The contractility of the myocardium exerts a major influence on the cardiac output. The strength of the cardiac contraction is called inotropic state of the heart. The factors that increase the strength of contraction are said to be positively inotropic and the factors that decrease the strength of contraction are said to be negatively inotropic.

Factors that are positively inotropic
- Sympathetic stimulation
- Digitalis
- Glucagon
- Caffeine and theophylline

Factors that are negatively inotropic
- Parasympathetic stimulation
- Hypoxia, hypercapnea and acidosis
- Loss of myocardium
  Drugs like propranolol, quinidine and barbiturate

4. Heart rate

Increase in heart rate increases cardiac output, and decrease in heart rate decreases cardiac output. However, a change in heart rate cannot significantly alter the cardiac output unless it is associated with a change in ventricular filling.

Factors Affecting Peripheral Resistance

1. Diameter of blood vessels

The decrease in vessel diameter (vasoconstriction) increases peripheral resistance and increases blood pressure. Vasodilation decreases peripheral resistance and decreases blood pressure. The diameter of the blood vessels depends mainly on the vasoconstrictor tone, which is the rate of discharge in the vasoconstrictor nerves (sympathetic tone). Increase in vasoconstrictor tone causes arteriolar constriction and increases blood pressure and, conversely, decrease in vasoconstrictor tone decreases blood pressure. When the wall of the blood vessel becomes stiff (less compliant), peripheral resistance increases and, therefore, blood pressure increases.

2. Viscosity

Viscosity of blood depends on the composition of plasma, total number of cells in the blood, and resistance of the cells to deformation and temperature.

Factors that increase viscosity
- Polycythemia
- Hyperproteinemia
- Hereditary spherocytosis
- Decreased temperature

Factors that decrease viscosity
- Anemia
- Hypoproteinemia
- Increased temperature

METHODS

Blood pressure is measured by two methods, direct and indirect.

Direct Method

Blood pressure is measured directly by placing a cannula in the lumen of the artery and connecting the cannula to a mercury manometer or a pressure transducer. This method is used for recording blood pressure in experimental animals. In humans, blood pressure can be measured directly during open thoracic surgeries. In clinical practice, blood pressure is measured by the indirect method.

Indirect Method (Sphygmomanometry)

The instrument used in this method is the sphygmomanometer. Therefore, the method of measurement is called sphygmomanometry.

Principle

The cuff of the sphygmomanometer is wrapped around the arm of the subject. The bag is then inflated until the air pressure in the cuff overcomes the arterial pressure and obliterates the arterial lumen. This is confirmed by palpating the radial pulse that disappears when the cuff pressure is raised above the arterial pressure. The pressure is then raised further by about 20 mm Hg and then slowly reduced. When the pressure in the cuff reaches just below the arterial pressure, blood escapes beyond the occlusion into the peripheral part of the artery and the pulse starts reappearing. This is detected by the appearance of sounds in the stethoscope and is taken as the systolic pressure. Subsequently, the quality of the sound changes and finally, disappears. The level where sound disappears is taken as the diastolic pressure. The sound disappears because the flow in the blood vessels becomes laminar.

Requirements

1. Sphygmomanometer
2. Stethoscope

Sphygmomanometer

The sphygmomanometer (Fig. 28.1) consists of a mercury manometer, cuff and air pump.

Mercury manometer The mercury manometer has two limbs. One limb is broader and shorter than the other. The broader limb is the reservoir for mercury. The narrow limb is graduated from 0 to 300 mm, with a smallest division of 2 mm Hg. The mercury reservoir is connected to a rubber tube.

Cuff The cuff is called a **Riva–Rocci cuff**. It consists of an inflatable rubber bag covered by non-distensible cotton fabric. Two tubes are attached to the bag, one transmits air pressure to the mercury manometer and the other is connected to the air pump. The width of the cuff is usually 12 cm. The length and width of the cuff are different for different age groups and body build. Roughly, the length of the rubber bag should be

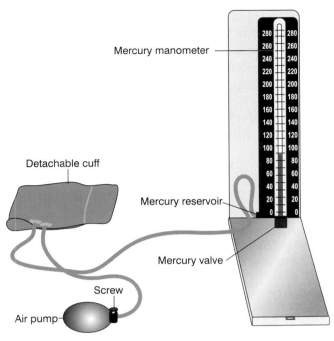

Fig. 28.1 Sphygmomanometer.

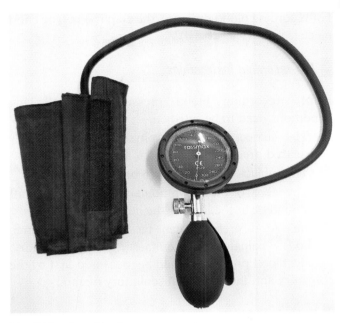

Fig. 28.2 Aneroid sphygmomanometer.

two-thirds and the width should be one-third of the mid-arm circumference of the subject.

The width of the cuff should be 12.5 cm for measuring BP in adults, 8 cm for children up to 8 years, 5 cm for children up to 4 years and 2 to 3 cm for newborns and infants.

Air pump It is a rubber hand bulb provided with a one-way valve at its free end and a leak valve arrangement at the other (Fig. 28.1). A rubber tube connects the air pump to the rubber bag. The rubber bag is inflated by turning the screw clockwise and repeatedly compressing the bulb. Deflation of the bag is achieved by turning the screw anti-clockwise.

Aneroid sphygmomanometer Nowadays, for students' practicals, the aneroid sphygmomanometer (Fig. 28.2) is preferred over the mercury manometer, due to chance of leakage in the mercury sphygmomanometer.

Stethoscope

There are two types of stethoscopes, the bell type and the diaphragm type. Modern stethoscopes are a combination of the bell and diaphragm types (Fig. 28.3A). The bell type chest piece detects low-pitched sounds like heart sounds, whereas high-pitched sounds such as aortic diastolic murmurs are better heard with the diaphragm of the stethoscope.

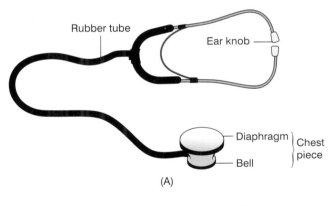

(A)

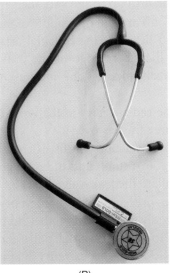

(B)

Fig. 28.3 Stethoscope. A. Diagram showing the parts; B: Diaphragm type of stethoscope.

For recording blood pressure, the diaphragm type chest piece is used (Fig. 28.3B).

Pre-recording Instructions

Before recording blood pressure, the following conditions need to be satisfied.
1. The subject should be physically and mentally relaxed, free from excitement and apprehension.
2. The subject should lie down or sit comfortably.
3. The 'zero' of the sphygmomanometer and the cuff should be at the level of the heart.

The blood pressure can be measured by three methods: palpatory, auscultatory and oscillatory. Ideally, blood pressure should be measured first by the palpatory and then by the auscultatory method.

Palpatory Method

Procedure

1. Check the level of the mercury column in the sphygmomanometer.

Note: Before recording the blood pressure, it should be ensured that the upper meniscus of the mercury coincides with the 'zero' of the mercury manometer. If the mercury column is higher than the zero level and cannot be readjusted, the difference should be noted and deducted from the final result. But, if the mercury column is below the zero level and cannot be brought up to the zero level, the apparatus should be discarded.

2. Expose the arm up to the shoulder.
3. Wrap the cuff around the middle of the arm (middle of the cuff lies over the brachial artery) in such a way that the lower edge of the cuff remains at a minimum distance of one inch above the cubital fossa.
4. Palpate the radial artery at the wrist by placing the middle three fingers over it.
5. Hold the rubber bulb in the other hand in such a way that your thumb and index finger remain free to manipulate the leak-valve screw.
6. Raise the pressure of the mercury manometer by repeatedly compressing the rubber bulb, and continue to feel the radial pulse simultaneously. Note the level of the mercury in the manometer scale where the pulse disappears.
7. Raise the mercury column to about 10 mm Hg above the point of disappearance of the pulse.

8. Reduce the pressure gradually by 2–4 mm Hg per second. However, reduction in this pressure may further be slowed if there is significant bradycardia. Note the mercury level where the pulse reappears.

Note: The pulse reappears at the same level where it had disappeared.

9. Reduce the pressure rapidly to the zero level.
10. Note your observation and express the result in mm Hg.

Note: The point of disappearance (or appearance) of the pulse is the blood pressure recorded by the palpatory method. This blood pressure is the systolic pressure.

Precautions

1. The subject should be mentally and physically relaxed.
2. The subject should lie down or sit comfortably for a minimum of five minutes before the recording.
3. The zero level of the mercury should be checked. If the mercury is not at the zero level, the difference should be noted and deducted from the result.
4. The arm of the subject should be completely exposed and kept at heart level.
5. The cuff should be tied neither very tightly nor loosely around the arm.
6. The width of the cuff should be according to the circumference of the arm to overcome the tissue resistance. The width of the cuff in adults is 12.5 cm. If a narrower cuff is used in adults, the recorded pressure will be falsely high. The narrower cuff is used for children.
7. The cuff and the equipment should be kept at the level of the heart to avoid the effect of gravity. The pressure in any vessel above the heart level is lower and in any vessel below the heart, higher.
8. The level of disappearance or reappearance of the pulse should be noted accurately.

Advantages

1. A stethoscope is not required for measuring BP.
2. As auscultation is not required, this method can be used by less experienced medical personnel.
3. Recording is not time-consuming.

4. It gives a rough indication of the systolic pressure before recording BP by the auscultatory method.
5. An auscultatory gap, if present, is not missed in the auscultatory method when the blood pressure is first recorded by the palpatory and then by the auscultatory method.

Disadvantages

1. This method records only the systolic pressure. Diastolic pressure cannot be determined.
2. The systolic pressure recorded is about 2–5 mm Hg less than the actual pressure.

Auscultatory Method

Procedure

1. Record blood pressure by the palpatory method as described above.
2. Raise the pressure to 30 mm Hg above the palpatory level, that is, 30 mm Hg above the level at which radial pulsation is no longer felt.
3. Place the diaphragm of the stethoscope lightly on the brachial artery in the cubital fossa, that is, over the upper part of the forearm medial to the tendon of the biceps (Fig. 28.4).
4. Lower the pressure at the rate of 2–4 mm Hg per second. Note the appearance of the sound, the

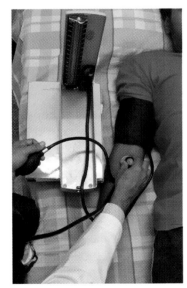

Fig. 28.4 Measurement of blood pressure by auscultatory method. Note that the sphygmomanometer is placed at the level of the heart; use a pile of books or any other suitable set-up to keep it at this level.

change in character of the sound and finally the cessation of the sound, while the pressure in the cuff is progressively lowered.

5. Note the level where the sounds are first heard as the systolic pressure, and the level where the sounds cease as the diastolic pressure.

> **Note:** When pressure in the cuff is progressively lowered, the sounds undergo a series of changes in their quality and intensity. These sounds are known as **Korotkoff sounds** (described by the Russian scientist Korotkoff in 1905). They are heard in five different phases (Fig. 28.5).

Phase I : Sudden appearance of faint tapping sounds which become gradually louder and clearer during the succeeding 10 mm Hg fall in pressure.

Phase II : The sound becomes murmurish in the next 10 mm Hg fall in pressure.

Phase III : The sound changes a little in quality but becomes clearer and louder in the next 15 mm Hg fall in pressure.

Phase IV : Sounds become muffled in character during the next 5 mm Hg fall.

Phase V : Sounds completely disappear.

Appearance of the sound is recorded as systolic blood pressure and disappearance of sound as diastolic blood pressure. In persons with severe hypertension and in children, muffling rather than the disappearance of the sound is taken as the diastolic pressure.

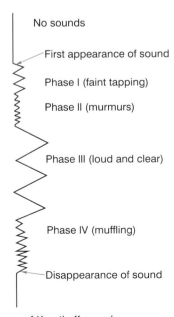

Fig. 28.5 Phases of Korotkoff sounds.

Precautions

1. The subject should be mentally and physically relaxed.
2. The size of the cuff should be proportionate to the circumference of the arm of the subject.
3. The zero reading of the manometer should be kept at the level of the heart.
4. Blood pressure should be detected first by the palpatory method before recording by the auscultatory method.
5. Pressure must be raised by 30 mm Hg above the palpatory level.
6. The cuff pressure should be decreased to the zero level between successive trials.
7. While reading the manometer, the eye should be at the level of the mercury column to avoid parallax.
8. If coarctation of the aorta is suspected, blood pressure should also be recorded in the thigh.

> **Note:** A cuff of greater width (about 18 cm) is used for measuring blood pressure in the thigh. The patient lies face downwards, the cuff is applied above the knee and auscultation is carried out over the popliteal artery.

Blood pressure should ideally be checked by the palpatory method before recording by the auscultatory method.

> **Note:** Blood pressure is checked by the palpatory method before the auscultatory method to include the **auscultatory gap** in the pressure range. In severely hypertensive patients, after the appearance of the sounds, occasionally the sounds disappear at a point below 200 mm Hg for a range of 20–50 mm Hg and then reappear and finally disappear at the level of diastolic pressure. The period of first (temporary) disappearance of sounds is called **silent gap** or auscultatory gap. The auscultatory gap is never missed if the pressure is measured first by the palpatory method because the auscultatory gap comes within the range of the systolic pressure recorded by the palpatory method. If the BP is directly measured by the auscultatory method, the auscultatory gap may be missed and the systolic value may be reported as lower than the actual value. The exact cause of the auscultatory gap is not known. It is thought to be due to the transient hyper-responsiveness of the vessel to compression.

9. The cuff and the equipment should be kept at the level of the heart to avoid the effect of gravity (Fig. 28.6).

Disadvantages

1. Unless followed by the palpatory method, the auscultatory method may miss the auscultatory gap.

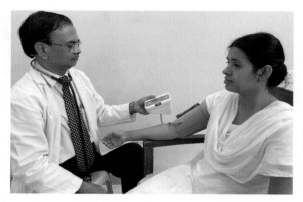

Fig. 28.6 Recording of BP using automatic BP monitor. Note that the cuff and the equipment are approximately at the level of the heart and the subject is seated on a wooden chair with hand rested on the arm of the chair and the trunk of the body kept straight but rested on the back of the chair.

2. Adequate experience needed for detecting sounds by the stethoscope.

Advantages

1. Gives accurate value for systolic pressure.
2. Detects diastolic pressure.

> **Special Notes**
> 1. Diastolic pressure recorded in the sitting posture is about 5 mm Hg more than in the supine posture.
> 2. Arm position above and below heart level gives lower and higher BP values, respectively.
> 3. If BP values are different between two arms, higher value should be used.

Oscillatory Method

Procedure

The procedure is the same as that in the palpatory method, but instead of palpating the artery, the oscillations of the mercury column in the sphygmomanometer are noted to record BP. The pressure in the cuff is raised and the appearance and disappearance of oscillations of the mercury column are noted while lowering the mercury column. The point of appearance of the oscillation gives the systolic pressure, and the point of disappearance of the oscillations gives the diastolic pressure.

Disadvantages

1. This method does not give accurate values for systolic and diastolic pressure.

2. Adequate experience needed to detect the exact level of the appearance and disappearance of oscillation.

DISCUSSION

Clinical Significance

Physiological Conditions Altering BP

1. **Age**   Blood pressure increases with age.
   In children : Systolic pressure is 90–119 mm Hg.
   Diastolic pressure is 50–79 mm Hg.
   In adults : Systolic pressure is 100–119 mm Hg.
   Diastolic pressure is 60–79 mm Hg.
   In elderly : The upper limit of systolic is considered to be 160 mm Hg, but diastolic pressure of 90 mm Hg or above is always considered abnormal.
2. **Gender**   BP is less in females due to the effect of progesterone, which relaxes the smooth muscles of the blood vessels. Also, cardiac vagal drive is relatively more in females compared to males. Therefore, the heart rate is comparatively less in females. Consequently, the systolic BP is less in females compared to males. This difference in females disappears after menopause.
3. **Eating**   BP increases after a meal. This may be due to increased body metabolism that increases the circulation.
4. **Sleep**   BP is less during sleep than in the waking state. This is because the human being is under constant stress which is absent in sleep.
5. **Emotion and excitement**   In emotional and excited states, increased sympathetic discharge increases the blood pressure.
6. **Exercise**   During exercise, the systolic pressure always rises because of increased cardiac output due to sympathetic stimulation which causes tachycardia and increased myocardial contractility. Diastolic pressure depends on the degree of exercise. Diastolic pressure increases in mild exercise due to vasoconstriction, remains unchanged or may even fall in moderate exercise, but always falls in intense exercise because of metabolic vasodilation and increased body temperature.
7. **Posture**   On immediate standing from the supine posture, BP decreases and then returns to normal or

increases due to correction by the baroreceptor reflex.
8. **Temperature**   BP decreases in a hot environment due to vasodilation and increases in a cold environment due to vasoconstriction.
9. **Pregnancy**   Increase in cardiac output due to increased blood volume increases systolic pressure during pregnancy, but diastolic pressure falls due to decreased peripheral resistance. Peripheral resistance decreases due to the effect of progesterone which relaxes the smooth muscle of blood vessels (causes vasodilation). Therefore, pulse pressure increases in pregnancy.

Pathological Conditions Altering BP

Blood pressure increases (hypertension) and decreases (hypotension) in different pathological conditions.

Pathophysiology of Hypertension

Hypertension is defined as sustained elevation of systemic arterial pressure. Usually, hypertension means rise in diastolic BP. Hypertension is broadly classified as essential and secondary.

Essential Hypertension

This is the commonest type of hypertension and is seen in 90 per cent of patients with hypertension. The cause of essential hypertension is not known, but is thought to be due to a hereditary defect that predisposes a person to hypertension.

Secondary Hypertension

This is the hypertension secondary to a disease elsewhere in the body. The following are the causes of secondary hypertension.
1. Adrenocortical diseases
   * Hyperaldosteronism
   * Cushing syndrome
   * Hypertensive form of congenital virilising tumour
2. Renal diseases
   * Glomerulonephritis
   * Pyelonephritis
   * Polycystic disease
   * Tumours of JG cells
3. Pheochromocytoma
4. Severe polycythemia
5. Oral contraceptives

Pathophysiology of Hypotension

Systolic pressure less than 90 mm Hg in adults is known as hypotension. Clinically, there are three types of hypotension: (1) chronic hypotension, (2) acute hypotension and (3) postural hypotension.

Chronic Hypotension

Chronic hypotension is characterised by persistent low blood pressure. Usually, the patients are asymptomatic, but sometimes they complain of lethargy, weakness and giddiness.

Causes

- Primary adrenocortical insufficiency
- Hypopituitarism
- Malnutrition and anemia
- Chronic diarrhea
- Prolonged bed rest

Acute Hypotension

The sudden fall of blood pressure is called acute hypotension. Usually, if severe, it is associated with fainting.

Causes

- Acute hemorrhage
- Acute diarrhea
- Severe vomiting
- Acute myocardial infarction
- Excessive diuresis
- Acute vasodilation

Postural Hypotension

If systolic blood pressure falls by 20 mm Hg or more when a subject assumes an erect posture (from the supine posture), the condition is called postural or orthostatic hypotension. This usually results from autonomic imbalance. It may be of chronic or acute variety.

Acute postural hypotension   This is due to temporary fall in blood pressure, which results in transient fainting. It is usually seen in the following conditions:

- Prolonged standing
- Rising from bed after a prolonged illness
- Strenuous physical exercise

Chronic postural hypotension   Chronic postural hypotension can be primary or secondary. Chronic primary postural hypotension is called idiopathic postural hypotension. The cause of this hypotension is not known. It usually occurs in the elderly and may be due to the degeneration of peripheral autonomic nerves. Chronic secondary postural hypotension has following causes:

- Polyneuropathy as seen in diabetes, amyloidosis and beriberi
- Autonomic neuropathy as seen in syringomyelia, tabes dorsalis and subacute combined degeneration of spinal cord
- Patients receiving sympatholytic drugs
- Surgical sympathectomy

Physiological Significance

Regulation of Blood Pressure

The mechanisms involved in regulation of blood pressure can be divided into two broad categories: (1) Short-term regulation and (2) Long-term regulation. Short-term regulation is mainly neural and long-term regulation is mainly hormonal.

Short-term regulation

Baroreceptor reflex   Baroreceptors are present in the carotid sinus and aortic arch, and respond to stretching. They detect any change in pressure in the vessels in which they are situated. Increase in blood pressure causes distension of the carotid sinus and aortic arch, which stretches the baroreceptors and increases the firing rate in the afferent nerves (IX and X cranial nerves). This leads to excitation of the nucleus tractus solitarius (NTS) in the medulla, which in turn inhibits the vasomotor centre via interneurons. The inhibition of the vasomotor centre decreases the sympathetic output and causes vasodilation, bradycardia, decrease in cardiac output and fall in blood pressure. The excitation of NTS also stimulates the vagus nerve, which decreases the heart rate and cardiac output.

Conversely, when blood pressure falls, less distension of the carotid sinus and aortic arch inhibits the receptors and decreases the discharge rate in the afferent nerves. Due to decreased activity in the IX and X cranial nerves, NTS is inhibited, which in turn causes disinhibition (stimulation) of the vasomotor centre, which increases sympathetic output. Inhibition of NTS also inhibits the vagus nerve. This finally results in vasoconstriction, tachycardia, increased cardiac output and increase in blood pressure. The baroreceptor reflex regulates blood pressure in the pressure range of 70–150 mm Hg.

Chemoreceptor reflex   Chemoreceptors are located in the aortic and carotid bodies. They respond to the change in chemical composition of blood, which occurs in conditions like hypoxia, hypercapnea and acidosis. Stimulation of these receptors results in bradycardia and vasoconstriction. This also causes pulmonary hyperventilation and secretion of catecholamines from the adrenal medulla, which increase heart rate. Therefore, the net effect of stimulation of chemoreceptors is no change in heart rate or mild tachycardia, and hypertension. Chemoreceptors regulate blood pressure in the pressure range of 40–70 mm Hg.

Cushing's reflex   In severe hypotension, blood flow to the brain decreases. Hypoxia and hypercapnea of vasomotor centre occur. This causes stimulation of vasomotor centre to the maximum, which results in intense vasoconstriction that attempts to bring the pressure back to normal. This response is called CNS ischemic response and is a life-saving mechanism when blood pressure falls below 40 mm Hg.

When intracranial pressure increases, blood flow to the vasomotor centre decreases due to compression of blood vessels. This stimulates the vasomotor centre and causes intense vasoconstriction, which results in increased blood pressure. This is called Cushing's reflex. The increase in blood pressure activates the baroreceptor reflex and causes bradycardia. Therefore, bradycardia rather than tachycardia is an outstanding feature of brain tumours.

Capillary fluid shift   When blood pressure increases, the hydrostatic pressure in the capillaries increases. This causes a shift of fluid from the intravascular compartment to the extravascular space. As a result, the circulating blood volume decreases and blood pressure falls to normal.

Stress relaxation   When blood pressure increases suddenly, the smooth muscles of the blood vessels relax in response to sudden stretching. This decreases the vascular tone and brings the pressure back to normal.

Hormonal mechanisms   Catecholamines are released from the adrenal medulla when sympathetic discharge increases, as in hemorrhage and hypotension. Norepinephrine is a potent vasoconstrictor. The renin–angiotensin system is also activated when blood pressure falls. Angiotensin II is a potent vasoconstrictor.

Long-term regulation

Long-term regulation is mainly achieved by hormonal mechanisms that involve changes in the fluid volume of the body. The kidneys also play a role in long-term regulation of BP.

Hormonal mechanism

1. **The renin–angiotensin system**   Fall in blood pressure releases renin from the JG cells of the kidney. Renin converts angtiotensinogen to angiotensin I, which is further converted to angiotensin II. Angiotensin II causes vasoconstriction and increases blood pressure. Angiotensin II also increases synthesis and secretion of aldosterone, which increases sodium and water reabsorption from the kidney, which in turn assists in restoration of pressure.

2. **Vasopressin (ADH)**   Decrease in extracellular fluid volume increases the release of ADH from the posterior pituitary. ADH increases water reabsorption from the kidneys and causes vasoconstriction.

3. **Catecholamines**   Stimulation of sympathetic fibres to the adrenal medulla causes the release of catecholamines. These hormones (especially norepinephrine) are potent vasoconstrictors.

Renal mechanism

When alteration in blood pressure occurs, the kidneys try to restore the pressure by changing the excretion of sodium and water. This mechanism is independent of other factors and is intrinsic to the kidneys.

OSPE

I.   Record the blood pressure of the given subject by the palpatory method.

   Steps
   1.   Inform the subject about the procedure and expose the arm.
   2.   Tie the cuff of the sphygmomanometer around the arm of the subject properly (not very tight nor loose) about 2.5 cm above the cubital fossa in such a way that the midpoint of the rubber bag of the cuff overlies the brachial artery.

3. Check that the mercury column of the sphygmomanometer is adjusted to the zero reading.
4. Keep the sphygmomanometer at the level of the heart of the subject.
5. Palpate the radial artery.
6. Raise the mercury column in the sphygmomanometer by raising the pressure in the cuff.
7. Mark the level of the mercury column for disappearance of the radial pulse.
8. Release the pressure in the cuff.

II. Record the blood pressure of the given subject by the auscultatory method.

Steps

1. Inform the subject about the procedure and expose the arm.
2. Tie the cuff of the sphygmomanometer around the arm of the subject properly (neither tight nor loose) about 2.5 cm above the cubital fossa, in such a way that the midpoint of the rubber bag of the cuff overlies the brachial artery.
3. Check that the mercury column of the sphygmomanometer is adjusted to the zero reading.
4. Keep the sphygmomanometer at the level of the heart of the subject.
5. Palpate the radial artery.
6. Raise the mercury column in the sphygmomanometer by increasing the pressure in the cuff and mark the level of disappearance of the radial pulse.
7. Raise the mercury column about 30 mm Hg above the palpatory level.
8. Place the diaphragm of the stethoscope medial to the tendon of the biceps where pulsation of the brachial artery is felt.
9. Slowly lower the mercury column by releasing the pressure in the cuff at the rate of 2–4 mm Hg per second and while decreasing the mercury column, auscultate for the appearance, change in quality and disappearance of the sounds.
10. Note the appearance of the sounds as systolic, and disappearance of the sounds as diastolic blood pressure.
11. Release the pressure from the cuff.

VIVA

1. Define blood pressure.
2. Define systolic and diastolic blood pressure and give their normal values.
3. What is mean arterial pressure and what is its significance?
4. What is pulse pressure and what is its significance?
5. What are the methods of measurement of blood pressure?
6. What are the conditions that must be satisfied before recording blood pressure?
7. Why are the zero level of the sphygmomanometer and the cuff kept at the heart level of the subject while recording blood pressure?
8. Why is the blood pressure ideally recorded by the palpatory method before recording by the auscultatory method?
9. What are the precautions for measuring blood pressure by the palpatory method?
10. Why is the pressure in the cuff raised by about 30 mm Hg above the palpatory level for recording blood pressure by the auscultatory method?
11. What is auscultatory gap and what is its significance?
12. What is the cause of the appearance, change in quality and disappearance of sounds at various phases of blood pressure measurement?
13. What is the ideal size of the cuff for different age groups?
14. What are the precautions taken for recording blood pressure by the auscultatory method?
15. What is the oscillatory method of measurement of blood pressure?
16. In which condition is the blood pressure measured in the lower limb and what is the size of the cuff used for this purpose?
17. What are the factors that affect blood pressure?
18. Why is the pressure lower in females?
19. Why is the pressure lower during sleep?
20. What is the mechanism of alteration of systolic and diastolic pressure during exercise?

21. What happens to blood pressure on immediately standing from the supine position?
22. What is the baroreceptor reflex and what is its significance?
23. What is essential hypertension?
24. What are the causes of secondary hypertension?
25. What are the causes of acute hypotension?
26. What is postural hypotension and what are the causes of postural hypotension?
27. What are the mechanisms of short-term regulation of blood pressure?
28. Why is bradycardia a feature of raised intracranial pressure?
29. What is the role of the renin–angiotensin system in the genesis of hypertension?

CHAPTER 29

Effect of Posture on Blood Pressure and Heart Rate

Learning Objectives

After completing this practical, you will be able to (MUST KNOW):

1. Record the effect of change in posture on heart rate and blood pressure (BP).
2. List the precautions to be taken while recording this effect.

3. Enumerate the changes in heart rate and BP response to standing.

You may also be able to (DESIRABLE TO KNOW):

1. Explain the compensatory mechanisms in response to standing.
2. Describe the physiological and clinical utility of this practical.

INTRODUCTION

Change in body posture affects the functions of the cardiovascular system. The changes are more marked when a person immediately stands up from the supine posture. The cardiovascular changes are different on immediate standing and on prolonged standing.

Cardiovascular Changes on Immediate Standing

Effect

When a person assumes an erect posture, the blood is pulled to the lower parts of the body due to the effect of gravity. About 200–500 ml of blood is immediately pulled in the capacitance vessels of the lower extremities. This decreases venous return, which results in decreased cardiac output. This is the cause of immediate fall in blood pressure on standing. The effects of a change in posture are more marked if it is done passively with the help of a tilting table, as the muscular activity of the act of standing is absent in passive tilt. The muscle activity after assuming the posture is also lower in passive tilting. The mean arterial pressure in the feet in the standing posture is 180–200 mm Hg and at the head level is 60–80 mm Hg, the venous pressure at feet level is 85–90 mm Hg and at the head level is 0.

Compensatory Mechanisms

The immediate compensatory mechanisms on standing are vasoconstriction, tachycardia and increased cardiac

output. These compensatory mechanisms are triggered by a fall in blood pressure and are mediated by the baroreceptor reflex. Decreased pressure in the carotid and aortic sinus decreases the rate of discharge from the baroreceptors, which in turn decreases stimulation of nucleus tractus solitarius (NTS). This in turn decreases vagal activity and increases sympathetic activity, which results in restoration of blood pressure (Fig. 29.1).

Cardiovascular Changes on Prolonged Standing

Effect

If the individual does not move (stands still) for a longer period, more than 500 ml of blood is pulled in the capacitance vessels of the lower extremities. This increases the capillary hydrostatic pressure in the lower limbs. The fluid from the intravascular compartment moves into the interstitial tissue spaces and accumulates there, as a result of which venous return to the heart significantly decreases. This decreases the stroke volume by up to 40 per cent. Therefore, cardiac output is considerably reduced, which decreases cerebral blood flow. The subject may become unconscious and fall. Fainting is a homeostatic mechanism to restore venous return, cardiac output and cerebral blood flow in the horizontal position by automatic change of posture.

Compensatory Mechanisms

The baroreceptor reflex restores blood pressure to normal. Activation of sympathetic fibres leads

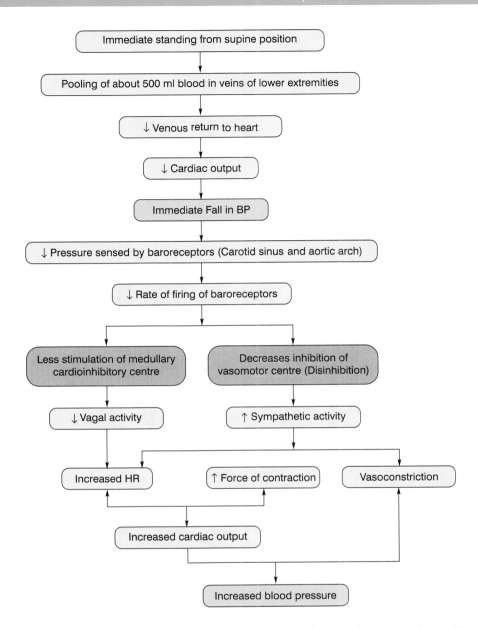

```
Immediate standing from supine position
                    ↓
Pooling of about 500 ml blood in veins of lower extremities
                    ↓
        ↓ Venous return to heart
                    ↓
        ↓ Cardiac output
                    ↓
        Immediate Fall in BP
                    ↓
↓ Pressure sensed by baroreceptors (Carotid sinus and aortic arch)
                    ↓
        ↓ Rate of firing of baroreceptors
```

Less stimulation of medullary cardioinhibitory centre | Decreases inhibition of vasomotor centre (Disinhibition)

↓ Vagal activity | ↑ Sympathetic activity

Increased HR   ↑ Force of contraction   Vasoconstriction

Increased cardiac output

Increased blood pressure

Fig. 29.1   Compensatory mechanisms activated by fall in BP in response to immediate standing from supine position.

to the release of catecholamines from the adrenal medulla. Catecholamines increase heart rate, cardiac output and blood pressure. The renin–angiotensin–aldosterone axis is also activated. Angiotensin II causes vasoconstriction and increases blood pressure. Aldosterone increases reabsorption of sodium and water from the kidneys and maintains blood volume and pressure. But, if the subject continues to stand for a much longer period, the compensatory mechanisms may fail and the subject may develop features of hypotension.

METHODS

Method to Measure the Effect of Posture on Heart Rate and BP

Principle

On resuming an erect posture, changes occur in the cardiovascular function. The change in heart rate and blood pressure is noted immediately on standing and after two, five and ten minutes of standing. These changes are compared with the heart rate and blood pressure recorded in the supine position prior to the change in posture.

Requirements

1. Sphygmomanometer
2. Stethoscope

Procedure

1. Ask the subject to lie down in the supine position on the couch, minimum for 5 minutes.
2. Tie the BP cuff properly at the proper position of the arm of the subject.
3. Record blood pressure and pulse rate in the supine position.
4. Do not remove the BP cuff; ask the subject to stand up, and immediately record the pulse rate and blood pressure of the subject.

> **Note:** The subject should stand with the support of the wall (leaning against the wall) to prevent the effect of muscle–heart reflex. The increase in heart rate due to contraction of skeletal muscles is known as **muscle–heart reflex**. If the subject stands without support, the muscles in the lower limb and trunk contract more, which affects the heart rate. Therefore, maximum possible relaxation should be achieved during the procedure by asking the subject to stand passively.

5. Record pulse rate and blood pressure two, five and ten minutes after standing (alternatively, pulse and BP can also be recorded every 2 min. for 10 min.).
6. Calculate pulse pressure, mean pressure and rate pressure product from the heart rate and blood pressure.
7. Enter your observation in a tabular form.

Observation

Enter your observation in a format as given in Table 29.1. Note that BP falls immediately on standing. Within 15–30 seconds, systolic pressure returns to normal (or remains slightly elevated), but diastolic pressure remains elevated and tachycardia persists.

Precautions

1. The subject should relax for 5 minutes before recording blood pressure and pulse rate in the supine position.
2. Pulse rate and blood pressure should be recorded as soon as the patient stands up (within 15 seconds if possible).

Table 29.1   Change in posture observation.

Posture	PR	SBP	DBP	PP	MP	RPP
Supine (after 5 min)						
On standing:						
1. Immediate						
2. After 2 min						
3. After 5 min						
4. After 10 min						

PR = Pulse rate; SBP = Systolic blood pressure; DBP = Diastolic blood pressure; PP = Pulse pressure; MP = Mean pressure; RPP = Rate pressure product (RPP = systolic pressure $\times$ heart rate $\times$ 10^{-2}).

3. The BP cuff should not be removed while changing the posture of the subject.
4. The subject should stand passively (leaning against the wall).

DISCUSSION

The immediate result of standing is that the cardiac output decreases due to pooling of blood in the lower extremities. Therefore, a fall in blood pressure is noted immediately (if possible within 15 seconds). The fall in pressure (through baroreceptor reflex) results in tachycardia, increased cardiac output and vasoconstriction. Therefore, within 15–30 seconds, the blood pressure reverts to normal. But, because of vasoconstriction, peripheral resistance increases, which in turn increases the diastolic pressure. Heart rate increases and systolic pressure remains normal or slightly raised.

Physiological Significance

A change in posture initiates changes in cardiovascular function, which can be detected by various tests. These changes reflect the integrity of the autonomous nervous system, because the compensatory mechanisms are dependent on the intactness of the reflex activities, especially the baroreceptor reflex. Therefore, the heart rate and blood pressure response to standing is among the important tests to assess autonomic functions. This test detects the efficiency of cardiovascular and autonomic functions.

Clinical Significance

Postural Hypotension

In some individuals, sudden standing causes a significant fall in blood pressure (fall in systolic pressure of more than 20 mm Hg and fall in diastolic pressure of more than 10 mm Hg), which results in fainting. This is called postural or **orthostatic hypotension**. It is usually seen in patients with autonomic neuropathy like diabetes or syphilis. It also occurs in patients receiving sympatholytic drugs. This is also seen in primary autonomic failure and sometimes in primary hyperaldosteronism, because the baroreceptor reflex is abnormal in these conditions.

Therapeutic Uses

Acute changes of postures are part of the practice of different asanas. Regular practice of change of postures (asanas) improves autonomic functions. Persons practising asanas regularly keep good health, as it improves their cardiac, respiratory, neuromuscular, autonomic, mental and physiological functions. Of late, asanas have become popular because of their beneficial effects. Lying down in prone position and asanas in prone posture are known to facilitate the functions of the respiratory apparatus and improve oxygenation.

Problems of Traffic Personnel

Traffic police personnel stand (without activity) for hours together. This causes accumulation of fluid in the lower parts of the body and may cause hypotension and pedal edema, and sometimes results in fainting. Therefore, instead of standing at one place, these people are advised to walk around so that the skeletal muscle pump activity increases the venous return and maintains cardiac output and blood pressure.

OSPE

Record the effect of standing, on blood pressure of the given subject and report your findings.

Steps
1. Give proper instructions to the subject.
2. Expose the arm of the subject.
4. Tie the BP cuff properly (not very tight or very loose) on the arm of the subject in such a way that the middle of the cuff lies over the brachial artery and lower edge of the cuff remains 1 inch above the cubital fossa.
5. Place the chest piece of the stethoscope on the brachial artery just below the cubital fossa, medial to the insertion of the biceps tendon; record systolic and diastolic pressure by appropriately inflating and deflating the pressure in the cuff.
6. Ask the subject to stand up and immediately record systolic and diastolic pressure.
7. Report your findings.

VIVA

1. *What are the physiological changes that occur on suddenly standing up and why?*
2. *What are the physiological changes that occur on prolonged standing and why?*
3. *Why should the pulse rate and blood pressure ideally be recorded within 15 seconds to record the immediate cardiovascular response to standing?*
4. *What is the significance of RPP (rate pressure product)?*
   Ans: As RPP is the product of heart rate and systolic BP, it reflects the myocardial work load. RPP is the index of myocardial oxygen demand and work stress. Chronically elevated RPP is a known cardiovascular risk.
5. *What is the physiological and clinical utility of this practical?*

CHAPTER 30

Effect of Exercise on Blood Pressure and Heart Rate and Cardiac Efficiency Tests

Learning Objectives

After completing this practical, you will be able to (MUST KNOW):

1. Describe the importance of study of the effect of exercise on blood pressure and heart rate.
2. List the types and degrees of exercise.
3. Record the effect of exercise on heart rate and blood pressure.
4. List the precautions of recording this effect.
5. Explain the effects of exercise on heart rate and blood pressure.
6. List the various cardiac efficiency tests for lower limbs and upper limbs.

7. List the indications and contraindications of cardiac efficiency tests.

You may also be able to (DESIRABLE TO KNOW):

1. Explain the differences between isotonic and isometric exercise.
2. Describe and explain the various effects of acute and chronic exercise on different body systems.
3. State the therapeutic uses of exercise in the treatment of lifestyle disorders.
4. Explain the physiological principle and basic methods of treadmill exercise and Master's step test.

EFFECT OF EXERCISE ON BLOOD PRESSURE AND HEART RATE

INTRODUCTION

Regular exercise improves health. Exercise affects all the body systems and improves the functioning of almost all the organs of the body. The body's response to exercise can be a short-term response to an acute exercise or a long-term response to chronic exercise. Long-term response to regular exercise makes the exercise easier and improves performance. What has been described in this chapter is the body's response to acute exercise—the short-term heart rate and blood pressure response to a single bout of exercise (acute exercise). The immediate response to acute exercise depends on the degree and type of exercise, and the exercise training that the individual has received. Exercise training means the regular practice of exercise for months or years together. The cardiovascular response to exercise is different in trained and untrained individuals.

Degree of Exercise

Depending on the rate of oxygen consumption, work done and rate of rise in heart rate, exercise is classified into three categories: mild, moderate and severe. The criteria of **WHO grading of exercises** are given in Table 30.1.

Mild exercise In this case, oxygen consumption is 0.5–1 litre per minute, work done is 150–350 watts, and rise in heart rate is about 25 per cent, that is, if the basal heart rate is 80, the heart rate will increase to about 100 per minute.

Table 30.1 WHO grading of exercise.

Grade (& Level) of Exercise	Heart rate (per minute)	O_2 consumption (L/min)	Relative load index (RLI) (% of maximum O_2 consumption)	Metabolic Equivalent Task (MET)
I (Mild)	<100	0.4–0.8	<25	<3
II (Moderate)	100–125	0.8–1.6	25–50	3.1–4.5
III (Heavy)	125–150	1.6–2.4	51–75	4.6–7
IV (Severe)	>150	>2.4	>75	>7

VO_2 max = Maximum oxygen consumption
MET = Oxygen consumption in multiples of basal oxygen consumption
RLI = Oxygen consumption as a percentage of VO_2 maximum

Moderate exercise In this case, oxygen consumption is 1–2 litres per minute, work done is 350–550 watts and rise in heart rate is about 50 per cent, that is, it rises from a basal heart rate of 80 to 120 per minute.

Severe exercise In this, oxygen consumption is more than 2 litres per minute, work done is more than 550 watts and rise is heart rate is about 75–100 per cent, that is, from a basal heart rate of 80 per minute, it increases to 150 per minute or more.

Types of Exercises

Exercise may be isotonic or isometric. Differences between isotonic and isometric exercises are given in Table 30.2.

Isotonic Exercise

In isotonic exercise, there is a change in muscle length and the exercise is **phasic in nature**. Common examples are walking, jogging and running.

Cardiovascular changes in isotonic exercise

◆ Heart rate increases proportionately with the severity of exercise.

Table 30.2 Differences between isometric and isotonic exercises.

	Isotonic exercise	Isometric exercise
1. Length of muscle	Shortening occurs	Remains same
2. Muscle tension	No change	Tension increases
3. External work	Work is done	No work done
4. Blood pressure	SBP increases moderately Change in DBP varies according to severity of exercise	SBP and DBP rise sharply
5. Cardiac parameters	C.O. increases significantly due to proportionate increase in both HR and SV	Change in SV is relatively less
6. Blood flow to exercising muscle	Blood flow to exercising muscle increases substantially	Blood flow to exercising muscle decreases due to compression of blood vessel by contracting muscle
7. Examples	Walking, jogging, running, cycling, swimming, dancing	Weight lifting (before lifting), pushing against wall

SBP = Systolic blood pressure; DBP = Diastolic blood pressure;
C.O. = Cardiac output; SV = Stroke volume

◆ Cardiac output increases markedly due to increase in heart rate and stroke volume.
◆ Systolic pressure increases.
◆ Diastolic pressure increases in mild exercise, does not change or decreases slightly in moderate exercise and always decreases in severe exercise.
◆ Blood flow to exercising muscle increases.

Isometric Exercise

Isometric exercise is the exercise in which there is no change in the length of the muscles. The exercising muscle remains contracted throughout the maneuver (e.g., pushing against the wall). Therefore, this type of exercise is tonic in nature.

Cardiovascular changes in isometric exercise

◆ Heart rate rises at the start of exercise. This is mainly due to decreased vagal tone. Increased discharge of cardiac sympathetic fibres may also contribute.
◆ Stroke volume changes relatively little.
◆ Systolic and diastolic pressures rise sharply.
◆ Blood flow to the exercising muscle decreases.

The cardiovascular response to isometric exercise is different, because the exercising muscles are tonically contracted during exercise. Peripheral resistance increases, which increases diastolic pressure significantly in isometric exercise.

METHODS

Method to Study the Effects of Exercise on Pulse Rate and BP

Principle

Cardiovascular functions alter during exercise. Pulse rate and blood pressure are recorded before and immediately after the exercise. The results are compared to study the effect of exercise on these parameters.

Requirements

1. Stethoscope
2. Sphygmomanometer

Procedure

1. Record the blood pressure (using sphygmomanometer) and the pulse rate of the given subject after 5 minutes of rest.

2. Ask the subject to perform spot jogging for a period of 5 minutes.

3. Record the pulse rate and blood pressure immediately, 2, 4, 6, 8 and 10 minutes after the exercise.

4. Calculate pulse pressure, mean pressure and rate pressure product and compare the pre- and post-exercise values.

> Note: Rate pressure product = Systolic pressure × Heart rate × 10^{-2}. RPP is a good index of myocardial function.

5. Record your observation in a tabular form.

Observation

Record your observation in the format given in Table 30.3. Note that heart rate and systolic pressure rise significantly immediately after exercise. As 5 minute spot jogging is a mild exercise, diastolic pressure also rises (or may not change). Pulse pressure changes accordingly. Also note that blood pressure returns to normal within 5–7 minutes of termination of exercise, whereas the heart rate takes a longer time to return to normal.

Precautions

1. The pre- and post-exercise heart rate and blood pressure should be recorded in the same position. Note: To eliminate the effect of posture on BP, it should be recorded in the standing position both before and after exercise. If BP is recorded in the supine or sitting posture before exercise, then post-exercise BP should also be recorded in the same position. As exercise is done in the erect posture, it is better to record BP in the standing posture.

2. The subject should be encouraged to exercise properly for five minutes.

3. For the first recording following exercise (immediately after exercise), blood pressure and pulse rate should be recorded as quickly as possible.

DISCUSSION

Effect of Acute Exercise

Cardiovascular Changes

Heart rate Heart rate increases and the degree of increase depends on the severity of the exercise. The maximum heart rate achieved during exercise decreases with age. In children, the heart rate can rise up to 200 beats per minute or more; in adults it seldom rises above this and in elderly subjects, it rarely goes beyond 150.

Cardiac output There occurs a marked increase in cardiac output. Cardiac output may increase even up to 25 litres per minute or more. Increase in cardiac output is due to increase in heart rate and stroke volume.

Systolic blood pressure Systolic pressure rises markedly. This occurs due to increased cardiac output.

Diastolic blood pressure Diastolic pressure may remain unchanged or may fall. This occurs due to decreased peripheral resistance, which is due to vasodilation in the exercising muscle.

Muscle blood flow Blood flow to the skeletal muscle increases due to vasodilation in the skeletal bed. There occurs vasoconstriction in the cutaneous and splanchnic circulation. So, the blood is diverted from the cutaneous and visceral circulation to the skeletal vascular bed.

Physiological Basis of Cardiovascular Changes

◆ **Cardiac output** increases due to increased heart rate and stroke volume. Tachycardia and increased stroke volume occur due to increased activity in the noradrenergic sympathetic nerves

Table 30.3 Exercise observation.

	PR	SBP	DBP	PP	MP	RPP
1. Basal (before exercise)						
2. Immediately after exercise						
3. Two minutes after exercise						
4. Four minutes after exercise						
5. Six minutes after exercise						
6. Eight minutes after exercise						
5. Ten minutes after exercise						

PR = Pulse rate; SBP = Systolic blood pressure; DBP = Diastolic blood pressure; PP = Pulse pressure; MP = Mean pressure; RPP = Rate pressure product.

to the heart. Sympathetic activity increases by psychic stimuli and stimulation of receptors in the muscles, joints and tendons. Inhibition of vagal tone also contributes to tachycardia. **Stroke volume increases** due to increased myocardial contractility by sympathetic stimulation and also due to increased venous return. **Venous return increases** due to sympathetic venoconstriction and increased skeletal muscle pump activity. Increased thoracic pump and mobilisation of blood from the splanchnic and cutaneous beds also contribute to increased venous return.

- The **systolic pressure increases** due to increase in cardiac output.
- The **diastolic pressure increases in mild exercise** due to sympathetic vasoconstriction. But in moderate exercise, diastolic pressure remains normal or falls and **in severe exercise it always falls**. This occurs due to vasodilation in the exercising muscle. The blood vessels in the skeletal vascular bed receive **sympathetic vasodilator fibres**. Therefore, vasodilation occurs in the skeletal bed. In addition, the systemic blood vessels also dilate in severe exercise due to: **(i)** rise in body temperature (thermal vasodilation), and **(ii)** deposition of metabolites like lactic acid, K^+ and CO_2 in the active tissues (metabolic vasodilation). Total peripheral resistance decreases due to vasodilation. Therefore, in spite of increased sympathetic activity diastolic pressure falls during severe exercise.
- **Muscle blood flow increases** to a great extent. This happens even before the start of exercise. The initial increase in blood flow is due to neural mechanisms and continued blood flow is due to local mechanisms. The **neural mechanism** is the activation of the sympathetic vasodilator system and a decrease in tonic vasoconstrictor discharge. The **local mechanisms** are accumulation of metabolites and rise in temperature in the active muscles. Vasodilation opens up many closed capillaries.

Respiratory Changes

- There is hyperventilation and increased oxygen supply to the tissues. Hyperventilation also removes excess CO_2 and heat produced by the active tissues.
- Respiratory minute volume increases linearly with work rate.
- Pulmonary blood flow increases and this increases perfusion of alveoli.

Other Changes

- The body metabolism increases.
- The body temperature increases.
- Catecholamine secretion from the adrenal medulla and glucocorticoid secretion from the adrenal cortex increase.
- Glycogenolysis is stimulated in the liver and skeletal muscles.
- Lipolysis occurs in prolonged aerobic exercise.

Effect of Regular Exercise (Training) on Health

On the Cardiovascular System

There is profound improvement in cardiovascular function. The basal heart rate decreases due to **increased vagal tone**. Stroke volume increases due to increased myocardial muscle mass. **A trained subject** achieves the required cardiac output during exercise mainly by increasing the stroke volume rather than by heart rate, whereas **an untrained individual** achieves the same cardiac output mainly by increasing the heart rate. The blood pressure is usually maintained within the normal range. Hypertension usually does not occur unless associated with some secondary pathology.

Regular exercise decreases cholesterol, TG and LDL and increases HDL. Decrease in bad lipids decreases the process of atherosclerosis and decreases cardiovascular risks in diabetes, hypertension, stroke and other lifestyle disorders.

On the Respiratory System

There is increase in breathing capacity and VO_{2max}. VO_{2max} is the product of maximal cardiac output and maximal oxygen extraction by the tissues. Both these parameters increase with training.

On the Skeletal Muscles

The size of the muscles and work capability increase. The number of mitochondria and the enzymes involved in oxidative metabolism increases. The number of capillaries increases, which increases extraction of oxygen.

On the Mind

Exercise improves memory and intellectual mental functions.

Clinical Significance

Exercise therapy   Exercise is becoming popular nowadays because of its visible therapeutic advantages in lifestyle disorders. It is regularly prescribed as part of treatment for patients suffering from cardiovascular diseases, especially hypertension and myocardial infarction. It has been seen that isotonic exercise (mild to moderate) performed regularly, decreases blood pressure significantly in otherwise resistant cases of hypertension. Exercise also improves cardiac performance in patients suffering from myocardial infarction, and prevents infarction in subjects at risk. Exercise also improves joint functions, and is therefore prescribed in patients suffering from chronic arthritis and degenerative joint diseases.

CARDIAC EFFICIENCY TESTS (OR, EXERCISE STRESS TESTING)

INTRODUCTION

Exercise Stress Testing

Measurements of cardiovascular functions during rest are poor predictors of cardiac performance as there is substantial cardiovascular reserve capacity. Exercise is currently used as the most convenient way of stimulating the myocardium to demand maximal blood flow so that even a moderate impairment of coronary blood flow capacity becomes detectable.

Physiological Basis

Cardiac efficiency tests (exercise tolerance tests or stress testing) are the procedures to assess the response of the cardiovascular system to a standardised exercise schedule. These tests are best methods for assessing the efficiency of the heart functions.

As described in the preceding section of this chapter, during exercise, there is a progressive increase in the heart rate and blood pressure and after the exercise is over, these parameters return back to the pre-exercise levels in few minutes. Thus, the ability to attain a peak rise and the magnitude of rise, and the ability to recover and the speed of recovery determine the cardiac efficiency of the individual. Therefore, these tests are called cardiac efficiency tests.

In a trained person, there is a greater increase in the HR and BP than in an untrained individual. During exercise, these values take a longer time to basal levels. This forms the basis of exercise tolerance tests. The response to physical exercise depends on the cardiac reserve (i.e., efficiency of the myocardial performance), skeletal muscle power, level of training, state of motivation and the status of nutrition. Hence, the cardiac efficiency tests are often used to assess physical fitness in an individual during recruitments to army, police force, fire-arm jobs, etc.

Indications for exercise testing
1. Evaluation of patients with chest pain.
2. Evaluation of functional capacity of the heart.
3. Evaluation of patients after myocardial infarction.
4. Evaluation of patients after coronary artery by-pass surgery.
5. Screening for latent coronary artery disease.
6. Evaluation of patients with valvular heart disease.
7. Evaluation of arrhythmias.

Contraindications to stress test
1. Impending or acute myocardial infarction
2. Unstable angina
3. Severe hypertension
4. Congestive heart failure
5. Severe aortic stenosis
6. Uncontrolled arrhythmias

METHODS

Basic Principle

The patient is made to exercise to 90% of his estimated maximal heart rate. The maximal heart rate is calculated from the age, sex, and physical training of the subject. The cardiac efficiency is tested by analysing the patient's ability to achieve the **target heart rate**.

The types of exercise stress testing can be divided into two broad categories: the dynamic lower extremity testing, and the dynamic upper extremity testing.

The lower extremity tests include treadmill, bicycle ergometry, and Master's step test and upper extremity testing includes arm ergometry.

Dynamic Lower Extremity Testing

1. Treadmill   Treadmill testing is a most widely used method for exercise testing. This includes simultaneous recordings of multiple leads of ECG in a computerised treadmill. The person exercises **until he achieves his target heart rate** or is unable to continue because of chest pain, dyspnea and intolerable fatigue. There are different protocols like Bruce protocol, Naughton protocol, and Balke and Ware protocol. In different protocols analyses of the heart rate achievement is different.

2. Bicycle ergometry This is used when a patient is unable to do treadmill exercise. It is the method of choice during radionuclide ventriculography and for dynamic testing during cardiac catheterisation.

3. Master's step test / Harvard step test

Procedure of Computerised Treadmill Testing

Requirements

Heavy-duty treadmill (e.g., GE T2100), computer system with requisite software (Cardiosoft), exercise ECG monitoring system (CAM 32), exercise blood pressure monitoring system (Suntech Tango), emergency resuscitation cart and trolley, couch for pre- and post-exercise recordings, sphygmomanometer and stethoscope (Fig. 30.1). Room temperature to be maintained at 20–22°C, consent forms and data sheets should be filled for recording all physiological parameters.

Personnel requirements Exercise Physiologist, General Physician (at least with MBBS degree), Multi-purpose Lab technician.

Pre-test Procedure

1. Instruct the participants to refrain from ingesting food, alcohol, caffeine, tobacco within 3 hours of testing and to avoid significant exertion or exercise on the day of the assessment.

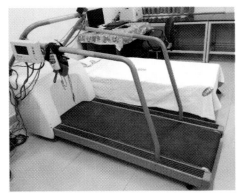

Fig. 30.1 The treadmill machine with all accessories. (*Courtesy*: CV Research Lab, JIPMER, Puducherry, India.)

2. Obtain a written informed consent from the participant explaining the entire procedure.

3. Obtain a thorough medical history, general physical examination, laboratory tests if required (blood glucose, lipid profile).

4. Record anthropometric parameters (height, weight, MBI).

5. Resting supine heart rate and blood pressure measurements, resting ECG recording, heart rate and blood pressure recording after five minutes of assuming standing posture.

Exercise Testing and Protocols

Computerised Treadmill Exercise stress ECG testing of healthy individuals is used to assess their cardio-respiratory fitness (CRF) by estimating their maximal oxygen consumption (VO_{2max}). This is based on the principle that the **heart rate response** of a healthy person subjected to a graded exercise of incremental work output, shows a linear relationship with his/her VO_{2max}. A graded exercise of incremental work output is devised in a treadmill by sequentially increasing the **treadmill speed and inclination**. The basic aim of graded exercise testing (GXT) is to determine the heart rate response of the subject to the given workload and use the total test duration result in validated prediction equations to predict VO_{2max}. Both maximal and sub-maximal intensity of GXT using treadmill can be performed to assess the CRF, however, maximal GXT provides a better estimate of VO_{2max}. The decision to use a maximal or sub-maximal exercise test depends largely on the reasons for the test, risk level of the client/patient, and availability of appropriate equipment and personnel.

The most commonly used GXT protocols are:

1. Bruce protocol In this protocol, the participant is subjected to a graded exercise of incremental stages (of treadmill speed and inclination), each lasting three minutes or until achieving steady state.

2. Modified Bruce protocol This protocol is similar to Bruce Protocol except for two additional stages of lesser workload at the start. This protocol is suitable for older individuals.

3. Bruce ramp protocol In this protocol, the incremental graded stages are of twenty seconds duration, thereby, providing no room for achieving steady state conditions.

Treadmill testing provides a familiar form of exercise and, if the correct protocol is chosen, can accommodate the least physically fit to the fittest individuals across the continuum of walking to running speeds. Nevertheless, a practice session might be necessary in some cases to permit habituation and reduce anxiety. Treadmills must be calibrated to ensure the accuracy of the test. In addition, holding on to the support rails should be discouraged to ensure accuracy of metabolic work output, particularly when VO_{2max} is estimated as opposed to directly measured. Extensive handrail use often leads to significant overestimation of VO_{2max}.

Expected cardiovascular changes during graded exercise

◆ Increase in heart rate, stroke volume, cardiac output, systolic blood pressure, mean arterial pressure and rate pressure product (RPP).
◆ Diastolic blood pressure usually shows an unequivocal response.
◆ Decrease in total peripheral resistance.

Normal ECG response to exercise

1. Minor and insignificant changes in P wave morphology.
2. Superimposition of the P and T waves of successive beats.
3. Increases in septal Q wave amplitude.
4. Slight decreases in R wave amplitude.
5. Increases in T wave amplitude (although wide variability exists among clients/patients).
6. Minimal shortening of the QRS duration.
7. Depression of the J point.
8. Rate-related shortening of the QT interval.

Exercise test termination criteria (ACSM criteria)

1. **Onset of angina** or angina-like symptoms
2. **Drop in SBP** of ≥ 10 mm Hg with an increase in work rate or if SBP decreases below the value obtained in the same position prior to testing
3. **Excessive rise in BP**: systolic pressure > 250 mm Hg and/or diastolic pressure > 115 mm Hg
4. **Shortness of breath**, wheezing, leg cramps, or claudication
5. **Signs of poor perfusion**: light-headedness, confusion, ataxia, pallor, cyanosis, nausea, or cold and clammy skin
6. **Failure of HR to increase** with increased exercise intensity

7. Noticeable change in heart rhythm by palpation or auscultation
8. Subject requests to stop
9. Physical or verbal manifestations of severe fatigue
10. Failure of the testing equipment

Post-test procedure

Post-exercise monitoring should continue in supine position for at least 6 min after exercise or until ECG changes return to baseline and significant signs and symptoms resolve. **ST-segment changes** that occur only during the post-exercise period are currently recognised to be an **important diagnostic part of the test**. HR and BP should also return to near baseline levels before discontinuation of monitoring.

Data Collection and Interpretation

At the end of the procedure, we arrive at the following data: Pre-exercise heart rate and blood pressure after five minutes supine rest and after five minutes of assuming standing posture, Maximal heart rate, Maximal RPP, Total treadmill exercise test time, Derived VO_{2max}, Cumulative METs (Metabolic Equivalents of Task), Cumulative Work Output achieved, Recovery heart rate and blood pressure.

VO_2 is calculated using the following formula:

$$\mathbf{VO_2} = HC + VC + RMR$$

where, HC (Horizontal component) = speed of the treadmill × 0.1,
VC (Vertical component) = speed of the treadmill × 1.8 x grade,
RMR (Resting metabolic rate) = 3.5 ml/kg/min.
Calculation of METs is given by the formula:

$$METs = VO2 / 3.5.$$

Cumulative METs is the METs calculated for each stage and successively added to the calculated METs value of the subsequent stage and this is continued until end of test.

Work output of exercise is calculated using the formula:

Work Output = body weight (kg) × vertical displacement (m) × total time (min)
where,
vertical displacement = percentage grade × speed of the treadmill m/min).

The work output is calculated for each stage and successively added to the calculated work output of the subsequent stage and this is continued until end of test.

Master's Step Test / Harvard Step Test

This method of exercise testing is routinely practiced in clinical physiology labs. In this, the subject walks up and down over a device (Master's step device / Harvard step device). Master's device is two steps high with total three steps, two of which are 9 inches above the floor and a top step 18 inches high (Fig. 30.2). The exercise is carried out for a prescribed number of ascents. The workload achieved in this test is usually too low to be of any significant clinical use. Therefore, after the advent of treadmill and bicycle ergometer, this method of exercise testing has lost its popularity and is seldom used in clinical set-ups now.

▌ Procedure

Record the basal pulse rate, then ask the subject to hop on each foot alternatively climbing on to each step. The subject steps on and off the steps 13 times a minute and the pulse rate is noted. The time of recovery is about 5 minutes. The test also used to be repeated with stepping rates of 18 or 24 times a minute, depending on the physical ability of the subject. If the heart is healthy, there should be little disturbance of breathing

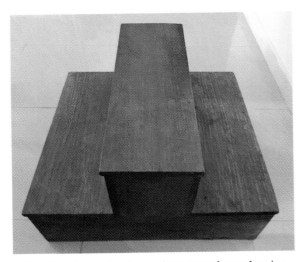

Fig. 30.2 Wooden device having three steps for performing Master's step test. Note that the two side steps are 9 inches high and the central step is 18 inches high.

and the pulse rate should not increase more than 10–20 beats per minute. The pulse rate should return to pre-exercise level in about a minute. Alternatively, Harvard step test is used.

Cardiac efficiency index is calculated by following formula.

$$\frac{\text{Duration of exercise in seconds (300)}}{\text{Sum of heart rate during the testing}} \times 100$$

In normal individuals, the cardiac efficiency index is nearly 100%, but is more in sports persons.

Efficiency index

Over 90%	Excellent.
81–90%	Good.
55–80%	Average.
Below 55%	Poor.

▌ Dynamic Upper Extremity Testing

▌ Arm Ergometry

This is sometimes used in patients with peripheral vascular disease or in orthopedic abnormalities. Arm ergometry is less sensitive than leg ergometry for eliciting exercise-induced ischemia.

Arm ergometry is done using **Mosso's ergograph** or **hand dynamometer** (details are described in Chapter 33).

DISCUSSION

▌ Exercise Test Response

Exercise responses are mainly assessed by ECG changes. When the heart rate increases with exercise, a number of predictable changes occur in normal ECG. The PR interval shortens, the P wave becomes taller, and the atrial repolarisation rate becomes prominent causing depression of PQ segment. This results in J point (junction between S wave and ST segment) depression, which is usually of short duration. The ST segment becomes upsloping and slightly convex and returns to baseline within 0.04 second after the J point. The abnormal changes in ECG are analysed with recordings obtained before, during and after the termination of the test and interpreted accordingly.

VIVA

1. What are the various types of exercise?
2. How do you determine the severity of exercise?
3. What are the differences between isotonic and isometric exercise?
4. What are the cardiovascular responses to acute exercise?
5. What are the causes of increased cardiac output in exercise?
6. What is the cause of systolic rise in blood pressure in exercise?
7. Why does diastolic pressure not change or decrease in moderate to severe exercise?
8. Why does heart rate take more time than blood pressure to come back to normal level following exercise?

    Ans: Heart rate increases in exercise due to increased sympathetic activity. Sympathetic activity takes time to return to normal, therefore the heart normalises slowly. BP returns to normal in 5–7 minutes due to muscle relaxation with stoppage of exercise, which produces vasodilation.

9. What are the effects of exercise on the respiratory system?
10. What are the benefits of performing regular exercise?
11. List the indications and contraindications for exercise stress testing.
12. Name the dynamic tests for upper extremity and lower extremity testing.
13. How is the exercise stress response interpreted?

CHAPTER 31

Nerve Conduction Study

INTRODUCTION

Nerve conduction study (NCS) is part of the electrodiagnostic procedures that help in establishing the type and degree of abnormalities of the nerves. NCS establishes diagnosis very early and more accurately then other electrodiagnostic techniques because of its sensitivity in detecting conduction slowing (or block), which is an early indicator of nerve entrapment or peripheral neuropathy, the problems most frequently encountered in neurology clinics. The principle of NCS is simple: apply shock at one point of the nerve and record the signal from another. But the complexity of NCS lies in the clinical application and interpretation of results. To interpret the result of nerve conduction studies, one should know the anatomical course of the nerve, the muscle supplied by the nerve, the normal conduction velocity of the nerve, the physiologic basis of the conduction of impulse in the nerves, the pathophysiologic responses of the nerve and muscle to dysfunction and the biological electrical signals.

Anatomical and Physiological Aspects

The conduction velocity of the nerve depends **on the fibre diameter, degree of myelination and the internodal distance**. As the axon increases in size, the myelin sheath becomes thicker and the internodal distance becomes longer. The conduction therefore becomes faster. The diameter of the nerve axons varies between 0.2 and 20 μ. The nerve fibres are classified as **myelinated and unmyelinated**. The myelinated axons are surrounded by Schwann cells, but there is no Schwann sheath in unmyelinated fibres. The junction between two Schwann cells is known as the node of Ranvier, where the axons remain uninsulated. The **internodal distance**, which is the distance between the two nodes of Ranvier, depends on the spacing of Schwann cells at the time of myelination during development. Proliferation of Schwann cells does not occur afterwards, but the internodal distance increases during the growth of the nerve. Thus, **the fibres myelinated early have a longer internodal distance, larger diameter and wider spacing** at the nodes of Ranvier.

Nerve fibres are classified into **groups A, B and C** depending on the fibre diameter (Table 31.1). **Group A fibres** contain both afferent and efferent myelinated somatic fibres of small, medium and large diameter (1–20 μ). They are subclassified into α, β, γ and δ in the order of descending diameter and conduction velocity. **Group B fibres** consist only of small preganglionic myelinated axons of the autonomous nervous system (1–3 μ). **Group C fibres** consist of small unmyelinated fibres, which are present in visceral afferents, pain and temperature afferents and preganglionic autonomic efferents (2–2.2 μm).

Impulse Conduction

The action potential originated in the axons is propagated in either direction from its site of origin. The conduction is continuous in unmyelinated and

Table 31.1   Classification of nerve fibres.

Fibre types	Fibre diameter (μm)	Conduction velocity (m/s)	Function
Aα	12–20	70–120	Somatic motor and proprioception
Aβ	5–12	30–70	Touch—pressure
Aγ	3–6	15–30	Motor to muscle spindle
Aα	2–5	12–30	Pain, cold and touch
B	< 3	3–15	Autonomic preganglionic fibres
C-dorsal root fibre	0.4–1.2	0.5–2	Somatic sensations
C-sympathetic fibre	0.3–1.3	0.7–2.3	Postganglionic sympathetic fibres

saltatory in myelinated fibres.

Myelinated Fibres

Conduction is much faster in myelinated fibres than in unmyelinated fibres. Myelin thickness is inversely related to internodal capacitance and conductance. Therefore, **conduction velocity increases** with increasing myelin in the axon.

As the myelin sheath becomes thinner, the internodal conductance and capacitance increase in conditions of **segmental demyelination or during remyelination**. This causes greater loss of local current before reaching the next node of Ranvier and fails to activate the nodes of Ranvier. This results in a **conduction block**. The segmental demyelination of smaller fibres may result in continuous conduction instead of saltatory conduction.

Unmyelinated Fibres

Impulse conduction in unmyelinated fibres is **much slower** than in myelinated fibres. The conduction velocity is slow due to the continuous nature of conduction. The conduction velocity further slows down in conditions of focal compression, which may occur due to demyelination or decrease in the diameter of the fibres.

Factors That Affect Nerve Conduction

A number of physiological and technical factors can influence the result of nerve conduction studies.

Physiological Factors

1. Temperature   Nerve temperature is the single most important factor that affects conduction velocity. The nerve conduction velocity is **directly related to intraneuronal temperature** which in turn depends on internal body temperature. Five per cent increase in conduction velocity occurs per degree Celsius rise of body temperature, from 30°C to 40°C. Conversely, a low temperature decreases the conduction velocity. For each degree Celsius fall in temperature, the latency increases by 0.3 ms and velocity decreases by 2.4 m/s. The change in conduction velocity due to alteration in body temperature is attributed to the effect of temperature on sodium channels in the nerves. Therefore, the laboratory temperature should ideally be maintained between 20°C and 25°C.

2. Age   Age significantly affects nerve conduction. The conduction velocity of nerves is **low in infants and children**. In neonates, it is nearly half of the adult values. It **attains the adult value by three to five years of age**, then remains relatively stable until sixty years of age, after which it starts declining at a rate of 1.5 per cent per decade. This is related to gradual loss of larger neurons with ageing.

3. Height   An **inverse relationship** exists between the height of the individual and the velocity of nerve conduction. This is because the shorter nerves conduct faster than the longer nerves of the same age group. **In tall subjects**, distal conduction slowing occurs due to greater axonal tapering and lesser myelination. Tall individuals are also subjected to more loss of large-sized axons with ageing because of higher metabolic stress related to supplying the more distal axon.

4. Limb   In the upper limb, conduction velocity is higher; this too is attributed to the length of the nerves.

The **factors that contribute** to the difference in conduction velocity of nerves between the upper and lower limbs are:

◆ Abrupt distal axonal tapering in the lower limbs.
◆ Shorter internodal distance in the lower limbs.
◆ Progressive reduction in axonal diameter in the lower limbs.
◆ Lower temperature of the feet compared to hands.

5. Gender   Gender is known to affect nerve conduction. In general, nerve conduction is more in males.

Technical Factors

Technical factors that affect nerve conduction may be due to a defect in the stimulating system or due to a defect in the recording system.

Stimulating system   Failure of the stimulating system may result in small responses or no response.

1. Faulty location of stimulator   The stimulator may be placed wrongly on the skin surface or the nerve may be stimulated submaximally. In such cases, the stimulator should be relocated close to the nerve and pressed firmly.
2. Fat or edema between stimulator and nerve: In some situations like obesity or edema, needle electrodes may be used, as the impulse may not reach the target properly.
3. Bridge formation between anode and cathode: An important source of failure of the stimulating systems, is the shunting of current between anode and cathode either by sweat or the formation of a bridge by the conducting jelly.

Recording system   Results may be erroneous if the recording system is defective, especially if the connection is faulty.

1. *Damage in the electrode wire*   The intactness of the recording system is tested by asking the subject to contract the muscle with the electrode in position. If there is a damage in the cable, the stimulus-induced muscle twitches cause movement-related potentials.
2. *Incorrect position of active or reference electrode*   An initial positivity preceding the peak of compound muscle action potential suggests incorrect positioning of the active electrode. The recorded potential is also distorted if the reference electrode is located in an active rather than a remote region in relation to muscle action potential.
3. *Wrongly connected preamplifier/Wrong settings of gain, sweep or filter*   Amplifier filters can change all the components (amplitude, latency and duration) of the recorded response.

METHODS

Method of Nerve Conduction Study

Principle

A nerve conduction study requires an external stimulation that initiates depolarisation simultaneously in all the axons of the nerve to produce a recordable response. The response is recorded by stimulating the nerve at two different points. Conduction velocity is determined by studying the difference in latencies of the responses, compared with the distance between the two points. Nerve conduction study involves the study of motor and sensory conduction.

Principles of motor nerve conduction

The measurement of motor nerve conduction study includes onset of latency, duration and amplitude of **compound muscle action potential (CMAP)** and nerve conduction velocity. The onset of latency is the time in ms from the stimulus artifact to the first negative deflection of CMAP (Fig. 31.1). This is achieved by stimulating the nerve at least at two points along its course. The motor nerve conduction velocity is calculated by measuring the **distance between two points of stimulation in mm, which is divided by the latency difference in ms** (Fig. 31.2). The nerve conduction velocity is expressed as m/s.

Principles of sensory nerve conduction

Similar to the motor nerve conduction study, the sensory nerve conduction measurement includes onset latency, amplitude, duration of **sensory nerve action potential (SNAP)** and nerve conduction velocity. Sensory nerve conduction can be measured orthodromically or antidromically. **In orthodromic conduction, a distal portion of the nerve, for example, digital nerve** is stimulated and SNAP is recorded at a proximal point along the nerve. **In antidromic sensory nerve**

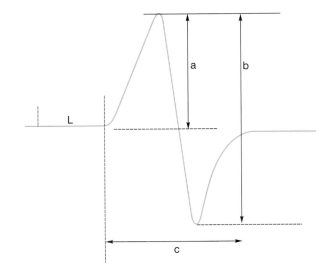

Fig. 31.1   Compound muscle action potential (CMAP) (L: Latency; a: Base-to-peak amplitude; b: Peak-to-peak amplitude; c: Duration of CMAP).

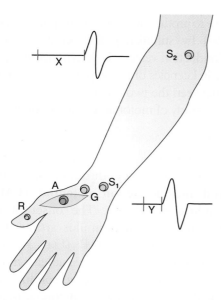

Fig. 31.2   Principle of motor neuron conduction. The conduction velocity is calculated by dividing the distance between the proximal (S2) and distal (S1) stimulating electrodes by the difference in the proximal (X) and distal latency (Y) (R: Reference electrodes; G: Ground electrode; A: Active recording electrode).

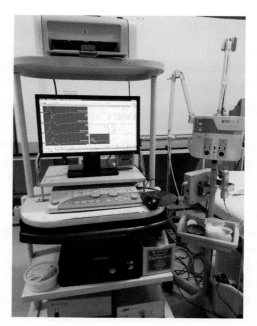

Fig. 31.3   Nerve conduction machine (preamplifier and oscilloscope). (*Courtesy:*   EP-EMG Lab, Physiology Department, JIPMER, Puducherry, India.).

conduction, the nerve is stimulated at a proximal point and the nerve action potential is recorded distally. The latency of orthodromic potential is measured from the stimulus artifact to the initial positive or subsequent negative peak. The **initial positive peak in SNAP having a triphasic appearance** is a feature of orthodromic potential. In antidromic potential, the initial positivity in SNAP is absent. The sensory conduction velocity is calculated by **dividing the distance (mm) between the stimulating and the recording site by the latency (ms)**. The **amplitude of SNAP** suggests the density of nerve fibres whereas the **duration** suggests the number of slow-conducting fibres.

Requirements

1.   Stimulator
2.   Stimulating and recording electrodes
3.   Preamplifier and oscilloscope of nerve conduction machine (Fig. 31.3).
4.   Electrode jelly
5.   Spirit

Procedure

1.   Clean the area and the skin overlying the nerve with spirit at the proximal and the distal ends.

2.   Fix the cup electrode on the skin overlying the muscle supplied by the nerve.
3.   Connect the electrodes to the oscilloscope through the preamplifier.
4.   Keep the sweep at 5 ms/cm.
5.   With the help of stimulating electrodes, stimulate the nerve first at the distal end (Fig. 31.4A) and observe the action potential on the oscilloscope.

Note: The stimulus artifact, which is due to current leak, appears at the beginning of the sweep. This is useful for noting the point of stimulus. The latent period is measured as the interval between the beginning of the stimulus artifact and the first deflection of the muscle potential.

6.   Then, stimulate the nerve at the proximal end and record the action potential (Fig. 31.4B). Note the latent period.

Note: The difference between the two latent periods gives the time taken by the impulse to travel from the proximal point to the distal point.

7.   Measure the distance between the points of stimulation.
8.   Measure the latent period of both distal and proximal action potentials (Fig. 31.5).
9.   Calculate the conduction velocity in m/s by the formula:

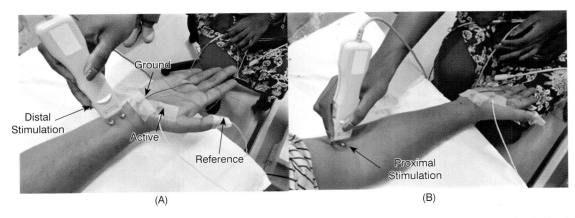

Fig. 31.4   Procedure of nerve conduction study. (A) Median nerve, stimulation of distal end; (B) Median nerve, proximal stimulation.

$$\text{Conduction velocity} = \frac{\text{Distance}}{\text{Difference in latent periods}}$$

Observation

Express the nerve conduction velocity in metres per second (m/s). In the recording shown in Fig. 31.5, the conduction velocity of the median nerve is 55.9 m/s. This is a normal nerve conduction report.

Precautions

1. The subject should be properly instructed and motivated to provide full cooperation.
2. The subject should be fully relaxed.
3. The room should be quiet and comfortable.
4. The subject should be grounded properly.

DISCUSSION

Recording of nerve conduction study is ordered in neurological practice to assess the velocity of conduction of impulses in the nerve. The important nerves tested are median, ulnar, radial nerves and brachial plexus in the upper limbs, and sciatic, femoral, common peroneal, tibial and sural nerves in the lower limbs.

Median Nerve

The median nerve (C5–T1) is a mixed nerve. It supplies the flexors of the forearm and the thenar muscles of the hand. It is sensory to the lateral aspect of the palm and the dorsal surface of the terminal phalanges. It has no innervation in the upper arm. In the forearm it supplies pronator teres, flexor carpi radialis, palmaris longus, flexor digitorum superficialis, flexor digitorum profundus, flexor pollicis longus and pronator quadratus. The nerve then passes through the carpal tunnel to enter the hand, where it supplies lumbricals I and II, opponens pollicis, flexor pollicis brevis and abductor pollicis brevis.

Median Entrapment Neuropathy

The entrapment (compression) neuropathy of the median nerve occurs commonly during its course in the carpal tunnel. In fact, the **carpal tunnel syndrome** is the **commonest entrapment neuropathy** seen in a neurology clinic. Pronator teres syndrome of the median nerve (entrapment of the nerve between the heads of the pronator teres, through which the nerve descends into the forearm from the arm) also occurs occasionally.

In these syndromes, the conduction of the median nerve decreases. The nerve conduction decreases distal to the site of compression.

Causes of Carpal Tunnel Syndrome

The common causes of carpal tunnel syndrome are:
- Rheumatoid arthritis
- Overuse of wrist (too much computer work)
- Hypothyroidism
- Acromegaly

Ulnar Nerve

The ulnar nerve arises from C7–T1 through the medial cord of the brachial plexus. It does not supply

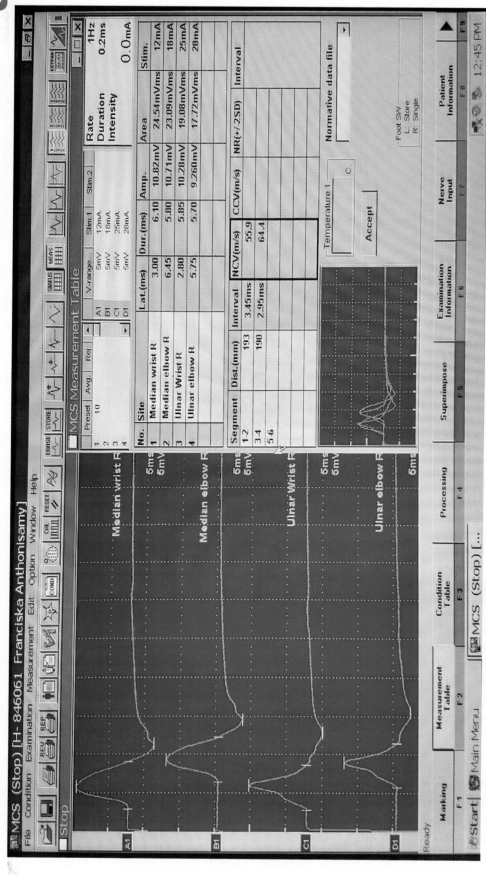

Fig. 31.5   Recording of CMAP of median nerve at distal end (A1 tracing); CMAP of median nerve at proximal end (B1 tracing); CMAP of ulnar nerve at distal end (C1 tracing); CMAP of ulnar nerve at proximal end (D1 tracing). Note the details of the values for latency, duration, amplitude and conduction velocity for each nerve on the right side of the recording display (CMAP: Compound muscle (nerve) action potential).

any muscle in the upper arm. It passes through the condylar groove in the elbow, to enter the forearm where it passes through the cubital tunnel. Here it supplies the flexor carpi ulnaris. Then it supplies the flexor digitorum profundus III and IV. At the wrist, it passes through Guyon's cannal where it bifurcates to form a superficial sensory and a deep motor branch. The motor branch supplies hypothenar muscles and abductor pollicis, medial half of flexor pollicis, interosseous and third and fourth lumbricals.

Ulnar Neuropathy

Ulnar nerve neuropathy can occur at the elbow, the distal forearm, and wrist.

Ulnar nerve lesion at the elbow

There are two vulnerable sites for lesion of the ulnar nerve in the elbow: the condylar groove and the cubital tunnel.

At condylar groove
◈ Repeated pressure
◈ Fracture of ulna
◈ Leprosy

At cubital tunnel
◈ Arthritis
◈ Ganglion

Ulnar nerve lesion in the distal forearm

The ulnar nerve in the distal forearm can be damaged by trauma or chronic repetitive ergonomic stress. It is usually associated with median and radial nerve involvement. The ulnar nerve may be compressed in the middle of the upper arm by the head during sleeping.

Ulnar nerve lesion at the wrist

1. **Lesion proximal to the branch to hypothenar muscles** This produces profound weakness of interossei and lumbricals, which is associated with mild hypothenar weakness. The sensations remain normal.
2. **Lesion distal to the branch to hypothenar muscles** This causes weakness of interossei and lumbricals, but not of the hypothenar muscles. The sensation remains normal.
3. **Lesion before the division of the superficial and deep branches** A lesion at this site causes weakness of the intrinsic muscles of the hand supplied by the ulnar nerve and impairment of sensation in the area of distribution of the superficial branch.
4. **Lesion of the superficial branch of the ulnar nerve** There is impairment of sensations in the areas supplied by the superficial branch. The motor conduction remains normal.

Radial Nerve

The posterior cord of the brachial plexus extends as the radial nerve. It has the root value of C5–T1. It supplies the triceps and then descends down in the spiral groove of the humerus. It supplies the brachioradialis and extensor carpi radialis and longus. In the proximal part of the forearm, it divides into the posterior interosseous and superficial radial nerves. The posterior interosseous nerve supplies the supinator, abductor pollicis longus, extensor carpi ulnaris, extensor digitorum, extensor digiti minimi, extensor pollicis longus and extensor indices. The superficial cutaneous nerve supplies the dorsum of the hand.

Radial Neuropathy

A lesion of the radial nerve causes wrist drop. The radial nerve may be affected in the axilla, behind humerus (retrohumeral), proximal forearm or distal forearm.

In axilla Lesion of radial nerve in the axilla usually occurs due to compression during sleep. There is weakness in all the muscles supplied by the radial nerve, including the triceps. The motor and sensory nerve conduction of the radial nerve reveals abnormality.

Retrohumeral lesion This is the commonest form of radial nerve palsies. It occurs due to compression as in Saturday night paralysis or following general anaesthesia.

In proximal forearm The posterior interosseous nerve is involved in the lesion of the radial nerve in the proximal forearm. Posterior interosseous nerve is a pure motor nerve. There is weakness in the extensors of the wrist and metacarpophalangeal joints. Motor conduction study reveals reduced CMAP. The radial sensory conduction remains normal.

In distal forearm This affects the superficial sensory nerve. Therefore, it results in pure sensory loss in the distribution of radial nerve. Motor conduction remains normal.

Brachial Plexus

The brachial plexus (C5–T1) carry the fibres that provide motor and sensory supply of the shoulder girdle, upper trunk and upper limb. It has two trunks (suprascapular and subclavian) and three cords (medial, posterior and lateral). The medial cord gives rise to the medial pectoral, the medial cutaneous nerve of the arm, and the medial cutaneous nerve of the forearm. The posterior cord gives rise to the superior subscapular, thoracodorsal and inferior subscapular nerves. The lateral cord forms the lateral pectoral nerve. The terminal branches of the brachial plexus form the musculocutaneous, axillary, radial, median and ulnar nerves.

Nerve conduction in the brachial plexus can be measured by stimulating at Erb's point. The **F waves** have been used in assessing conduction in the proximal portion of the nerves, plexus or roots. The brachial plexus is involved in brachial neuritis, thoracic outlet compression syndrome, radiation induced plexopathy, and the obstetric and congenital brachial plexus palsy in newborns.

Femoral Nerve

The femoral nerve has the root value of L2–4. It innervates the extensors of the knee. It carries sensation from the anteromedial thigh, medial leg and foot. In its intraabdominal course, it supplies the iliopsoas muscle. It emerges from the pelvis under the inguinal ligament and divides into the anterior and posterior branches. The anterior division supplies the anterior and medial thigh, and the posterior division supplies the knee and hip joint and quadriceps muscle and terminates as the saphenous nerve.

Femoral Neuropathy

Causes

1. Diabetes mellitus
2. Vertebral tumours
3. Compression of inguinal ligament during prolonged surgery in lithotomy position

In femoral neuropathy, the motor conduction abnormalities include decreased conduction velocity and small CMAP amplitude. Compression at the level of the inguinal ligament results in conduction block which can be detected by stimulating the femoral nerve above and below the inguinal ligament and comparing the CMAP.

Saphenous Nerve

This is a purely sensory nerve. It is the largest and longest branch of the femoral nerve. Any lesion of the saphenous nerve, which occurs in laceration injuries or during surgery for varicose veins, results in sensory impairment in the medial aspect of the knee, leg and foot. There is no defect in motor conduction.

Sciatic Nerve

The sciatic nerve is the largest nerve of the body. It has medial and lateral trunks. The medial trunk below the popliteal fossa continues as the tibial nerve and the lateral trunk continues as the common peroneal nerve. Sciatic neuropathy commonly results from fracture dislocation of the hip joint, hip replacement surgery, prolonged compression during anaesthesia or sitting in an awkward position, or sometimes during gluteal injection. Electrophysiological evaluation involves motor conduction studies of the peroneal and posterior tibial, and sensory conduction of the sural and superficial peroneal nerve.

Common Peroneal Nerve

The common peroneal nerve winds around the neck of the fibula and descends down to divide into the superficial and deep peroneal nerves. The superficial peroneal nerve innervates the peroneus longus and peroneus brevis, and then supplies the lateral and dorsal portion of the lower leg and dorsum of the foot. The deep peroneal nerve supplies the muscles of the anterior compartment.

Common Causes of Common Peroneal Nerve Lesions

Neuropathy usually occurs due to compression of the common peroneal nerve as it winds around the fibula. It usually occurs in:

1. Plaster cast
2. Tight bandage
3. Fracture neck of fibula
4. Habitual crossing of legs

Nerve conduction studies reveal defects in both motor and sensory conduction.

Tibial Nerve

This is the continuation of the medial trunk of the sciatic nerve below the popliteal fossa. It supplies both heads of the gastrocnemius, soleus and tibialis posterior muscle. It descends and passes through the tarsal tunnel and supplies the intrinsic foot muscles.

Tibial Neuropathy

The tibial nerve is frequently affected in leprosy. Lesion of the tibial nerve results in the weakness of plantar flexors, invertors and intrinsic foot muscles. The nerve is also involved in tarsal tunnel syndrome.

Nerve conduction reveals impairment in both motor and sensory conduction. The tarsal tunnel syndrome is diagnosed by demonstrating a conduction block and latency prolongation across the tarsal tunnel.

Sural Nerve

The sural nerve is the root value of S_1 and S_2. It is derived from both the tibial and peroneal nerves. It is a purely sensory nerve. It innervates the posterolateral part of the distal leg and the lateral aspect of the foot. In sural neuropathy, there is abnormality in sensory conduction.

VIVA

1. *What is the importance of nerve conduction study in clinical medicine?*
2. *How does myelination affect conduction velocity of the nerves?*
3. *How do you classify nerve fibres?*
4. *What are the factors that affect nerve conduction?*
5. *What is the principle of nerve conduction?*
6. *What is the course and innervation of the median nerve?*
7. *What are the common sites and causes of median neuropathy?*
8. *What are the effects of median neuropathy at different sites?*
9. *What is the course and innervation of the ulnar nerve?*
10. *What are the common sites and effects of ulnar neuropathy?*
11. *What are the effects of ulnar neuropathy at different sites?*
12. *What is the course and innervation of the radial nerve?*
13. *What are the common sites and causes of radial neuropathy?*
14. *What are the effects of radial neuropathy at different sites?*
15. *What is the course and innervation of the femoral nerve?*
16. *What is the common site of lesion of the femoral nerve?*
17. *What are the causes and effects of femoral neuropathy?*
18. *What is the course and innervation of the common peroneal nerve?*
19. *What are the common sites and causes of common peroneal neuropathy?*
20. *What are the effects of common peroneal neuropathy?*
21. *What is the course and innervation of the tibial nerve?*
22. *What are the common sites and causes of lesion of the tibial nerve?*
23. *What are the effects of tibial neuropathy?*
24. *What is the F wave and what is its significance?*
    Ans: The F wave is recorded from the muscle. When a supramaximal stimulus is given, an action potential travels up the motor nerve and ventral root to the motor neuron, and is reflected back down to the muscle, causing a delayed muscle contraction.
25. *What is the H reflex and what is its significance?*
    Ans: An **H reflex** is recorded in the soleus muscle using a submaximal stimulus. The action potential travels in the proprioceptive sensory fibre within the nerve, and through the dorsal root and a monosynaptic reflex arc, it reaches the motor neuron, resulting in a late muscle contraction. This is sensitive for detecting S_1 radiculopathy.

CHAPTER 32

Electromyography

Learning Objectives

After completing this practical, you will be able to (MUST KNOW):
1. Explain the importance of performing EMG in clinical physiology.
2. List the uses of EMG.
3. Describe the types and features of motor unit potentials.
4. List factors that affect motor unit potentials.

5. Describe the principle and precautions of recording EMG.

You may also be able to (DESIRABLE TO KNOW):
1. Explain insertional activity.
2. List the different types and common causes of spontaneous activity.

INTRODUCTION

Electromyography (EMG) refers to the **recording of action potentials of muscle fibres** firing singly or in groups, near the needle electrode in a muscle. The muscle action potential when recorded by a needle usually has **three phases**. The rise time and fall of muscle action potential depends on the distance of the recording electrode from the muscle fibres.

Each muscle is composed of thousands of muscle fibres and each fibre is a complex multinucleated cell of variable length and diameter. Each muscle fibre receives a nerve twig from a motor neuron in the anterior horn of the spinal cord. A single motor neuron and the group of muscle fibres innervated by it is are together known as a **motor unit** (Fig. 32.1). The rate and pattern of firing of muscle fibres of a motor unit depend on the stimuli that approach through the nerve. **A denervated muscle** exhibits unstable membrane potential and fires spontaneously (without stimulation).

Motor Unit Potential

The motor unit potential (MUP) is the **sum of the action potentials produced in the muscle supplied by an anterior horn cell**. The muscle fibres discharge synchronously near the needle electrode. Therefore, the MUP has higher amplitude and longer duration than the action potential produced by a single muscle fibre. The MUPs can be characterised by their **firing pattern and appearance**. With mild contraction, the firing rates of MUPs are normally 5–15 Hz. With additional firing during muscle contraction, there is recruitment of MUPs. The recruitment of MUPs

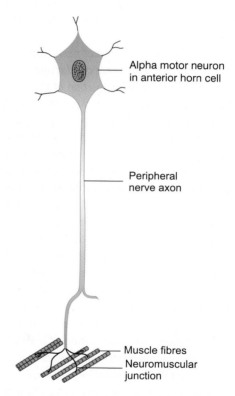

Alpha motor neuron in anterior horn cell

Peripheral nerve axon

Muscle fibres
Neuromuscular junction

Fig. 32.1 Schematic representation of a typical motor unit.

depends on the size principle. According to the **size principle**, the motor neurons are recruited in the order of size from small to large.

Features

The MUP is characterised by its duration, number of phases, amplitude and rate of rise of first component (Fig. 32.2).

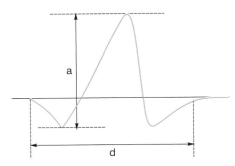

Fig. 32.2 Normal motor unit potential (a: amplitude; d: duration).

Duration

The duration is measured from the initial take-off to the point of return to the baseline. It varies from 5–15 ms. It is shorter in children and longer in elderly subjects.

The duration of MUP is a measure of:

- Conduction velocity
- Length of muscle fibre
- Membrane excitability
- Synchrony of different muscle fibres of a motor unit

Phases

Usually **MUP is triphasic**, that is, positive, negative and positive. The **phase** is defined as the portion of the MUP between the departure and the return to the baseline. An MUP with more than four phases is called a polyphasic MUP. Normally, the polyphasic potentials do not exceed 5–15 per cent of the total MUP population. Presence of more polyphasic potentials indicates desynchronisation or dropout of muscles.

Amplitude

Amplitude is measured from the maximum peak of the negative phase to the maximum peak of the positive phase. **The amplitude depends on**:

- Size of the muscle fibres
- Density of the muscle fibres
- Synchrony of firing
- Proximity of the needle to the muscle fibre
- Type of muscles examined
- Muscle temperature
- Age of the subject

Rise Time

The rise time of MUP is the duration from the initial positive to the subsequent negative peak. The usual rise time is less than 500 µs. If it is more than 500 µs, the increased resistance and capacitance of the intervening tissue could be accountable.

Factors That Affect MUP

Technical factors

- Type of needle electrode
- Characteristics of recording surface
- Electrical characteristics of cable
- Preamplifier and amplifier
- Method of recording

Physiological factors

- Age of the patient
- Muscle examined
- Temperature

METHODS

Electromyography Method

Principle

A resting muscle does not show recordable electrical potential. If allowed to contract, it does. With increased force of contraction, the amplitude of the potential increases.

Requirements

1. Cathode ray oscilloscope (CRO)
2. Preamplifier and amplifier (Same as described in Chapter 31, *refer* Fig. 31.3)
3. Recording electrodes
4. Electrode paste
5. Spirit

Recording electrodes There are different types of recording electrodes. They are broadly divided into **needle electrodes and surface** electrodes.

The different types of needle electrodes are:

1. Concentric needle electrodes
2. Monopolar needle electrodes
3. Single fibre needle electrodes
4. Macro needle electrodes

The concentric needle electrodes are the most commonly used electrodes in clinical practice. A concentric needle electrode consists of 24–26-gauge needle with a fine wire in its lumen. The recording area of the tip of the needle is 125×580 μm². In this electrode, the shaft of the needle is considered as the active electrode, thus, reducing the surrounding muscle noise. The monopolar needle electrode is a solid, 22–30-gauge teflon-coated needle with a bare tip. The MUP recorded by a monopolar electrode is slightly higher in amplitude and longer in duration.

Procedure for Surface EMG

1. Clean the skin overlying the muscle with spirit.
2. Fix a set of three electrodes on the skin over the muscle (one for ground, and the other two for recording EMG) with a small amount of electrode paste. The electrode paste minimises the skin–electrode resistance.
3. Connect the electrodes through the preamplifier to the oscilloscopes.
4. Observe the resting potentials in the oscilloscope.
5. Ask the subject to contract the muscle, and observe the potentials.

Procedure for Needle EMG

1. Clean the skin overlying the muscle with spirit. Fix the ground electrode.
2. Insert the concentric needle electrode into the muscle to be tested.
3. Observe the potentials in the oscilloscope during insertion.
4. Ask the subject to contract the muscle, and observe the potentials.
5. Move the needle in different directions in the muscle and record the potential.

Observation

The following activities are observed during recording EMG.
1. Insertional activity
2. Spontaneous activity
3. Voluntary activity

Precautions

1. The subject should be properly instructed and motivated to provide full cooperation.
2. The subject should be fully relaxed.
3. The room should be calm and comfortable.
4. The subject should be grounded properly.

DISCUSSION

Motor Unit Potentials

Types

1. Short-duration MUP
2. Long-duration MUP
3. Polyphasic MUP
4. Mixed pattern MUP
5. Doublets MUP

Short-duration MUPs are usually low- amplitude MUPs (Fig. 32.3C). They have rapid recruitment with minimal effort. These are found in diseases associated with the loss of muscle fibres. Short-duration MUPs are commonly seen in:
1. Myopathies (endocrine and metabolic)
2. Neuromuscular junction disorder
3. The early stages of reinnervation after nerve damage.

Long-duration MUPs are generally associated with high amplitude and poor recruitment (Fig. 32.3B). Long-duration MUPs are commonly seen in:
1. Motor neuron disease
2. Neuropathies

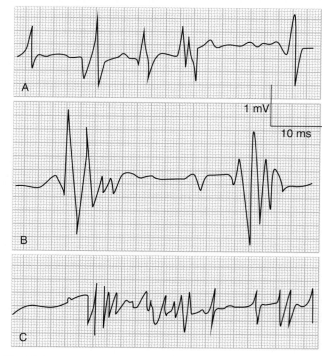

Fig. 32.3   Motor unit potentials. (A) Normal; (B) Neurogenic (MUPs are larger, prolonged and polyphasic); (C) Myopathic (MUPs have low amplitude).

3. Chronic myositis

When there are more than four phases in MUP, they are called **polyphasic**. They are commonly seen in:

i) Myopathies where there is regeneration of fibres and increased fibre density and

ii) Neurogenic diseases where there is regeneration of axons.

In a mixed pattern of MUPs, short-duration MUPs, long-duration MUPs and polyphasic MUPs occur. This pattern is seen in both myopathies and neuropathies.

Normally, MUPs are discharged as a single potential in a semi-rhythmic fashion. In some diseased conditions, the rhythm of MUPs is disturbed and occurs in bursts of two or more at an interval of 10–30 ms. These are called **doublets, triplets or multiplets** depending on the number of bursts. This is commonly seen in:

1. Hyperventilation
2. Motor neuron disease
3. Muscle ischemia

Insertional Activity

When a needle is introduced into the muscle, normally there is a brief burst of electrical activity. This is due to mechanical damage of the muscle by the needle. It appears as positive or negative high-frequency spikes in clusters.

Alteration of Insertional Activity

Increased insertional activity is seen in:

1. Denervated muscles
2. Myotonia
3. Familial

Decreased insertional activity is seen in:

1. Periodic paralysis (during the attack)
2. Myopathies (in which muscle is replaced by connective tissue and fat)
3. Insertional activity is lower in calf muscles

Spontaneous Activity

Normally, there is no spontaneous electrical activity (after the decay of insertional activity). However, some kind of spontaneous activity is recorded in the end plate zone, which appears as monophasic negative waves of less than 100 µV and duration of 1–3 ms. The end plate potentials are known as end plate noise. The end plate spikes occur due to mechanical activation of the nerve terminals by the needle. The abnormal spontaneous activities are:

❖ Fibrillations
❖ Fasciculations
❖ Complex repetitive discharges (CRD)
❖ Cramp potentials

Fibrillations

Fibrillations are spontaneously occurring action potentials from a single muscle fibre. These fire regularly at a rate of 1–15 Hz with amplitudes of 20–200 µV and duration of 1–5 ms when recorded by a concentric needle. Fibrillations are biphasic or triphasic waves with initial positivity (this differentiates it from end plate spike).

Causes

1. Neurogenic diseases
   • Anterior horn cell disease
   • Axonal neuropathy
2. Diseases of neuromuscular junction
   • Myasthenia gravis
   • Botulism
3. Myogenic diseases
   • Myositis
   • Muscle trauma

Fasciculations

Fasciculation potentials are spontaneous activities generated by a number of muscle fibres belonging to whole or a part of motor unit. They occur randomly and irregularly at variable rates of 1–500 per minute. Their size and shape depend on motor units from which they arise and on the distance of recording electrode from the motor unit.

Causes

1. Physiological
   • Benign fasciculations
   • Muscle cramps
2. Neurological
   • Root compression
   • Amyotrophic lateral sclerosis
   • Syringomyelia

Complex Repetitive Discharge

This refers to repetitive and synchronous firing of a group of muscle fibres. They have amplitudes of 50 μV – 1 mV, duration of 50–100 ms and frequency of 5–100 Hz.

Causes
1. Polymyositis
2. Poliomyelitis
3. Spinal muscular atrophy
4. Chronic neuropathies

Cramp Potentials

During muscle cramp, the spontaneous discharges of potential occur at 40–60 Hz, usually with abrupt onset and cessation.

Causes
1. Salt depletion
2. Chronic neurogenic atrophy
3. Pregnancy
4. Also seen in normal persons

VIVA

1. What are the clinical uses of electromyography?
2. What is the motor unit potential (MUP)?
3. What are the factors that affect MUPs?
4. What is the principle of EMG?
5. What are the types of needles used in EMG recording?
6. What are the precautions taken for EMG recordings?
7. What are the different types of activities recorded in EMG?
8. What are the different types of MUPs?
9. What are the features of short-duration MUPs? In what conditions are they seen?
10. What are the features of long-duration MUPs? In what conditions are they seen?
11. What are the features of polyphasic MUPs? In what conditions are they seen?
12. What are the features of mixed MUPs? In what conditions are they seen?
13. What is doublet or multiplet MUPs? In what condition is it seen?
14. What is insertional activity? What are the conditions in which insertional activities increase and decrease?
15. What is spontaneous activity? What are the different types of spontaneous activity?
16. What are the features and causes of fibrillation?
17. What are the features and causes of fasciculation?
18. What are the features and causes of complex repetitive discharge?
19. What is cramp potential? In what conditions is it seen?

CHAPTER 33

Mosso's Ergography and Use of Handgrip Dynamometer

Learning Objectives

After completing this practical, you will be able to (MUST KNOW):

1. State the importance of performing this practical in human physiology.
2. Define ergography.
3. Perform Mosso's ergography and use handgrip dynamometer to study the hand-muscle performance and the phenomenon of fatigue.
4. List the precautions to be taken for Mosso's ergography.
5. Calculate the work done.

6. List the factors that affect fatigue and work done.
7. Name the sites of fatigue in human beings.

You may also be able to (DESIRABLE TO KNOW):

1. Explain the factors that affect the performance.
2. Explain the effect of venous and arterial occlusion and motivation on work done.
3. Explain the sites of fatigue in humans.

MOSSO'S ERGOGRAPHY

INTRODUCTION

Ergography is the recording of an ergogram. It was first described by Mosso, and is therefore called Mosso's ergography. An **ergogram** is a recording of the voluntary contractions of the skeletal muscles of a human being on a moving kymograph. Mosso's ergography is done to **assess the performance** (the ability to work) of the flexors of the fingers of the hand. It is also performed to study the **phenomenon of fatigue** in human skeletal muscles.

Factors That Affect Performance

1. **Age** Young adults can perform better than children and elderly individuals.
2. **Gender** Men can perform voluntary contractions better.
3. **Height** Usually taller people perform better.
4. **Physical build** Persons with sound physical build can perform better than the obese or very thin.
5. **Training** A physically trained individual can always perform better than untrained persons.
6. **Race** Europeans and Caucasians perform better than Asians.
7. **Motivation** Encouragement and motivation stimulate the reward system in the brain and increase the performance.

Factors That Affect Fatigue

◈ The degree of work
◈ The duration of work

In Mosso's ergography, fatigue is affected by:

1. *The weight to be lifted* When the weight to be lifted increases, fatigue occurs early.
2. *The frequency of contractions* Fatigue occurs early when the frequency of contractions increases.
3. *Motivation* Encouragement delays fatigue.
4. *Blood supply to the exercising muscle* Venous and arterial occlusion accelerate fatigue.

The **factors that cause muscle fatigue** are the following:

◈ Depletion of nutrients (oxygen, creatine phosphate, ATP)
◈ Depletion of neurotransmitters
◈ Accumulation of metabolites

METHODS

Ergography Method

Principle

The subject contracts the flexors of the fingers against resistance, using Mosso's ergogram, till the finger is fatigued. The work done is calculated to study the effect of various factors on the performance.

Requirements

1. Mosso's ergograph Mosso's ergograph (Fig. 33.1) is the apparatus (laboratory set-up) used to record an ergogram. In Mosso's ergograph, there is an arrangement for fixing the fingers and forearm in the appropriate holders. A cord passing over a pulley and carrying a load of 3 kg at one end is attached to a sliding plate. The sliding plate is connected through a sling to the finger, the flexors of which are being studied. The metal plates also carry a writing lever which writes on a slow-moving drum. When the middle finger is flexed, the load is lifted and the distance through which the load is lifted is marked by the writing lever on the drum.

2. Metronome This instrument (Fig. 33.2) is used in experiments requiring an interrupter adjusted from 40 to 200 contacts/min. The frequency of interruption is adjusted by sliding the clip on a sideways-movable metal plate in front of a graduated scale. The position of the clip on the scale gives the frequency at which the sound is delivered.

3. Electrical kymograph
4. Sphygmomanometer
5. A set of 500 g weights

Procedure

1. Give proper instructions to the subject.
2. Insert the index and the ring finger of the subject into the fixed-tube holders, leaving the middle finger to pull the load (Fig. 33.3).
3. Set the metronome to oscillate once in two seconds.
4. Connect the sling to the middle finger.
5. Ask the subject to lift the load by maximal contraction of the flexors of the middle finger and repeat lifting the load every two seconds along with the metronome oscillations.
6. Ask the subject to continue (lifting the load) till the load can no longer be lifted.

Note: The record of the contractions obtained in the drum is called an ergogram.

7. Allow the subject to rest for 15 minutes.
8. After rest ask her to repeat the same procedure till she is fatigued.

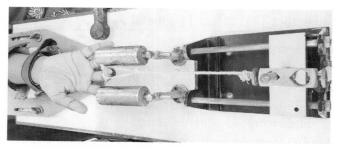

Fig. 33.1 Mosso's ergograph. Note the arrangement for the arm fixing clamp and finger-holder.

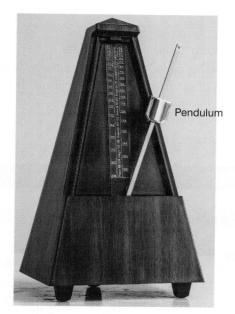

Pendulum

Fig. 33.2 Color shot of a vintage metronome, on gray background. (*Source:* Shutterstock/Konstantin Kolosov.)

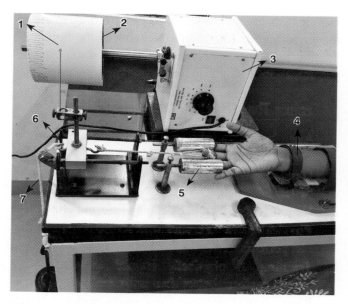

Fig. 33.3 Procedure of Mosso's ergography. Note the various parts of the ergograph (1: Writing point of the lever; 2: Drum; 3: Kymograph; 4: Arm fixing clamp; 5: Finger holder; 6: Pulley; 7: Cord connected to weights). With middle finger pulling the weight, the lever writes on the kymograph.

9. When she can no longer lift the weight encourage her (to study the effect of encouragement) to continue the effort and record the ergogram.
10. Allow the subject to rest for 15 minutes, following which obtain the ergogram after venous occlusion.

Note: Venous occlusion is obtained by tying the BP cuff around the arm of the subject and raising and maintaining the pressure to 40 mm Hg. This occludes the veins in arms.

11. Allow the subject to rest for 15 minutes following which obtain the ergogram after arterial occlusion.

Note: Arterial occlusion is obtained by raising the pressure to 200 mm Hg and keeping the BP cuff inflated till the experiment is over. This occludes both veins and arteries.

12. Study the ergogram of each condition and calculate the work done (as described below) for each.

Precautions

1. The subject should be instructed properly to give her maximum effort.
2. The subject should move the finger (contract the flexors of the middle finger) according to the oscillations of the metronome.
3. The subject should continue to do the work till she is unable to lift the load.
4. Fifteen minutes of rest should be provided between all the procedures (encouragement, venous occlusion and arterial occlusion).
5. To study the effect of encouragement and motivation, the subject should be properly and adequately encouraged to give maximum performance.
6. For obtaining venous occlusion, the BP cuff pressure should be raised to 40 mm Hg and should be maintained at the same pressure till the subject is fatigued.
7. For obtaining arterial occlusion, the BP cuff pressure should be raised to 200 mm Hg and should be maintained at the same pressure till the subject is fatigued.

Calculation

Calculate the work done for each ergogram by the formula:

$$W = F \times S$$

where,

W is the work done (in kg m),
F is the load (in kg), and
S is the total distance (in metres) through which the load is lifted. S is the sum of all the vertical amplitudes in each ergogram, that is, total length of all vertical lines.

Observation

Study the amplitude of contractions and the time of onset of fatigue. Work done improves with encouragement and decreases with venous and arterial occlusion (Fig. 33.4).

1. Motivation and encouragement increase the amplitude of contractions and delay the onset of fatigue.
2. Venous occlusion decreases the amplitude of contractions and shortens the onset of fatigue.
3. Arterial occlusion further decreases the amplitude of contractions and brings on early onset of fatigue.

DISCUSSION

Mosso's ergography is performed to study the work done by the flexors of the fingers and to study the phenomenon of fatigue in human skeletal muscles.

Encouragement

Encouragement and motivation increase the performance of the subject. The exact mechanism of motivation increasing the performance is not known. The **prefrontal cortex** is part of the reward system in the brain which on stimulation increases the bar pressing in experimental animals. It is possible that, in human beings too, encouragement stimulates the **frontal lobe** of the cortex, which increases the activity in the motor cortex. This in turn stimulates the flexor muscles by increasing the activity in the corresponding motor neurons.

Venous Occlusion

Venous occlusion decreases the work done due to **accumulation of metabolites** in the muscle. Metabolites like lactic acid and so on are removed from the tissue by the veins. Accumulation of metabolites decreases muscle performance.

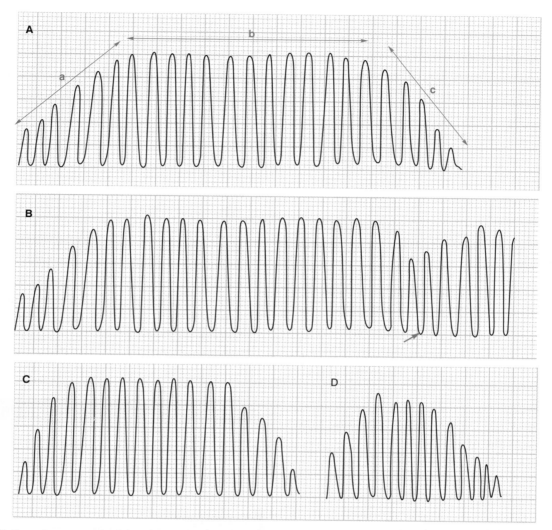

Fig. 33.4 (A) Normal ergogram (a: rising phase; b: plateau phase; c: falling phase); (B) Effect of encouragement (arrows indicate the starting of encouragement prior to which is the normal recording); (C) Effect of venous occlusion; (D) Effect of arterial occlusion.

Arterial Occlusion

Arterial occlusion decreases the work done maximally because it **prevents the supply of nutrients** to the muscle. Nutrients, especially oxygen, are essential for metabolic oxidation in the tissues to provide energy (ATP). Therefore, intact blood supply to the muscle is a minimum for its functioning. The sphygmomanometer pressure that occludes the artery also occludes the veins. So, arterial occlusion is accompanied by venous occlusion. Therefore, work done decreases maximally.

Sites of Fatigue in Human Beings

In human beings, the first site of fatigue is the CNS as is proved by the fact that encouragement enhances performance and prolongs onset of fatigue. This can be demonstrated by **Merton's experiment**. The next site of fatigue is the muscle followed by neuromuscular junction, as rest helps in continuation of work. The nerve is theoretically unfatiguable.

HANDGRIP DYNAMOMETER

INTRODUCTION

The handgrip dynamometer is used for exercise of upper limb muscles, especially of the hand and forearm.

METHOD

Handgrip Dynamometer Method

Requirement

Handgrip dynamometer This uses a spring to measure the maximum isometric contractions of hand and forearm muscles. The device has a handle and a graduated pressure scale on a circular metal plate (Fig. 33.5). The results are read manually from the scale.

Procedure

1. Explain the procedure of use of the instrument to the subject. Ask the subject to seat comfortably with arms at the sides and elbows slightly bent.

Note: The dominant hand should be used for the exercise to get a maximum grip of it.

2. Ask the subject to pull and squeeze and note the tension developed (Fig. 33.6).
3. Instruct the subject to make two more trials with a pause of about a minute between the trials to avoid fatigue. Calculate the mean of these readings. This is called T_{max} (**maximal isometric tension**).

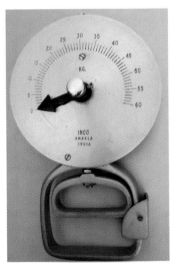

Fig. 33.5   Handgrip dynamometer (spring type).

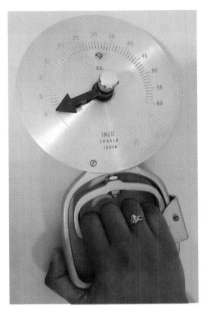

Fig. 33.6   Procedure of testing muscle strength (work done) by using handgrip dynamometer.

Note: The scale needs to be reset to zero after each test.

4. Determine the endurance time for 60–80% of Tmax. This is the time of the onset of fatigue after starting the exercise on the dynamometer.
5. After a rest of 2–3 minutes, measure the endurance time for 60–80% of T_{max}, first after occlusion of veins and then after occlusion of arteries with a BP cuff on the upper arm.

Observation and Discussion

Factors affecting T_{max}

T_{max} depends on age, gender, muscle strength, hand dominance, time of the day, nutrition, sensitivity to fatigue and pain. There may be slight difference in values between the two hands.

Venous occlusion decreases the performance due to accumulation of metabolites and arterial occlusion considerably decreases work done and facilitates early onset of fatigue due to decreased nutrition supply to muscle. Encouragement and motivation enhance the performance.

VIVA

1. What is the use of Mosso's ergography in physiology?
2. What is an ergogram?
3. What are the precautions taken for Mosso's ergography?
4. What are the factors that affect performance (the work done)?
5. What are the causes of fatigue?
6. What are the factors that delay and facilitate fatigue?
7. How does encouragement improve physical performance?
8. Why does venous occlusion decrease the performance?
9. Why does arterial occlusion decrease the performance maximally?
10. What is the primary site of fatigue in human beings?
11. How can you prove the primary site of fatigue in an intact muscle?
12. What are the neurotransmitters that delay fatigue?
    Ans: Dopamine and norepinephrine.

CHAPTER 34

Visual and Auditory Reaction Times

Learning Objectives

After completing this practical, you will be able to (MUST KNOW):

1. Define reaction time, visual reaction time and auditory reaction time.
2. To determine the reaction time to visual and auditory stiamuli.

3. List the factors affecting visual reaction time and auditory reaction time.
4. Understand the physiological importance of learning visual reaction time and auditory reaction time.

INTRODUCTION

Reaction time (RT) is a measure of the quickness with which an individual responds to a stimulus. RT plays an important role in our daily lives as its practical implications have great consequences. Factors that can affect the average human RT include age, gender, left or right hand, central versus peripheral vision, practice, fatigue, fasting, breathing cycle, personality types, exercise, and intelligence of the subject.

Definition and Concept

RT is defined as the interval of time between the presentation of the stimulus and appearance of appropriate voluntary response in the subject. Welford had described three types of RT.

1. Simple RT Here there is one stimulus and one response.

2. Recognition RT Here there is some stimulus that should be responded to and others that should not get a response.

3. Choice RT Here there are multiple stimuli and multiple responses.

Human RT works by having a developed nervous system that recognises the stimulus. The neurons then relay the message of sensory stimulation to the brain, which travels from the brain to the spinal cord, and then reaches the person's hands and fingers. The motor neurons then instruct the hands and fingers to react in a particular way. The accepted figures for mean simple

RTs for healthy adults have been about 190 ms for light stimuli (visual RT) and about 160 ms for sound stimuli (auditory RT).

Factors Affecting RT

RT in response to a situation can significantly influence our lives due its practical implications. Fast RTs can produce rewards (e.g., in sports) whereas slow RT can produce grave consequences (e.g. driving and road safety matters). Factors that can affect RT include age, gender, left or right hand, central versus peripheral vision, level of practice, fatigue, fasting, breathing cycle, personality types, exercise, and intelligence status of the subject.

METHODS

Manual Method of Determination of VRT and ART

Principle

Reaction time is the time interval between the application of an adequate stimulus and the voluntary motor response to it. It varies with the complexity of reflex and interrelated sensory pathways associated with the course of the impulse as it travels to the centre.

Requirements

1. Two tapping keys (K1, K2)
2. Signal marker

3. Short-circuiting key
4. Bulb
5. Low-voltage current (6V DC mains)
6. Kymograph with drum

Procedure

Visual reaction time (VRT)

1. Set up a circuit with two tapping keys (termed as K1 and K2), electromagnetic signal maker and a bulb, connected in series to the 6V DC mains current source.
2. Place the kymograph to record the movement of the signal marker.
3. Instruct the subject to press the tapping key K1.

Note: The subject should be given some training to be alert and to release the key the moment the bulb is lit up.

4. Without making any sound, the examiner gently presses K2 to light the bulb.

Note: The event is marked on the drum with the signal marker as Event 1 (E1). The subject as instructed releases K2, which is marked on the drum as Event 2.

5. Record a time tracing below the event recordings by using a tuning fork of 100 Hz and calculate VRT from the time interval between E1 and E2.

Auditory reaction time (ART)

1. Remove the bulb from the circuit. Instruct the examiner to press the tapping key K2 to produce the sound.
2. Instruct the subject to press the tapping key K1.

Note: The subject should be alert and release the key the moment he hears the tapping sound.

3. The event is marked on the drum with the signal marker as Event-1.
4. The subject is instructed to release K2, which is marked on the drum as Event 2 (E2).
5. Calculate ART from the time interval between E1 and E2.

Precautions

1. The subject should not face the examiner.

Note: The subject should respond to the visual and auditory stimuli and not to the movement of the examiner's hand.

2. The subject should remain alert through the procedure.
3. The examiner's key should be released without making any noise for VRT.

NORMAL VALUE

Visual reaction time   : 200–400 ms
Auditory reaction time : 100–200 ms

Note: Normally, VRT is more than ART because visual responses involves chemical mechanisms for information processing, mainly for the conversion from a photon to a bioelectric stimuli, which takes a lot longer than the conversion from a pressure wave to bioelectric stimuli.

DETERMINATION OF RT USING SOFTWARE

The reaction time tests are done using Inquisit 4.0 computer software released in 2013 by Millisecond Software in Seattle, Washington.

During the visual RT (VRT) task, in the centre of the white background screen, the participant gets presented a black fixation cross that is followed after variable time intervals by a target stimulus that is, red circle. The subject is asked to concentrate on the fixation cross and press the "space bar" key as quickly as possible once the red circle (target stimulus) appears on the screen.

In a simple auditory RT (ART) task after variable time intervals, the sound is played for 30 s to the participant through the speakers. The task is to press the space bar as soon as the sound is presented. The subject is thoroughly acquainted with the procedure and practice trials need to be given before taking the test.

By default, the time intervals are randomly chosen from 2000 ms, 3000 ms, 4000 ms, 5000 ms, 6000 ms, 7000 ms, 8000 ms. For each stimulus, five readings are taken, and the respective fastest RT for each stimulus is recorded. The readings are taken during a fixed time and in a quiet secluded room.

DISCUSSION

Physiological Significance

As reaction time is defined as the interval of time between the presentation of the stimulus and appearance of appropriate voluntary response in a subject, a number of external environmental stimuli of different modalities influence it. There are various sensory modalities and the human body responds to various stimuli with different speeds. This plays an important role in routine life activities as well as in an emergency, as for example, while driving any vehicle, it is necessary to apply the brakes as quickly as possible when required. Reaction time becomes an important component of information processing, as it indexes speed of stimulus processing and response programming.

Reaction time has mainly **two components:**

1. Mental processing time   It is the time required by the responder to perceive, identify and analyse a stimulus, and decide the proper motor response.

2. Movement time   It is the time required to perform a movement after deciding how to respond.

In simple reaction time, there is one stimulus and one response. **In recognition reaction time**, there are some stimuli that should be responded to and others that should not get a response. In choice reaction time, there are multiple stimuli and multiple responses.

In simple reaction time, the stimulus and the response are one; so to complete a task, only identification of the stimulus and its proper response are required. But in choice reaction time, the stimulus and the appropriate response are multiple; after identification of the stimulus among the many stimuli, one response out of the many responses has to be verified. Therefore, in choice reaction time, the task involves more mental process, which would require more time. Thus, the choice auditory reaction time would be more than simple auditory reaction time.

The reaction time can be decreased with practice and training. It can also be decreased by alertness and concentration. The reaction time is prolonged with advancing age, fatigue, distractions and muscular weakness.

VIVA

1. Define reaction time, visual reaction time and auditory reaction time.
2. Give the normal values of visual reaction time and auditory reaction time.
3. Explain why ART is less than VRT?
4. List the factors affecting visual reaction time and auditory reaction time.
5. Explain the application of visual reaction time and auditory reaction time in daily life.

CHAPTER 35

Electroencephalogram

Learning Objectives

After completing this practical, you will be able to (MUST KNOW):

1. Define EEG.
2. Name EEG waves and rhythms.

3. Understand the basic principle of EEG recordings.
4. List the uses of EEG.
5. Appreciate clinical application of EEG in common epilepsies and other neurological disorders.

INTRODUCTION

Electroencephalogram (EEG) is the *record of spontaneous electrical activities generated in the cerebral cortex* which are picked up from brain's surface through electrodes placed on designated sites in the scalp. These electrical activities reflect the electrical currents that flow in the extracellular spaces in the brain. These electrical currents reflect the **summated effects of innumerable excitatory and inhibitory synaptic potentials** upon the cortical neurons. These spontaneous activities of cortical neurons are greatly influenced by the afferent inputs arising from the thalamus and brainstem reticular formation. These afferent impulses entrain the cortical neurons to produce most of the characteristic rhythmic EEG waves.

Electroencephalography is the procedure of recording EEG. **Electroencephalograph** is the sensitive device that records EEG. EEG is the best diagnostic tool available for assessing the abnormalities of electrical activities of the brain. Therefore, EEG is very helpful in diagnosing epilepsies and for studying sleep and sleep disorders.

Specialities in EEG Recording

Hans Berger, a German psychiatrist in 1929 for the first time demonstrated that electrical activities of the human brain could be recorded using external electrodes on the scalp, which he termed as electroencephalogram (EEG). As the EEG waves are of very low voltage, they require more amplification before recording.

1. **EEG leads** may be bipolar (comparing the potentials between two active leads) or unipolar (measuring the potential changes at a single lead against a reference lead placed on the ear or nose or chin).
2. EEG electrodes are solder or silver-silver chloride discs of 0.5 cm diameter.
3. Recording is done with the subject preferably in the recumbent position with his head and neck supported to ensure that the posterior electrodes are secure.
4. Usually, four leads are attached to the scalp by means of adhesive material on standard skull locations on each side.
5. A **multi-channel pen recorder** is used to record the activities from the **eight or more leads simultaneously**.
6. The EEG waves are analysed manually or by using a computer.

EEG Waves

EEG waves are described in terms of their frequency, which usually ranges from 1 to 30 Hz, and amplitude, which ranges from **20 to 100 μV**. The characteristics of EEG waves vary according to the state of consciousness.

1. When the **individual is fully alert** (sensory inputs are maximum), the waves are mostly of **high frequency and low amplitude** with as many units asynchronised.
2. When the person is **minimally alert** as in deep sleep (least sensory input), the waves are of **low frequency and high amplitude, and synchronised**.

3. Absence of EEG waves indicates brain death.

EEG Wave Patterns and Rhythms

EEG **wave patterns** are classified into **four types**: α, β, θ and δ according to their frequency. The characteristic features of the various EEG rhythms are as follows:

Alpha Rhythm

Frequency ranges from **8 to 13 Hz** and amplitude from **50 to 100 μV** (Fig. 35.1).
- This is the most prominent EEG rhythm seen in a **normal adult at rest** (awake but relaxed) with eyes closed.
- It is found in the posterior half of the brain, especially **in the parieto-occipital regions**.

Alpha block

The alpha rhythm **disappears once the subject opens his eyes** and engages in mental effort such as mental arithmetic. The regular alpha rhythm is replaced by irregular low-voltage activity. This phenomenon is known as alpha block or **desynchronisation**. This is also called arousal or **alerting response**.

Factors affecting α wave frequency

Frequency of alpha rhythm is decreased by hypoglycemia, hypothermia, high arterial pressure and low levels of glucocorticoids.
1. High blood glucose, increased body temperature, low arterial pressure and high levels of glucocorticoids increase frequency of alpha rhythm.

Beta Rhythm

Frequency of beta waves ranges from **13 to 30 Hz** with low amplitude ranging from **5–10 μV**.
- This is seen in adults, when the **eyes are open**.
- These waves appear **in posterior regions**. Beta rhythms are sometimes seen in the frontal regions regardless of whether the eyes are closed or open.

Theta Rhythm

Frequency of theta waves ranges from **4 to 8 Hz** with large amplitude.
- Usually, theta rhythm is **seen in normal children**.
- It also occurs **during moderate sleep**.
- It may sometimes appear in adults when they are severely disappointed or depressed.

Delta Rhythm

Frequency of delta waves ranges from **0.5 to 4 Hz** and amplitude from **20 to 200 μV**.
- Delta rhythm occurs normally **during deep sleep**.
- Its appearance in an alert state in adult suggests a serious organic brain damage.

EEG Rhythms in Infants and Children

The EEG recordings in children show wide range of patterns.
- Usually, **in awakened infants**, there is **fast beta rhythm**.
- The rhythm speeds up during childhood and **theta rhythm appears**.
- As the child matures, the theta rhythm is replaced by **faster alpha rhythms**.

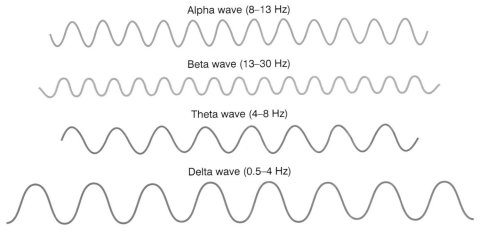

Alpha wave (8–13 Hz)

Beta wave (13–30 Hz)

Theta wave (4–8 Hz)

Delta wave (0.5–4 Hz)

Fig. 35.1 EEG waves.

◈ The **alpha rhythm of adults** gradually appears **during adolescence**.

◈ The theta rhythm is prominent in the temporal or parietal region, while alpha rhythms are in the occipital region.

METHODS

Method to Record an EEG

Principle

EEG reflects spontaneous brain electrical activities recorded from the surface of the scalp. It measures changes in electric potentials caused by a large number of electric dipoles generated in neural networks, either excitatory (EPSP) or inhibitory (IPSP) potentials. When these potentials get summed up spatially or temporally, they become strong enough to be picked up by the electrodes placed on the surface (of the scalp) by the principle of volume conduction. The signals picked up by special bio-electric sensors are of very low amplitude and hence amplified and then converted into a set of numeric values (analog to digital conversion), which accurately represent the original bio-electric signal. The converted signal can then be displayed in the form of traces, stored on magnetic disk, printed, or processed in several ways.

Requirements

A **computerised EEG System with Video monitoring** is desirable for better EEG recording and analysis, for example, Galileo video-assisted EEG system (Fig. 35.2). The **hardware** used is BE light (EB Neuro) and the **software** used for acquisition is Galileo Suite (EB Neuro). A schematic diagram of the hardware is shown in Fig. 35.3.

Procedure

Preparation of the subject

The electrodes (gold / silver) are applied to the scalp surface with the help of **conductive paste** (Ten20 paste), and can be held in place by adhesives, suction, or pressure from caps or headbands. To maintain a constant relationship between the location of the electrode and the underlying cerebral structures, a **system of electrode placement** is necessary. Although

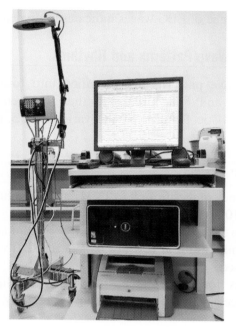

Fig. 35.2   EEG machine with all its accessories. (*Courtesy:*   Neurophysiology Lab, Physiology Department, JIPMER, Puducherry, India.)

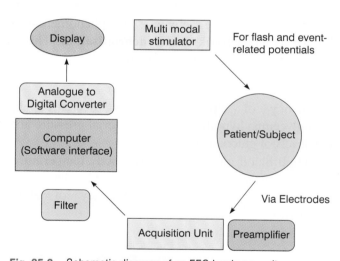

Fig. 35.3   Schematic diagram of an EEG hardware unit.

other systems like Gibbsian, Michigan and Houston have been used successfully, the great majority of EEG labs throughout the world utilise the **10–20 International system of Electrode Placement**.

Standard electrode placement uses **21 electrodes** in accordance with 10–20 International Federation of Societies for EEG and Clinical Neurophysiology in 1958. This system is based on percentages of the total head size; the anatomical landmarks for measurement are the nasion, the inion, **the left and right pre-auricular points** (tragus).

Position of the electrodes

Electrodes are placed based on anatomical landmarks of the scalp:

a) The electrode placement should be symmetrical in the sagittal plain and more strictly on the landmarks.

b) Electrodes should be spaced equally along the anteroposterior and transverse axis of the head.

c) The designation of position of electrodes should be in terms of brain area, e.g., frontal, parietal, temporal, occipital, etc.

Electrode nomenclature

F – Electrode over frontal lobe

T – Electrode over temporal lobe

C – Electrode over central area

Fp – Electrode over frontopolar

O – Electrode over the occipital lobe

P – Electrode over the parietal lobe

Z – Midline electrodes

Odd numbers refer to electrodes over the left hemisphere while even numbers refer to electrodes over the right hemisphere (Fig. 35.4).

International 10-20 system of measurement

Measure the distance from nasion to inion on the sagittal line

Mark 50% (of nasion–inion distance) perpendicular to the tape: **Cz**

Measure and mark 10% up from nasion on the sagittal line: **Fpz**; 10% up from inion: **Oz**

Measure and mark 20% from Fpz towards **Cz** on the sagittal line: **Fz**

20% anteriorly on the sagittal line from **Oz** towards **Cz** on the sagittal line: **Pz**

Measure the distance from the left and right pre-auricular points (tragus) on the coronal line: (A1 and A2)

Measure and mark 50% (of the inter-tragal line) perpendicular to the tape: **Cz**

Measure and mark 10% up from the pre-auricular point: **T3** on the left and **T4** on the right

Measure the head circumference connecting the 4 points: **Fpz** anteriorly, **T4** on the right, **Oz** posteriorly and **T3** on the left)

Measure 5% of the head circumference on either side of **Fpz**: **Fp1** on the left and **Fp2** on the right

Measure 5% of the head circumference on either side of **Oz**: **O1** on the left and **O2** on the right

Measure 10% of the head circumference on either side of **T3**: **F7** anteriorly and **T5** posteriorly on the left side

Measure 10% of the head circumference on either side of **T4**: **F8** anteriorly and **T6** posteriorly on the right side

On the coronal line between **T3** and **Cz** (20% of the inter-tragal line): **C3** on the left side and **C4** in between **Cz** and **T4** on the right side

EEG software

The acquisition unit transmits the data to the software in the computer like the Galileo NT in this case. The acquired data is sampled and displayed as a digital polygraph in the window of the software which is customisable according to the requisites of the investigator.

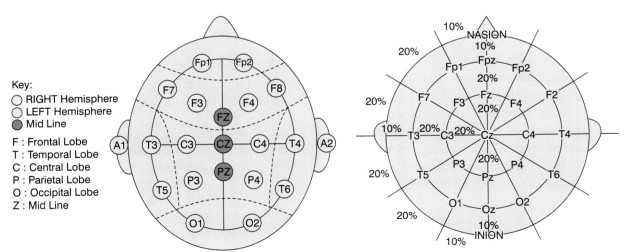

Fig 35.4 International 10–20 system of electrode placement.

Important terminology in EEG recordings

Sensitivity   Sensitivity is defined as the ratio of input voltage to pen deflection. It is expressed in microvolts per millimetre (µV/mm). A commonly used sensitivity is 7 µV/mm, which, for a calibration signal of 50 µV, results in a deflection of 7.1 mm. Sensitivity of the EEG equipment for routine recording should be set in the range of 5–10 µV/mm of pen deflection.

Filters   These selectively restrict frequency domain of a signal.

◆ **High pass filters** allow high frequency to pass through while eliminating the rapidly changing low frequencies (low frequency filters) and are set at 0.5 Hz.

◆ **Low pass filters** allow low frequencies to pass through while eliminating the rapidly changing high frequencies (high frequency filters) and are set at 70 Hz.

Filtering can be done electronically by resistors, capacitors, amplifiers while it can be done digitally by mathematical algorithms.

Notch filter   The 50 Hz (notch) filter can prevent the signals from distortion or attenuation by electrical line noise; it therefore should be used only when other measures against 50 Hz interference fail.

Epoch   Digital display of 10 seconds/page, should be utilised for routine recordings.

Montage   The representation of the EEG channels is referred to as a montage (Fig. 35.5).

◆ **Bipolar montage** Each channel represents the difference between two adjacent electrodes. The entire montage consists of a series of these channels.

◆ **Referential montage** Each channel represents the difference between a certain electrode and a designated reference electrode (normally ear / vertex reference electrode; A1 on the left side and A2 on the right side).

◆ **Average reference montage** The outputs of all the amplifiers are summed and averaged, and this averaged signal is used as the common reference for each channel.

◆ **Laplacian montage** Each channel represents the difference between an electrode and a weighted average of the surrounding electrodes.

Instructions to subject (or patient)

◆ Ask the subject to come after a hair wash with oil-free scalp (to avoid sticky scalp).

◆ For activating procedures, give proper instruction; for example, sleep deprivation in night (3–4 hour of sleep only is advisable).

◆ Avoid caffeinated drinks before the procedure.

◆ Discuss with the clinician regarding withholding drugs before procedure, especially sedatives, antidepressants, antipsychotics, antiepileptics, and instruct the subject accordingly.

Procedure

1. Instruct the subject to lie down on the couch comfortably and relax. It is advisable to have the head end of the bed elevated to have proper access to the scalp for electrode placement (Fig. 35.6).

2. Apply the reference electrodes on the earlobes and the ground electrode above the bridge of the nose. Place the sensitive electrodes on the scalp as per the "10–20" system as describe above. Connect them to the electrode board and ensure there are no loose connections.

3. *Sensitivity calibration*   Calibration of the machine should be done to ensure that an input of 50 µV gives a pen deflection of 7 mm.

4. Ask the subject to close his eyes and make a test recording.

> **Note:** Normally, alpha rhythm is recorded. Records are taken simultaneously from multiple analogous areas of the scalp for at least 20-minute period.

5. *Effect of opening the eyes*   Ask the subject to open his eyes.

> **Note:** The alpha rhythm is immediately replaced by desynchronisation, i.e. by fast, irregular activity. Ask the subject to close his eyes, the alpha rhythm reappears.

6. *Photic stimulation*   As the record is running, deliver light flashes at the rate of 25/sec for 5 seconds, first with eyes closed, then with eyes open.

> **Note:** Normally, there may be no change, but in diseases like epilepsy, delta rhythm may appear. In some cases, an attack of epilepsy may be precipitated.

7. Note the images in the video, in case of an epilepsy attack. Correlate EEG waves with flickering television to ensure the result in an attack of epilepsy.

8. *Effect of hyperventilation*   Ask the subject to deep-breathe for 3 minutes.

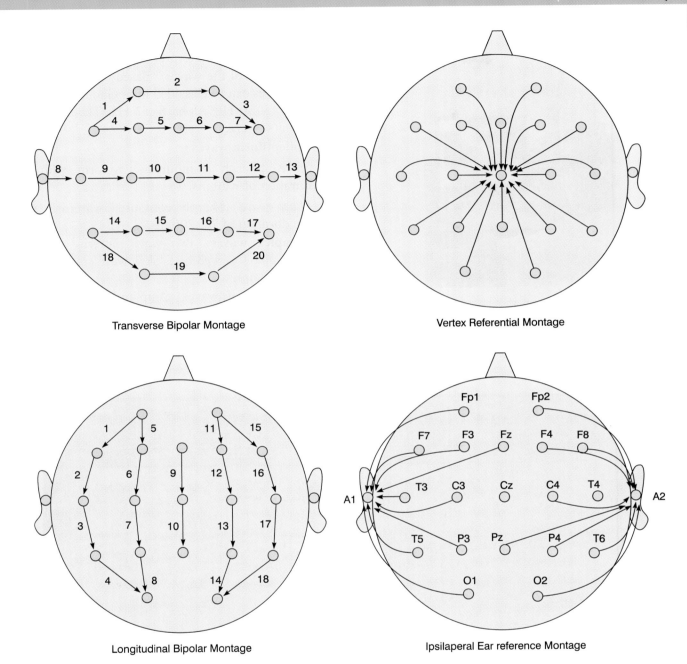

Transverse Bipolar Montage

Vertex Referential Montage

Longitudinal Bipolar Montage

Ipsilaperal Ear reference Montage

Fig. 35.5   Recording montages.

Note: Normally, the frequency of alpha waves decreases by low PCO_2 and the record may show theta or delta rhythm. An attack of epilepsy may be precipitated along with abnormal patterns of waves, which may be correlated with the video recording of the seizure movements.

Precautions

1. Avoid kinking of wires; this prevents physical damage to these sensitive wires
2. Clean electrodes properly after use; this prevents corrosion

3. Prepare the skin properly before placing the electrodes; this decreases the impedance.
4. Apply conducting (Ten20) paste judiciously; it should be adequate for conduction of the signal but not in excess, because excess of it would result in salt-bridge artifact which should be avoided.

Observation

Carefully note, read and analyse the EEG waves of all the tracings as recorded for each electrode (Fig. 35.7).

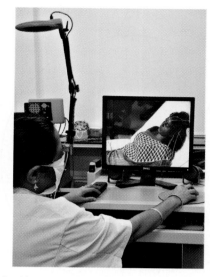

Fig. 35.6   Position of the patient while placing the electrodes on the scalp. This picture of the subject is shown on the computer screen, which is transmitted from the video clip of the system. (*Courtesy:*   Ms. Bharathi Balakumar, Senior Technical Officer, Physiology Dept., JIPMER, Puducherry, India.)

EEG analysis

What to look for and interpret in an EEG montage?

1. **Frequency of the waves**   Based on the frequency the waves can be classified into: Gamma > 30 Hz, Beta 13–30 Hz; Alpha 8–12 Hz; Theta 4–7 Hz; Delta < 4 Hz.

2. **Epileptiform waves**

   Spike   Sharply contoured waveform with the duration of <70 ms.

   Sharp wave   Sharply contoured waveform with the duration of 70–200 ms.

3. **Complex waves**   Two wave patterns together, e.g., spike followed by a 'slow wave spike' – 'slow wave' complex.

4. **Amplitude of waves**   Amplitude is the size of the waveforms (μV), often measured peak to peak. Amplitude can be reported as a numerical range (20 to 40 μV) or in descriptive terms as low (0 to 25 μV), moderate (25 to 75 μV), or high

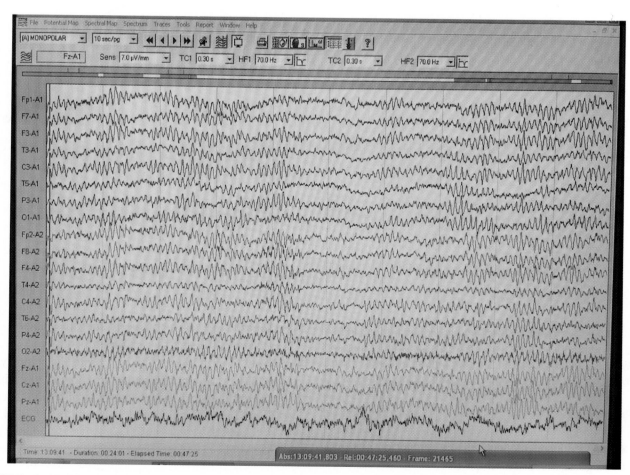

Fig. 35.7   EEG waves as originally recorded on the computer screen. Note the waves against each electrode, demarcated on the extreme left side against each tracing.

(>75 µV) amplitude. Some pathological conditions are associated with enormous amplitudes of hundreds of microvolts, such as hypoarrhythmia, a chaotic pattern seen in severe infantile epilepsy. The degree to which the original waveform signal is amplified in the computer is called gain.

5. **Polarity** Electrical signals approaching an electrode sensed as positive deflection and spreading away from it as negative deflection. Polarity reversal helps in localising the focus of epileptiform discharge.

6. **Phase** Refers to that part of the waveform that begins in one direction (up or down) then changes its direction in the next turn. Depending upon the turns, the waves can be classified as monophasic, biphasic and triphasic.

7. **Rhythmicity** Refers to the appearance of uninterrupted monomorphic waveforms. Based on rhythmicity, it can be classified into rhythmic, irregular and semi-rhythmic patterns.

8. **Reactivity** The degree of changes that occur in an EEG in response to an exogenous or endogenous stimulation. The test for reactivity is routine in EEG recording. The stimulus includes opening and closing of eyes, arithmetic calculations and orientation questions.

9. **Activation** It is the appearance of a particular pattern in response to an activating procedure. Activation procedures are done to induce epileptiform waves during interictal phase to aid in diagnosis. The commonly used activation procedures are sleep deprivation, hyperventilation and photic stimulation.

10. **Synchrony** Simultaneous occurrence of similar waveforms over each hemisphere is called synchrony of waveforms. Normal EEG activity is usually synchronous over the left and right hemispheres, both for relatively continuous background activities and more sporadic waveforms (e.g., "K complexes," the large amplitude biphasic slow waves seen in stage 2 sleep, should have simultaneous onset over both hemispheres). Loss of synchrony is observed in damage to the corpus callosum, severe disorders of cortical function. Lack of synchrony can also indicate that the location where the waveform appears first may be closer to the origin of that activity, and thus help with the localisation of abnormal or epileptiform activity.

11. **Symmetry** Comparing waveform patterns based on their spatial distribution in the left and right hemisphere.

EEG artifacts

Biological artifacts These include ECG artifacts, eye movement artifacts (blink, side-to-side movement, eyelid flutter and slow roving eye movement during drowsy state), muscle artifacts, pulse artifacts, respiratory movement artifacts, glossokinetic (tongue movement-induced) artifacts, tremor-induced head movement, sweat artifact, and induced artifacts.

Technical artifacts These include artifacts caused due to electrical interference (50 Hz electrical line artifact), excess paste use (salt bridge artifact), electrode pop out from scalp.

Instrumental artifacts These include portable air pumps, monitoring devices in ICU, respirator, lights and lamps, fans, air conditioner, pneumatic boots, heating and cooling blankets, electric beds, intravenous infusion pumps, feeding delivery systems, elevators, computers, telephones, diathermy, dialysis machine and X-ray equipment.

Quantitative EEG

The numerical data analyses of EEG to provide supportive diagnosis for the clinical condition forms the basis of quantitative EEG. The waves can be analysed by using Fast Fourier Transform analysis (FFT), power spectral analysis or wavelet analysis. Increased abnormal electrical activity as in an epileptic focus or decreased conductance as in brain injury can be picked by alterations in power spectrum confined to a topographic area.

DISCUSSION

The electroencephalogram (EEG) represents the electrical activity of the brain as recorded from electrodes placed on the scalp. EEG is an important tool used by neurophysiologists, neurologists and neurosurgeons as it is a non-invasive technique, and in conjunction with imaging techniques like CT scan and MRI, it is effective in **diagnosing abnormal electrical activities** in the brain causing seizure disorders. EEG is also effectively used in diagnosing **sleep disorders** as it forms an essential component of **polysomnography**.

Other uses in the clinical setting include diagnosis of **encephalopathy**, monitoring of comatose patients in ICU for confirming **brain death**.

Clinical Applications of EEG

- To confirm seizure activity
- To study sleep physiology and diagnose sleep disorders—polysomnography
- In encephalopathies—generalised slowing, burst suppression
- To confirm brain death in comatose patients—absent electrical activity (electrically silent / near silent)
- To monitor the depth of anaesthesia. Used to decide the optimal dose of anaesthesia
- To monitor prognosis in seizure disorders
- To monitor the effectiveness of antiepileptics
- Used for EEG biofeedback

In recent days, EEG is widely used as one of the tools to **intra-operatively monitor** the depth of anaesthesia, to assess burst suppression and extent of cortical excision in epileptic surgery. Also, EEG signals are also used as **Neuro feedback/Bio feedback** inputs suggesting the effectiveness of specific brainwave entrainment procedures.

Limitations of EEG Studies

- Preparing the subject is a tedious process
- Technical expertise needed for signal acquisition
- Poor signal-to-noise ratio
- Poor spatial resolution compared to imaging techniques
- Does not use signals from deeper layers of brain

Diagnosis of Epilepsies and Other Problems

Epilepsy (seizure or fit) is defined as the intermittent disorder of cerebral function associated with a sudden uncontrolled discharge of cerebral neurons, which may or may not be accompanied by loss of consciousness. The epileptogenic focus in the cerebral cortex discharges irregular slow waves or sometimes, high-voltage waves that can be recorded in the EEG.

There are **two main groups** of epilepsy:

A. **Generalised seizures** with loss of consciousness associated with generalised synchronous EEG discharge from both hemispheres; e.g., grand mal and petit mal epilepsies.

Grand mal epilepsy is characterised by immediate loss of consciousness followed by sustained contraction of limb muscles (*tonic phase*) and then jerky movements due to rhythmic contraction-relaxation of limb muscles (*clonic phase*). In EEG, **fast activities** are recorded in tonic and slow activities in clonic phase.

Petit mal epilepsy (absence seizure) manifests in the form of short-lived loss of consciousness with mild or no motor activity. EEG recording shows **doublets consisting of a spike and a dome**. Three such doublets occur typically per second.

B. **Focal epilepsy**, the manifestations of which depend on the site of the cortex from which the discharge occurs, e.g., temporal lobe epilepsy and Jacksonian (motor cortex) epilepsy.

Though EEG confirms the type of epilepsy, EEG recording between the attacks may be normal.

Intracranial Space-Occupying Lesion

Cerebral tumours do not directly produce abnormal electrical activity. They compress adjoining neurons and suppress their normal rhythms that manifests as **irregular or slow waves**. This helps in localising cerebral tumours. Fluid collection such as subdural hematoma can suppress neurons and produce local abnormal EEG waves.

Diagnosis of Sleep Disturbances

Analysis of sleep, and diagnosis of sleep disorders are accomplished with the help of EEG.

Brain Death

EEG can confirm brain death when it shows no electrical activity more than 2 microvolts, at a sensitivity of 2 microvolts/mm for at least 30 seconds. Also, it should show no reactivity to intense somatosensory stimuli.

Definition and Meaning

According to the American Academy of Neurology guidelines, brain death is clinically equivalent to the **irreversible loss of all brain stem functions**, which refers to the impossibility of recovery, regardless of any medical intervention. However, patients with brain death could be maintained physiologically for prolonged periods in the intensive care units.

Criteria for Diagnosis of Brain Death

Brain death **can be assessed** by doing physical examination, apnea test, and ancillary tests.

I. Physical examination

This includes the response to pain and assessment of brain stem reflexes. Loss of eye response and motor reflexes in response to deep pain stimuli occur in brain death. Brain death can be confirmed if **brain stem reflexes are lost**, including:

◆ **CN II** Loss of light reflex, pupils should be mid-dilated 4 to 9 mm, and not reactive to light.
◆ **CN III, IV, VI** Eye motion is lost in reaction to head movement (Doll's eyes).
◆ **CN V, VII** Loss of corneal reflex.
◆ **CN VIII** Loss of oculovestibular reflex (caloric test)—with irrigation of each by 60 ml of ice water, the eye will not move towards the irrigated ear.
◆ **CN IX** Loss of gag reflex.
◆ **CN X** Loss of cough reflex

II. Apnea test

The apnea test is used to assess the brain's ability to drive pulmonary function in response to the rise of CO_2. During the test, oxygen should be supplemented using a cannula connected to the endotracheal tube at 6 l/min. In the case of loss of respiratory drive, CO_2 is expected to rise 5 mmHg every minute in the first 2 minutes, then by 2 mmHg every minute. The rise of CO_2 more than 20 mmHg above baseline is consistent with brain death.

III. Ancillary tests

Two types of ancillary tests are considered if there is uncertainty of diagnosis or if apnea test cannot be performed.

A. For detection of cessation of cerebral blood flow

◆ **Cerebral angiography** Four vessel angiography is considered the gold standard.

◆ **Transcranial ultrasound** This is used to assess pulsations of middle cerebral arteries, vertebral and basilar arteries bilaterally.
◆ **Computed tomogram (CT) brain angiography and MR angiography** This shows cessation of cerebral blood flow.
◆ **Radionuclide brain imaging** This can be done using a ^{99m}Tc-isotope tracer, then imaging by SPECT brain scintigraphy. The absence of a tracer in the brain circulation (the hollow skull phenomenon) is consistent with brain death.

B. For detection of loss of bioelectrical activity of the brain

◆ **Electroencephalogram (EEG)** This can confirm brain death when it shows no electrical activity more than 2 microvolts, at a sensitivity of 2 microvolts/mm for at least 30 seconds.
◆ **Somatosensory evoked potentials** Patients with brain death show no SEP in response to bilateral median nerve stimulation, and no BAEP in response to auditory stimuli.

Implications

It is crucial to differentiate brain death from other forms of severe brain damage, which can cause vegetative states when some of the brain functions are maintained, and recovery can occur even after prolonged periods, especially in patients with traumatic brain injuries. Another essential topic that evolved in parallel with brain death is the need of obtaining organs for transplantation. According to the "dead donor rule," organ procurement can occur only after death. So, for patients who are brain dead, the procurement of viable organs is allowed, even if they still have some circulatory and pulmonary functions.

VIVA

1. *Define EEG.*
2. *What are EEG waves and rhythms?*
3. *What is the basic principle of EEG recording?*
4. *List the precautions observed during EEG recording.*
5. *List the uses and applications of EEG.*
6. *What is the definition of brain death and what are the criteria to detect brain death?*

CHAPTER 36

Autonomic Function Tests

After completing this practical, you will be able to (MUST KNOW):

1. Describe the importance of performing autonomic function tests (AFTs) in clinical physiology.
2. List the functions of ANS.
3. Enumerate the major differences between the sympathetic and parasympathetic systems.
4. List the various autonomic function tests.
5. Perform various non-invasive AFTs.
6. Explain the principle of AFTs.

7. List the precautions taken for doing AFTs.
8. State the normal values of AFTs.
9. Name the conditions in which there is alteration in AFTs.

You may also be able to (DESIRABLE TO KNOW):

1. Explain the differences between the parasympathetic and sympathetic functions.
2. Explain the physiological basis of AFTs.
3. Explain the mechanism of alteration in AFTs.

INTRODUCTION

The autonomic nervous system (ANS) regulates the activity of the smooth muscle, cardiac muscle and certain glands. The ANS has traditionally been described as a specific motor output portion of the peripheral nervous system. However, to maintain homeostasis, the functioning of the ANS depends on a continuous flow of sensory input from visceral organs and blood vessels into the CNS. Therefore, the ANS has two main components, general visceral sensory (afferent) neurons and general visceral motor (efferent) neurons. The ANS maintains internal homeostasis of cardiovascular, thermoregulatory, gastrointestinal, genitourinary, exocrine and pupillary functions. It was originally thought that the ANS functions autonomously, but actually it is under the control of different centres in the brain, especially the hypothalamus and medulla oblongata which receive inputs from the limbic system and other regions of the cortex.

Autonomic functions can be evaluated by a number of invasive and non-invasive tests. The non-invasive tests can be readily performed and used to confirm the diagnosis of autonomic neuropathy whereas invasive tests require complex procedures and are used for localisation of the site of lesion. This chapter describes the different non-invasive tests to used assess autonomic functions.

Many of these autonomic function tests are affected by age, gender, race and environment. Therefore, every laboratory should establish its own control values.

Anatomical and Physiological Considerations

Functional Anatomy

1. The ANS is divided into the **sympathetic and parasympathetic** systems.
2. Both the divisions of the ANS have preganglionic and postganglionic neurons.
3. **Preganglionic neurons** are myelinated and cholinergic. The **postganglionic neurons** are unmyelinated and cholinergic in the parasympathetic division, and adrenergic in the sympathetic division, except the fibres that innervate the sweat glands and blood vessels in the skeletal muscles (sympathetic vasodilator system).
4. Cell bodies of the sympathetic preganglionic neurons lie in the intermediolateral grey horns of twelve thoracic and the first three lumbar segments of the spinal cord (Fig. 36.1A). The cell bodies of the parasympathetic preganglionic neurons lie in four cranial nerve nuclei (III, VII, IX and X) in the brainstem and lateral grey horns of the 2–4 sacral segments of the spinal cord (Fig. 36.1B).

5. Sympathetic preganglionic neurons synapse with postganglionic neurons in the paravertebralsympathetic chain of ganglia. The parasympathetic preganglionic neurons synapse with the postganglionic neurons, which are present very close to the viscera, sometimes in the viscera.

6. The gastrointestinal system is richly innervated by the ANS and the innervation has been regarded as the **enteric nervous system**, the third division of the ANS.

Physiological Considerations

Most organs of the body receive dual innervation from the ANS. Usually, one division causes facilitation and the other causes inhibition of functions of the organs.

1. Cholinergic neurons release acetylcholine as neurotransmitter whereas adrenergic neurons release norepinephrine or epinephrine.

2. The effect of parasympathetic stimulation is usually short-lived as acetylcholine is degraded rapidly, whereas the effect of sympathetic stimulation lasts long and has widespread effect.

3. Cholinergic receptors are divided into muscarinic and nicotinic types whereas adrenergic receptors are broadly categorised into α and β.

4. The parasympathetic division regulates activities that conserve and restore body energy; the sympathetic division prepares the body for emergency situations (fight or flight response), and causes loss of body energy.

5. The autonomic reflexes adjust the activities of smooth muscles, cardiac muscles and glands.

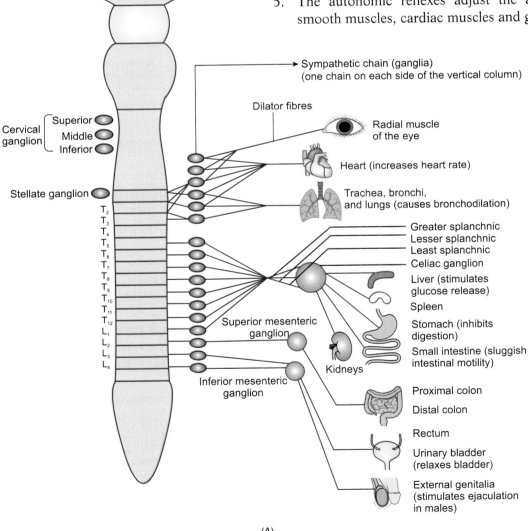

(A)

Fig. 36.1 The autonomic nervous system. (A) The sympathetic system; (B) The parasympathetic system. Note that preganglionic fibres are small in sympathetic and long in parasympathetic. The postganglionic fibres are long in the sympathetic, which are close to the organs or in the organs in the parasympathetic. (*Continues ...*)

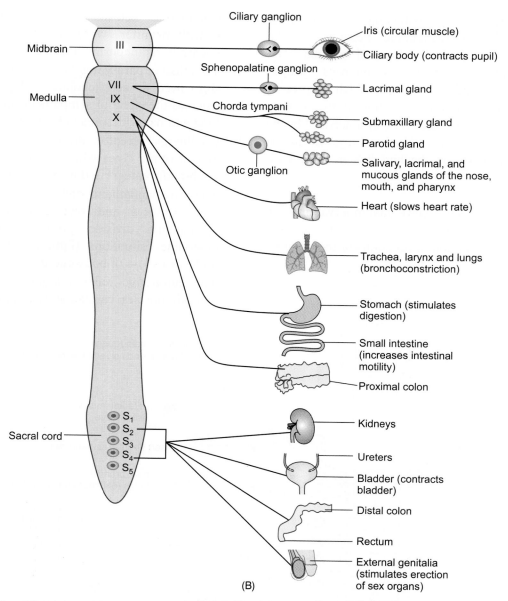

Fig. 36.1   The autonomic nervous system. (A) The sympathetic system; (B) The parasympathetic system. Note that preganglionic fibres are small in sympathetic and long in parasympathetic. The postganglionic fibres are long in the sympathetic, which are close to the organs or in the organs in the parasympathetic. (*Source:*   Prasad J. 2019. *Textbook of Pharmacology*, 2nd edition. Hyderabad: Universities Press.)

6. The autonomic reflexes consist of receptors, sensory neurons, centre of integration, autonomic motor neurons and visceral effectors.

7. The hypothalamus controls and integrates the functions of both the divisions of the ANS. The control by the cortex occurs mostly during emotional states, especially by the limbic cortex.

Autonomic Function Tests (AFTs)

A list of AFTs has been described by various authors. But the commonly used tests are:

Cardiovascular Function Tests

1. Heart rate and blood pressure (BP) response to standing
2. Heart rate and BP response to passive tilting
3. Heart rate response to deep breathing
4. Valsalva ratio
5. BP response to isometric handgrip
6. Cold pressor test

Sweat Tests

1. Sympathetic skin response

2. Quantitative sudomotor axon reflex test (QSART)

Vasomotor Tests

1. Laser Doppler Velocimetry for skin blood flow measurement with inspiratory gasp
2. Valsalva maneuver
3. Cold pressor test

Only the conventional or classical autonomic function tests (CAFT) that can easily be performed and reproduced are described in this chapter.

METHODS

Heart Rate and BP Response to Standing

Principle

Immediately on standing (from the supine position) blood pressure falls by 20 mm Hg and heart rate increases usually from 10 to 20 beats. These changes occur within 5–15 seconds.

Requirements

1. A multichannel polygraph with provision to record beat-to-beat variation in heart rate.
2. NIBP monitor or a servoplethysmo-manometer (Finapres).

Note: Though ideally polygraph and NIBP should be used, this test can also be performed with a sphygmomanometer and an ECG machine, which are routinely used clinically.

Procedure

1. Ask the subject to lie down in the supine position.
2. Connect the ECG electrodes from the subject to the polygraph and connect the pulse cap of the NIBP on one finger of the subject, or tie the cuff of the NIBP around the arm of the subject.
3. Ask the subject to relax completely for a minimum period of 10 minutes.
4. Record basal heart rate and blood pressure from the polygraph and NIBP.
5. Ask the subject to stand up and immediately note the change in heart rate and blood pressure from the monitoring screen of the polygraph and NIBP.
6. Record blood pressure and heart rate serially for 1–3 minutes after standing.

7. Determine the **30 : 15 R–R ratio** from the ECG recording of the polygraph.

Note: The longest R–R interval (slowest heart rate) occurring about 30 beats after standing divided by the shortest R–R interval (fastest heart rate) which occurs at about 15 beats after standing, gives the 30 : 15 R–R ratio.

Precautions

1. The subject should relax completely in the supine position for 10–20 minutes for recording basal blood pressure and heart rate.
2. When the subject stands up he should lean (passive standing) against the wall to avoid the effect of muscular effort of active standing on heart rate and blood pressure.
3. The change in heart rate and blood pressure should be observed within 15 seconds of standing.

Heart Rate and BP Response to Passive Tilting

Principle

The cardiovascular response to change in position is tested by tilting (passively) using a tilt table. The early responses are similar but not identical to those on standing. The early response to tilt, which occurs in 30–60 seconds, reflects the autonomic cardiovascular reflexes, but the changes that occur after 30–60 seconds reflect neurocardiogenic reflex.

Requirements

1. Tilt table
2. ECG electrodes
3. NIBP
4. Multichannel polygraph

Procedure

1. Ask the subject to lie down on the tilt table.
2. Connect ECG electrodes to the polygraph and connect the NIBP.
3. Ask the subject to relax for 10 minutes.
4. Record baseline heart rate, and blood pressure.
5. Position the head side of the tilt table to an inclination of 80° (80° head-up tilt) from the horizontal.

6. Immediately record heart rate and blood pressure and then record at one-minute intervals for three minutes.

Note: Heart rate and blood pressure response to passive tilt with head-down (head-down tilt) can also be recorded.

Precautions

1. The subject should be instructed properly regarding the maneuver.
2. The subject should be completely relaxed for a minimum of 10 minutes before recording basal heart rate and ECG.
3. The changes in heart rate and blood pressure to tilt should be recorded accurately.

Valsalva Ratio

Principle

The Valsalva ratio is a measure of the change of heart rate which takes place during a brief period of forced expiration against a closed glottis or mouthpiece (Valsalva maneuver). During and after the Valsalva maneuver there will be changes in cardiac vagal efferent and sympathetic vasomotor activity, resulting from stimulation of the carotid sinus and aortic arch baroreceptors and other intrathoracic stretch receptors.

Requirements

1. A mercury manometer
2. Nose clip
3. Mouthpiece
4. Electrocardiograph

Procedure

1. Give proper instructions to the subject regarding how to exhale forcefully into the manometer and maintain the pressure at 40 mm Hg.

Note: The subject may be allowed to practise the procedure till he is capable of doing it properly.

2. Ask the subject to lie down in a semi-recumbent or sitting position.
3. Close the nostrils with the help of the nose clip.
4. Put a mouthpiece into the mouth of the subject and connect the mercury manometer to it.

5. Switch on the ECG machine for continuous recording.
6. Ask the subject to breathe forcefully into the mercury manometer and then ask him to maintain the expiratory pressure at 40 mm Hg for 10–15 seconds.
7. Record ECG changes throughout the procedure, and 30 seconds before and after the procedure.
8. Repeat the procedure three times with a gap of five minutes between the maneuvers.
9. Calculate the Valsalva ratio and take the largest ratio of the three (which represents the best performance) for consideration.

Note: The Valsalva ratio is calculated by dividing the longest interbeat interval after the maneuver by the shortest interbeat interval during the maneuver.

Precautions

1. The subject should be instructed properly.
2. The subject should be allowed to practice the maneuver before the actual performance.
3. The subject should maintain the pressure constantly at 40 mmHg throughout the maneuver (10–15 seconds).
4. The procedure should be repeated three times and the best of the three should be taken for consideration.

Heart Rate Response to Deep Breathing

Principle

Heart rate increases during inspiration due to decreased cardiac vagal activity and decreases during expiration due to increased vagal activity. This is detected by recording the heart rate while the subject is breathing deeply.

Requirements

1. ECG apparatus with electrodes
2. ECG jelly

Procedure

There are two methods for determining heart rate variation with breathing. One method uses a single deep breath whereas the other method uses deep breathing at a rate of six breaths per minute. Usually, the method using six breaths per minute is used to determine heart rate variation with respiration.

1. Provide proper instructions to the subject.
2. Ask the subject to lie down comfortably in the supine position with the head elevated to 30°.
3. Connect ECG electrodes for recording lead II ECG.
4. Ask the subject to breathe deeply at a rate of six breaths per minute (allowing 5 seconds each for inspiration and expiration).
5. Record maximum and minimum heart rate with each respiratory cycle.
6. Determine the expiration to inspiration ratio (**E : I ratio**).

> **Note:** The E : I ratio is the mean of maximum R–R intervals during deep expiration to the mean of minimum R–R intervals during deep inspiration. The E : I ratio can also be calculated following a single deep breathing.

▌Precautions

1. The subject should be instructed properly to perform six breaths per minute.
2. The subject should be relaxed and comfortable before performing the test.

BP Response to Isometric Handgrip

▌Principle

Sustained handgrip against resistance causes an increase in heart rate and blood pressure. These responses are detected using ECG and blood pressure monitors.

▌Requirements

1. ECG electrodes and ECG machine
2. NIBP monitor/sphygmomanometer

▌Procedure

1. Give proper instructions to the subject regarding the test.
2. Ask the subject to lie down in a semirecumbent position.
3. Connect ECG electrodes for lead II recording and NIBP monitor/sphygmomanometer for blood pressure measurement.
4. Record basal heart rate and blood pressure.

5. Ask the subject to maintain a pressure of 30 per cent of the maximum activity for about 5 minutes.
6. Record the heart rate and change in diastolic pressure.

> **Note:** Change in diastolic pressure is defined as the difference between the last value recorded before the release of handgrip pressure and the mean resting value calculated by averaging the last 3 minutes of recording before commencing isometric exercise.

▌Precautions

1. The subject should be instructed properly.
2. The basal diastolic blood pressure should be recorded.
3. The subject should maintain a pressure of 30 per cent of the maximum activity for about 5 minutes.
4. The diastolic blood pressure before the release of the grip should be recorded.

Cold Pressor Test

▌Principle

Submerging the hand in cold water results in rise in systolic and diastolic pressure, which is detected by a blood pressure monitor or sphygmomanometer.

▌Requirements

1. NIBP monitor/sphygmomanometer
2. Ice cold water (just below 4°C).

▌Procedure

1. Give proper instructions to the subject regarding the test.
2. Record the blood pressure.
3. Take very cold water (at or below 4°C) in a container.
4. Ask the subject to submerge one of his upper limbs in the cold water for 60 seconds.
5. Record blood pressure at 30 and 60 seconds of submersion of the limb.

▌Precautions

1. The subject should be instructed to be mentally prepared to submerge his limb for one minute in the cold water.

2. The temperature of the cold water should be 4°C or less.

3. The subject should dip his limb in ice-cold water for one minute (not less than 30 seconds).

Sympathetic Skin Response

Principle

Sympathetic skin response (SSR) or Galvanic skin response (GSR) assesses the integrity of peripheral sympathetic cholinergic (sudomotor) function by evaluating the changes in resistance of skin to electrical conduction.

Requirements

1. EMG equipment/polygraph with provision to record EMG
2. Electrodes

Procedure

1. Give proper instructions to the subject regarding the test.
2. Connect the electrodes from the hand or feet of the subject to the EMG machine or the polygraph.

Note: Connect the active electrode on the palm or sole and the reference electrode over the dorsum of the respective body part. Disc electrodes with electrode gel are used.

3. Set the low frequency filter at 0.1 or 0.5 Hz and high frequency filter at 500–1000 Hz.
4. Set the apparatus to obtain the gain to record potential of 0.5–3 mV and set the sweep to record 5 seconds after the stimulus.
5. Provide a stimulus in the form of startling sound and record the response.
6. Record the SSR potentials, their amplitude and latency.

DISCUSSION

The assessment of autonomic function is an important part of the evaluation of the peripheral and central nervous system. Abnormalities of autonomic function lead to different clinical entities like orthostatic hypotension, sexual dysfunction, diarrhea, incontinence, dryness of mouth, and so on. Autonomic function tests are performed to confirm the clinical diagnosis of autonomic neuropathies and to assess the intactness of the sympathetic and parasympathetic pathways.

Heart Rate Response to Standing

On changing the posture from supine to standing, the heart rate increases immediately, usually by 10–20 beats per minute. On standing the heart rate increases until it reaches a maximum at about the 15th beat, after which it slows down to a stable state at about 30th beat. The ratio of R–R intervals corresponding to the 30th and 15th heart beat is called the 30 : 15 ratio. The 30 : 15 ratio is a measure of parasympathetic function. This ratio decreases with age. In young individuals, a ratio less than 1.04 is considered abnormal.

The blood pressure changes on standing are studied to assess the integrity of the sympathetic system. Immediately on standing, blood pressure falls but this activates the baroreceptor reflex and blood pressure returns to normal within 15 seconds. When systolic pressure falls by 20 mm Hg or more or diastolic pressure by 10 mm Hg or more on standing, orthostatic hypotension is said to be present.

Heart Rate Response to Tilting

Heart rate response to **head-up tilt** is especially useful in the diagnosis of multisystem atrophy and patients suffering from recurrent unexplained syncope. On changing from the recumbent to the upright position on a tilt table, there is pooling of about 30 per cent venous blood in the peripheral compartment. This decreases cardiac filling pressure and stroke volume by 40 per cent. The heart rate rises immediately due to withdrawal of parasympathetic activity and afterwards due to increased sympathetic activity.

Heart Rate Response to Deep Breathing

The variation of heart rate with respiration is known as sinus arrhythmia. Inspiration increases and expiration decreases heart rate. This is primarily mediated by parasympathetic innervation of the heart. Pulmonary stretch receptor, cardiac mechanoreceptors and baroreceptors contribute to sinus arrhythmia. The difference between the maximum and minimum heart rate during deep breathing is called **deep breath difference (DBD)**. DBD is more than 15 beats per minute in normal individuals. It assesses the parasympathetic activity. DBD decreases with age.

Normal Values of DBD

10–40 years	> 18 beats per minute
41–50 years	> 16 beats per minute
51–60 years	> 12 beats per minute
61–70 years	> 8 beats per minute

Normal Values of E : I Ratio

16–20 years	> 1.23
21–25 years	> 1.20
26–30 years	> 1.18
31–35 years	> 1.16
36–40 years	> 1.14
41–45 years	> 1.12
46–50 years	> 1.11
51–55 years	> 1.09
56–60 years	> 1.08
61–65 years	> 1.07
66–70 years	> 1.06

Clinical Conditions With Abnormalities in DBD

- Multisystem atrophy
- Progressive autonomic failure
- Diabetes
- Autonomic neuropathy
- Uremic patients
- CNS depression
- Hyperventilation
- Pulmonary diseases

Sinus arrhythmia is abolished by parasympathetic block but not by sympathetic dysfunction. This indicates that HR response to deep breathing is purely a vagal function. In fact, HR response to deep breathing is a classical parasympathetic function test.

Valsalva Ratio

The Valsalva ratio is a measure of parasympathetic and sympathetic function. For the response to occur in the Valsalva maneuver, parasympathetic acts as afferent and efferent and sympathetic as part of the efferent pathway. Therefore, the Valsalva ratio assesses more of parasympathetic (cardiovagal) function.

Valsalva Maneuver

The Valsalva maneuver has **four phases** (Fig. 36.2).

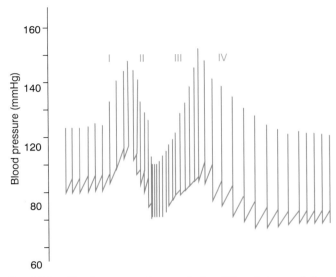

Fig. 36.2   Blood pressure changes during different phases (I, II, III, IV) of the Valsalva maneuver.

Phase I   Phase I consists of the onset of strain. In this phase, there occurs transient increase in blood pressure, which lasts for a few seconds. This is due to increased intrathoracic pressure and mechanical compression of the great vessels. However, the heart rate does not change much.

Phase II   This is the phase of straining. In the early part of this phase, venous return decreases, which decreases cardiac output and blood pressure. This change persists for 4 seconds. In the later part of this phase, blood pressure returns towards normal, which occurs due to increased peripheral resistance as a result of sympathetic vasoconstriction. However, the heart rate increases steadily throughout this phase due to vagal withdrawal (in the early phase) and sympathetic activation (in the later phase).

Phase III   This phase occurs following the release of strain in which there occurs a transient decrease in blood pressure lasting for a few seconds. This is caused by mechanical displacement of blood to the pulmonary vascular bed, which was under increased intrathoracic pressure. There is little change in heart rate.

Phase IV   This is the phase that occurs with further release of strain. The blood pressure slowly increases and the heart rate proportionately decreases. It occurs 15–20 seconds after release of strain and lasts for about a minute or more. The cardiovascular changes occur due to increase in venous return, stroke volume and cardiac output.

Calculation of Valsalva Ratio

Valsalva ratio (VR) is the ratio of longest R–R interval during phase IV to the shortest R–R interval during phase II.

$$VR = \frac{\text{Longest R–R interval during phase IV}}{\text{Shortest R–R interval during phase II}}$$

Normal Value

A Valsalva ratio of more than 1.45 is considered to be normal. When it is 1.2–1.45, it is borderline, and if it is less than 1.2, is regarded as abnormal.

Valsalva ratios in different age groups are:

10–40 years > 1.5	51–60 years > 1.40
41–50 years > 1.45	61–70 years > 1.35

Factors That Affect Valsalva Ratio

- Age
- Sex
- Position of patient
- Expiratory pressure
- Duration of strain
- Practice of yogic techniques

Clinical applications

1. Changes in the Valsalva maneuver occur due to changes in cardiac vagal efferent and sympathetic vasomotor activity, which are stimulated by the carotid sinus and aortic arch baroreceptors and other intrathoracic stretch receptors.
2. Failure of heart rate to increase during strain suggests a sympathetic dysfunction and failure of heart rate to slow down after the strain suggests parasympathetic dysfunction.
3. If the cardiovascular response to the Valsalva maneuver is abnormal but that to cold pressure test is normal, the lesion is thought to be present in the baroreceptors or their afferent nerves. Such abnormalities occur commonly in diabetes, other neuropathies, multisystem atrophy and autonomic failure.

BP Response to Isometric Handgrip

In the isometric handgrip (IHG) test, there is a rise in heart rate and blood pressure. These cardiovascular responses to isometric exercise are mediated mainly by influence of cardiovascular centres and partly by metabolic or mechanical changes or both, in response to contraction of the muscles that activate small fibres in the afferent limb of the reflex arch. The normal response is **rise in diastolic pressure of more than 15 mm Hg** and rise in the heart rate by about 30 per cent. The blood pressure rise is due to increased sympathetic activity and heart rate rise is due to decreased parasympathetic activity and increased sympathetic activity. This response is not influenced by age. The BP response to IHG is a pure sympathetic response, and is considered as the best among sympathetic function tests.

Cold Pressor Test

Submerging hands in ice-cold water increases systolic pressure by about 20 mm Hg and diastolic pressure by 10 mm Hg. The afferent limb of the reflex pathway consists of somatic fibres whereas the efferent pathway consists of the sympathetic fibres. Though this test is a classical sympathetic function test, it requires standardisation for the age and gender as the rise in BP is not equal in all subjects and there are variations.

OTHER TESTS

Standing to Lying Ratio (SLR)

Heart rate (RR interval) response to lying down from standing posture is assessed by continuous recoding of ECG.

- Following lying from standing position, **increase in venous** return produces **reflex bradycardia**.
- Ratio of **longest RR interval in standing to shortest RR interval in lying down** is calculated as SLR.
- Value of SLR **below 1** is considered as abnormal.

Tests for Sudomotor Functions

Sympathetic Skin Response

Sympathetic skin response (SSR) helps in studying the functions of **peripheral sympathetic cholinergic (sudomotor) fibres** by evaluating the changes in resistance of skin in response to electrical stimuli.

- SSR is age dependent and is present in both hands and feet till the age of 60.
- Composition of surface electrodes, stimulus frequency, skin temperature, and mental state of the subject affect the parameters of SSR.
- The latency and amplitude of SSR are measured.
- The amplitude of SSR in hand is 1.6 mV and in feet is 2.1 mV.
- SSR is helpful in diagnosing multisystem atrophy, progressive autonomic failure, diabetes, uremic patients and alcoholic neuropathy.

Thermoregulatory Sweat Test (TST)

Assessment of **sweating response to heat** also assesses sudomotor functions.

- The subject's body temperature is raised to by 1°C by exposing to heat of the electric heater.
- Sweating response is studied by demarcating the area of sweating with the help of iodide starch or quinizarin powder that changes the colour of the moist skin.
- Absence of sweating in TST indicates sympathetic pre- and post-ganglionic lesions.

Quantitative Sudomotor Axon Reflex Test

Quantitative sudomotor axon reflex test (**QSART**) is a measure of regional autonomic function by Ach-induced sweating.

- In this test, Ach is injected intradermally and the sweat production rate is assessed.
- Reduced or absence of sweating indicates post-ganglionic lesion of sudomotor fibres (sympathetic fibres concerned with sweating).

Tests for Pupillary Functions

Pupillary function tests assess the function of sympathetic nerve supplying iris. Two tests usually performed are: cocaine test and adrenaline test.

Cocaine Test

Dilation of pupil is observed following instillation of 4% cocaine on both eyes. Cocaine prevents reuptake of norepinephrine at adrenergic nerve endings. Therefore, pupils dilate in response to cocaine, but, Horner's pupils do not.

Adrenaline Test

Instillation of 1:100 or 1% noradrenaline on eyes dilate Horner's pupil more than normal pupil. This is due to the mechanism of denervation hypersensitivity of Horner's pupil.

Tests for Bladder Function

Cystometrogram (CMG) is performed to detect autonomic dysfunctions of urinary bladder.

- CMG reveals decreased ability of bladder to accommodate urine.
- Absence of accommodation to filling indicates autonomic dysfunction.
- Also, contraction of bladder muscle is poor in response to the act of micturition (evacuation).

Spectral Analysis of HRV and BRS

Recently, spectral analysis of heart rate variability (HRV) and baroreflex sensitivity (BRS) have evolved as a sensitive tool for assessing integrity of sympathetic and parasympathetic functions, determining the **sympathovagal balance and for assessing CV risks**. (Details are given in next two chapters)

AFTs to Assess Sympathetic and Parasympathetic Functions

AFTs for Assessment of Sympathetic Functions

1. BP response to standing/tilt
2. Cold pressor test
3. Isometric hand-grip
4. Galvanic/sympathetic skin response
5. Thermoregulatory sweat test
6. Tachycardia ratio
7. Valsalva ratio
8. NE spillage test
9. LF, LFnu and LF-HF ratio of HRV

AFTs for Assessment of Parasympathetic Functions

1. **Resting heart rate**   Basal heart rate is a good index of parasympathetic functions as heart rate in resting conditions is a measure of vagal tone. Resting HR more 75 indicates poor vagal tone and is considered as a CV risk.
2. 30:15 ratio
3. E:I ratio
4. Valsalva ratio
5. Bradycardia ratio
6. Baroreceptor reflex sensitivity
7. Standing to lying ratio
8. HF and HFnu of HRV

Concept of Reactivity and Activity Tests and CAFTs

Reactivity Tests

Tests that are based on stimuli or disturbances such as change in position (standing, lying, dipping finger in cold water, handgrip against resistance,

Valsalva maneuver etc.) are called **reactivity tests**. Accordingly, they are grouped as *sympathetic and parasympathetic reactivity tests*.

Activity Tests

Tests that are performed without disturbing the subject (subject at rest usually lying on couch in a comfortable room for 15 to 20 min) are called **activity tests**.

1. Recording of Resting HR and BP, and HRV analysis are examples.

2. Accordingly, they are grouped as **sympathetic and parasympathetic activity tests**.

3. **Resting heart rate is a parasympathetic test and resting BP is a sympathetic test.**

CAFTs

CAFTs refer to conventional autonomic function tests. HR and BP response to standing, HR response to deep breathing, isometric handgrip, cold pressor test and Valsalva maneuver are CAFTs.

VIVA

1. *What are the divisions of ANS?*
2. *What are the postganglionic cholinergic fibres in the sympathetic system?*
3. *What are the functions of the sympathetic and parasympathetic divisions of ANS?*
4. *List the classical or conventional autonomic function tests (CAFT).*
5. *How do you assess cardiovascular response to standing? Why is the 30 : 15 ratio significant?*
6. *What is the significance of cardiovascular response to standing?*
7. *What are the precautions taken for testing cardiovascular response to standing?*
8. *How do you assess cardiovascular response to passive tilting?*
9. *What is the difference between cardiovascular response to standing and cardiovascular response to passive tilting?*
10. *What is the Valsalva ratio? What is its significance?*
11. *What is the normal value of the Valsalva ratio in different age groups?*
12. *What are the factors that affect the Valsalva ratio?*
13. *What is the procedure for the Valsalva maneuver?*
14. *What is the principle of the Valsalva maneuver?*
15. *What are the precautions taken while performing the Valsalva maneuver?*
16. *How do you assess heart rate variation with deep breathing? What is the principle of this test?*
17. *What is the normal value of deep breathing difference (DBD) and E : I ratio in different age groups?*
18. *What is sinus arrhythmia?*
19. *What are the conditions that alter DBD?*
20. *What is isometric hand-grip test? What is its principle?*
21. *What is the cold pressure test? What is its significance?*
22. *What is sympathetic skin response (SSR)? What is its significance?*
23. *What are the factors that affect SSR?*
24. *What is the most sensitive AFT?*

   Ans: Spectral analysis of heart rate variability (HRV) is the most sensitive AFT. LF–HF ratio of HRV indicates sympathovagal balance of the individual. However, HRV is not an accurate test, especially for diagnosis of autonomic dysfunctions. HRV help in future prediction of cardiovascular (CV) problems and CV risk stratification.

25. *What are the best sympathetic AFTs.*

   Ans: BP response to IGH, SSR and QSART are the best sympathetic function tests. However, BP response to IHG is considered to be the best among them due to its consistent result and easy recording & reproducibility.

26. *What is the best parasympathetic AFT.*

   Ans: HR response to deep breathing is the best parasympathetic function test. Resting heart is a good index of vagal tone.

CHAPTER 37

Spectral Analysis of Heart Rate Variability

Learning Objectives

After completing this practical, you will be able to (MUST KNOW):

1. Define and explain heart rate variability (HRV).
2. List the different components (time domain and frequency domain) of HRV.
3. State the physiological importance of each HRV component.
4. Explain the principle of HRV recording.
5. Explain the concept of sympathovagal balance.
6. Explain the importance of HRV in health and disease.

You may also be able to (DESIRABLE TO KNOW):

1. Describe the different methods of HRV measurement.
2. Explain the time domain and frequency domain indices of HRV.
3. State the importance of HRV recording in assessing sympathovagal balance.
4. Explain the significance of HRV recording from other autonomic function tests.
5. Explain the clinical utility of HRV analysis.

INTRODUCTION

Heart rate variability (HRV) is the cardiac beat-to-beat variation (variation in cardiac cycle length), a physiological phenomenon that occurs mainly due to variation in cardiac activity during the respiratory cycle (**respiratory sinus arrhythmia**) at rest, though the circadian rhythm, environmental factors and exercise also contribute to it. Variation in cardiac cycle length (the physiological basis of HRV) will be appreciated from presentation of 2.5 seconds of heart beat recordings, as depicted in Fig. 37.1.

Resting heart rates can vary, some have rates of 100 beats/min while others beat at only 60 beats/min for no obvious reason. The rate of the heart and its beat-to-beat variations are dependent on the rate of discharge of the primary pacemaker, the SA node, which is influenced by

autonomic activities that are controlled in a complex way by a variety of reflexes, central irradiations and cortical factors. As SA nodal discharge is largely controlled by parasympathetic (vagal) influence, and sinus arrhythmia is primarily due to alteration in vagal tone in inspiration and expiration, **HRV is mainly influenced by vagal activity**, though both the divisions of ANS influence it. Recently, HRV has been proposed as the most sensitive indicator of autonomic function, especially for the assessment of sympathovagal balance, the balance between the sympathetic and parasympathetic activity of the individual at any given time. The state of sympathovagal balance is used for the prediction of many cardiovascular (CV) dysfunctions and other dysfunctions affecting cardiovascular function, its main use is in the CV risk stratification. However, the use of HRV analysis is limited in the diagnosis and management of CV and other diseases.

Technical Aspects

HRV can be quantified in the time and frequency domains. The time domain measures include the usual tools of assessment of variation, as is performed in statistics. The time domain is easier to assess but finer aspects of variations are not appreciated. In a short period, the overall magnitude of HRV is assessed well but the individual contributions of various factors are not elucidated.

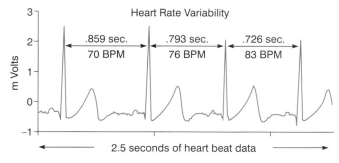

Fig. 37.1   Variation in cardiac cycle length during heart beats, as presented in three consecutive beats here.

On the other hand, variations in instantaneous heart rate can be assessed spectrally. That is, **an R–R tachogram** is plotted using the R–R intervals in the five-minute lead II ECG. The R–R tachogram is considered as a non-periodic signal which is transformed to its frequency spectrum using the **Fast Fourier Transform (FFT) algorithm or autoregressive (AR) modelling**. The biggest advantage of this complex mathematical transformation is that the distribution of magnitude of variation in different frequency bands corresponds to the activity of different physiological systems. The entire frequency spectrum, 0.0–0.4 Hz, is divided as follows.

HRV Components

The power spectrum of HRV in mammals usually reveals three spectral components (Fig. 37.2):
1. A high-frequency band (HF) 0.15–0.4 Hz
2. A low-frequency band (LF) 0.04–0.15 Hz
3. A very low-frequency band (VLF) 0.0–0.04 Hz

The HF component is caused by vagal activity during the respiratory cycle. The inspiratory inhibition of vagal activity is evoked centrally in the cardiovascular centre and this explains why the heart rate fluctuates with respiratory frequency. In addition, peripheral reflexes arising from the thoracic stretch receptors contribute to this so-called respiratory sinus arrhythmia (RSA). RSA is clearly abolished by atropine or vagotomy and the power of the HF component is used as an index of vagal modulation of cardiac function.

The LF component of HRV is characterised by an oscillatory pattern with a period of 10 seconds. This rhythm originates from self-oscillation in the vasomotor part (sympathetic component) of the

baroreflex loop as a result of negative feedback, and it is commonly associated with synchronous fluctuations in blood pressure, the so-called Mayer waves. Though LF component mainly represent cardiac vagal drive, it has some parasympathetic contribution.

The VLF component accounts for all other heart rate changes, including those associated with thermoregulation and humoral (especially, the renin–angiotensin mechanism) and local factors.

Power Spectrum Analysis of HRV

The power spectrum of HRV is analysed by two methods: FFT and AR modelling.

Fast Fourier Transform

Any non-periodic electrophysiological signal can be described as the sum of sine waves, and this decomposition is called the Fast Fourier Transform (FFT). This is an efficient algorithm, which, with some improvements and modifications, is still in use in many applications such as voice analysis and vibration studies analysis of short-term HRV (SHRV). FFT algorithms impose some constraints on the signal to be analysed because an evenly sampled, infinite, stationary time series is required.

Autoregressive Modelling

An alternative method to the FFT is the autoregressive (AR) identification algorithm combined with power spectral estimation for the assessment of SHRV. This method fits the data to a prior defined model and estimates the parameters of the model. The power spectrum implied by the model is then computed.

FFT and AR modelling share a common goal: the estimation of the power spectrum of a signal. FFT-based methods are also called non-parametric methods because the time domain prior to spectral analysis is greatly simplified.

The **FFT and AR algorithms** are the most commonly used tools to study the SHRV. The final step in SHRV analysis is the application of power spectrum estimation methods to characterise the frequency components associated with vagal and/or sympathetic outflow. AR methods are parametric because they require prior information of the system under study. Thus, it was suggested that **FFT-based methods are still the best choice** for the assessment of SHRV in

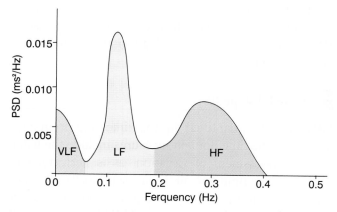

Fig. 37.2   Distribution of VLF, LF, and HF in HRV power spectrum. Note that in this picture, the TP was 920 ms², of which VLF was 70 ms², LF was 400 ms² and HF was 450 ms².

comparative studies, where no previous knowledge of the system is available. In addition, FFT algorithms are readily available in many languages, even in commercial statistical packages. Once the basic spectral content of the system is known and an initial model of the signal can be formulated, AR algorithms should be a better choice because they provide better frequency resolution and avoid the problems of spectral leakage.

The electrocardiogram (ECG) is the most appropriate signal to study SHRV because it offers the most accurate representation of electrical cardiac events. In particular, the QRS complex of the ECG sharply defines the onset of ventricular electrical depolarisation and is the closest approach used to time the occurrence of pacemaker potentials, which in turn are modulated by the autonomic outflow.

HRV Indices

HRV analysis has two components: time domain and frequency domain. The HRV assessed by calculating indices is based on statistical operations on R–R intervals (**time domain analysis**) or by spectral analysis of an array of R–R intervals (**frequency domain analysis**). Both methods require accurate timing of R waves. The analysis can be performed on short ECG segments (lasting 0.5–5 minutes) or on 24-hour ECG recordings. The analysis of the five to ten minutes of ECG recording is called short-term HRV and of the 24-hour ECG recording is called long-term HRV.

Time Domain Analysis

Two types of HRV indices are distinguished in time domain analysis. Beat-to-beat or short-term variability (STV) indices represent fast changes in heart rate. Long-term variability (LTV) indices are slower fluctuations (fewer than 6 per minute). Both types of indices are calculated from the R–R intervals occurring in a chosen time window (usually between 0.5 and 5 minutes). An example of a simple STV index is the standard deviation (SD) of beat-to-beat R–R interval differences within the time window. Examples of LTV indices are the SD of all the R–R intervals, or the difference between the maximum and minimum R–R interval length within the window. With calculated heart rate variability indices, respiratory sinus arrhythmia contributes to STV, and baroreflex- and thermoregulation-related heart rate variability contributes to LTV.

Frequency Domain Analysis

Since spectral analysis was introduced as a method to study heart rate variability, an increasing number of investigators have preferred this method over time domain analysis for calculating heart rate variability indices. The main advantage of the spectral analysis of signals is that one can study the signal's frequency-specific oscillations. Thus both the amount of variability and the oscillation frequency (number of heart rate fluctuations per second) can be obtained. Spectral analysis involves decomposing the series of sequential R–R intervals into a sum of sinusoidal functions of different amplitudes and frequencies by the FFT algorithm. The result can be displayed (power spectrum) with the magnitude of variability as a function of frequency. Thus, the power spectrum reflects the amplitude of the heart rate fluctuations present at different oscillation frequencies.

Measurement of HRV

Time Domain Methods

The variation in heart rate may be evaluated by a number of methods. Perhaps the simplest to perform are the time domain measures. In these methods, either the heart rate at any point in time or the intervals between successive normal complexes are determined. In a continuous ECG record, each QRS complex is detected, and the so-called normal-to-normal (N–N) intervals (all intervals between adjacent QRS complexes resulting from sinus node depolarisation or in the instantaneous heart rate) are determined. Simple time domain variables that can be calculated include the mean N–N interval, mean heart rate, difference between the longest and shortest N–N interval, the difference between night and day heart rates and so on. Selected time domain measures of HRV are listed in Table 37.1.

Statistical Methods

From a series of instantaneous heart rates or cycle intervals, particularly those recorded over longer periods, traditionally 24 hours, more complex statistical time domain measures can be calculated. These may be divided into **two classes**: (1) Those derived from direct measurements of the N–N intervals or instantaneous heart rate and (2) those derived from the differences between N–N intervals. These variables may be derived from the analysis of the total ECG recording or may

Table 37.1 Selected time domain measures of HRV.

Variable	Description	Physiological significance
SDNN (ms)	Standard deviation of all normal to normal (NN) intervals.	Overall vagal modulation of cardiac functions from beat to beat
RMSSD (ms)	Square root of the mean of the sum of the squares of the differences between adjacent NN intervals.	Vagal modulation of cardiac functions on short-term basis
SDNN index (ms)	Mean of the standard deviations of all NN intervals for all 5 min segments of the entire recording.	Same as SDNN
NN50 count	Number of pairs of adjacent NN interval differing by more than 50 ms in the entire recording.	Short-term variability of vagal modulation
pNN50 (%)	NN50 count divided by the total number of all NN intervals.	Short-term variability of vagal modulation

be calculated using smaller segments of the recording period. The most commonly used measures derived from interval differences include: **SDNN**, the standard deviation of all N-N intervals; **RMSSD**, the square root of the mean squared differences of successive N–N intervals; **NN50**, the number of interval differences of successive N–N intervals greater than 50 ms; and **pNN50**, the proportion derived by dividing NN50 by the total number of N–N intervals (Table 37.1). All of these measurements of the short-term variation estimate high-frequency variations in heart rate and are thus highly correlated.

Geometrical Methods

A series of **N–N intervals** also can be converted into a geometric pattern such as the sample density distribution of N–N interval durations, sample density distribution of difference between adjacent N–N intervals, Lorenz plot of N–N or R–R intervals and so on. A simple formula that judges the variability on the basis of the geometric and/or graphics properties of the resulting pattern is used. The HRV triangular index measurement is the integral of the density distribution (that is, the number of all N–N intervals) divided by the maximum of the density distribution. The main advantage of the geometric methods lies in their relative insensitivity to the analytical quality of the series of N–N intervals. The main disadvantage is the need for a reasonable number of N–N intervals to construct the geometric pattern.

The methods expressing overall HRV and its long- and short-term components cannot replace each other. The selection of the method used should correspond to the aim of each particular study.

Frequency Domain Methods

Various spectral methods for the analysis of the tachogram have been applied since the late 1960s.

Power spectral density (PSD) analysis provides the basic information about how power (variance) distributes as a function of frequency. Independent of the method used, only an estimate of the true PSD of the signal can be obtained by proper mathematical algorithms.

Methods for the calculation of PSD may be generally classified as **non-parametric and parametric**. In most instances, both methods provide comparable results.

The advantages of the non-parametric methods are: (1) the simplicity of the algorithm used (FFT in most of the cases and (2) the high processing speed.

The advantages of parametric methods are: (1) smoother spectral components that can be distinguished independently of pre-selected frequency bands, (2) easy post-processing of the spectrum with automatic calculation of low- and high-frequency power components and easy identification of the central frequency of each component and (3) an accurate estimation of PSD even on a small number of samples on which the signal is supposed to remain stationary.

The basic disadvantage of parametric methods is the need for verification of the suitability of the chosen model and of its complexity (that is, the order of the model). Selected frequency domain measures of HRV are listed in Table 37.2.

Spectral Components of Frequency Domain

Short-Term Recordings

Three main spectral components are distinguished in a spectrum calculated from short-term recordings of 5 to 10 minutes: **VLF, LF and HF**. The distribution of the power and the central frequency of LF and HF are not fixed but may vary in relation to changes in autonomic modulations of the heart period. The physiological explanation of the VLF component is less clearly defined and the existence of a specific process attributable to these heart period changes might even be questioned. The non-harmonic component, which does not have coherent properties and is affected by algorithms of baseline or trend removal, is commonly accepted as a major constituent of VLF. Thus VLF assessed from short-term recordings (≤5 minutes) is a dubious measure and should be avoided when the PSD of short-term ECGs is interpreted.

The measurement of VLF, LF and HF power components is usually made in **absolute values of power** (milliseconds squared). LF and HF may also be measured in normalised units, which represent the relative value of each power component in proportion to the total power minus the VLF component (Table 37.2). The representation of LF and HF in normalised units (LF nu and HF nu) emphasises the controlled and balanced behaviour of the two branches of the autonomic nervous system. Moreover, the normalisation tends to minimise the effect of the changes in total power on the values of LF and HF components. Nevertheless, **normalised units** should always be quoted with absolute values of LF and HF power in order to describe completely the distribution of power in spectral components. The LF–HF ratio provides a better indicator of spectral powers.

Long-Term Recordings

Spectral analysis may also be used to analyse the sequence of N–N intervals of the entire 24-hour period, recorded by Holter monitoring. The result then includes an ultra-low frequency (ULF) component, in addition to the VLF, LF and HF components. The slope of the 24-hour spectrum can also be assessed on a log–log scale by linear fitting the spectral values. Frequency domain measures are summarised below.

METHODS

Method to Determine Spectral Indices of HRV

Principle

Beat-to-beat variation in SA nodal discharge as recorded by ECG is computed and analysed by the software to determine the spectral indices of HRV.

Requirements

1. All equipment as required for ECG recording
2. Computer with software for HRV analysis

Procedure

There are two types of HRV recordings: the short-term 5-minute HRV recording and the 24-hour (day–night) long-term HRV recording. As the short-term HRV recording is usually performed for research and clinical investigations, we shall describe its procedure as given in the Task Force Report on HRV.

1. Ask the subject to lie down comfortably in the supine position in the laboratory (5 min rest).

Table 37.2   Selected frequency domain measures of HRV.

Variable	Frequency range	Description analysis of short-term recordings (5 min.)	Physiological significance
TP (ms^2)	Approximately <0.4 Hz	The variance of NN intervals over the temporal segment.	Overall vagal potency of cardiacmodulation, i.e., the heart rate variability
VLF (ms^2)	0–0.04 Hz	Power in very low frequency range.	Integrity of renin-angiotensin system
LF (ms^2)	0.04–0.15 Hz	Power in low frequency range.	Mainly, cardiac sympathetic drive
LF-normalised (LFnu)		LF power in normalisedunits LF/ (Total Power – VLF) x 100	Cardiac sympathetic modulation, independent of other powers of modulation
HF (ms^2)	0.15–0.4 Hz	Power in high-frequency range.	Cardiac parasympathetic drive
HF-normalised (HFnu)		HF power in normalised units HF/ (Total Power – VLF) x 100	Cardiac parasympathetic modulation, independent of other powers of HRV
LF/HF		Ratio LF [ms^2] / HF [ms^2]	Sympathovagal balance

TP: total power; nu: normalised unit

2. Place the ECG electrodes on the limbs of the subject and connect the leads to the machine for lead II ECG recording (Fig. 37.3).

3. Acquire the ECG signals at a rate of 1000 samples/second during supine rest using a data acquisition system such as BIOPAC MP 100 (BIOPAC Inc., USA) (minimum 250 Hz sampling rate).

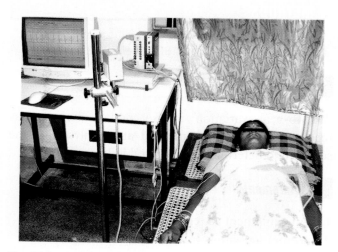

Fig. 37.3   System of HRV recording. Note that the Lead II ECG signals are recorded at a rate of 1000 samples/second during supine rest using a data acquisition system (BIOPAC MP 100).

Note: The raw ECG signal and the R–R intervals are acquired on a moving time base.

4. Transfer the data from BIOPAC to a Windows-based PC loaded with software for HRV analysis, such as AcqKnowledge software 3.8.2.

5. Remove ectopics and artifacts from the recorded ECG.

6. Extract the R–R tachogram from the edited 256-second ECG using the R wave detector in the AcqKnowledge software and save it in the ASCII format which is later used offline for short-term HRV analysis (the R–R tachogram should have a minimum of 288 R–R intervals) (Fig. 37.4).

7. Perform HRV analysis using the HRV analysis software version 1.1 (Biosignal Analysis group, Finland).

Note: Mean R–R is measured in second(s). Variance, defined as power in a portion of the total spectrum of frequencies, is measured in milliseconds squared (ms^2). Mean R–R is measured in seconds (s).

Different spectral indices (TP, LF, HF, LF nu, HF nu and LF/HF ratio) and the time domain indices (mean R–R, SDNN and RMSSD) are calculated as described below.

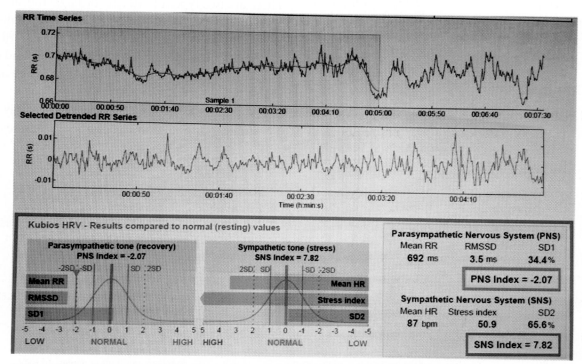

Fig. 37.4   R-R tachogram obtained from continuous ECG recordings for HRV analysis. Note that 300 R-R intervals (30 to 330) were selected from R-R interval time series (upper R-R tracing). Lower R-R tracing represents selected R-R intervals. Also note the PNS index and SNS index of the sympathetic and parasympathetic drive respectively.

Calculation of Time Domain Indices

In a continuous ECG record, each QRS complex is detected and the so-called normal to normal (N−N) intervals (that is, all intervals between adjacent QRS complexes resulting from sinus node depolarisation) or instantaneous heart rate is determined. Simple time domain variables that are calculated include the mean R–R, standard deviation of normal to normal interval (SDNN) and square root of the mean squared differences of successive normal to normal intervals (RMSSD) of HRV.

Calculation of Frequency Domain Indices

Frequency domain variables that are usually calculated include total power (TP), low frequency (LF) component, LF component expressed as normalised unit (LF nu), high-frequency (HF) component, HF component expressed as normalised unit (HF nu) and LF/HF ratio. Normalising spectral powers are calculated by the following formulae:

1. LF nu = LF/(TP − VLF) × 100
2. HF nu = HF/(TP − VLF) × 100
3. LF/HF ratio = Ratio of LF to HF spectral powers

Precautions

1. The subject should take light breakfast if the recording is done in the morning. The stomach should not be full and heavy.
2. The room temperature should be comfortable and constant for all recordings.
3. The subject should not have taken coffee, tea and soft drinks at least one hour prior to recording.
4. No smoking and alcohol two hours prior to recording.
5. Patient should not be disturbed throughout the recording.
6. All ectopics should be removed from the ECG tachogram.
7. Take all the precautions of ECG recording (refer Chapter 26).

Observation and Analysis

Meticulously study and analyse the entire recording of HRV graph. Note the time domain and frequency domain results and assess the Poincaré plots (Fig. 37.5).

DISCUSSION

Physiological Significance

HRV analysis is used to precisely assess the efficiency of vagal control of the individual, as it reflects the heart rate variability that occurs mainly due to sinus arrhythmia. Due to inspiratory inhibition of the vagal tone, the heart rate shows fluctuations with a frequency similar to the respiratory rate. The inspiratory inhibition is evoked primarily by central irradiation of impulses from the medullary respiratory to the cardiovascular centre. Respiratory sinus arrhythmia can be abolished by atropine or vagotomy as it is parasympathetically mediated.

HRV Analysis for Assessment of Sympathovagal Balance

HRV, that is, the degree of heart rate fluctuations around the mean heart rate, can be used as a mirror of the cardio-respiratory control system. It is a valuable tool to investigate the sympathetic and parasympathetic function of the autonomic nervous system. SA nodal activity at any particular time is determined by the balance between vagal activity, which slows it, and sympathetic activity, which accelerates it. Generally, if the rate is lower than the intrinsic rate of the pacemaker, it implies predominant vagal activity, while high heart rates are achieved by increased sympathetic drive. The **HF component of HRV** indicates the **cardiac vagal drive** of the individual. Increased HF power (or more specifically, increased HF nu) represents increased vagal drive and **decreased HF power (decreased HF nu) represents decreased vagal drive to the heart**.

The **LF component of HRV** mainly indicates the **cardiac sympathetic drive** of the individual. **Increased LF power (or more specifically, increased LFnu) represents increased sympathetic drive** while decreased LF power (decreased LF nu) represents decreased sympathetic drive.

The **sympathovagal balance** is assessed by the LF–HF ratio. Increased **LF–HF ratio reflects increased sympathetic activity**, while decreased LF–HF ratio indicates increased parasympathetic and decreased sympathetic activity.

The relationship between vagal stimulation frequency and the resulting change in heart rate is hyperbolic, with changes in frequency at low heart rates having a much greater effect, which does not directly control the

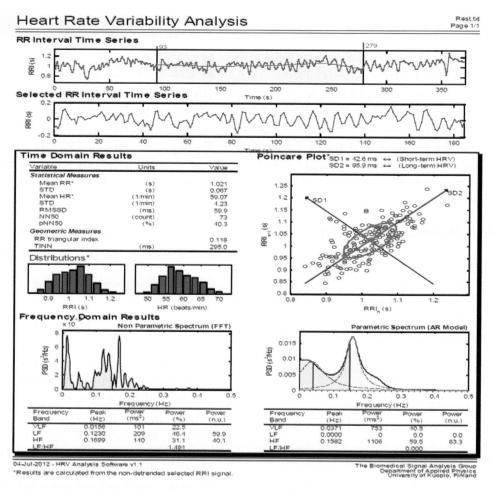

Fig. 37.5 Graph of the entire recording of HRV. Note the time domain and frequency domain results (parametric and non-parametric) and observe the Poincaré plots.

heart rate, but regulates the interval between successive beats. The effect of vagal stimulation is rapid. Vagal stimulation releases the neurotransmitter acetylcholine, which inhibits the pacemaker potentials. Sympathetic responses differ from vagal effects in that they develop much more slowly. Hence, responses with longer latency are likely to be mainly sympathetic.

Peripheral vascular resistance exhibits intrinsic oscillations with a low frequency. These oscillations can be influenced by thermal skin stimulation and are thought to arise from thermoregulatory peripheral blood flow adjustments. The fluctuations in peripheral vascular resistance are accompanied by fluctuations with the same frequency in blood pressure and heart rate and are mediated by the sympathetic nervous system. Hence, analysis of HRV also indicates the tone of sympathetic outflow and therefore reflects the individual's state of sympathetic function and susceptibility to sympathetic dysfunction.

Importance of LF–HF Ratio and Sympathovagal Balance

The HF component of HRV, which indicates the cardiac vagal drive to the heart, represents parasympathetic activity. The LF component of HRV, which mainly indicates the cardiac sympathetic drive, represents sympathetic activity. In healthy individuals, **HF constitutes about 60%**, and LF constitutes about 40% of the total power **(TP) of HRV**. Therefore, **LF–HF ratio less than 1 indicates good cardiovascular health**. However, LF–HF ratio in normal population varies from 0.5 to 1.5. The sympathovagal balance is assessed by the LF–HF ratio. Increased LF–HF ratio reflects increased sympathetic activity (Fig. 37.6), which is invariably associated with decreased TP, while decreased LF–HF ratio indicates increased parasympathetic and decreased sympathetic activity, which is invariably associated with increased TP (Fig. 37.7).

Clinical Applications

Though there is considerable discussion regarding the physiology of HRV, it is well correlated and studied in many physiological and pathological conditions:

1. **Total power (TP) of HRV** indicates the magnitude of heart rate variability. Decreased TP (decreased

overall cardiac vagal modulation) has been implicated with future adverse cardiovascular (CV) morbidities and mortalities.

2. Decreased HRV (decreased total power of HRV) is observed in many cardiovascular disease conditions and generally indicates poor prognosis in these conditions.

Frequency domain results

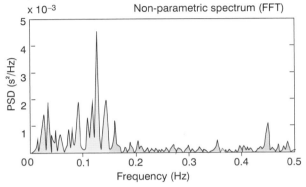

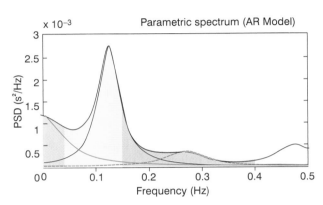

Frequency band	Peak (Hz)	Power (ms²)	Power (%)	Power (n.u.)
VLF	0.0332	22	15.4	
LF	0.1250	89	62.7	74.0
HF	0.1602	31	22.0	26.0
LF/HF			2.852	

Frequency band	Peak (Hz)	Power (ms²)	Power (%)	Power (n.u.)
VLF	0.0000	61	21.1	
LF	0.1270	189	65.9	64.6
HF	0.2734	37	13.0	12.7
LF/HF			5.077	

Fig. 37.6 Frequency domain indices of HRV analysis of a subject having increased sympathetic activity. *Refer* Fig. 37.2 for PSD of VLF, LF and HF of HRV. Note that as depicted in parametric spectrum, LF Power (ms²) is significantly increased (189 ms²) compared to HF Power, which is grossly reduced (37 ms²) and LF–HF ratio is increased to 5.077. Also, total power is only 287 (VLF 61 + LF 189 + HF 37).

Frequency domain results

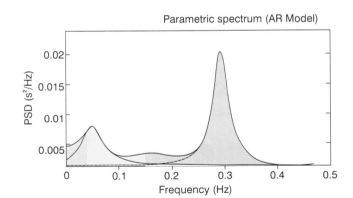

Frequency band	Peak (Hz)	Power (ms²)	Power (%)	Power (n.u.)
VLF	0.0254	247	15.2	
LF	0.0527	312	19.2	22.7
HF	0.3145	1063	65.5	77.3
LF/HF			0.293	

Frequency band	Peak (Hz)	Power (ms²)	Power (%)	Power (n.u.)
VLF	0.0000	0	0.0	
LF	0.0508	557	30.0	28.4
HF	0.3105	1301	70.0	66.3
LF/HF			0.428	

Fig. 37.7 Frequency domain indices of HRV analysis of a subject having more parasympathetic activity. *Refer* Fig. 37.2 for PSD of VLF, LF and HF of HRV. Note that as depicted in parametric spectrum, HF Power (ms²) is significantly increased (1301 ms²) compared to LF Power, which is much less (557 ms²) and LF–HF ratio is decreased to 0.428. Also, total power is 1858 (VLF 0 + LF 557 + HF 1305), which is quite high and reflects increased HRV, an indicator of good CV health.

3. Much before the onset of clinical symptoms of the cardiovascular disease, alterations are observed in HRV, indicating that HRV could be used as a sensitive tool in the prediction of CV health. However, more research is required to establish the predictive value of HRV in CV dysfunctions.

4. Presently, HRV is used as a prognostic tool in conditions like post-myocardial infarction and cardiac transplantation.

5. The most important application of HRV analysis is the surveillance of post-infarction and diabetic patients.

6. HRV gives information about the sympathetic–parasympathetic autonomic balance, and used as tool for assessment of autonomic imbalance.

7. As HRV analysis is used to assess the state of sympathovagal balance of the individual, it can be used to determine the individual's susceptibility to developing autonomic dysfunctions in conditions like prehypertension and hypertension.

8. Decreased HRV is well correlated with the risk of sudden cardiac death in patients with heart disease.

9. Improvement in HRV and CV health are observed in interventions like exercise, yoga and relaxation exercises. Hence, this can be used in future research works for holistic improvement of health.

The clinical applicability is still limited for lack of established normative data of HRV for different ages, genders and ethnic groups due its demanding technical and mathematical comprehensibility. However, with increasing use of automation and computers in medicine, the clinical applicability of HRV is bound to increase rapidly.

VIVA

1. What do you mean by HRV? What is its physiological importance?
2. What is sinus arrhythmia? What is its contribution to HRV?
3. What are the frequency distribution curves in HRV as recorded in a parametric spectrum (AR model)?
4. What are the time domain and frequency domain indices of HRV?
5. What do the time domain and frequency domain indices of HRV represent?
6. What are the methods of HRV measurement?
7. What is the importance of HF nu?
8. What is the importance of LF nu?
9. What is the LF–HF ratio and what is its importance?
10. What is sympathovagal balance? What is its importance in health and disease?
11. What is the importance of TP of HRV and how does it predict the CV health of the individual?
12. What is the application of HRV analysis in clinical medicine?
13. What are the limitations of HRV analysis?

CHAPTER 38

Blood Pressure Variability and Baroreflex Sensitivity

Learning Objectives

After completing this practical, you will be able to (MUST KNOW):

1. Understand the concept of blood pressure variability (BPV).
2. Learn the principle of measurement of BPV.
3. Apprehend the application of BPV in health and disease.
4. Define baroreflex sensitivity (BRS) and give the normal value.

5. Know the basic principle and method of BRS measurement.
6. Outline the role of BRS in assessing CV health of an individual.

You may also be able to (DESIRABLE TO KNOW):

1. Describe the principle and application of BPV and BRS.
2. Appreciate the application of BRS in clinical physiology and research.

BLOOD PRESSURE VARIABILITY

INTRODUCTION

Like heart rate variability recorded by continuous ECG tracings and analysed by spectral HRV analysis, serial blood pressure variability (BPV) recorded by continuous pulse pressure tracing of arterial pressure waves provides the evaluation of the hemodynamic conditions. As the hemodynamic parameters change rapidly from moment to moment, a single pressure pulse measurement does not provide sufficient information. Therefore, continuous measurement of pressure pulse tracings of BP (pressure pulse waves) provides the information of beat-to-beat variation in BP.

Among non-invasive methods, finger cuff technology is considered to be the best one as it provides such continuous and non-invasive monitoring of BP and other hemodynamics parameters. The finger cuff method using Finapres is a superior method as it detects changes in cardiac preload, cardiac hemodynamics, cardiac output and peripheral circulation, in addition to beat-to-beat heart rate variability.

Physiological Aspects

Though spectral indices of BPV are useful in determining the type, degree and quality of disturbances in many CV diseases, the finapres recordings have been established as gold-standard in detecting the hemodynamic turbulence in hypertension and circulatory disorders. The important CV parameters recorded in the latest version of finapres are:

1. Heart rate and heart rate variability
2. Systolic blood pressure and its variability
3. Diastolic blood pressure and its variability
4. Mean arterial pressure and its variability
5. Mid-cardiac cycle pressure
6. Delta-systolic pressure
7. Rate-pressure product
8. Stroke volume
9. Left-ventricular ejection time
10. Maximum slope of ejection
11. Cardiac output
12. Pulse interval (inter-beat interval)
13. Mid-interval and delta-interval
14. Total peripheral resistance
15. Baroreceptor-reflex sensitivity

Except vessel diameter and wall thickness, ventricular wall thickness, and size of cardiac chambers and orifices, finapres records almost all the hemodynamics parameters required for studying functional abnormalities of cardiovascular systems. Among all the BPV parameters, baroreceptor reflex sensitivity (BRS) has been considered as the most vital one in the assessment of CV function and dysfunction, and CV risks in health and various clinical disorders.

METHODS

Finapres Recording of BPV

FINAPRES represents recording from finger arterial pressure (FINger Arterial PRESsure). In Finapres, arterial pressure waveform measurement is done at the level of the finger using a finger cuff. Finapres was introduced in the early 1980s.

- As it provided a reliable non-invasive measurement of the beat-to-beat blood pressure variation, it was appreciated widely.
- The first-generation FinapresTM device was developed by Wesseling et al., which was based on the principle of **volume-clamp method** invented by the Czech physiologist Jan Peñáž.

Principle

Finapres measurement is based on the principle of 'development of the dynamic or pulsatile unloading of the finger arterial walls' using an inflatable finger cuff with built-in photo-electric plethysmograph. The dynamic unloading is ensured by "A fast pneumatic servo system and a dynamic servo setpoint adjuster that assure arterial unloading at zero transmural pressure and consequent full transmission of arterial blood pressure to cuff air pressure". Pressure pulse waveforms obtained from the finger arteries provide the derivation of parameters such as heart beats, pulse rate, cardiac output, systolic, diastolic and mean pressure from beat-to beat of cardiac pumping.

Procedure

1. Explain the procedure in detail and get consent of the patient/subject. Anthropometric measurements, viz., height and weight of the subject are made. Ask the subject to lie down on the couch and rest for 10 min.
2. Connect the blood pressure cuff (arrow of the cuff over brachial artery) and tie the front-end box over the wrist of the same arm (Fig. 38.1).
   - Use the cuff size guide to choose the appropriate finger cuff.
   - The appropriate cuff should be attached to the middle phalanx of any of the middle 3 fingers preferably the middle finger.
   - If the cuff does not fit to 3 fingers, thumb can be used.

3. Connect the metal plug first to the front-end box so that the red dot in the plug faces upwards followed by the air plug.
4. *Steps with finometer*   Usually for BPV recording, FINAPRES or FINOMETER is used.
   - Switch on the finometer and the desktop. Select finometer research and press the mark button
   - Then click to enter subject details/describe the subject using the buttons provided on the finometer. Describe gender, age, height and weight of the subject
   - Then press configure and wait for the barometric pressure to buffer around 800 mmHg.
   - Then choose height correction so that both brachial and finger height sensors are maintained at 0 cm when placed together and press mark. (Either 0 or within +/−2)
5. Attach the brachial and finger sensors to the BP cuff and finger cuff respectively.
6. Go back to finometer to 'describe subject' and confirm.
7. *With software*   The usual software used is Beat-scope Easy.
   - Open the software and press start: Enter the subject id in the window and press start.
   - Then press/choose Physiocal & RTF cal menu in the finometer and press down to come to step.
   - Wait for 2 min. for the physiological calibration to run. After 2 min., press the same button, following which Return to Flow (RTF) calibration will be done.
   - Come back to the desktop and switch off the physiocal and wait for a minute following which the physiocal will switch on again and needs to be switched off.
8. Start the timer and recordings to be made for a minimum of 10 min. After 10 min., press stop and wait for 30 sec. for the measurement to get stored.
   - Click File > Save to > Other location > choose a specific folder to be saved
   - Again click File > Export > BRS > Save to the same folder (Label as BRS)
9. Disconnect the brachial and finger height sensors.
   - While disconnecting the finger cuff, first, the air tube should be disconnected followed by the metal tube. Remove the finger cuff with care. Remove the front-end box and the BP cuff

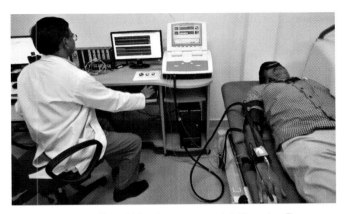

Fig. 38.1 Recording of blood pressure variability using Finapres with subject lying down in supine posture with brachial cuff and finger cuff tied at appropriate position. (*Courtesy:* Cardiovascular Research Lab, Physiology Dept., JIPMER, Puducherry, India.)

respectively.

– Switch off the finometer by pressing both the arrow buttons simultaneously.

10. *Analysis*   Open the saved text document and copy the values. Open an excel sheet and Paste the values in the excel removing the semicolons.

– After physiocal, the values of all the parameters are obtained by averaging all the values obtained. Similarly, BRS analysis is done in another excel sheet.

BAROREFLEX SENSITIVITY

INTRODUCTION

As integrity of baroreceptor reflex or, baroreflex sensitivity (BRS) reflects the status of sympathovagal balance or imbalance.

❖ BRS assesses the reciprocal increase of sympathetic activity and reduction of parasympathetic (vagal) activity, which is the precursor for development of many CV diseases. The measurement of BRS is a reliable tool for CV disease risk stratification.

❖ Also, assessment of BRS is an ideal measure of determination of autonomic tone of CV functions and circulatory homeostasis.

Therefore, BRS evaluation provides valuable information in clinical management, especially prognostic evaluation, risk stratification and assessment of treatment of many cardiac diseases.

BRS Definition and Calculation

BRS is defined as the **change in interbeat interval (IBI) in milliseconds per unit change in BP**. For example, when the BP rises by 10 mmHg and IBI increases by 100 ms, BRS would be $100/100 = 10$ ms/mmHg.

Though from this definition, it appears that there is no direct relation of BRS to the BP buffering capacity of the baroreflex, but rather it focuses more on the reflex effect on sinus node, it accurately reflects the alteration in IBI which is the result of influence of parasympathetic and sympathetic tones or a combination thereof.

Physiological Basis and Importance of BRS

The baroreceptor reflex system plays a critical role in short-term regulation of BP. Arterial baroreceptors distributed in the wall of the carotid sinus and aortic arch provide the information on alterations in blood pressure continuously to the central nervous system.

Vago-Sympathetic Assessment

Baroreflex responses mediated by vagal and sympathetic efferents exhibit significant differences in the time of onset of their action and the time delay in execution of effects.

❖ Following an immediate and considerable rise in arterial pressure, parasympathetic activation occurs faster and this produces an immediate response usually between 200 and 600 ms, whereas cardiac and vasomotor sympathetic stimulation occur after a gap of 2–3 seconds and the peak effect of responses reaches more slowly.

❖ Also, sympathetic-mediated alteration in venous return takes still longer time (more sluggish response) in fulfilling the baroreflex control of BP.

❖ Therefore, the potency of baroreflex to control heart rate and BP on a beat-to-beat basis is mediated principally through vagal activity rather than through sympathetic activity.

❖ Further, baroreflex modulation of heart rate is greatly influenced by respiration, the process known as sinus arrhythmia.

❖ Inspiration decreases baroreceptor stimulation of vagal efferents (motoneurons) and expiration increases vagal activity (activates baroreceptor stimulation of vagal motoneurons). This is called **the respiratory gate of vagal activity**.

◆ Within the physiological limit of BP, baroreceptors constantly exert inhibitory effects on sympathetic efferent activity. Many neural, humoral, behavioral, and environmental factors influence the functioning of the baroreceptor reflex.

METHODS

Assessment of BRS

▌ *Principle*

In the BPV method, the brachial artery pressure measured is the reconstructed pressure from the finger pressure, estimated via generalised waveform inverse modelling and generalised level correction. The baroreceptor reflex sensitivity (BRS) and other CV parameters are measured by continuous BPV method using Finapres, using **volume clamp technique of Penaz** and the **Physiocal criteria of Wesseling**.

▌ *Brief Procedure*

If BRS is recorded by Finapres, the procedure of measurement is same as for Blood Pressure Variability, as described above.

1. The subject is instructed to lie down on the couch for 15 min. and then the brachial cuff of Finapres

is tied around the mid-arm, 2 cm above the cubital fossa (Fig. 38.1).

• The finger cuff of appropriate size (small, medium or large) is tied around the middle phalanx of the middle finger, depending on the finger width. For the height correction, two sensors are placed, one at the heart level and another at the finger level.

• The BPV recording is obtained following connection of cables of the cuffs to the Finometer, after minimum of ten minutes of supine rest.

2. The 'return to flow calibration and the Physiocal' is done for the level correction between the brachial and finger pressure during the initial 5 minutes of the recordings.

3. Following this, continuous BP recording is done for a period of 10 minutes (Fig. 38.2).

4. The BRS is recorded as small star-like shining dots on pressure-pulse wave tachogram (Fig. 38.3).

▌ *Results*

The important parameters obtained from the reconstructed brachial pressure tachogram are: Heart rate (HR), Systolic BP, Diastolic BP, Mean arterial pressure (MAP), Rate-pressure product (RPP), Interbeat interval, Left ventricular ejection

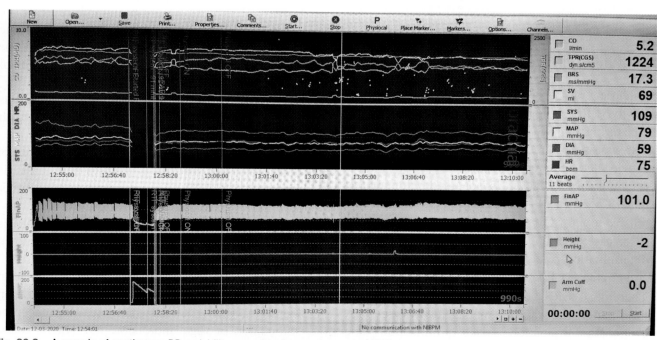

Fig. 38.2   A sample of continuous BP variability recording for assessment of BRS.

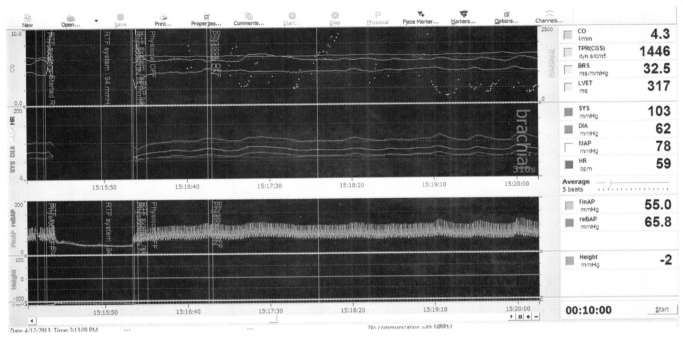

Fig. 38.3   BP variability recording by Finapres, in a normal healthy (Control) subject. Note that the SBP was 103 mmHg, DBP was 62 mmHg and BRS was 32.5 ms/mmHg. BRS is recorded as small star-like shining dots on pressure-pulse wave tachogram.

time (LVET), Stroke volume, Cardiac output, Total peripheral resistance (TPR), Baroreflex sensitivity (BRS) and many other cardiac parameters except data about chamber wall thickness and valvular orifices.

Normal Value and Variations

The reports of G. K. Pal *et al.* have demonstrated that BRS in the normal healthy Indian population varies from 20 to 40 ms/mmHg (Fig. 38.3). Values of BRS

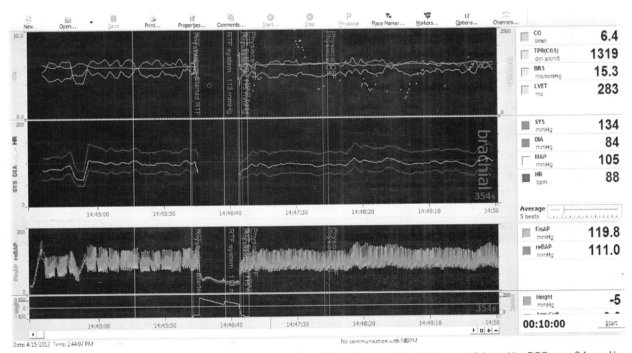

Fig. 38.4   BP variability recording by Finapres, in a prehypertensive subject. Note that the SBP was 134 mmHg, DBP was 84 mmHg (prehypertension range) and the BRS was 15.3 ms/mmHg. The BRS was considerably less due to BP in prehypertension range.

between 14 to 19 are seen in prehypertension and prediabetes (Fig. 38.4) and values of 13 or less are considered as a significant CV risk.

DISCUSSION

Physiological Applications of BRS

CV diseases are usually associated with the impairment of baroreflex activity and associated with imbalance in sympatho-vagal outflow from the CNS to the heart and blood vessels, resulting in persistent sympathetic activation.

- Chronic baroreflex-mediated sympathetic activation contributes to progression of the underlying disease process and promotes end-organ damage.
- Blunted baroreflex gain is reported to be predictive of increased CV risk in patients suffering from hypertension, myocardial infarction and heart failure.

Clinical Applications of BRS

Cardiovascular (CV) diseases are often accompanied by an impairment of baroreflex mechanisms, often with a reduction of central inhibitory activity, resulting in an imbalance in sympathovagal outflow to the heart and blood vessels, lasting vagal withdrawal and chronic adrenergic activation. Quantification of arterial baroreflex sensitivity (BRS) is a source of valuable information for the assessment of neural cardiovascular regulation in normal and diseased states.

1. BRS provides prognostic information in coronary artery disease (CAD) and myocardial infarction (MI), as documented from experimental observations and also confirmed in human studies. The major reports are that baroreflex regulation of

heart rate and BP is considerably decreased and the risk of developing cardiac complications is inversely related to BRS.

2. The first human study emphasising the clinical implication of BRS was ATRAMI study (Autonomic Tone and Reflexes After Myocardial Infarction) that analysed the utility of BRS in risk stratification of myocardial infarction patients.
   - In ATRAMI study, decreased BRS (<3 ms/mmHg), was established as a significant predictor of cardiac death with the relative risk of 2.8 (95% CI 1.40–6.16), independent (statistically adjusted) of other established risk factors.

3. Later, the importance of BRS analysis was evidenced in heart failure, hypertension and other CV diseases.

4. BRS has recently been reported to be reduced in prehypertension, prediabetes and in the early part of many metabolic disorders.

5. BRS has been used as an important tool in CV risk stratification in many cardiovascular and metabolic disorders.

6. BRS has been recently used to assess the prognosis of cardiac diseases and therapeutic responses that have direct or indirect CV dysfunctions, and in the assessment of implantable cardioverter defibrillator (ICD) implantation, cardiac resynchronisation therapy (CRT), etc.

7. BRS is an important marker of sympathovagal balance. Hence, alteration in BRS is used extensively in the assessment of the degree of sympathovagal imbalance.

8. BRS is reported to be a better marker of sympathovagal balance or imbalance compared to other methods of autonomic assessments including HRV. Therefore, measurement of BRS is very useful in clinical research.

VIVA

1. *What is the meaning and concept of blood pressure variability (BPV)?*
2. *What is the principle of measurement of BPV?*
3. *List the CV parameters recorded in BPV measurement.*
4. *Define baroreflex sensitivity (BRS)?*
5. *What is the normal value of BRS?*
6. *What is the basic principle of BRS measurement?*
7. *What is the physiological basis of BRS in assessing the CV health of an individual?*

CHAPTER 39

Brainstem Auditory Evoked Potential

Learning Objectives

After completing this practical, you will be able to (MUST KNOW):
1. Define brainstem auditory evoked potentials (BAEPs).
2. State the physiological basis of generation of BAEP waveforms.
3. List the physiological factors that affect BAEP waveforms.

4. Trace the auditory pathway.
5. List the normal characteristics of different BAEP waveforms.
6. correlate the changes in waveforms with common diseases that affect the auditory pathway.

INTRODUCTION

Brainstem auditory evoked potentials (BAEPs) constitute an objective hearing test. These are the potentials recorded from the ear and the scalp in response to a brief auditory stimulation. The evoked potentials that appear following transduction of the acoustic stimulus by the ear cells create an electrical signal that is carried through the auditory pathway to the brainstem and from there to the cerebral cortex. When the signal travels, it generates action potential in all the fibres. These action potentials can be recorded at several points along the auditory pathway and even from the surface of the body. BAEPs assess conduction of the impulse through the auditory pathway up to the midbrain.

Uses of BAEP   Clinically, BAEPs are used:
1. To assess hearing in uncooperative patients and very young children.
2. To detect degree of hearing loss in infants.
3. To assess the functions of the midpart of the brainstem.

Anatomical and Physiological Considerations

Auditory Pathway

The axons of the spiral ganglion, which innervate hair cells of the ear, form the cochlear nerve. The first order of neurons terminates in the cochlear nuclei in the medulla from where the second order of neurons arises and ends in the superior olivary nucleus. The third order of neurons originates from the superior

olivary nucleus and ascends the lateral lemniscus to project onto the inferior colliculus which is the centre for auditory reflexes. From the inferior colliculi, many fibres project to the medial geniculate body in the thalamus and from there to the primary auditory cortex (area 41) (Fig. 39.1).

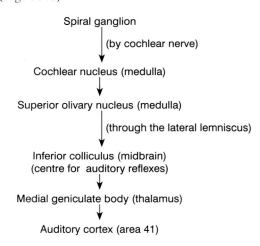

Spiral ganglion
↓ (by cochlear nerve)
Cochlear nucleus (medulla)
↓
Superior olivary nucleus (medulla)
↓ (through the lateral lemniscus)
Inferior colliculus (midbrain)
(centre for auditory reflexes)
↓
Medial geniculate body (thalamus)
↓
Auditory cortex (area 41)

Fig. 39.1   Auditory pathway.

Physiological Basis of BAEPs

BAEPs are recorded within 10 ms after acoustic stimulus is given. A series of potentials are generated corresponding to sequential activation of different parts of the auditory pathway, that is, peripheral, pontomedullary, pontine and midbrain portions of the pathway.

Waves of BAEP

Five or more distinct waveforms are recorded within 10 ms of the auditory stimulus. These waveforms are named wave I, II, III, IV and V (Fig. 39.2). If the recording continues, a few more positive and negative waves are recorded.

These peaks are considered to originate from the following anatomical sites:

1. Waves I and II—cochlear nerves
2. Wave III—cochlear nucleus
3. Wave IV—superior olivary complex
4. Wave V—nuclei of lateral lemniscus
5. Waves VI and VII—inferior colliculus

Factors That Affect BAEP

1. Age The latency of BAEP is affected by age, especially in early childhood. Latency is age-dependent up to two years. The effect of age is more pronounced in premature infants. Older adults have slightly longer I to IV interpeak latency compared to younger individuals.

2. Sex Women have shorter latency and higher amplitude of BAEPs.

3. Height The height of the subject has no direct correlation with latency or amplitude of BAEPs.

4. Temperature Increased body temperature decreases the latency and decreased temperature increases the latency of BAEP.

5. Drugs Barbiturates and alcohol prolong the latency of wave V. These drugs affect latency by decreasing the body temperature instead of directly acting on the auditory pathway.

6. Hearing loss Hearing deficit affects BAEPs. Therefore, hearing tests, especially to detect conductive deafness and examination of the ear to diagnose ear block by cerumen, should be done prior to recording BAEPs.

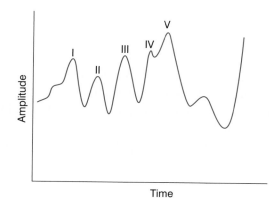

Fig. 39.2 Brainstem auditory evoked potential recorded in a normal individual.

METHODS

Methods of Recording BAEPs

Principle

A brief auditory stimulation generates action potentials in the auditory pathway. These potentials are recorded from the ear and vertex as BAEPs.

Requirements

1. Recording electrodes
2. Amplifier and average (EP-EMG machine) (Fig. 39.3)
3. Electrode paste
4. Earphone

Procedure

1. Place the recording electrode on both the ear lobes or on the mastoid process (Fig. 39.4).
2. Place the reference electrode on a point slightly in front of the vertex.
3. Place the ground electrode on a point in front of the reference electrode.
4. Connect the recording electrodes to the amplifier.
5. Use amplifications of 2,00,000–5,00,000.

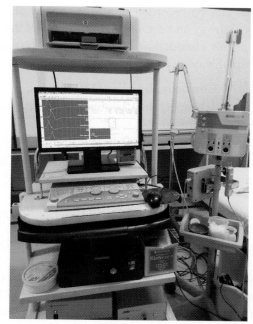

Fig. 39.3 Evoked potential-Electromyogram (EP-EMG) machine with all its accessories. (*Courtesy*:   Physiology EP-EMG Lab, JIPMER, Puducherry, India).

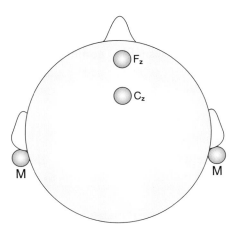

Fig. 39.4 Sites of placing electrodes for recording BAEP (M [mastoid process] for active electrode, C_z for reference and F_z for ground electrode).

6. Set the low filter at 100 Hz and high filter at 3000 Hz.
7. Give a brief click stimulus of 0.1 ms duration.

> **Note:** The stimulus applied is usually a square wave pulse. The pulse can move towards or away from the ear. The earphone movement towards the ear is called condensation phase stimulus and away from the ear is called rarefaction phase stimulus. The amplitude of the waveforms is affected by the type of stimulus; for example, wave I amplitude is greater with rarefaction stimulus. The clicks are usually presented 10–70 times per second. Waveforms are poorly defined at faster rates. Therefore, slower or intermediate rates are preferred. The click rate of 11–31 Hz is commonly used in clinical practice. Stimulus intensity is usually kept within 40–70 dB. Some laboratories keep stimulus intensity at 60 dB above the hearing threshold.

8. Observe the recording of potentials from both the ears (Fig. 39.5).
9. Repeat 2–3 times and see that recordings are superimposed to check the reproducibility.

> **Note:** The BAEP repetition should be superimposed almost exactly.

Precautions

1. The subject should be properly instructed and motivated to provide full cooperation.
2. The subject should be fully relaxed, otherwise hypnotics can be used to achieve maximum relaxation.
3. The room should be quiet and comfortable.
4. The skin of the scalp and mastoid should be grease-free.

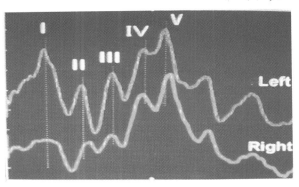

Fig. 39.5 Brainstem auditory evoked potentials recorded from both right and left sides.

DISCUSSION

Normal BAEP Waveforms

Wave I

Characteristics

1. This is the first prominent upgoing peak in the ipsilateral ear recording channel. It is reduced or absent from the contralateral ear recording channel.
2. It appears 1.4 ms after the stimulus.
3. The amplitude of this wave can be increased by using horizontal montage, external canal needle electrode or nasopharyngeal electrode, by increasing the stimulus intensity or by decreasing the stimulus rate.

Clinical application As it originates from the eighth nerve, this wave is preserved in patients who have only central problems. But, those who have peripheral hearing impairment have reduced or absent wave I (wave II to V remain relatively normal).

Wave II

Characteristics

1. This is a poorly defined wave.
2. It appears as a small peak following wave I. It may appear in the downgoing slope of wave I or in the upgoing slope of wave III.
3. It is more prominent in the contralateral channel recording where it has a slightly prolonged latency compared to the ipsilateral recording.

Clinical application It is absent in lesions of the eighth nerve.

Wave III

Characteristics

1. This is a prominent upgoing peak.
2. It is smaller and appears earlier in the contralateral channel.
3. It may sometimes appear as a bifid wave (with two peaks).

Clinical application   It is reduced or absent in lesions of the cochlear nucleus.

Wave IV

Characteristics

1. This is a very small wave, which usually appears in the upgoing slope of wave V.
2. Sometimes it may be absent or may appear as a very small wave at the peak of wave V, giving it a bifid appearance.

Clinical application   It is absent in lesions of the superior olivary nucleus.

Wave V

Characteristics

1. This is the most prominent peak in BAEP.
2. It appears 5.5 ms after the stimulus.
3. It starts usually above the baseline immediately following wave IV.

Clinical application   It disappears in diseases affecting the lateral lemniscus and the inferior colliculi.

Measurement of BAEP Waveforms

The following parameters are measured for analysing the waveforms of BAEPs:

1. Absolute latency and amplitude
2. Interpeak latencies
3. Amplitude ratio of V/I
4. Inter-ear–interpeak difference

Absolute Latency and Amplitude

The absolute amplitude is measured as the height (expressed in μv) from the peak of the wave to the trough of that wave. The absolute latency is measured as the distance (expressed in ms) from the beginning of the first wave to the peak of that wave.

Interpeak Latencies

The interpeak latencies (IPLs) commonly measured are I–V, I–III and III–V. This is measured as the distance between the peak of both the waves (expressed in ms).

I–V interpeak latency

1. The normal value is 4.5 ms.
2. It represents conduction from the proximal part of the eighth nerve through the pons to the midbrain.
3. It is slightly less in females and more in elderly men.
4. It is prolonged in:
   • Demyelination
   • Degenerative diseases
   • Hypoxic brain damage

I–III interpeak latency

1. The normal value is about 2.5 ms.
2. It measures conduction from the eighth nerve across the subarachnoid space into the core of the lower pons.
3. It is prolonged in:
   • Inflammation or tumour of the eighth nerve
   • Diseases at the pontomedullary junction
   • Guillain–Barré syndrome

III–V interpeak latency

1. The normal value is about 2.4 ms.
2. It measures conduction from the lower pons to the midbrain.
3. It is prolonged in prolongation of I–V IPL. The isolated prolongation III–V IPL is not considered significant.

Amplitude Ratio of V/I

Wave I is generated outside and V is generated inside the CNS. Therefore, the V/I ratio compares the relationship of the signal amplitude.

Normal value   The ratio is normally between 50 per cent and 300 per cent.

Clinical implication   If the ratio is less than 50 per cent, this suggests small wave V, which indicates a central impairment of hearing. If the ratio is more than 300 per cent, this suggests small amplitude of wave I, which indicates peripheral hearing impairment.

Clinical Applications

The changes in brainstem auditory evoked potentials have been correlated with diseases at different levels of the auditory pathway. BAEP is usually helpful in localising the lesions in the brainstem. It is useful in diagnosing diseases like cerebellopontine angle tumour, intrinsic brainstem tumour, multiple sclerosis, coma, brain death and strokes affecting the brainstem (thrombosis of vertebrobasilar system). It is also useful in pediatrics for assessing auditory function in children whose hearing cannot be tested behaviourally.

VIVA

1. What are the different waveforms seen in the recording of BAEP and how are they generated?
2. Trace the pathway for audition.
3. What are the physiological factors that affect BAEP?
4. What are the precautions observed during recording of BAEP?
5. What should be the stimulus intensity and duration for recording BAEP?
6. By what means can wave I of BAEP be improved in amplitude?
7. In what condition is wave I reduced or absent?
8. What is the cause of wave II in BAEP and in what diseases may it be absent?
9. In which conditions may wave III be absent?
10. What is the significance of wave V and in which conditions is it altered?
11. What does I–V interpeak latency represent and in what conditions is it prolonged?
12. What does I–III interpeak latency represent and in what conditions is it prolonged?
13. What does III–V interpeak latency represent and in what conditions is it prolonged?
14. What is the significance of the V/I ratio?
15. What is the clinical utility of recording BAEP in children?

CHAPTER 40

Visual Evoked Potential

Learning Objectives

After completing this practical, you will be able to (MUST KNOW):

1. Describe the significance of performing this practical in clinical physiology.
2. Define visual evoked potentials (VEPs).
3. State the physiological basis of VEPs.
4. List the factors that influence VEP.
5. List the pre-test instructions given to the subject prior to recording the VEP.

6. State the principle of recording of VEP.
7. List the precautions taken during the recording of VEP.

You may also be able to (DESIRABLE TO KNOW):

1. Describe the normal waveforms of the VEP.
2. List the abnormalities of VEP waveforms.
3. Name the diseases associated with different abnormalities.

INTRODUCTION

Visual evoked potentials (VEPs) are electrical potential differences recorded from the vertex in response to visual stimuli. The VEPs represent the mass response of the cortical and possibly subcortical areas. Normal VEPs indicate the intactness of the entire visual system. A normal cortical response is recorded when the entire visual pathway is normal. Responses become abnormal if there is any defect in any part of the visual system. Therefore, VEPs can only detect the abnormality, but cannot exactly localise the site of the lesion in the visual pathway.

Anatomical and Physiological Consideration

Layers of the Retina

The retina has ten layers. The outermost layer is the pigment epithelium. The rods and cones lie next to the pigment layer. They synapse with the inner nuclear or bipolar cells, which in turn project to the ganglion cell layer. The axons of the ganglion cells form the optic nerve. The rods and cones are the receptors that are stimulated by light impulses and the information is conveyed through the bipolar and ganglion cells to the visual pathway.

Visual Pathway

Fibres in the optic nerves terminate in the lateral geniculate body via the optic chiasma, which in turn project to the visual cortex through optic radiation. (for details of the visual pathway, refer Chapter 43.)

Physiological Basis of VEPs

The P_{100} waveform of VEPs is generated in the occipital cortex by activation of the primary visual cortex and activation of areas surrounding the visual cortex by thalamocortical fibres. The retinal ganglion cells are of three types: X, Y and W. The X cells are small ganglion cells that mediate the function of the cone system (colour vision). They have small-diameter axons and small receptive fields. They are concentrated in the central portion of the visual field (central retina) and exhibit lateral inhibition. They provide the substrate for pattern VEPs via the geniculate pathway. The Y cells are large ganglion cells that mediate functions of the rod system. Their axons have a large diameter with a large receptive field. They are concentrated in the peripheral visual field (peripheral retinal location) and provide the substrate for flash VEPs via the extrageniculate pathway. The VEPs primarily represent the activity originating in the central visual field, which is connected to the surface of the occipital cortex. The activities originating from the peripheral retina are directed to the deeper regions of the visual cortex, which attenuates the VEPs (on peripheral retinal stimulation only). The central part of the retina (fovea centralis) has greater cortical representation in the visual cortex and activities in the central visual field magnify the VEPs.

The Waveforms of VEPs

The VEPs consist of a series of waveforms of opposite polarity. The negative waves are denoted by N and positive waves by P, which is followed by the approximate latency in ms. The commonly seen waveforms are N_{75}, P_{100}, and N_{145} (Fig. 40.1). The peak latency and peak-to-peak amplitudes of these waves are measured. Generally the peak latency, duration and amplitude of P_{100} are measured. The normal values of parameters of P_{100} are:

Latency (ms)   : 100
Amplitude (μv)   : 11
Duration (ms)   : 60

N_{75} mainly results from foveal stimulation and originates in area 17.

P_{100} originates in area 19.

N_{145} reflects the activity of area 18.

Factors That Influence VEP

1. Age The amplitude of P_{100} is high in infants and children, and is almost double the adult value. The adult value is reached in 5–7 years. After 50 years, the amplitude decreases.

2. Gender P_{100} latency is longer in men, which may be due to bigger head size in men. However, the P_{100} amplitude is greater in women, which may be due to hormonal influence.

3. Drugs Drugs that cause miosis (pupillary constriction), for example, pilocarpine, increase the P_{100} latency, which is due to decreased area of retinal illumination. The mydriatics decrease P_{100} latency.

4. Eye dominance The duration and amplitude of P_{100} is shorter if recorded by stimulating the dominant eye compared to the non-dominant eye. This is attributed to the neuroanatomic asymmetries in the human visual cortex.

5. Eye movement The amplitude of P_{100} is decreased by eye movement but the latency remains unaffected.

6. Visual acuity With decreased visual acuity, the amplitude of P_{100} is decreased, but the latency remains normal.

METHODS

Method of Recording VEP

Principle

The stimulation of the visual pathway generates activities in the visual cortex. A visual stimulus is presented to the subject for a selected number of times, and the cerebral responses are amplified, averaged by a computer and displayed on the oscilloscope screen or printed out on paper.

There are different methods of VEP measurement:

⬥   Pattern reversal VEP
⬥   Flash VEP
⬥   Goggle VEP

The pattern reversal VEP is most commonly used for adult patients who can follow the light. The flash VEP is used for infants and people who have very poor visual acuity or are in coma and the goggle VEP is used for children.

Requirements

1.   Standard disc EEG electrodes
2.   Preamplifier and amplifier (*refer* Fig. 39.2)
3.   Oscilloscope
4.   Electrode paste

Procedure

For best results, proper instructions should be given to the subject and a thorough eye examination should be conducted.

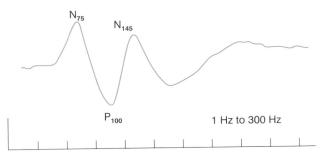

Fig. 40.1   Visual evoked potentials recorded from full-field mono-ocular stimulation.

Pretest instructions

1. The subject should be told about the procedure of the test to get full cooperation.
2. The subject should avoid applying hair spray or oil after the last hair wash.
3. If the subject uses optical lenses, these glasses should be worn during the test.
4. The subject should be instructed not to use any miotic and mydriatics 12 hours before the test.
5. The full ophthalmological examination should be carried out to determine the visual acuity, the pupillary diameter and the field of vision.
6. If there is any field defect, the electrodes may be placed laterally (in addition to midline electrodes). This is done because the field defects alter the potential field distribution of P_{100}.

Steps

1. Prepare the skin by abrading and degreasing.
2. Place the recording electrode at O_Z (Fig. 40.2) using conducting jelly or electrode paste.
3. Place the reference electrode at F_{PZ} or 12 cm above the nasion.
4. Place the ground electrode at the wrist.
5. Keep the electrode impedance below 5 kΩ.
6. Use amplification ranging between 20,000–1,00,000 to record pattern shift visual evoked potentials (PSVEPs).
7. Set low-cut filters at 1–3 Hz and high-cut filters at 100–300 Hz.

Note: The filter setting should be kept constant.

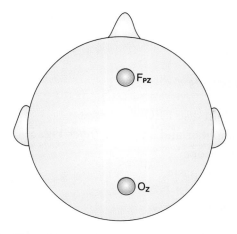

Fig. 40.2   Sites of placing electrodes for recording VEP (reference electrode at the point F_{PZ}, recording electrode at O_Z and the ground electrode at wrist).

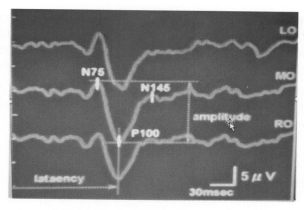

Fig. 40.3   Visual evoked potentials (LO: Left occipital; MO: Mid-occipital; RO: Right occipital).

8. Keep the sweep duration at 250–500 ms.
9. Stimulate visual pathways by different photic stimulation and record the response (Fig. 40.3).
10. Compare the obtained tracing, with the normal one (as given in Fig. 40.1).

Precautions

1. The subject should be instructed properly.
2. The skin of the scalp should be grease-free.
3. Mydriatics and miotics should not be used for minimum of 12 hours before the test.
4. Visual acuity, pupillary diameter and field of vision must be checked before starting the test.
5. Additional lateral electrodes should be used if there is any visual field defect.
6. Electrode impedance should be kept below 5 kΩ.
7. Amplification ranging should be between 20,000 and 1,00,000, for recording pattern shift VEP.
8. Filter setting should be kept constant.
9. The subject should not sleep during the procedure.

DISCUSSION

For recording VEPs, the eyes are tested one at a time. Each eye projects to the occipital cortex through the optic chiasma. Therefore, unilateral VEP abnormality is obtained by full-field mono-ocular stimulation, which is likely to be due to pre-chiasmal lesion. If the pattern shift visual evoked potential (PSVEP) is abnormal bilaterally, it becomes difficult to locate the anatomical site of the defect.

N_{20} : Generated by VPL nucleus of the thalamus, the primary sensory cortex.

Tibial SEPs

Tibial SEPs are recorded from the posterior tibial nerve. The important waveforms are N_8, N_{22}, N_{28} and P_{37}.

N_8 : Generated by the tibial or sciatic nerve.

N_{22} : Generated by the dorsal grey matter of the lumbar spinal cord.

N_{28} : Generated by the cervical spinal cord.

P_{37} : Generated by the primary sensory cortex.

Factors That Affect SEPs

Age In infants and children, N_9 and N_{13} potentials of median SEPs occur early. In elderly individuals, most of the latencies are longer by about 10 per cent after the age of 55. The interpeak latencies are shorter with increasing age, which indicates slowing of conduction in peripheral nerves in old age.

Gender Women have shorter central conduction time.

Temperature Peripheral nerve conduction decreases with decrease in limb temperature. With change in body temperature, conduction in the peripheral portion of the pathway is more affected than in the central portion. The temperature and latency have a linear relationship.

Sleep The amplitude of the peak component of N_{20} decreases in sleep than in the awake state (waking).

Drugs SEPs are resistant to various drugs. Therefore, sedatives like diazepam can be used if needed. The patient can continue to take them, if already advised by the physician, while recording SEPs. Sedatives are used in uncooperative patients.

METHODS

Method of Recording SEPs

Principle

The stimulation of sensory nerves generates action potentials that are carried in the ascending pathways to the sensory cortex, from where these are recorded as SEPs; they are usually recorded from the large conducting fibres in the sensory pathway.

Requirements

1. Electrodes
2. Amplifier (EP-EMG machine) (*refer* Fig. 39.2)
3. Averager
4. Oscilloscope
5. Electrode paste

Procedure

Pretest instructions

1. Give proper instructions to the subject to get maximum cooperation.
2. Ensure that the subject is fully relaxed in the supine position with head supported (to relax the neck muscles).
3. Use mild hypnotics, if needed, to ensure relaxation.
4. Ensure that the room is quiet and comfortable.
5. Prior to recording, obtain information about the nerve (features of nerve injury, and so on).

Steps in brief

(SEPs recorded from the posterior tibial nerve are described here). Place the ground electrode about 5 cm above the medial malleolus. Stimulate the posterior tibial nerve just posterior to the medial malleolus, and the recording electrode at various points on the body as depicted in Fig. 41.1.

Precautions

1. Provide proper instruction and motivation to the subject, to provide full cooperation.
2. Ensure that the subject is fully relaxed, otherwise hypnotics can be used to achieve maximum relaxation.
3. Ensure that the room is quiet and comfortable.

Observation

Study the latency and amplitude of N_8, N_{22}, P_{37} and N_{45} from the recorded tracings. For example, P_{37} and N_{45} can be studied from C_Z–F_Z recording (Fig. 41.2).

DISCUSSION

Median SEPs

The following parameters are measured for analysis of median SEPs.

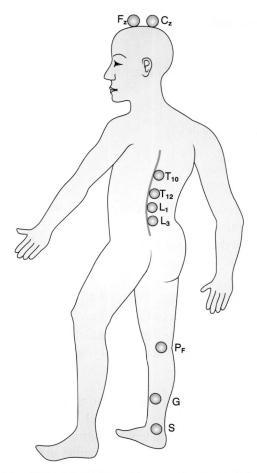

Fig. 41.1   Sites of placing electrodes for recording posttibial SEP (S: Stimulating electrode; G: Ground electrode; F_z, C_z, T_{10}, T_{12}, L_3 and P_F (popliteal fossa): Recording electrodes).

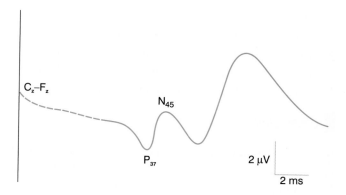

Fig. 41.2   Normal waveforms of SEP (C_z–F_z) of posterior tibial nerve.

1. Latency
2. Amplitude
3. Interpeak latency

Amplitude and Latency

The amplitude and latency of N_9, N_{11}, N_{13}, N_{18}, N_{20} and P_{25} waveforms are measured. These latencies are prolonged and the amplitudes are reduced in diseases at different parts of the sensory pathway that they represent.

Interpeak Latency

The two important interpeak latencies (IPL) are clinically significant. These are N_9–N_{11} and N_{13}–N_{20} IPL.

N_9–N_{11} IPL represents the conduction time from the brachial plexus to the spinal cord. Therefore, this is delayed by any lesion between the brachial plexus and the spinal cord.

N_{13}–N_{20} IPL represents central sensory conduction time. Therefore, this is delayed in any condition that affects the central sensory pathway, that is, the pathway from the spinal cord to the cortex.

Tibial SEPs

Like median SEPs, the latency and amplitude of N_8, N_{22} and P_{37} are measured. The two important interpeak latencies (IPL) are clinically significant. These are N_8–P_{37}, and N_{22}–P_{37} IPL. The N_8–P_{37} IPL is used to measure the conduction time in both peripheral and central pathways. The N_{22}–P_{37} IPL is used to measure the conduction time in the central pathway, that is, from the lumbar spinal cord to the sensory cortex.

Clinical Applications of SEPs

SEPs have good correlation with impairment of joint position and vibration sensation but not with pain and touch. For an abnormality in SEP to occur, a significant degree of sensory impairment must take place. In general, latency abnormalities are more pronounced in demyelinating diseases, and amplitude abnormalities are more common in ischemic lesions. A combination of latency and amplitude abnormalities is seen in compressive lesions. Thus, SEPs are helpful in the diagnosis of the nature and degree of sensory abnormalities in demyelinating diseases, vascular lesions, infections of the spinal cord and brain like acute transverse myelitis, Pott's paraplegia, degenerative diseases like cervical and lumbar spondylosis, and nutritional myopathies.

VIVA

1. What is somatosensory evoked potential (SEP)?
2. What is the sensation actually assessed by SEPs and why?
3. Trace the pathway of proprioception.
4. What are the different waveforms of median SEPs and how are they produced?
5. What are the different waveforms of tibial SEPs and how are they produced?
6. What are the factors that affect SEPs?
7. What are the pretest instructions given before recording SEPs?
8. What is the principle of recording SEPs?
9. What are the precautions taken for recording SEPs?
10. What is the information obtained from amplitude and latency of SEPs?
11. Which interpeak latencies of median SEPs are clinically important and what do they actually represent?
12. What is the clinical significance of the study of SEPs?

CHAPTER 42

Motor Evoked Potential

Learning Objectives

After completing this practical, you will be able to (MUST KNOW):
1. Define motor evoked potentials (MEPs).
2. Differentiate between sensory evoked potentials and MEPs.
3. Trace the pathway for the corticospinal tract.
4. Explain the principle of recording MEPs.
5. List the common abnormalities of MEP recordings.
6. List the clinical uses of MEPs.

INTRODUCTION

The sensory evoked potentials (visual, auditory and somatosensory) are recorded from the cerebral cortex or from the sensory pathways following the application of sensory stimulation, whereas motor evoked potentials (MEPs) are recorded from the muscles (as EMG responses) following stimulation of the motor cortex or spinal cord. MEPs can be recorded by two types of stimulations, electrical and magnetic. The MEPs recorded following transcranial electrical stimulation is painful. Therefore, magnetic stimulation (by using magnetic stimulator) of the cortex is done to record MEPs. The MEPs are higher in amplitude and easier to record in contrast to other evoked potentials.

Anatomical and Physiological Considerations

Corticospinal Tract

Refer Chapter 55.

Physiological Basis

Transcranial stimulation can be carried out by electrical or magnetic stimulation.

Electrical stimulation This is done using a bipolar or unipolar montage. For transcranial stimulation, anodal stimulation is preferred over cathodal stimulation. The MEPs are restricted to the muscles contralateral to the side of cortical stimulation. Cortical stimulation excites the pyramidal cells in the cortex, which in turn stimulate the corticospinal fibres. The spinal cord can be stimulated by high-voltage electrical stimulation either in the cervical or lumbar region. For spinal cord stimulation, cathodal stimulation is preferred. Electrical stimulation of the spinal cord stimulates the peripheral motor axons close to the spinal cord and the muscle innervated by the axon.

Magnetic stimulation Magnetic stimulation is more advantageous than electrical stimulation as it is painless and can stimulate the deep structures.

METHODS

Method for Recording MEPs

Principle

Motor evoked potentials are recorded as EMG responses from the muscles by stimulating the motor cortex or the spinal cord.

Requirements

1. Magnetic or electrical stimulator
2. Electrodes

Procedure

Pretest instructions

1. Remove all magnetic objects like watches and so on from the patient and the operator, and keep them at a minimum distance of 50 cm from the stimulator.

2. Enquire about cardiac pacemaker, cochlear device, and so on, because electrical or magnetic stimulations are contraindicated in patients with such devices.

3. Electrical stimulation should not be performed in patients with craniotomies. However, magnetic stimulations can be carried out in such patients.

4. Elicit the history of epilepsy from the subject as transcranial stimulation must be avoided in epileptic patients.

5. Enquire about the use of hypnotics, anticonvulsants and anxiolytics by the patient as these drugs affect the MEPs.

Important steps

1. Brief the subject about the test.

2. Place the magnetic stimulator on the vertex according to the direction of current flow needed to stimulate the specific area of the cortex, and record the MEP from the target muscle (Fig. 42.1). Butterfly stimulators are used for deep penetration of the pulses beneath the scalp and for recording MEPs from the upper limb and hand muscles.

3. For recording of MEPs from the target muscles, place the surface EMG electrodes over the muscle.

4. Use magnetic stimulation for stimulating spinal roots and peripheral nerves, and record the MEPs from the target muscle.

5. Increase the stimulator output gradually in steps of 10–20 per cent.

6. Ask the subject to slightly contract the target muscle for cortical stimulation and relax the target muscle for spinal stimulation.

7. Record the central motor conduction time (CMCT) by detecting the difference in the latencies between cortical and spinal stimulation (Fig. 42.1 A and B).

Measurement of CMCT

Central motor conduction time (CMCT) is measured by subtracting the latency of MEP on spinal stimulation from that on cortical stimulation. The latency difference is then compared with the distance between two stimulating electrodes.

Precautions

All the pre-test instructions can be taken as precautions for recording MEPs.

DISCUSSION

Normal Values

The normal values of central motor conduction (ms) of various muscles are:

Muscle	Latency	CMCT
Deltoid	10.6 ± 1.0	4.9 ± 0.5
Biceps	11.6 ± 1.2	4.9 ± 0.5
Thenar	20.1 ± 1.8	6.4 ± 0.3
Tibialis anterior	26.7 ± 2.3	13.2 ± 0.7
Anal sphincter	22.8 ± 3.6	13.3 ± 2.3

MEP Abnormalities

Two major MEPs abnormalities are:

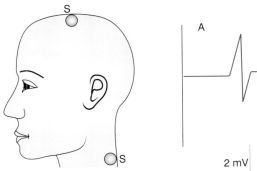
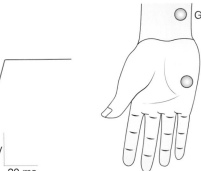
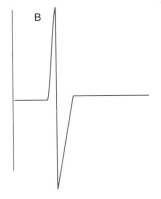

Fig. 42.1 Sites for placing electrodes for recording MEP (S: Stimulating electrodes; G: Grounding electrode; R: Recording electrode placed on abductor digiti minimi; A: Response to cortical or scalp stimulation; B: Response to spinal or neck stimulation).

1. Prolongation of CMCT   This indicates a slowing down in the central pathways. Significant increase in CMCT is found in demyelinating conditions like multiple sclerosis.

2. Inexcitability of motor pathways   This occurs in:
   a) Degeneration or damage to the corticospinal tract.
   b) Motor neuron disease.

Clinical Applications

The central motor conduction studies are used as a valuable tool for diagnosis and prognosis of various neurological diseases. This is especially important in the diagnosis of demyelinating diseases, stroke, degenerative diseases, hereditary ataxia, acute transverse myelitis, encephalitis and Parkinson's disease.

VIVA

1. What do you mean by MEPs?
2. How does MEP differ from EMG?
3. What is the physiologic basis of EMG?
4. What are the types of stimulations given for MEP recordings? What are the differences between them?
5. What is the principle of MEP recording?
6. What are the MEP abnormalities?
7. What is the physiological basis of different MEP abnormalities?
8. What is the physiologic significance of MEPs in clinical physiology?

CHAPTER 43

Perimetry

Learning Objectives

After completing this practical, you will be able to (MUST KNOW):

1. Appreciate the importance of perimetry in clinical physiology.
2. Define field of vision, visual axis, isopters, meridians and blind spot (scotoma).
3. Read the perimeter chart.
4. State the principle of perimetry.
5. Chart the field of vision by using a perimeter.
6. List the precautions for perimetry.
7. Explain the extent of visual field in different quadrants.

8. List the factors that affect field of vision.
9. Trace the visual pathway.
10. Name the visual field defects with lesions at various levels of the visual pathway.

You may also be able to (DESIRABLE TO KNOW):

1. Name and describe different perimeters.
2. Describe a perimeter chart.
3. Explain physiological and pathological blind spots.
4. Explain the effect of lesions of the visual pathway.

INTRODUCTION

Perimetry is the method of accurate **charting of peripheral field of vision**, using a perimeter. A **perimeter** is the instrument used to determine the field of vision. Clinically, the field of vision is determined at the bedside of the patient by the confrontation method (as described in Chapter 55). The confrontation method gives a rough idea of the field of vision. Perimetry is performed to detect the exact nature and extent of defects in the field of vision. The defects in the field of vision occur due to lesions at various levels of the visual pathway.

The Visual Pathway

Visual fibres originate in the nerve cell layer in the retina (from bipolar and ganglion cells). The neurons travel as optic nerves to the optic chiasma where partial decussation of the fibres takes place. The fibre coming from the temporal side of the retina (that receives information from the nasal half of the visual field), remain uncrossed and the fibre emerging from the nasal hemiretina (that receives information from the temporal half of the visual field) cross to the opposite side at the **optic chiasma**. Thus, the **optic tract** contains fibres from the temporal hemiretina of the same side

and nasal hemiretina of the opposite side. This means that the left optic tracts carry the fibres from the left halves of both retina and the right optic tract from the right halves of both the retina. In the optic tract, the fibres, before crossing, ascend in the optic chiasma for a short distance, which is known as **von Willebrand's knee**. Most fibres in the optic tract terminate in the **lateral geniculate body** of the thalamus, from where the second order of neurons originates and ascend the **geniculocalcarine pathway** to reach the **visual cortex**. Few fibres from the optic tract enter the superior colliculus, from where the fibres project to the pretectal area that mediates visual reflexes (Fig. 43.1). The fibres originating from the lateral geniculate body form a loop at their origin called **Meyer's loop**.

Field of Vision

The portion of the external world visible to the eye when the gaze is fixed at a particular point is called the field of vision. The visual field depends mainly on the size and colour of the object used for mapping the field. In the temporal side of the fixation point at about 12°–15°, a **scotoma** (blind spot) is located where perception of light does not occur. This is called **physiological scotoma** and it corresponds to the **optic disc** in the retina, which does not contain rods and cones. It measures approximately 7.5° in height and 5.5° in width. The visual fields of both

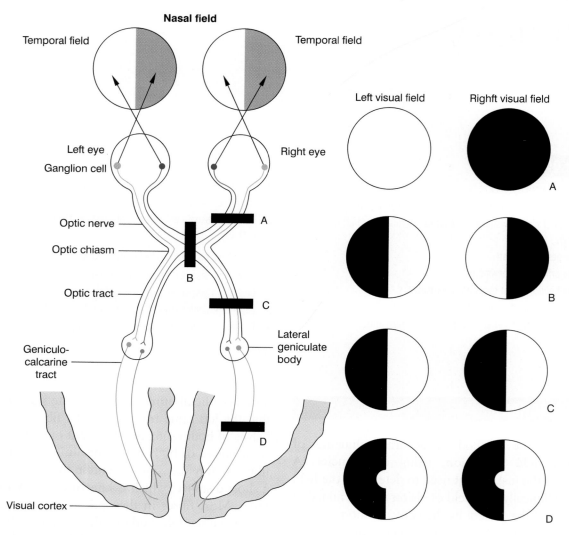

Fig. 43.1   Effects of lesions at various levels of the visual pathway (A: Lesion of the right optic nerve produces blindness in the right eye; B: Lesion of the optic chiasma produces bitemporal hemianopia; C: Lesion of the right optic tract produces left homonymous hemianopia; D: Lesion of the right geniculocalcarine tract produces left homonymous hemianopia with macular sparing).

the eyes overlap in their medial part to form the area of binocular vision, in which objects are seen by both the eyes. The extent of visual field is described under the discussion section.

METHODS

Method of Perimetry

Principle

The part of the external world visible to a person when he fixes his gaze on an object is called the field of vision. The method of charting the field of vision is

called perimetry. The field of vision charted with one eye (the other eye closed) gives the field of vision for that eye. One eye is covered while the other is fixed on a central point. A small target is moved towards this central point along the selected meridians. Along each meridian, the location where the object becomes first visible is plotted in degrees, and is repeated in all meridians. Determination of the visual field by the **confrontation method** is described in Chapter 55 (2nd cranial nerve).

Requirements

1. **Perimeter**   Perimeter is the instrument that accurately maps the field of vision. There are different types of

perimeters available. The commonly used perimeters are Priestley–Smith's perimeter, Lister's perimeter and Student's perimeter (a simple hand perimeter). The most commonly used perimeter in physiology laboratories is the Lister's perimeter.

Lister's perimeter   This consists of a broad concave metal arc which can be rotated around its centre, clockwise or anticlockwise (Fig. 43.2). The metallic arc is graduated in degrees. There is a groove in one limb of the metallic arc, into which a test object is fitted. The concavity of the arc faces the subject. The arc rotates through various angles on a pivot in any direction along with the test object. There are two metallic chin rests. At the back of the perimeter, there is an arrangement for fixing the perimeter chart.

Priestley–Smith's perimeter is also used in many laboratories (Fig. 43.3).

2. Perimeter chart   The centre of the chart (Fig. 43.4) corresponds to the visual axis. The concentric circle around the centre denotes the point of equal visual acuity called isopters and is marked in degrees (at 10° intervals) from the central fixation points. Perimeter charts contain lines through the centre of the circle denoting various meridians in

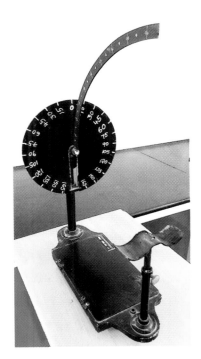

Fig. 43.3   Priestley–Smith's perimeter.

degrees. These radii (meridians) are marked at 15° intervals. A black oval dot present on the horizontal meridian (15° on either side of the central fixation point) corresponds to the normal blind spot. For comparison with the normal field of vision, right and left visual fields are marked on the chart as dotted lines. For mapping the visual field, the chart is fixed to the back of the perimeter.

3. Test objects   Test objects of different colours and diameters are used. Usually, the size of the test objects is 3, 5, 10, 15 and 20 mm. The test object is fitted into a carrier, which moves in a groove in one limb of the metal arc. The test object moves with a knob, which causes movement of a pin on the back of the metal arc. The most commonly used object is white and 5 mm in size.

▌ *Procedure*

1. Read the perimeter chart.
2. Give proper instructions to the subject.
3. Ask the subject to sit on a stool comfortably in front of the perimeter.
4. Arrange the perimeter in such a way that the concavity of the arc faces the subject.
5. Ask the subject to sit straight and rest his chin on one of the chin rests.

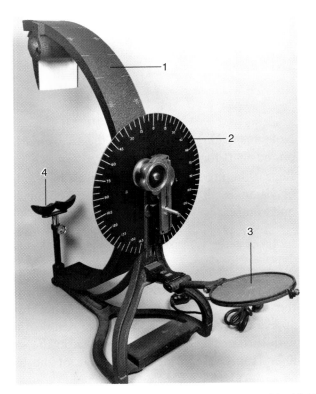

Fig. 43.2   Lister's perimeter (1: Metallic arc; 2: Removable shield; 3: Chart plate; 4: Chin rest).

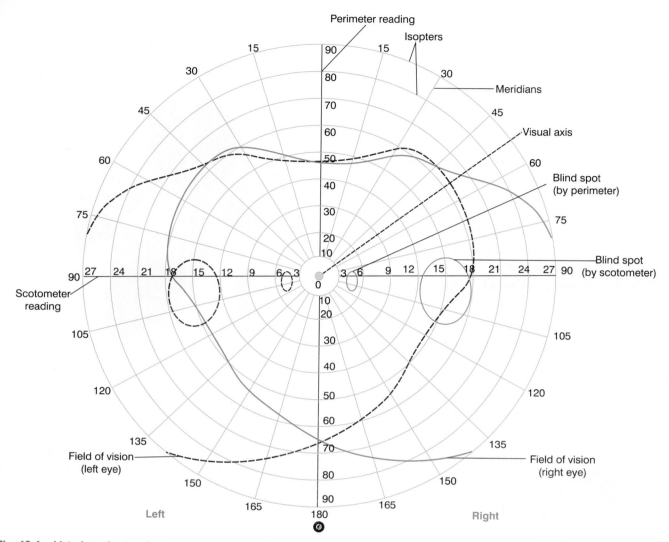

Fig. 43.4   Lister's perimeter chart.

Note: When the field of vision of the right eye is to be tested, the subject should rest his chin on the left chin rest. This brings his right eye in line with the fixation point.

6. Focus the eye to be examined on the fixed object which is a white object of 5 mm size placed at the centre of the metallic arc.

Note: It should be emphasised that the subject's gaze should be fixed at the object throughout the maneuver.

7. Fix the metallic arc in one meridian.
8. Move the test object (which is fixed to the carrier along the arc) gradually from the periphery (90°) towards the central fixation point and ask the subject to indicate when he first sees the object, and note the point.

9. Note this reading in degrees on the arc by marking on the chart for that meridian.
10. Repeat the procedure at 15° intervals till the field of vision is plotted in all meridians of the four quadrants.

Note: The blind spot is marked along the horizontal meridian in the temporal quadrant.

11. Mark the point of disappearance by bringing the test object towards the centre after initial appearance in the field and point of reappearance with further movement of the object in the same line. This gives an idea of the size of the blind spot.
12. Repeat the whole procedure in the opposite eye on the same chart.

Observation

Observe the obtained field of vision and compare it with the normal visual field depicted in the chart. Note the site and size of the blind spot.

Precautions

1. Provide proper instructions to the subject.
2. Before mapping the field of vision, study the perimetry chart thoroughly.
3. While testing for one eye, ensure that the other eye is closed.
4. Fix the eye on the central fixation point.
5. Repeat the procedure at 15° intervals till the field of vision is plotted in all meridians.
6. Do the mapping in a clockwise direction.
7. Mark the blind spot along the horizontal meridian in the temporal quadrant.
8. Test the field of vision for both the eyes separately.
9. Ensure that there is adequate illumination throughout the procedure.
10. Ask the subject to remove his glasses, if he normally uses them, otherwise the field of vision will be restricted.

DISCUSSION

The visual field of each eye is the portion of the external world visible in that eye. The visual field theoretically should be circular, but actually is restricted by the nose medially and roof of the orbit superiorly. Mapping of visual fields is one of the important tests in clinical neurology to detect different diseases of the brain, especially of those that affect the visual pathway.

The visual field is divided into the peripheral and central field of vision. The peripheral field of vision is mapped by perimetry whereas the **central field of vision** is mapped with the help of a *tangent screen (Bjerrum's screen)* in which a white target is moved across a black screen.

Factors That Affect Field of Vision

The field of vision depends on:

1. Colour of the object Visual acuity is better for a white object than coloured objects. Thus the field of vision is better delineated with a white object. Roughly, the field of vision obtained by using blue and yellow objects is less by 10° and that by using red and green objects is less by 20° from the visual field obtained by a white object.

2. Size of the object The larger the size of the object the better is the visual acuity. However, an object of a standard size is used in perimetry.

3. Brightness of the object Brightness, contrast and illumination affect visual acuity and therefore the field of vision.

4. Illumination Poor illumination decreases the visual field.

Normal Field of Vision

The normal field of vision with a white object of 5 mm size is:

Temporal 100° (since there is no anatomical obstruction on the temporal side of the eyes, the extent of the field of vision in this quadrant is more).

Inferior 75° (maxilla of the cheek provides anatomical obstruction and reduces the extent of the field in this quadrant.)

Superior 60° (supraorbital margin provides anatomical obstruction and reduces the extent of the field in this quadrant.)

Nasal 60° (nasal bridge provides anatomical obstruction and reduces the extent of the field in this quadrant.)

Visual Field Defects

A defect in the same side of both visual fields is called a homonymous defect and a defect in half of the visual field is called hemianopia. A defect in the opposite sides of the visual field is called heteronymous defect (Fig. 43.1).

Complete Blindness

This occurs due to lesion of the optic nerves. If the lesion is on one side, it causes blindness of that eye.

Heteronymous Hemianopia

The lesions that affect optic chiasma, for example, tumours of pituitary gland expanding the sella turcica causes this defect. Bitemporal hemianopia is seen commonly whereas binasal hemianopia occurs rarely.

Homonymous Hemianopia

The lesion of the optic tract causes this defect. Lesion of the right side of the optic tract produces left homonymous hemianopia and lesion of the left optic tract produces right homonymous hemianopia.

Homonymous Hemianopia With Macular Sparing

The lesion in the geniculocalcarine tract causes this defect. The macular sparing (loss of peripheral vision with intact macular vision) occurs because the macular representation is separate from that of the peripheral field and is large relative to that of the peripheral fields. Therefore, the lesion in the occipital cortex must extend to large areas to affect peripheral as well as macular vision.

VIVA

1. What is perimetry?
2. What is the use of perimetry in ophthalmology and neurology?
3. What are the different types of perimeters?
4. What are the precautions taken for doing perimetry?
5. Why is the visual field not circular?
6. What are the factors that affect field of vision?
7. Trace the visual pathway.
8. What are the visual field defects produced by lesions at various levels in the visual pathway?
9. How is central field of vision determined?
10. What is blind spot? How is it detected?
11. What is scotoma?

CHAPTER 44

Visual Acuity

Learning Objectives

After completing this practical, you will be able to (MUST KNOW):

1. Explain the importance of determining visual acuity in clinical medicine.
2. Define visual acuity.
3. List the factors that affect visual acuity.
4. Determine the visual acuity for distant and near vision.
5. List the precautions taken for determining visual acuity.
6. Define myopia and hypermetropia.
7. Name the type of lens used to correct the defects of visual acuity for distant and near vision.

INTRODUCTION

Visual acuity is defined as the resolving power of the eyes, that is, the extent to which the eye can perceive the details and contours of an object. It can be explained in terms of minimum separable distance, that is, the smallest gap by which two lines can be separated and still be seen as two separate lines. Visual acuity is the function of cones. It is tested separately for distant vision and near vision.

Factors Affecting Visual Acuity

Visual acuity is mainly affected by **three factors**: optical factors, retinal factors and stimulus factors.

Optical Factors

The image-forming mechanism is the primary factor that determines visual acuity. Optical aberrations and defects of the image-forming mechanism decrease the visual acuity.

Retinal Factors

Visual acuity is the function of the cones. Cones are more in number at the centre (densely packed in the fovea centralis) than in the periphery of the retina. Therefore, visual acuity is maximal at the fovea and less in the periphery of the retina.

Stimulus Factors

The main stimulus factors are the **size and colour of the object**.

Size of the object   Size of the object and its distance from the eye affect visual acuity. Visual acuity is directly proportional to the visual angle (VA).

$$VA = \frac{\text{Size of the object}}{\text{Distance of the object from the eye}}$$

Colour of the object   Visual acuity is better for white objects than for coloured objects. Visual acuity also depends on the brightness of the stimulus, contrast between the stimulus and the background, and the length of time the subject is exposed to the stimulus.

METHODS

Test for Distant Vision

Principle

A series of letters of varying sizes are constructed in such a way that the top letter is visible to normal eyes at 60 metres, and the subsequent lines at 36, 24, 18, 12, 9, 6, and 5 metres respectively. Visual acuity is recorded according to the formula $V = d/D$, where V is the visual acuity, d is the distance at which the letters are read, and D is the distance at which the letters should be read.

Requirements

Snellen's chart   Snellen's letters are depicted on a cardboard (Fig. 44.1) with eight rows of black letters of

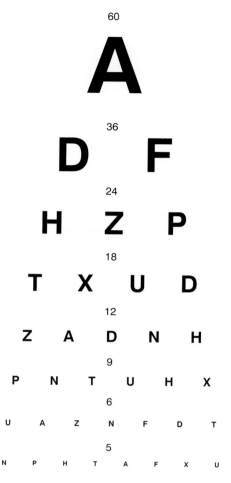

Fig. 44.1 Snellen's chart.

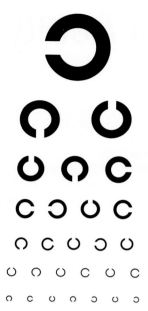

Fig. 44.2 Landolt ring chart.

different fonts. The topmost line can be read by a normal subject at a distance of 60 metres and subsequent lines at 36, 24, 18, 12, 9, 6, and 5 metres respectively.

For uneducated or illiterate persons, **Landolt ring chart** is used (Fig. 44.2).

Procedure

1. Provide proper instructions to the subject.
2. Ask the subject to sit at a distance of 6 metres from the chart ($d = 6$).
3. Ask him to close one of his eyes and read the chart with the other eye.
4. Note up to which line the subject is able to read comfortably.
5. Ask him to repeat the procedure with the other eye.

Precautions

1. Provide proper instructions to the subject.

2. Ascertain if the subject knows the letters (language) written on the Snellen's chart.
3. Ensure that the Snellen's chart is well-lit.
4. Ensure that the patient sits exactly at a distance of 6 metres from the chart.
5. Test each eye separately.
6. If the subject wears glasses, test the visual acuity with and without them.

Observation

If only the top letter of the chart is visible, the visual acuity is 6/60. If the subject can read the lowest line, the visual acuity is 6/5, that is, he has better than normal vision. Normal visual acuity is 6/6. Accordingly visual acuity is expressed as 6/6, 6/9, 6/12, 6/18, 6/24, and 6/36, respectively, depending on the line up to which the subject can read. If his visual acuity is less than 6/60, that is, the subject cannot read the top line from a distance of 6 metres, he should move closer until he can read the top letter. If the top letter is visible at 2 metres, the visual acuity is expressed as 2/60. If the acuity of vision is less than 1/60, the subject is asked to count fingers held up (**finger counting method**) or to perceive hand movement (**hand movement method**). If the subject cannot count the finger or perceive hand movement, a light is focused in front of his eyes and he is asked whether he perceives the light (**light perception method**).

Test for Near Vision

Principle

The visual acuity for near vision is tested by reading Jaeger's chart at ordinary reading distance. This consists of letters of various sizes based on the principle of *Printer's point system*.

Requirement

Jaeger's chart: This chart (Fig. 44.3) consists of letters of various sizes on the Printer's point system. The smallest point is N5 and the largest point is N36.

Procedure

1. Provide proper instructions to the subject.
2. Ensure that the room is well-lit and the subject sits comfortably.
3. Hold Jaeger's chart at a distance of 10–12 inches from the subject's eyes.
4. Ask the subject to read the letters of the different sizes.
5. Note the smallest type of the letters that the subject can read comfortably.
6. Repeat the test separately for each eye with the other eye closed.

Precautions

1. It should be ascertained that the subject knows the language in which the letters are written.
2. The room should be adequately lighted.
3. The Jaeger's chart should be kept at a distance of about 25 cm from the subject.
4. The test should be performed with both eyes open. It should also be performed separately for each eye with the other eye closed.

Observation

Express the result by noting the smallest size of letters that the subject can read.

DISCUSSION

The visual acuity of a normal person is 6/6, that is, the subject should be able to read up to the seventh line. If his visual acuity is less than 6/6, it is considered to be reduced. For correction of the acuity of vision, concave lenses are prescribed after doing a thorough postmydriatic examination of the eye.

If the subject wears glasses, the type of lens used should be mentioned. The examiner can detect the type of lens by holding the lens in front of the eye and looking at an object through it. By moving the lens side to side if the object moves in the opposite direction, the lens is convex; and if the object moves in the same direction, the lens is concave. Concave lenses are used for myopia and convex lenses for hypermetropia.

For young children, simple pictures constructed on a chart on the basis of Snellen's principle can be

N5
When I was ten years old, my father had a small estate near Satara where he used to take us during the holidays. It was situated in rough and uncultivated country side where wild animals were often seen. Once we heard that there was a panther in the surroundings who was killing the cattle and attacking the villagers. Father had warned me not to wander for from home in the evenings. I had made friends with a your villager called Ramu.

N6
Ramu used to drive the cattle to graze and bring them back to shelter at the end of the day. He was lean and of a short build and was barely fifteen. He used to be my companion whenever I meet him winding his way home. One afternoon, just about five o'clock, early in the month of March, chance brought us together.

N8
As there had been considerable variation in the series of Jaeger's test types produced by different printers, a new series of standard graduated test types for near vision has been recommended by the Faculty of Opthalmologist of England in which Times Roman types are used with standard spacing.

N10
The eye to be examined is anaesthetised with 1% solution in anaethine and the instrument is lightly pressed against the eye in the suspected area. If there is a solid tumour, the pupil remains dark. Then the instrument is placed on another region when the pupil is found to be read.

Fig. 44.3   Jaeger's chart.

used. Another test used for children is the *Sheridan–Gardiner* test in which Snellen's letters are matched with different types of objects. For illiterate persons the 'E' test is effective.

Myopia

Myopia or short-sightedness is an error of refraction in which parallel rays of light coming from a distant object are focused in front of the retina. The person cannot see distant objects. It is corrected by using concave lenses.

Hypermetropia

Hypermetropia or long-sightedness is an error of refraction in which parallel rays of light coming from distant object are focused behind the retina. Thus the person cannot see near objects. It is corrected by using convex lenses.

VIVA

1. Define visual acuity.
2. What are the factors that affect visual acuity?
3. What is visual angle? How does it affect visual acuity?
4. How do you test visual acuity for distant vision?
5. How do you test visual acuity for near vision?
6. What are the precautions for the tests of visual acuity?
7. What is the Sheridan–Gardiner test? What is its significance?
8. What is myopia? How do you correct it?
9. What is hypermetropia? How do you correct it?

CHAPTER 45

Colour Vision

Learning Objectives

After completing this practical, you will be able to (MUST KNOW):

1. Explain the clinical importance of performing the test of colour vision.
2. Test the colour vision by using Ishihara chart.
3. Give the function of cone systems.
4. Trace the pathway of colour vision.

5. Classify and define different types of colour blindness.

You may also be able to (DESIRABLE TO KNOW):

1. Name the theories of colour vision.
2. Explain different types of and the mode of transmission of colour blindness.
3. Describe other methods of detecting colour vision.

INTRODUCTION

The human eye has the ability to respond to all wavelengths of light from 400 to 700 nm. This is called the visible part of the spectrum. The sense of colour is perceived by cones. There are **three types of cone systems**: red, green and blue. There are also **three types of cone pigments**: cyanolabe, chlorolabe and erythrolabe showing highest response to specific parts of the spectrum. Each cone shows maximum absorption of light at a particular wavelength. Due to differential stimulation of the three types of cones by different wavelengths of light, the human eye perceives all the colours. For example, the wavelength of 580 nm stimulates red cones maximally and we perceive the colour red. It also stimulates the green cones to some extent and therefore we see the colour orange. Likewise, the wavelength of 535 nm stimulates green cones and the wavelength 445 nm stimulates blue cones maximally, therefore, we perceive the colours green and blue.

There are **three primary colours**—red, green and blue—each responding maximally to the light of certain wavelengths. When colours are mixed in appropriate amounts, the object looks white. Therefore, for any colour, there is a complementary colour which, when properly mixed with a specific colour, produces white.

Pathway of Colour Vision

Neurons carrying colour vision in the optic nerve pass through the **optic tract** to reach the parvocellular part of the **lateral geniculate body** (LGB) of the thalamus. From parvocellular laminas of the LGB, fibres project to blob regions in layer four of the **visual cortex**. Blobs are the clusters of cells arranged in a mosaic in the visual cortex and are concerned with colour vision.

Mechanism of Colour Vision

There are **two mechanisms** of colour vision, the retinal and the cortical.

The Retinal Mechanism

The retinal mechanism of colour vision is based on **Young and Helmholtz's theory**. According to this theory, the perception of the three primary colours is possible due to the presence of three types of cone systems in the retina, each containing a specific pigment which is maximally sensitive to one type of primary colour.

The Cortical Mechanism

The colour-sensitive ganglion cells project to the cells of the lateral geniculate body (single opponent cells), which in turn project to the cells of the primary visual cortex (double opponent cells). The cortical cells in turn project to area 18. It is believed that different colours are perceived by the activities in the primary visual cortex and the cortical association areas.

METHODS

Ishihara's Chart Method

There are different methods of detecting colour vision. However, the Ishihara chart is routinely used for this purpose.

Principle

Colour vision is tested by using Ishihara's chart, which consists of lithographic plates where numericals are drawn in coloured spots amidst other parts of different colours and sizes. The subject reads the number and traces the pathway by appreciating the colour. The colour of these plates is such that they are liable to be confused with spots in the background by people with defective colour vision.

Requirements

Ishihara's chart This consists of lithographic plates in which numerals are written in different colour spots (Fig. 45.1). The colour of these spots is such that they are liable to be confused with spots in the background by people with defective colour vision. These plates are so constructed that a person with colour vision defect will read a different number from a normal person.

Procedure

1. Give proper instructions to the subject.
2. Ask the subject to sit comfortably in a well-lit room.
3. Instruct the subject to read the numbers or trace the lines in each plate of the book.
4. Note if he reads the number or traces the pathway properly.

Precautions

1. The room should be adequately lit.
2. All the plates of the book should be read.
3. While reading the plates, a maximum of 5–10 seconds should be allowed per plate.

Other Methods

There are two other methods of testing colour vision: Edridge–Green lantern test and Holmgren's wool-matching test.

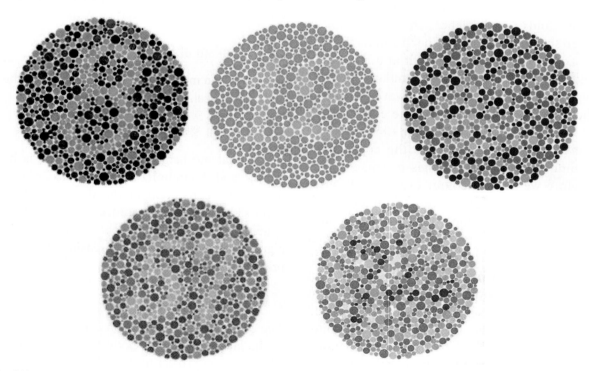

Fig. 45.1 Lithographic plates of Ishihara's chart.

Edridge-Green Lantern Test

In this test, different colours are shown by a lantern and the subject is asked to name the colours. The lantern contains the following colours: pure red, red of different intensities, yellow, green, signal green, blue and purple. The subject sits in a dimly illuminated room 6 metres away from the lantern. He names the colour of the light, focused through the glass fixed on a rotating disc in the lantern. This test is usually employed for railway recruitment.

Holmgren's Wool-Matching Test

In this test, the subject is asked to perform a series of colour-matching from a collection of wools of different colours. There are three sets of coloured wools: test colours, match colours and confusing colours. The subject matches different colours of all the three groups.

DISCUSSION

Clinical Significance

The test for intactness of colour vision is performed routinely as part of the health check for recruitment to a government job or admission to any professional course. Intact colour vision is mandatory for selection for posts related to driving, traffic services, railways and armed forces. Defect in the perception of colour is called **colour blindness**.

Types of Colour Blindness

Colour blindness is classified into three types:

1. Trichromats Trichromats are of two types: protanomaly and deuteranomaly. The person is less sensitive to one of the primary colours.

2. Dichromats Dichromats are of three types: protanopia, deuteranopia, and tritanopia. The person perceives two primary colours.

3. Monochromats The person perceives only one primary colour.

The suffix "anomaly" represents colour weakness and the suffix "anopia" represents colour blindness. The prefixes "prot", "deuter" and "trit" represent red, green and blue colour defects. For example, protanomaly means weakness of perception of red and protanopia means blindness for red. A trichromat has all the three cone systems but one system may be weak (**protanomaly or deuteranomaly**). A dichromat is an individual having only two cone systems, with one cone system absent. Depending on the absence of a cone system, a subject can be **protanopic, deuteranopic or tritanopic**. A monochromat is a person having only one cone system, with two systems absent.

Colour blindness is inherited as an **X-linked recessive**. This occurs due to an abnormal gene on the X chromosome. Women are carriers but suffer from the disease only when both X chromosomes carry the defective gene.

VIVA

1. What is the clinical significance of the test of colour vision?
2. What is the chart used for detecting colour blindness? What is its principle?
3. What do you mean by colour blindness? How do you classify it?
4. What is the mode of transmission of colour blindness?
5. What are the theories of colour vision?
6. What is the pathway for colour vision?
7. What are the other methods of detecting colour vision? What is the principle behind each of these methods?

CHAPTER 46

Hearing Tests

Learning Objectives

After completing this practical, you will be able to (MUST KNOW):

1. Elucidate the importance of performing this practical in clinical physiology.
2. Name the hearing tests.
3. State the principles of the tuning fork test.
4. Perform and interpret the tuning fork tests.
5. List the precautions to be taken for tuning fork tests.

6. Differentiate conductive deafness from neural deafness.

You may also be able to (DESIRABLE TO KNOW):

1. Trace the auditory pathway.
2. State the attributes of sounds.
3. State the principles of audiometry and BAEP.
4. Explain the abnormalities of hearing tests.

INTRODUCTION

Hearing tests are commonly performed by audiologists to detect the type and degree of hearing loss for prescribing hearing aids. Hearing tests also help neurologists establish the extent of lesions, especially if the brainstem is involved in the pathological process.

Anatomical and Physiological Considerations

Auditory Pathway

Refer Chapter 39 and Fig. 39.1 for details.

Physiological Basis

Characteristics of sound   Perception and interpretation of speech is a complex phenomenon. There are four attributes of sound: frequency, intensity, direction and pattern. The sound waves are sensed by the hair cells of the cochlea and the impulses are transmitted to the auditory cortex by a very complex pathway. The actual perception and interpretation of most aspects of sound take place in the auditory cortex.

Frequency   The frequency of the sound stimuli is detected by the basilar membrane. Sharpening of frequency occurs in the hair cells and auditory neurons. The cells in the auditory cortex respond only to a narrow range of sound frequency. The frequency of the nerve impulses is related to the intensity of the stimulus.

Intensity   Intensity of the sound is coded as early as with the receptors. The outer hair cells respond to weaker stimuli because of the lower threshold of the cilia of the outer hair cells that are embedded in the tectorial membrane. In the auditory cortex, there are neurons that are maximally sensitive to a specific intensity of the stimulus.

Direction   The direction of sound is judged by the difference in time and intensity at which it arrives at the two ears. Though the direction of sound is detected by the superior olivary nucleus, the auditory cortex is essential for perception of the direction of sound.

Pattern   The pattern of a sound is the sequence in which different components of the sound appear. This property of sound is recognised by the auditory cortex alone.

Hearing Tests

A number of hearing tests have been described to detect hearing loss:

1. Watch test
2. Tuning fork test
3. Audiometry
4. Recording of brainstem auditory evoked potentials (BAEP)

The commonly used hearing tests in clinical practice are tuning fork tests.

METHODS

Watch Test

Principle

Sound is sensed by the hair cells in the ear and conducted via auditory pathways to the auditory cortex. A defect in either perception or conduction of sound can lead to hearing loss.

Requirement

1. Wrist watch

Procedure

1. Ask the subject to close his eyes.
2. Ask him to plug one ear with a finger.
3. Slowly bring a watch from a distance to his opened ear and ask him when he hears the sound.
4. Note the distance at which the subject hears the sound of the wrist watch.
5. Repeat the same in the other ear.
6. Compare the result with a normal subject.

Disadvantages

1. It detects only gross hearing impairment.
2. It cannot detect the nature and degree of hearing loss.

Tuning Fork Tests

Tuning fork tests are based on the principle that sound is conducted to the ear by the air (air conduction). Therefore, deafness can be detected by testing air conduction or by directly stimulating the bone that conducts sound.

There are **three types of tuning fork tests**: Rinne's test, Weber's test and Schwabach test. For all these tests, tuning fork (512 Hz) is required. Tuning forks of higher frequency like 512 Hz or 256 Hz produce more sound than vibration, whereas tuning forks with lower frequency produce more vibration than

sound. Therefore, **512 Hz or 256 Hz** tuning forks are preferred for hearing tests (Fig. 46.1).

Rinne's test

Principle

Rinne's test compares hearing ability through the mediums of bone and air; that means there is comparison of bone conduction with air conduction of the same ear.

Procedure

1. Give proper instructions to the subject.

Note: Instruct him to raise the finger when he stops hearing the sound of the vibrating tuning fork.

2. Hold the stem of the tuning fork between the thumb and the index finger in such a way that the fingers do not touch the blades of the tuning fork (Fig. 46.2A).
3. Make the tuning fork vibrate by suddenly stroking the blades of the fork against the hypothenar eminence (Fig. 46.2B) or the thigh.
4. Immediately place the base of the vibrating tuning fork on the mastoid process (Fig. 46.2C) of one side and ask the subject to raise his finger when he ceases to hear the sound (Fig. 46.2D).
5. Once he stops hearing, hold the vibrating tuning fork very close to his ear (Fig. 46.2E) and ask him whether he hears the sound. When he stops hearing it, bring the tuning fork close to your ear to

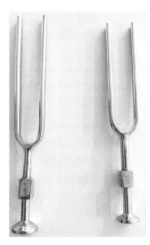

Fig. 46.1   Tuning forks for hearing tests. The longer one is 256 Hz and the shorter one is 512 Hz.

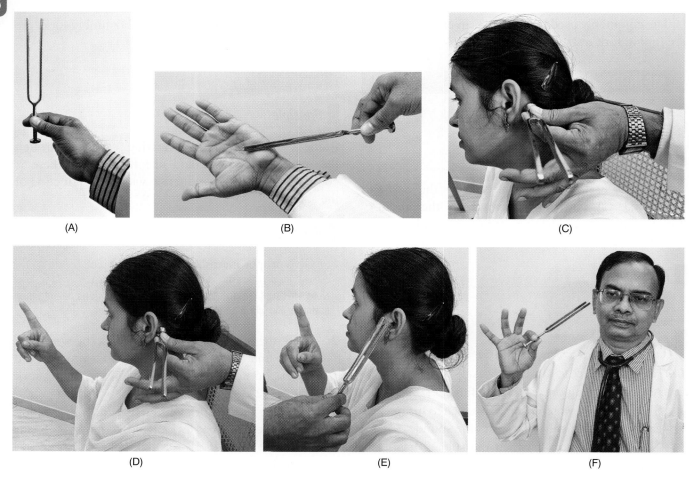

Fig. 46.2 Methodology for Rinne test. (A) The tuning fork is held properly; (B) It is made to vibrate; (C) The vibrating tuning fork is placed on the mastoid process;(D) The subject is asked to raise her finger immediately after she ceases hearing; (E) The vibrating tuning fork is kept close to the subject's ear, and she is asked to raise her finger once she ceases hearing; (F)The tuning fork is brought to the examiner's ear to confirm if vibrating sounds have actually stopped.

confirm whether the vibrating sounds have actually stopped (Fig. 46.2F).

6. Record your observation.

Precautions

1. Proper instructions should be given to the subject.
2. The tuning fork should be held by the stem, taking care not to touch the blades.
3. To start the vibration in the tuning fork, the fork should be stroked against the hypothenar eminence or the thigh, not against the table or any hard surface as the loud sound produced will disturb others and may damage the tuning fork.
4. If the subject stops hearing the sound, the vibrating tuning fork should be taken close to the examiner's ear (taking the examiner as normal) for comparison.

Weber's Test

Principle

Weber's test compares bone conduction of both the ears.

Procedure

1. Give proper instructions to the subject.
2. Make the tuning fork vibrate by hitting the blades of the fork against the hypothenar eminence or the thigh.
3. Place the base of the vibrating tuning fork on the vertex of the skull (Fig. 46.3) or on the forehead of the subject (Fig. 46.4).
4. Ask the subject to indicate whether he hears equally on both sides or if the sound is better heard in one ear.

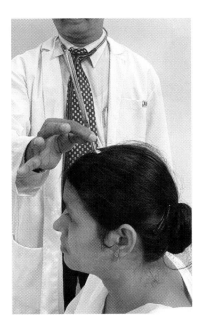

Fig. 46.3   Methodology for Weber test. The vibrating tuning fork is placed on the centre of the vertex of the skull, and the subject is instructed to indicate whether she hears equally on both sides or if the sound is better heard in one ear.

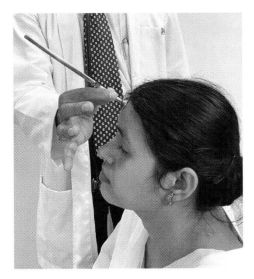

Fig. 46.4   Another methodology for Weber test. The vibrating tuning fork is placed on the centre of the forehead of the subject, and the subject is instructed to indicate whether she hears equally on both sides or if the sound is better heard in one ear.

Precautions

1. Proper instructions are to be given to the subject (subject should understand the procedure of the test).
2. To make the tuning fork vibrate, the blades of the fork should be hit against the hypothenar eminence or the thigh.

Schwabach Test

Principle

This test compares the bone conduction of the subject with that of the examiner.

Procedure

1. Give proper instructions to the subject.
2. Make the tuning fork vibrate.
3. Place the vibrating tuning fork over the subject's mastoid process (Fig. 46.5A).
4. Ask the subject to raise his finger when he stops hearing the sound (Fig. 46.5B).
5. Immediately bring the tuning fork and place it on your mastoid process to check if you still hear the sound (Fig. 46.5C).

Precautions

1. Proper instructions should be given to the subject.
2. Once the subject stops hearing the sound, a comparison should be made with the examiner by placing the tuning fork on his mastoid process.

Interpretation of the results of hearing tests is summarised in Table 46.1.

Audiometry

Principle and Brief Procedure

Audiometry is an objective and accurate method to assess the degree of deafness and frequency range at which it manifests. This is done by using an audiometer which is an electroacoustic device. The test is conducted in a soundproof room. One ear is tested at a time with the help of an earphone. The subject flashes a light when a sound is heard. At each frequency the threshold intensity is determined and plotted against a graph as a percentage of normal hearing. The audiometer provides pure tones of different frequencies at various levels of loudness or intensity from an oscillator connected via an amplifier to the earphones. Routinely, the audiometer provides a minimum of 7 tones (250, 500, 1000, 2000, 3000, 4000 and 8000 Hz). The intensity of each tonal frequency can be increased. The lowest decibel at which the patient hears the tone is called the

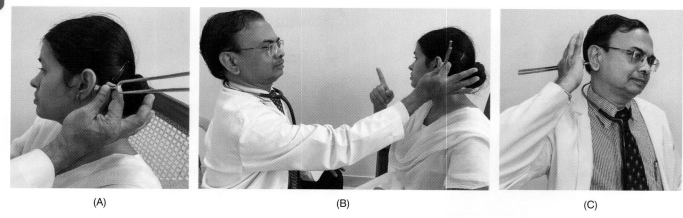

(A)   (B)   (C)

Fig. 46.5   Methodology for Schwabach test. (A) The vibrating tuning fork is placed on the mastoid process; (B) The subject is asked to raise her finger immediately after she ceases hearing; (C) The examiner places the same tuning fork on his mastoid process to confirm if the sounds are still audible.

Table 46.1   Observation and inference of hearing tests.

Name of the test	Observation	Inference
Rinne's test	i) Air conduction is greater than bone conduction (Rinne-positive) ii) Bone conduction is greater than air conduction (Rinne-negative) iii) Both air and bone conduction are absent iv) Air conduction is greater than bone conduction in the defective ear (Rinne-false positive)	i) Normal ii) Conduction deafness iii) Complete nerve deafness iv) Partial nerve deafness
Weber's Test	i) Sound is heard equally in both ears ii) Sound is better heard in the defective ear (lateralised to the defective ear) iii) Sound is better heard in the healthy ear (lateralised to the healthy ear)	i) Normal ii) Conduction deafness in the defective ear iii) Partial nerve deafness in the defective ear
Schwabach Test	i) Bone conduction of the subject is equal to the bone conduction of the examiner ii) Bone conduction of the subject is better than the bone conduction of the examiner iii) Bone conduction of the subject is worse than the bone conduction of the examiner	i) Normal ii) Conduction deafness in the subject iii) Partial nerve deafness in the subject

threshold. A graph is plotted showing the audiometric threshold as a function of frequency discrimination. This graph is called an audiogram.

Brainstem Auditory Evoked Potential (BAEP)

This is the most accurate method to differentiate organic deafness from functional deafness, and determine the exact site of hearing loss. The details of BAEP are described in Chapter 39.

DISCUSSION

Rinne's Test

This test compares bone conduction with air conduction of the same ear. If the hearing is normal, the subject will hear the sound of the vibrating fork by air conduction even after he has ceased hearing by bone conduction, because air conduction is better than bone conduction. This is called **Rinne-positive.** In conduction deafness, vibrations in the air are not heard after bone conduction is over, that is, bone conduction is better than air conduction. This is **Rinne-negative.** In total nerve deafness, no sound is heard in either case. In partial nerve deafness, the Rinne's test becomes **false positive** (Table 46.1).

Weber's Test

Normally, sound is heard equally in both ears. If sound is heard better in the defective ear, the hearing loss is due to conduction deafness. If the sound is louder in the normal ear, the hearing loss in the defective ear is due to nerve deafness.

Schwabach Test

If the subject is normal, bone conduction of the subject is equal to bone conduction of the examiner.

In conduction deafness, bone conduction is better than normal. In nerve deafness, bone conduction is worse than normal.

OSPE

I.   Perform Rinne test on the given subject.

Steps

1. Give proper instructions to the subject. Instruct him to raise the finger when he stops hearing the sound of the vibrating tuning fork.
2. Hold the stem of the tuning fork between the thumb and the index finger in such a way that the fingers do not touch the blades of the tuning fork and make the tuning fork vibrate by stroking the blades of the fork against the hypothenar eminence.
3. Immediately place the base of the vibrating tuning fork on the mastoid process of one side of the subject and ask him to raise his finger when he ceases to hear the sound.
4. Once he stops hearing, hold the vibrating tuning fork very close to his ear and ask him whether he hears the sound.
5. When he stops hearing it, bring the tuning fork close to your ear to confirm whether the sound has actually stopped.
6. Repeat on the other side (if asked to do on both the sides) and report.

II. Perform Weber's test on the given subject.

Steps

1. Give proper instructions to the subject.
2. Hold the stem of the tuning fork between the thumb and the index finger in such a way that the fingers do not touch the blades of the tuning fork and make the tuning fork vibrate by stroking the blades of the fork against the hypothenar eminence.
3. Immediately place the base of the vibrating tuning fork on the vertex of the skull or on the forehead of the subject.
4. Ask the subject to indicate whether he hears equally on both sides or if the sound is better heard in one ear.
5. Report his findings.

III. Perform Schwabach test on the given subject.

Steps

1. Give proper instructions to the subject. Instruct him to raise the finger when he stops hearing the sound of the vibrating tuning fork.
2. Hold the stem of the tuning fork between the thumb and the index finger in such a way that the fingers do not touch the blades of the tuning fork and make the tuning fork vibrate by suddenly stroking the blades of the fork against the hypothenar eminence.
3. Immediately place the base of the vibrating tuning fork on the mastoid process of one side of the subject and ask him to raise his finger when he ceases to hear the sound.
4. Once he stops hearing, immediately place the vibrating tuning fork on your mastoid process to assess if the sounds have actually stopped.
5. Repeat on the other side (if asked to perform on both sides) and report.

VIVA

1. What are the uses of hearing tests in clinical medicine?
2. What are the attributes of sound?
3. What are the different hearing tests?
4. What are the principles of hearing tests?
5. What are the tuning fork tests?

6. How do you perform Rinne's test? What are the precautions for this test?

7. How do you perform Weber's test? What are the precautions of this test?

8. How do you perform the Schwabach test? What are the precautions of this test?

9. What is the principle of audiometry?

10. What is BAEP? What is its use in diagnosis of hearing loss?

11. What is the significance of the Rinne test? What do you mean by Rinne-positive and Rinne-negative?

12. How do you differentiate nerve deafness from conduction deafness by using Weber's test?

13. What is the significance of the Schwabach test?

14. How are the observations of the hearing tests interpreted?

Ans: Interpretation of tuning fork tests is performed as given in the tabular form above.

CHAPTER 47

Examination of Taste and Smell

Learning Objectives

After completing this practical, you will be able to (MUST KNOW):

1. Describe the importance of examination of taste and smell in clinical physiology.
2. Name the primary tastes.
3. Explain the distribution of receptors for primary tastes in the tongue.
4. Name the cranial nerves that carry the sensations of smell and taste.
5. Examine the sensations of smell and taste.

6. List the precautions taken while performing the practical.
7. Name the conditions that alter the sensations of taste and smell.

You may also be able to (DESIRABLE TO KNOW):

1. Trace the auditory pathway.
2. Trace the pathway for taste and smell.
3. Explain the physiological bases of the abnormalities associated with taste and smell.

INTRODUCTION

The sensations of smell and taste are very basic to our existence as they are closely associated with ingestive behaviours. The olfactory nerve carries the sensation of smell from the nasal mucosa to the olfactory cortex of the brain. Facial, glossopharyngeal and vagus nerves carry the sensation of taste from the receptors in the tongue to the postcentral gyrus of the cortex.

Taste

Taste receptors are present in the taste buds that are distributed in the papillae of the tongue and the mucous membrane of the oral cavity. The seventh cranial nerve carries the sensation of taste from the anterior two-thirds of the tongue, the ninth cranial nerve carries the sensation of taste from the posterior third of the tongue, and the tenth cranial nerve carries the sensation from the pharyngeal region.

Primary Tastes

There are **four primary tastes**: sweet, sour, salt and bitter. Receptors for these tastes are different and are distributed in different parts of the tongue.

Sweet   Receptors for the sweet taste are present mainly in the tip of the tongue.

Salt   Receptors for the salt taste are present mainly in the centre of the dorsum of the tongue.

Sour   Receptors for the sour taste are distributed mainly in the lateral portions of the tongue.

Bitter   Receptors for the bitter taste are distributed primarily at the back of the tongue.

Taste Pathway

The first order of neurons carries the sensation from the receptors in the seventh, ninth and tenth cranial nerves to the nucleus tractus solitarius (NTS) in the medulla.

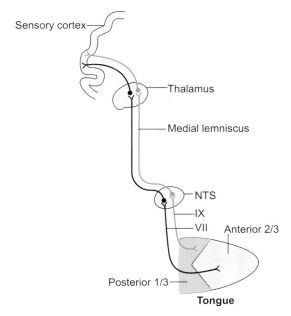

Fig. 47.1   Pathway for taste sensation (NTS: Nucleus tractus solitarius; IX: Ninth cranial nerve; VII: Seventh cranial nerve).

The second order of neurons arises from the NTS. They ascend the medial lemniscus to relay in the thalamus. The third order of neurons arises from the thalamus and projects to the lower part of the postcentral gyrus (Fig. 47.1).

Smell

The sensation of smell is more developed in animals (macrosmatic) and less developed in humans (microsmatic). Receptors are present in the olfactory mucosa. This is the only part of the central nervous system, which is exposed to the external world.

Olfactory Pathway

The first-order neurons carrying the sensation pierce the cribriform plate of the ethmoid bone to reach the olfactory bulb. In the olfactory bulb, they synapse with the dendrites of the mitral and tufted cells to form the olfactory glomeruli. The glomeruli also receive inputs from the granule cells which can modulate the output from the olfactory bulb. The second-order neurons (axons of the mitral cells) form the olfactory tract that divides into the medial and lateral pathways. The fibres in the lateral division project to the olfactory lobe of the same side to terminate in the centres for olfaction (prepyriform cortex, amygdala and preamygdaloid areas). The fibres in the medial division project to the opposite olfactory tubercle from where they go to the dorsomedial nucleus of the thalamus and the orbitofrontal cortex (Fig. 47.2).

METHOD

This is described in Chapter 55 (under Method of Examination of Olfactory Nerve and Facial Nerve).

DISCUSSION

The physiological significance and clinical importance of examination of taste and smell are described in Chapter 55.

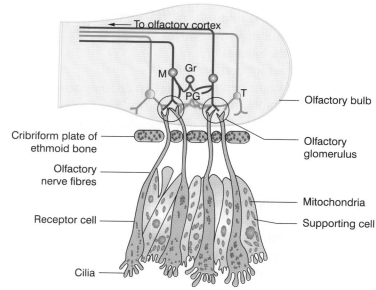

Fig. 47.2 Olfactory receptor cells and the olfactory pathway.

VIVA

1. *What are the primary tastes?*
2. *What is the distribution pattern of receptors for primary tastes in the tongue?*
3. *What is the pathway for the taste sensation?*
4. *What are the abnormalities of taste sensation?*
5. *What is the pathway for the sensation of smell?*
6. *What are the abnormalities of the sensation of smell?*

CHAPTER 48

Semen Analysis

INTRODUCTION

Semen analysis is the most important test for evaluation of male fertility. It is routinely ordered in clinical practice to know if infertility is due to a defect in the semen. It is also performed after vasectomy to check the completeness of the surgical procedure. It reflects the activity of the testes and accessory sex organs.

Features of Normal Semen

Volume   : 2–5 ml per ejaculation
Motility   : > 60% of sperms should be actively motile (within 3 hours of collection)
Count   : > 40 million/ml is considered normal
Liquefaction : Should liquefy within 30 minutes
Morphology   : > 70 per cent should have normal morphology
pH   : Normal pH 7.2–7.7
Fructose   : Fructose normally present

METHODS

Method for Analysis of Semen

Principle

Analysis of freshly collected sample of semen gives information about male fertility, which is detected by examining the sample under the microscope.

Requirements

1. Microscope
2. Viscometer
3. Neubauer's chamber and WBC pipette
4. Freshly collected sample of semen

Procedure

1. Collect semen from the person after a period of sexual abstinence for a minimum of two days.
2. Perform semen analysis 30 minutes after collection of the sample.

Note: Immediately after collection, semen coagulates and liquefies after 15–20 minutes. Therefore, the sample is examined 30 minutes after collection. Semen contains fibrinogen which is converted to fibrin by an unknown mechanism on exposure to atmosphere, and coagulates the sample. Plasmin is also present in semen and is activated in 30 minutes and liquefies the sample.

3. Measure the volume of the sample.
4. Observe whether the sample has been uniformly liquefied.
5. Examine the motility and morphology of the sperm, first under the low-power and then under the high-power objective of the microscope.
6. Count the sperm by using Neubauer's chamber and the WBC pipette.

Note: Seminal fluid is drawn up to the 0.5 mark of the WBC pipette and then diluted up to the 11 mark by using 4% sodium bicarbonate in 1% phenol. Then the Neubauer's chamber is charged and sperm count is done in WBC squares. N×50 (for details of calculation and steps of counting, see Chapter 9) gives the sperm count in mm³ of fluid. N×50,000 gives the sperm count per ml of fluid.

7. Determine the pH of the sample.
8. Determine the viscosity of the sample by using the viscometer.
9. Estimate the sugar (fructose) content of the sample by appropriate biochemical tests.

Precautions

1. The sample should be collected after a minimum of 48 hours of abstinence.
2. The sample should be taken for analysis 30 minutes after collection.
3. The analysis should ideally be done within 6 hours of collection. If the analysis is likely to be delayed, the sample should be stored in the refrigerator, and before analysis, the temperature of the sample should be brought to normal room temperature.
4. While counting sperms, all the precautions of hemocytometry should be followed.

Observations

Note your observation under the following heads:
1. Volume
2. Motility
3. Count
4. Liquefaction
5. Morphology
6. pH
7. Fructose content

DISCUSSION

Volume

A low volume might suggest an anatomical or functional defect or an inflammatory condition of the genital tract.

Motility

In a normal sample, at least 60 per cent of the sperms should show good forward motility within the first three hours of collection of the specimen. Motility less than 60 per cent is considered subnormal and less than 40 per cent suggests infertility.

Count

Sperm count below 20 million/ml indicates sterility. A count between 20–40 million per ml indicates borderline cases of infertility.

Liquefaction

Delayed liquefaction of more than 2 hours suggests inflammation of the accessory glands or enzyme defects in the secretory products of the glands. Liquefaction occurs due to the presence of plasmin in the prostatic fluid.

Morphology

Normally 70 per cent of the sperms should have normal morphology. Abnormalities of more than 30 per cent indicate pathology. The abnormalities may be found in the form of abnormal shapes and poorly formed head or tail. Abnormal sperms may have bifurcated tail, bifid head, spirally coiled tail or absence of head.

pH

pH below 7.0 indicates that the semen primarily contains prostatic fluid, which may be due to congenital absence of the seminal vesicles or excessive secretion of the prostatic fluid.

Fructose

Sugar is usually present in the semen. Its absence indicates obstruction or absence of the ejaculatory ducts or seminal vesicle.

Clinical Application

Semen count is mandatory in the investigation of infertility. A normal report of semen analysis does not guarantee fertility. However, grossly reduced sperm count and motility or presence of large numbers of abnormal sperms definitely suggests that the person is sterile.

VIVA

1. *What is the normal composition of the semen?*
2. *What is the importance of semen analysis in clinical practice?*
3. *When is a person considered infertile?*
4. *Why is there a need for abstinence of 48 hours before collecting the sample?*
5. *Why should the analysis be done after 30 minutes of collection of the sample?*
6. *Why should the analysis be done ideally within 6 hours of collection of the sample?*
7. *What is the mechanism of coagulation and liquefaction of seminal fluid?*
8. *What is normal sperm count?*

CHAPTER 49

Pregnancy Diagnostic Tests

Learning Objectives

After completing this practical, you will be able to (MUST KNOW):

1. Describe the clinical significance of pregnancy diagnostic tests (PDTs).
2. Name the different pregnancy diagnostic tests.
3. State the principles of biological and immunological PDTs.
4. Compare the merits and demerits of various PDTs.
5. Explain the role of various hormones in the maintenance of pregnancy.

INTRODUCTION

Most laboratory tests of pregnancy are based on **demonstration of human chorionic gonadotropin (hCG)** in the urine of the pregnant woman. As hCG in the urine appears within two weeks of pregnancy, it provides an early diagnosis of pregnancy. The tests are classified into **biological tests, immunological tests and other tests**.

The biological tests are not routinely performed in clinical practice as these are time-consuming and expensive, and interpretation of these tests requires knowledge of the histological study of the gonadal tissues. **Immunological tests are usually carried out** to diagnose pregnancy as these tests can be performed in less time and they detect pregnancy as early as the seventh day of gestation. However, recently, **ultrasonographic detection** of pregnancy has virtually replaced the other tests of pregnancy.

METHODS

The main principle behind all tests of pregnancy is that hCG is excreted in the urine of pregnant women as early as 8–12 days after conception. Detection of hCG in the urine permits early diagnosis of pregnancy.

In biological tests, the urine of the pregnant woman is injected into female animals and its action on ovarian morphology is studied to confirm the presence of pregnancy. Various types of biological tests are available and include the following:

- Ascheim–Zondek test
- Kupperman test
- Friedman test
- Hogben test
- Galli–Mainini test

In immunological tests, hCG is detected in the urine or serum of the pregnant woman by reaction with specific antibodies to hCG.

Ascheim–Zondek Test

Procedure

Immature female mice weighing 6–10 g (20–30 days old) are used. The urine is injected intraperitoneally or subcutaneously into five mice in varying doses (0.2–0.4 ml) thrice daily for two days. The abdomen is opened after 100 hours and ovarian changes are observed. A positive test is indicated by enlarged and hyperemic ovaries, and the presence of recent corpus luteum.

Accuracy

The accuracy rate of this test is about 90 per cent.

Disadvantages

1. It takes at least one week to give the report.
2. Large numbers of animals are required for the test.
3. It is expensive.
4. Knowledge of histology is essential to detect the corpus luteum in sections of the ovary.
5. Microscopic study is required to interpret the results.

Kupperman Test

Procedure

Immature female rats are used for this test. The urine of the pregnant woman is injected subcutaneously. Positive test is indicated by marked hyperemia of the ovaries after 6 hours of injection.

Accuracy

This test gives an accurate result of up to 90 per cent.

Disadvantages

1. The test is expensive.
2. It requires animals.
3. It requires skill/experience

Friedman Test

Procedure

Adult female rabbits are used for this experiment. Urine (15 ml) from the pregnant woman is injected intravenously into the rabbit. A positive test is indicated by the presence of fresh corpus luteum and corpus hemorrhagica in the ovary, 36–48 hours after the injection.

Disadvantages

1. The test is expensive.
2. It requires animals.
3. It needs experience.

Hogben Test

Procedure

Adult female toads (Xenopus laevis) are used for the experiment. The urine of the pregnant woman is injected into the lymph space. Positivity is indicated by ovulation (extrusion of eggs) within 18 hours of injection.

Disadvantages

1. The test requires animals.
2. It needs experience.

Galli–Mainini Test

Procedure

Male toads (Bufo bufo) are taken for this experiment. The urine of the pregnant woman is injected into the toad. Positive test result is indicated by the release of sperms which are collected from the cloaca of the test animal 3 hours after injection.

Immunological Test

Principle

The hCG secreted from the syncytiotrophoblast has antigenic properties. Its presence in the serum or in the urine can be detected by using specific antibodies against hCG.

Procedure

Selection of time The approximate level of hCG in urine for sensitivity is **1.5–3.5 IU/ml** in the slide test and 0.2–1.2 IU/ml in the tube test. This concentration of hCG is usually reached after the **eighth day of pregnancy**. Therefore, the test can be performed any time after the eighth day of pregnancy. It is ideally performed after 14 days of missed period.

Collection of urine The patient is advised to restrict water intake from the evening and the first urine sample the next morning is collected in a clean container. The test should be performed within 12 hours of collection of urine. The specific gravity of the urine should be at least 1.015 and it should be protein-free.

Brief Methodology When the urine containing hCG is added to the hCG antisera, the hCG will combine with its antibody and neutralise the antibody. If the hCG-coated tanned red cells or latex particles are then added, no agglutination occurs. A **positive test is indicated by no agglutination**. If the urine to which hCG antisera is added does not contain hCG, the antibody will remain available to agglutinate with the added hCG-coated particle (tanned red cells or latex particles), then **agglutination occurs**, which is *negative for pregnancy*.

Tests performed The two standard immunological tests performed are:

1. Latex agglutination inhibition (LAI) test: **Gravindex test**

2. Hemagglutination inhibition (HAI) test: **Pregnosticon test**

The materials are supplied **in kits** containing all the reagents needed for the test.

Inference

LAI test

The test is done on a slide and the result is observed after 2 minutes. **Positive pregnancy is suggested by the absence of agglutination**, and negative test is suggested by the presence of agglutination.

HAI test

The test is done in a test tube and the observation is taken after 2 hours. A positive pregnancy test is indicated by the formation of a **sharply demarcated brown ring** at the bottom of the tube; the negative test is suggested by the absence of the ring.

Accuracy

The LAI test is 98 per cent accurate. The HAI test is 99 per cent accurate.

Advantages

1. The result is available in a short time.
2. It is simple to perform.
3. It is more accurate than biological tests.

Other Tests

Radioimmunoassay

This is a more sensitive method and can be used to detect the presence of hCG in the serum as early as 7–10 days following fertilisation. The assay can detect even 0.003 IU/ml of the β subunit and 0.001 IU/ml of the α subunit of hCG in the serum. However, it has limited availability in developing countries.

Ultrasonography

The gestational ring is detected by ultrasound as early as the fifth week of pregnancy. The real-time method detects cardiac pulsation by the tenth week and fetal movement by the twelfth week.

Advantages

1. It is non-invasive.

2. It gives the details of morphology of the fetus.
3. It detects abnormalities if present.
4. It gives details about the amount of liquor present.
5. It is easy to repeat.
6. It takes less time.

DISCUSSION

Clinical Significance

Pregnancy diagnostic tests are performed for **early detection of pregnancy**. Early pregnancy tests detect **tiny amounts of hCG in urine**. The hCG appears in the urine at **7–10 days** of fertilisation. Several test kits are available, especially for immunological tests. Though these tests are sensitive and accurate and are used in many hospitals, **false negative and false positive results** can occur. A **false negative result** (the test is negative but the woman is pregnant) may occur from testing too early or from an ectopic pregnancy. A **false positive result** (the test is positive but the woman is not pregnant) may be due to excess protein or blood in urine or hCG production from other sources like choriocarcinoma and hydatidiform mole. Thiazide diuretics, steroids and thyroid drugs may also affect the outcome of the tests.

Hormones of Pregnancy

hCG

The chorion of the placenta secretes hCG. It mimics the luteinising hormone (LH). The primary function of hCG is to rescue the corpus luteum from degeneration and to stimulate continued production of estrogen and progesterone, which is necessary to prevent menstruation and facilitate attachment of the embryo and fetus to the lining of the uterus. hCG appears **as early as the sixth day** after fertilisation in blood and the eighth day after fertilisation in urine, the peak being reached at the ninth week of pregnancy; the level then sharply decreases during the fourth and fifth months.

hCS

hCS is human chorionic somatomammotropin secreted from the placenta. It helps in preparing the mammary glands for lactation, enhances growth of the fetus by increasing protein synthesis, causes nitrogen, potassium and calcium retention, causes lipolysis and decreases glucose utilisation. Decreased concentration of hCS is a sign of placental insufficiency.

Relaxin

Relaxin is secreted from the placenta. It relaxes the uterus and helps in continuation of pregnancy. In the latter part of pregnancy, it relaxes the pubic symphysis and dilates the uterine cervix.

Progesterone

Progesterone is secreted by the corpus luteum during early pregnancy and later by the placenta. It relaxes the uterus and helps in continuation of the pregnancy. Along with estrogen, it maintains the endometrium during pregnancy and prepares the mammary glands for lactation.

Estrogen

Estrogen is secreted by the corpus luteum in the earlier stages and later by the placenta. The secretion of estrogen is less in early pregnancy, but the concentration increases towards term. Estrogen prepares the mammary glands for lactation and the mother's body for parturition.

VIVA

1. *Name the different pregnancy diagnosis tests.*
2. *What is the principle of biological tests for the detection of pregnancy?*
3. *What is the principle of immunological tests for the detection of pregnancy?*
4. *Why are immunological tests preferred to biological tests?*
5. *What are the advantages of immunological tests?*
6. *What are the advantages of radioimmunoassay for the detection of pregnancy?*
7. *What are the advantages of ultrasonography in the detection of pregnancy?*
8. *What are the hormones secreted by the placenta during pregnancy?*
9. *What are the functions of different hormones during pregnancy?*

CHAPTER 50

Birth Control Methods

Learning Objectives

After completing this practical, you will be able to (MUST KNOW):
1. Classify contraceptives used for males and females.
2. Name the temporary and permanent methods of contraception in males and females.
3. Explain the mechanism of action of OCP and IUCD.

4. List the merits and demerits of each intrauterine contraceptive device.
5. Remember the merits and demerits of other types of contraceptives.

You may also be able to (DESIRABLE TO KNOW):
1. Describe the mechanisms, merits and demerits of different types of contraceptives.

INTRODUCTION

India is a highly populous nation. One of the major problems India is facing in recent years is birth control. In April 1976, India formulated its first 'National Population Policy', and 'National Population Policy–2000' is the latest in the series. All these policies primarily aim at reducing the birth rate. When **birth control procedures** work prior to implantation of the fertilised egg, they are called **contraceptives**, and when work after implantation (cause death of the embryo), they are termed as **abortifacients**.

Classification of Birth Control Methods

Contraceptive methods are classified into the following categories (Fig. 50.1):
1. Barrier methods
   – Physical methods   – Chemical methods
2. Intrauterine devices   3. Hormonal methods
4. Post-conceptional methods 5. Permanent methods
   They may also be classified as temporary and permanent methods.

METHODS

Physical Methods

In Males

Condom is the most widely used barrier device in male. It prevents the sperms from being deposited in

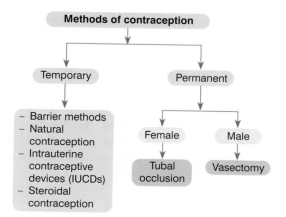

Fig. 50.1   Methods of contraception.

the vagina. The biggest advantage is that it provides **protection against sexually transmitted diseases**.

In Females

Diaphragm is the most commonly used vaginal barrier. A **spermicidal jelly** is usually used along with the diaphragm. Another female barrier device is the **vaginal sponge**.

Chemical Methods

Various spermicidal agents like foams, creams and suppositories are inserted manually into the vagina before intercourse. These act as 'surface-active agents' that attach themselves to sperms and decrease their oxygen uptake and kill them. They are not usually used due to their high failure rate.

Intrauterine Devices

Intrauterine devices (IUDs) are the most effective contraceptive devices for a parous lady (who has borne at least one child).

Types

The IUDs are of **three generations**:
1. **First-generation IUD**
   - Lippes Loop
2. **Second-generation IUD**
   - **Earlier devices**—Copper-7; Copper T-200
   - **Newer devices**—Copper T variants (T-Cu 220C; T-Cu 380A; T-Cu 380Ag)
3. **Third-generation IUD** (with hormonal preparation)
   - **Progestasert**—a T-shaped device filled with 38 mg of progesterone.
   - **Levonorgestrel-20 (LNG-20)**—a T-shaped IUD releasing 20 mcg of levonorgestrel, a synthetic steroid.

Mechanism of Action

IUD works by several mechanisms.
1. Usually, they work after fertilisation has occurred but before implantation is completed. The presence of these small objects in the uterus brings about uterine changes that *interfere with the endometrial preparation* for acceptance of the blastocyst. Thus, implantation is prevented.
2. They also act as a **foreign body** in the uterine cavity causing cellular and biochemical changes in the endometrium and the uterine fluid, which impair the viability of the gamete. Therefore, the chance of fertilisation is reduced.
3. **Copper facilitates cellular reaction** in the endometrium, alters the composition of cervical mucus, impairs sperm motility and impairs capacitation of the sperm.
4. Hormone-releasing devices increase the viscosity of cervical mucus by releasing progesterone. They **thicken the mucus**, and thus prevent entry of the sperm into the uterus. They also make the endometrium unfavourable for implantation.

Merits and Demerits

The merits and demerits of IUDs are summarised in Table 50.1.

Hormonal Contraceptives

1. **Oral contraceptive pills**
   - Combined pill
   - Progestogen-only pill
   - Post-coital pill
   - Once-a-month pill
   - Male pill
2. **Depots** (slow-releasing formulations)
   - Injectable preparations
   - Subcutaneous implants
   - Vaginal rings

Oral Contraceptive Pills (OCPs)

Presently, OCPs contain 30–35 mcg of estrogen and 0.5 to 1 mg of progesterone. The pill is given for 21 days from the 5th day of the cycle. Oral contraceptives are based on the principle that estrogen and progesterone **inhibit pituitary gonadotropin release**, thereby **preventing ovulation**. Progesterone-only pill affects the composition of the cervical mucus, reducing

Table 50.1 Merits and demerits of IUDs (Cu devices and hormone-releasing IUDs).

Advantages	Disadvantages
Inexpensive: Cu-T distributed free of cost through government channels	Require motivation
Simplicity in techniques of insertion and most cost-effective of all methods	Limitation in its use
Prolonged contraceptive protection after insertion (5–10) years and suitable for the rural population of developing countries	Adverse local reactions manifested by menstrual abnormalities, PID, pelvic pain and heavy periods. The effects are less with third generation of IUDs
Systemic side effects are nil. Suitable for hypertensives, breastfeeding women, and epileptics	Risk of ectopic pregnancy
Reversibility to fertility is prompt after removal	

the ability of the sperm to pass through the cervix, and inhibit the estrogen-induced proliferation of the endometrium, making it inhospitable for implantation.

Side effects of OCPs

Though OCPs are 100% effective in preventing pregnancy, there are risks of few side effects, especially when consumed for many years.

- *Cardiovascular side effects* **Myocardial infarction, cerebral thrombosis, venous thrombosis** and **hypertension** have been reported. These side effects are more seen in aged (more than 35 years) woman and in smokers.
- *Carcinogenesis* Increased risk of cervical cancer and breast neoplasia have been reported. Hepatic tumours occur rarely.
- *Metabolic side effects* OCPs **decrease HDL** and alter blood coagulability. These two factors **facilitate atherosclerosis** and proneness to myocardial infarction and stroke. They also cause **glucose intolerance** and insulin resistance.
- *Miscellaneous* Other side effects include cholestatic jaundice, breast tenderness, weight gain and migraine.

Depots

Subcutaneous implants are contraceptive (progestogen) capsules (Norplant) implanted beneath the skin, which release hormone slowly and last for five years. Injectable forms (intra-muscular injection of progestogen substance like Depo-Provera every three months) are also available. Vaginal ring containing levonorgestrel has been found to be effective.

Post-conceptional pills

Contraceptives can be used **within 72 h** after intercourse (post-coital contraception).

1. These pills interfere with ovulation, transport of the conceptus to the uterus, or implantation.
2. Usually, high dose of estrogen, or two large doses (12 h apart) of a combined estrogen-progestin oral preparation are prescribed.
3. Most effective with fewer side effects is the pill RU 486 (mifepristone), which antagonises progesterone activity by binding competitively with progesterone receptors in the uterus.
4. This causes the endometrium to erode and the contractions of the Fallopian tubes and myometrium to increase.

Other Methods

The Rhythm (Safe Period) Method

The rhythm method is the **abstinence from sexual intercourse during the fertile period** of the cycle (near the time of ovulation).

1. In 28 days regular cycles, normally ovulation occurs between 12th and 16th day (usually on 14th day). Functionally sperm can survive for two days and ovum for 3 days.
2. Therefore, unprotected intercourse should be avoided during the **fertile period** of the cycle, which will fall between 2 days before and 3 days after ovulation i. e. from 10th day to 19th day of the cycle. Rest of the period in the cycle is considered to be **safe period**.
3. However, the day of ovulation is not always fixed even in regular cycles and cycle length is also not always regular. Moreover, only the **length of luteal phase is constant**, which is 14 days from the day of ovulation, and practically it is difficult and tedious to know the day of ovulation.
4. Therefore, in practice, **shortest cycle minus 18 days gives** the first day of fertile period and **longest cycle minus 10 days** gives the last day of fertile period. For example, if the duration of shortest cycle is 25 days (25 − 18 = 7th day) and duration of longest cycle is 32 days (32 − 10 = 22nd day), the unprotected intercourse should be **avoided between 7th and 22nd day** of any cycle.
5. However, pregnancy has been documented due to intercourse on any day of the cycle. Therefore, it is believed that no period in any cycle, even during the bleeding phase is absolutely safe.

Coitus Interruptus

In this method, during fertile period, the male partner withdraws penis from vagina before ejaculation. Thus, sperm is not deposited in the female genital tract in the fertile period.

Breastfeeding

Till the mother continues to breast-feed the baby, ovulation does not occur. This is because prolactin secreted during lactation produces **lactational amenorrhea** by inhibiting GnRH secretion.

Family Planning Operations

Government of India encourages people of India with different incentives to opt for family planning operation after a couple are blessed with a child ('we two-ours one' policy). It is done either by male or female sterilisation.

Male Sterilisation

Male sterilisation is performed by **vasectomy**. In vasectomy, bilateral ligation of the vas deferens is performed instead of sectioning the vas because recanalisation can be taken up in future whenever needed. However, antibodies developed against spermatozoa following vasectomy cause infertility following restoration of patency of the vas.

Female Sterilisation

Female sterilisation is performed by **bilateral tubal ligation**. Tubal recanalisation can also be performed later whenever needed.

VIVA

1. What are the contraceptives usually used for males and females?
2. What are the temporary and permanent methods of contraception in males and females?
3. What is the mechanism of action of OCP and IUCD?
4. List the merits and demerits of each intrauterine contraceptive device.
5. List the merits and demerits of other types of contraceptives?
6. What are the mechanisms, merits and demerits of different types of contraceptives?

CHAPTER 51

History Taking and General Examination

Learning Objectives

After completing this practical, you will be able to (MUST KNOW):

1. Describe the importance of general examination in clinical physiology.
2. List the parameters (signs) to be examined in general examination.
3. Examine and elicit different signs in general examination.
4. List the common causes of abnormalities of these signs.

You may also be able to (DESIRABLE TO KNOW):

1. Explain the physiological basis of development of abnormal signs.
2. Correlate the abnormal signs with the pathophysiology of the disease processes.

INTRODUCTION

A detailed history taking and a thorough and detailed general examination is an essential part of the clinical examination of a patient and should be performed prior to any systemic examination. If meticulously performed, the history taking and general examination provides adequate clues to the diagnosis.

History Taking

History taking is an important part of the clinical examination of a patient. This is done prior to general physical examination. History taking includes:

1. Name, age and address
2. Marital status, religion
3. Personal, occupational and social history (including history of smoking and alcohol intake)
4. History of past illness
5. Family history (of similar or related problems or illness, especially in first-degree relatives)
6. History of present illness
7. Treatment history (and use of drugs)
8. Presenting complaints
9. For women: Menstrual and obstetric history

General Examination

Requirements

1. Patient's examination should be conducted in a comfortable, private and quiet area.

2. Preferably, examination should be done in daylight as skin changes are better appreciated in natural light. Artificial light should be avoided.
3. Usually patients will be apprehensive to be examined, especially when the environment is unfamiliar. Reassure the patient about the need for the examination for diagnosing the disease.
4. A thorough general examination requires the subject to be adequately exposed. The patient should be asked to undress maximally.
5. If a male doctor examines a female patient, especially if the private parts are to be examined, always a chaperone/female attender/female nurse should be present. This is done to reassure the patient and to protect the doctor from accusations of immodesty.
6. If covered areas and private parts need to be examined as part of the clinical examination, there should be no hesitation to unclothe these parts and examine properly.
7. Only the area being examined should be exposed at the time. The body parts just examined should be covered as the examiner proceeds to the next.
8. The subject/patient should stand on the examiner's right-hand side, as it is easy to examine the abdominal viscera, jugular vein, apex beat from the right side.
9. Regular attention should be given to the patient's comfort, especially while examining an elderly subject, such as adjustment of pillow, which

usually gets disturbed during examination. This would help in reassuring the patient.

10. A quick assessment of patient's illness should be made. If the patient is very sick, the detailed examination may be postponed till the acute problem has been attended. The examination should not distress the already ill patient.

Steps of Examination

The general examination begins the moment the patient is seen. It should be done without unnecessary embarrassment and discomfort to the patient. It should preferably be performed in daylight. General examination is carried out under the following headings:

1. General appearance
2. Mental state and intelligence
3. Consciousness and cooperation
4. Build
5. Development (height, weight and sexual maturity)
6. State of nutrition
7. Pallor (anemia)
8. Icterus (jaundice)
9. Cyanosis
10. Clubbing
11. Edema
12. Lymphadenopathy
13. Skin condition
14. *Vital signs* Temperature, pulse, respiration, blood pressure

GENERAL APPEARANCE

Look at the subject, and observe whether he looks healthy, unwell or ill. If he looks ill, assess the severity of the illness: whether the patient is ill, very ill or in distress.

MENTAL STATE AND INTELLIGENCE

One should assess the mood of the patient and should try to study his/her mind. This is detected by observing the way the patient describes his emotional state.

The patient's level of intelligence is one of the important pieces of information to be obtained from the interview. This helps to determine the treatment that is most suitable. An approximate assessment of intelligence is obtained from the educational and occupational history and from an assessment of his general knowledge.

CONSCIOUSNESS AND COOPERATION

It is important to ascertain the level of consciousness of the patient. The level of consciousness can be clear sensorium, drowsiness, stupor, semicoma and coma. If he is fully conscious, assess whether he is cooperative enough to provide all information.

BUILD

Build is the skeletal structure of a person. It is assessed in relation to the age and sex of the individual as compared to a normal person. It should be observed whether the patient is tall or short, lean or fat, and muscular or asthenic.

DEVELOPMENT

Height

The height of each patient should be measured to find out whether he is of average height for that age and sex. If he is too tall or short, details of the **measurement of span** (from the tip of the middle finger of one side to the tip of the middle finger of the other side of outstretched upper limbs), **upper segment** (crown to the pubic symphysis), and the **lower segment** (pubic symphysis to foot) should be taken.

> Note: Normally, in adults, the arm-span is equal to the height of the person and the upper segment is equal to the length of the lower segment.

Weight

The weight should be recorded preferably on an empty stomach, without shoes and with minimum clothing. It should be ascertained whether the patient's weight is normal for age and sex or if he is overweight or underweight.

Body Mass Index

Body mass index (BMI) is an important index of physical development of an individual. It is assessed by the **Quetlet formula,**

$$BMI = \frac{Weight\ (in\ kg)}{Height\ (in\ metres^2)}$$

Though there are many other anthropometric indices such as waist circumference, waist–hip ratio, waist–height ratio, skin fold thickness, neck circumference, etc., BMI is the commonly used parameter for assessment of **adiposity and cardiovascular (CV) risk** of the person, as degrees of obesity have traditionally been calculated by the level of BMI. As the Asian population is more prone to CV risks even at lower range of BMI, compared to European, African, American and other populations, the BMI range for grading obesity in Asian population is different.

BMI range for Asian population is as follows:
Normal BMI : 18.5–22.99 (below 18.5 is underweight)
Overweight (Preobese) : 23–27.49
Obesity : 27.5 or above

Sexual Development

Effort should be made to assess the development of secondary sexual characteristics.

In males, secondary sexual characteristics develop between 13 and 18 years. Hair grows on the face, trunk, axillae and pubic region. The pubic hair develops with the upper border convex upwards and may extend up to the umbilicus. Laryngeal growth results in thick voice. Considerable muscular development occurs.

In females, secondary sexual characteristics develop between 11 and 15 years. There is development of breasts, and the female distribution of fat gives the characteristic curves of the body. Hair also grows in the axillae and pubis. The pubic hair exhibits an upper margin, which is concave upwards.

NUTRITION

Assessment of the nutritional state of a patient is an important part of the general examination. It is done by taking dietary history, and by performing physical examination including anthropometric measurements. The physical examination includes measurement of the bulk of the muscles and body fat (**skinfold thickness**). **Anthropometric measurements** include recording of height and weight. It is performed to ascertain whether the patient is well nourished or malnourished. **Malnutrition** may be due to starvation, maldigestion of food or malabsorption of nutrients from the gastrointestinal tract.

PALLOR

Pallor is paleness of the skin. It depends on the thickness and quality of the skin, and the amount and quality of the blood in the capillaries. Thus, pallor is seen in persons with thick or opaque skin, in conditions where blood flow in the capillaries is diminished, such as shock, or when the hemoglobin content in the blood is decreased. Pallor is usually detected by examining the lower palpebral conjunctiva (Fig. 51.1).

Note: The tip and dorsum of the tongue, soft palate, palms and nails should also be examined to assess pallor.

The degree of pallor is expressed as **plus 1 to plus 3** (Fig. 51.2).
Pallor : 0 (no anemia)
Pallor : + (mild anemia)

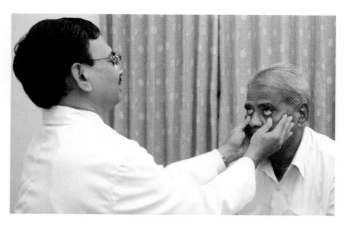

Fig. 51.1   Detection of pallor. Note that the lower eyelids are retracted down to assess the paleness of the lower palpebral conjunctiva.

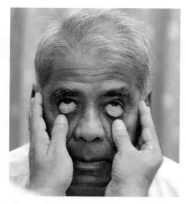

Fig. 51.2   Note the pallor as + (mild anemia) in this subject.

Pallor : ++ (moderate anemia)

Pallor : +++ (severe anemia)

JAUNDICE

Jaundice is the yellow discolouration of the sclera (Fig. 51.3), skin and mucous membranes of the body, which occurs due to the presence of excess bilirubin in the blood. Normal serum bilirubin concentration is 0.2 to 0.8 mg/100 ml of blood. When the bilirubin level exceeds 2 mg per cent, jaundice appears clinically (Fig. 51.4). Hyperbilirubinemia between 0.8 and 2 mg% is called **subclinical or latent jaundice**.

Types

Jaundice is classified clinically into **three types**: prehepatic, hepatic and post-hepatic.

Prehepatic Jaundice

Prehepatic jaundice occurs due to excessive destruction of red cells. Therefore, it is also called **hemolytic jaundice**. Jaundice is usually mild to moderate and bilirubin is mostly unconjugated. Fecal stercobilinogen and urinary urobilinogen are increased. Excretion of bilirubin in urine is absent (**acholuric jaundice**) because the excess unconjugated bilirubin in the blood combines with albumin and therefore cannot be filtered in the kidneys. The *van den Bergh test is indirect positive*.

Hepatic Jaundice

This usually occurs due to hepatitis or damage to the cells of the liver. Therefore, it is also called hepatic or

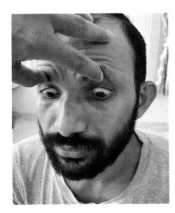

Fig. 51.3 Method of detection of icterus. Note that the upper eyelids are retracted upwards and the subject is asked to look downward to assess the yellow discolouration of the sclera.

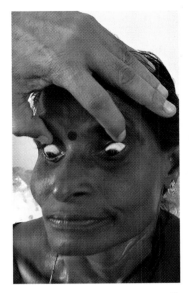

Fig. 51.4 A patient having jaundice. Note the yellow discolouration of the sclera.

hepatocellular jaundice. Jaundice is usually moderate to severe and may be associated with bleeding disorders. Bilirubin is both conjugated and unconjugated. Fecal stercobilinogen and urinary urobilinogen are normal or raised. Bilirubins exhibit a *biphasic reaction to the van den Bergh test.*

Post-hepatic Jaundice

This occurs due to obstruction in the biliary tract. Therefore, it is called **obstructive jaundice**. Because of obstruction, no bilirubin reaches the intestine. Hence, fecal stercobilinogen and urinary urobilinogen are absent. The bilirubin is conjugated and appears in the urine. The *van den Bergh test is direct positive.*

Causes of Yellow Discolouration of Skin

1. Jaundice
2. Carotenemia
3. Hemochromatosis
4. Picrates
5. Mephacrine

CYANOSIS

Cyanosis is the bluish discolouration of the skin and mucous membranes of the body due to the presence of **reduced hemoglobin in more than 5 g%** in the blood.

Physiological Basis

Hemoglobin in the arterial blood is 95 per cent saturated with oxygen. Therefore, about 14.25 g (taking 15 g% of hemoglobin as the standard) in the arterial blood is oxyhemoglobin and only 0.75 g is reduced hemoglobin in a normal adult. In mixed venous blood, about 70 per cent of hemoglobin is saturated with oxygen. Hence, 10.5 g of the 15 g per cent of hemoglobin in the venous blood is oxyhemoglobin and 4.5 g is reduced hemoglobin. The amount of reduced hemoglobin in capillary blood is assumed to be the mean of arterial and venous content of the reduced hemoglobin. Thus, in a normal individual at rest, capillary blood contains 2.6 g% (0.75 + 4.5/2) of reduced hemoglobin. The colour of normal skin and mucous membrane is therefore pink. ***When the concentration of reduced hemoglobin is more than 5 g per cent,*** the skin and mucous membrane become blue because of the dark colour of the reduced hemoglobin. The presence of excess of other hemoglobin complexes like methemoglobin and sulfhemoglobin in the blood also produces cyanosis because of their dark colour.

> Note:
> 1. Patients suffering from severe anemia with hemoglobin content less than 5 g per cent may not show cyanosis (as the total hemoglobin is less than 5 gm per cent).
> 2. Cyanosis may not be seen in carbon monoxide poisoning, because carboxyhemoglobin prevents reduction of oxyhemoglobin and the colour of carboxyhemoglobin is cherry red.

Types

Cyanosis is of **three types**: peripheral, central and mixed. There is another special category of cyanosis, called differential cyanosis.

Peripheral Cyanosis

This occurs due to slowing of the flow of blood through the tissues, thereby allowing more time for removal of oxygen by the tissues.

Causes

1. Decreased cardiac output, for example, heart failure
2. Local vasoconstriction, for example, extreme cold
3. Venous obstruction, for example, superior venacaval obstruction
4. Increased viscosity of blood, for example, polycythemia

Central Cyanosis

When reduced hemoglobin concentration is more than 5 g% due to mixing of arterial blood with venous blood, or inadequate oxygenation of the arterial blood, central cyanosis results. In the early stage, cyanosis manifests in the palate, tongue and inner side of the lips. When the amount of reduced hemoglobin becomes very high, cyanosis appears in different peripheral sites too.

Causes

I. Due to admixture of venous and arterial blood This occurs in the right to left shunt in which venous blood bypasses the pulmonary circulation and directly enters into the systemic circulation. It is seen in:

i) Fallot's tetralogy
ii) Pulmonary arteriovenous fistula
iii) Patent truncus arteriosus
iv) Transposition of great vessels

II. Due to inadequate oxygenation of arterial blood

1. Low atmospheric oxygen, for example, high altitude
2. Inadequate ventilation, for example, lung collapse, airway obstruction
3. Decreased gaseous exchange through the pulmonary membrane, for example, hyaline membrane disease

Mixed Cyanosis

In this type of cyanosis, both central and peripheral mechanisms operate. The most common example is chronic cor pulmonale due to emphysema.

Differential Cyanosis

This is a condition where cyanosis appears only in one half of the body. For example, in patent ductus arteriosus with reversal of shunt due to pulmonary hypertension, cyanosis is seen only in the lower limbs; both upper limbs are spared.

CLUBBING

Bulbous enlargement of soft parts of the terminal phalanges with over-curving of the nails both transversely and longitudinally is called clubbing.

Detection

Clubbing is diagnosed by the presence of any of the following five signs.

1. Fluctuation test (Nail bed fluctuation)   Normally, the nail bed fluctuates very slightly. Fluctuation increases in clubbing. This is elicited by assessing fluctuation of the nail base. The examiner holds the base of the nail from both sides and gently presses the tip of the nail (Fig. 51.5) to elicit nail bed fluctuation, if present. Alternatively, fluctuation test can be elicited by firmly holding and fixing the finger of the patient with the middle fingers and thumbs of the examiner and testing the nailbed flocculation by pressing from both sides alternatively with the index fingers (Fig. 51.6).

2. Curving of nails   In clubbing, the nails curve in both transverse and longitudinal directions. The curving is due to hypertrophy of nail bed tissue.

3. Profile sign   The presence of a transverse ridge at the root of the nail due to thickening of fibroelastic tissue is called profile sign.

4. Schamroth's sign   When two fingers are held together with their nails facing each other, a space is seen at the nail folds (Fig. 51.7). This space is lost in clubbing (positive Schamroth's sign).

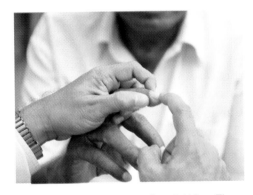

Fig. 51.5   Fluctuation test for assessing clubbing. The examiner holds the base of the nail and gently presses the tip of the nail to assess fluctuation of the nail bed.

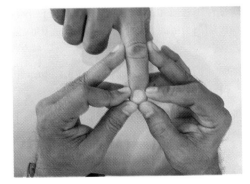

Fig. 51.6   Alternative method of fluctuation (nail bed fluctuation) test for assessing presence of clubbing.

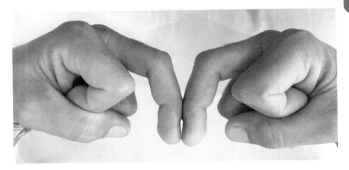

Fig. 51.7   Normal space is seen at the nail folds, when nails are apposed facing each other. This is negative Schamroth's sign.

5. Base angle   In a normal finger the angle between the base of the nail and the adjacent portion of the dorsum of the terminal phalanx is an obtuse angle of about 160°. In clubbing, this angle gets obliterated in the outward direction and becomes 180° or more. This is best viewed vertically from the side.

Physiological Basis

The exact physiological basis of clubbing is not known. It may be due to any of the following causes:

1. Dilatation of AV anastomosis   In clubbing, the AV (arteriovenous) anastomotic channels increase in the fingers (the cause is not known). This causes hypertrophy of tissues in the nail bed.

2. Increased pressure gradient   An increase in pressure gradient between the radial artery and digital artery causes edema and increased cellularity of the connective tissue in the finger. This predisposes the finger to clubbing.

3. Capillary stasis   Capillary stasis results from back pressure, which may cause clubbing.

4. Vitamin deficiency and hormonal disorders   These are thought to be involved in the genesis of clubbing.

Causes

A. Bronchopulmonary diseases
   1.   Bronchiectasis
   2.   Lung abscess
   3.   Bronchogenic carcinoma
   4.   Emphysema
B. Cardiac diseases
   1.   Congenital cyanotic heart disease
   2.   Subacute bacterial endocarditis

C. Gastrointestinal diseases
1. Ulcerative colitis
2. Biliary cirrhosis of liver
D. Endocrine disorders
1. Thyrotoxicosis
2. Acromegaly
E. Hereditary

Degrees of Clubbing

First degree   When only increased fluctuation of the nail bed is present, it is first degree clubbing.

Second degree   When curving of nail is present in addition to increased fluctuation of nail bed, there is second degree clubbing.

Third degree   If increased fluctuation, increased curving and obliteration of base angle of the nails are present together, there is third degree clubbing.

Fourth degree   A combination of the above changes plus subperiosteal thickening of the wrist and ankle bones with the presence of definite transverse ridge at the root of the nails show that there is fourth degree clubbing.

EDEMA

Edema is swelling of the skin and subcutaneous tissues due to accumulation of free fluid in excess in the interstitial tissue space.

Types

Edema is classified as localised or generalised and pitting or non-pitting.

Method of Detection

Edema is diagnosed by pressing the skin against the bones in the dependent parts (Fig. 51.8), which leaves a pit or depression in the case of pitting edema (Fig. 51.9). Edema may be non-pitting as seen in filariasis.

Common Causes

A. Cardiac causes
1. Congestive heart failure
2. Constrictive pericarditis

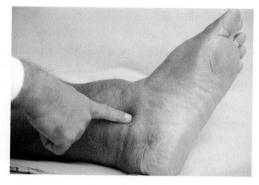

Fig. 51.8   Assessment of edema. Note that the skin against the medial malleolus (dependent part of this subject) is pressed for about 20 seconds.

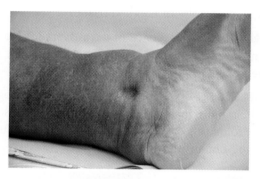

Fig. 51.9   Pitting edema. Note the presence of pit (depression) in the ankle following putting pressure over the area.

B. Hepatic causes
1. Cirrhosis of liver
2. Carcinoma of liver
C. Renal causes
1. Nephrotic syndrome
2. Acute nephritis
D. Anemia and hypoproteinemia

Special Features

Cardiac edema   It is usually seen in the dependant parts of the body. Dyspnea at rest is one of the associated features.

Hepatic edema   Edema is prominent on the abdomen. Ascites is one of the associated features.

Renal edema   Edema first appears in the face. Puffiness of the lower eyelid in the morning is a characteristic feature.

Anemia and hypoproteinemia   Edema is generalised from the beginning. Severe pallor is one of the associated features.

Physiological Basis

Edema occurs due to **excess accumulation of fluid in the interstitial tissue space**. Interstitial fluid is formed by filtration through the capillary walls. The capillary wall is regarded as a semi-permeable membrane. The main driving forces causing filtration of fluid through the capillaries are hydrostatic pressure within the capillaries and oncotic pressure (osmotic pressure exerted by the plasma proteins). Hydrostatic pressure favours filtration whereas oncotic pressure opposes it. Therefore, when **hydrostatic pressure increases or oncotic pressure decreases**, there is excess filtration of fluid into the interstitial tissue space. Normally, the fluid from the interstitial space is removed by the lymphatics. When excess filtration of fluid occurs, the lymphatics cannot remove all the fluid and more fluid accumulates in the interstitial tissue space. This leads to formation of edema.

Physiological Mechanisms

In Cardiac Failure

In congestive cardiac failure, edema develops in dependent parts of the body due to the following mechanisms.
1. Decreased cardiac output decreases blood volume and pressure, which **increases renin release** from the kidney. Renin forms angiotensin II which **increases aldosterone secretion** from the adrenal cortex. Aldosterone increases reabsorption of sodium and water from the kidney. This increases total body sodium and water, which results in edema formation.
2. Decreased cardiac output also **stimulates sympathetic activity** which causes renal vasoconstriction. Constriction of the renal artery causes release of renin which activates the renin–angiotensin–aldosterone axis.
3. In congestive cardiac failure, due to failure of the right ventricle (backward failure), pressure in the systemic veins increases. This **increases hydrostatic pressure** in the capillaries, which results in edema formation.

In Nephrotic Syndrome

The main cause of edema formation in nephrotic syndrome is the **loss of protein in the urine**. Protein passes from the glomerulus into the tubular fluid, which results in proteinuria. Loss of protein from the kidney decreases oncotic pressure because of hypoproteinemia and results in edema formation.

In Cirrhosis of Liver

In cirrhosis of liver, there is loss of liver tissue. There is decrease in the synthesis of protein by the liver. This results in **hypoproteinemia** which causes decreased oncotic pressure and edema formation.

In Anemia and Hypoproteinemia

In anemia, hypoxia of capillaries increases capillary permeability, which results in edema formation. However, the main cause of edema in anemia is hypoproteinemia.

LYMPHADENOPATHY

The neck, axilla, inguinal region and supratrochlear areas of both the sides should be examined thoroughly to check for enlargement of lymph nodes. The lymph nodes in the neck should be examined by standing behind the subject and with the patient's head slightly flexed. The glands should be examined in proper order starting from the submental group and proceeding to the submandibular, cervical, posterior auricular and the occipital groups. Lymph nodes in the axilla should also be examined by standing behind the subject and with the patient's arm slightly abducted. In the axilla, anterior, posterior, apical and lateral groups of lymph nodes are examined. The lymph nodes in the inguinal region are examined in a supine position with thigh extended.

Procedure of Examination

Lymph nodes are palpated to check their size and shape, consistency, mobility and tenderness.

1. **Size and shape**   The size of the enlarged lymph node is expressed in centimetres in its longest diameter. The surface of the enlarged nodes may be smooth, irregular or lobulated. Malignant lymph nodes are often irregular.

2. **Consistency**   Lymph nodes are often elastic and rubbery. They are firm in tuberculosis, firm and shotty in syphilis, and hard in carcinoma.

3. Mobility Nodes may be mobile or fixed. In benign conditions, nodes are usually separated and mobile. In tuberculosis, the nodes are often matted. In malignant conditions, the nodes are usually fixed to the skin and surrounding tissues.

4. Tenderness While palpating the lymph nodes, the patient may complain of pain or may grimace during palpation, which indicates that the lymph nodes are tender. Usually lymph nodes are tender in inflammatory conditions and non-tender (painless) in malignant diseases.

Causes

A. Neoplastic

   I. Hematologic
1. Lymphomas (Hodgkin and non-Hodgkin)
2. Acute leukemia
3. Chronic lymphocytic leukemia

   II. Non-hematologic
1. Carcinoma of breast
2. Carcinoma of lungs

B. Inflammatory

   I. Infections
1. Tuberculosis
2. Syphilis
3. Filariasis
4. Infectious mononucleosis

   II. Connective tissue diseases
1. Systemic lupus erythematosus
2. Sarcoidosis

C. Endocrine diseases
1. Hyperthyroidism
2. Addison's disease

D. Drugs
1. Carbamazepine
2. Cephaloridine
3. Meprobamate
4. Phenylbutazone
5. Phenytoin

THE SKIN

The skin is examined carefully, preferably in daylight and the maximum surface of body should be exposed.

The skin is examined for the colour, pigmentation, eruptions and secondary lesions.

Colour of the Skin

Pallor of the skin is seen in anemia. Yellow skin is seen in jaundice. Blue skin is seen in cyanosis.

Pigmentation

The skin looks white in albinisim. Patches of white and black pigments are seen in vitiligo. The skin is dark in Addison's disease.

Eruptions

Different skin eruptions like macules, papules, vesicles, pustules and petechiae occur in different clinical conditions.

Secondary Lesions

Scales, crusts, excoriations, fissures, ulcers and scars occur in different conditions.

VITAL SIGNS

There are **four vital signs** that must always be checked in general examination. These are temperature, pulse, respiration and blood pressure. Usually it is referred to as in routine practice as **'BPTPR'**

Temperature

Body temperature is usually recorded by using a clinical thermometer. The thermometer is placed either in the mouth or in the axilla for at least one minute. The thermometer can also be placed in the rectum, especially in infants and collapsed patients. The body temperature is usually expressed in Fahrenheit or in Centigrade.

Normal Value

The normal body temperature at rest is 98–99°F (36.6–37.2°C).

Febrile	: >37.2°C (99°F or above)
Mild fever	: 37.2– 38.3°C (99–101°F)
Moderate fever	: 38.3–40°C (101–104°F)
High fever	: 40–41.2°C (104–106°F)

Hyperpyrexia : > 41.6°C (>107°F)
Subnormal   : < 36.6°C (<98°F)
Hypothermia : < 35°C (< 95°F)

Fever

Increase in the diurnal variation of body temperature by more than 1°C (1.5°F) or rise of temperature above the maximum normal temperature is called fever.

Types

Typically, **three classical types** of fever are seen in clinical practice. These are **continued, remittent and intermittent fever**.

Continued fever The temperature remains high throughout the day and at no time does it touch the baseline, and the diurnal variation of temperature is not more than 1°C. This is commonly seen in:

◆ Typhoid
◆ Subacute bacterial endocarditis
◆ Urinary tract infection
◆ Brucellosis
◆ Glandular fever

Remittent fever The temperature remains raised throughout the day and at no time does it touch the baseline, but the diurnal variation is more than 2°C.

Intermittent fever Fever is present only for several hours during the day and remits to normal for the rest of the day. Intermittent fever may be quotidian, tertian, quartan or irregular intermittent.

◆ **Quotidian** When the paroxysm of intermittent fever occurs every day.
◆ **Tertian** When the paroxysm of fever occurs on alternate days.
◆ **Quartan** When two days intervene between consecutive attacks.
◆ **Irregular intermittent** Paroxysm of fever occurs irregularly.

Causes

1. Infections
   Bacterial
   Viral
   Rickettsial
   Fungal
   Parasitic
2. Immunologic
   Rheumatic fever
   Rheumatoid arthritis
   Other collagen diseases
3. Neoplastic
   Carcinoma of any organ
   Leukemia
4. Metabolic
   Gout
   Porphyria
   Addison's disease
5. Physical agents
   Heat stroke
   Radiation sickness
6. Drug-induced fever

Hypothermia

Hypothermia is a condition in which body temperature decreases below the normal range.

Causes

1. Prolonged exposure to cold
2. Myxedema
3. Hypopituitarism
4. Hypoglycemia
5. Hypnosedative poisoning

Physiological Effects

Hypothermia causes bradycardia, hypotension and shallow respiration and, in severe cases, confusion, stupor and coma. The brain is probably protected by the low temperature.

Pulse

Count the radial pulse for a minute when the subject is at rest. Examination of pulse is not only performed as part of the examination of the cardiovascular system, but also routinely in general examination as it provides information about the functioning of the heart. It is palpated by three middle fingers with the patient's forearm semipronated and wrist slightly flexed. The pulse is examined for rate, rhythm, volume, character and condition of the arterial wall. A normal pulse rate is 60–100 per minute, regular in rhythm, and normal in volume and character. The arterial wall is neither thickened nor tortuous. (*Details of the procedure and abnormalities of pulse are given in* Chapter 27).

Respiration

The rate of respiration is counted for a minute. It should preferably be counted when the subject's attention is distracted from his breathing. Rhythm and type of respiration are also noted. The normal rate of respiration in an adult is 12–20 per minute. (*Details of change in respiration in different conditions are given in Chapter 52*).

Blood Pressure

The blood pressure is recorded by a sphygmomanometer, first by the palpatory and then by the auscultatory method. The normal range of blood pressure in adults:

Systolic : 100–119 mm Hg

Diastolic : 60–79 mm Hg

(*Details of blood pressure recording and the conditions affecting blood pressure are given in Chapter 28*).

VIVA

1. What is the importance of general examination in clinical medicine?
2. What are the parameters that are looked for in general examination?
3. How do you assess the development of the subject?
4. How do you assess the nutritional status of the subject?
5. Where do you look to confirm pallor clinically?
6. What is jaundice?
7. Where do you look to detect jaundice clinically?
8. What are the types of jaundice and how do you differentiate them?
9. What are the causes of the yellow colour of the skin?
10. What is cyanosis?
11. What are the types of cyanosis and how do you differentiate them?
12. What is the physiological basis of cyanosis?
13. What is clubbing?
14. What are the causes of clubbing?
15. How do you detect clubbing?
16. Define edema.
17. What are the types of edema and what are their causes?
18. What is the physiological basis of edema in heart failure, nephrotic syndrome and cirrhosis of the liver?
19. Which regions of the body are specially checked for lymph node enlargement? Why?
20. What are the common causes of lymphadenopathy?
21. What are the vital signs?
22. What is the normal body temperature?
23. What is fever?
24. What are the types of fever?
25. How do you differentiate between various types of fever?
26. What are the common causes of fever?
27. What is hypothermia?
28. What are the causes of hypothermia?
29. What is the importance of examination of pulse in general examination?
30. What is the normal rate of respiration in adults?
31. What is the normal systolic and diastolic pressure in adults?

CHAPTER 52

Clinical Examination of the Respiratory System

Learning Objectives

After completing this practical, you will be able to (MUST KNOW):

1. Trace the different lines, prominences, lung fissures and borders on the surface of the chest.
2. Perform a clinical examination of the respiratory system, proceeding in the proper sequence.
3. List the different abnormalities of the shape of the chest.
4. Name the different types and causes of abnormal respiration.
5. State the causes of unilateral and bilateral restriction of chest movements.

6. State the causes of increased and decreased vocal fremitus.
7. List the rules of percussion.
8. List the differences between vesicular and bronchial breath sounds.

You may also be able to (DESIRABLE TO KNOW):

1. Explain the common abnormalities observed in different parameters of examination of the respiratory system.
2. Explain the differences between vesicular and bronchial breathing.
3. Describe the types and causes of bronchial breathing.
4. List the reasons for production of different bronchial breath sounds.

INTRODUCTION

Clinical examination of the respiratory system is performed to assess the functional status of the respiratory tract and lungs. It should be carried out meticulously and methodically in a patient suffering from lung disease. The clinical examination can provide sufficient information to diagnose the exact nature of pathology in the lungs. For interpretation and correlation of the findings of the clinical examination with the disease process, one should have knowledge of the functional anatomy of the lungs.

Anatomical Landmarks

Different Lines

The different lines that are drawn on the chest (Fig. 52.1) for denoting areas of clinical examination of the respiratory system are as follows:

1. Midsternal line   This is a vertical line drawn through the centre of the sternum and xiphoid.

2. Midclavicular line   This is a vertical line, parallel to the midsternal line, which extends downwards from the centre of each clavicle. The centre of the clavicle is located between the middle of the suprasternal notch

and the tip of the acromion.

3. Anterior axillary line   This is a vertical line extending downwards from the anterior axillary fold.

4. Posterior axillary line   This is a vertical line extending downwards from the posterior axillary fold.

5. Midaxillary line   This is a vertical line originating at a point midway between the anterior and posterior axillary line.

6. Midspinal line   This is a vertical line that passes through the centre of the back as defined by the spinal processes. This is called **vertebral line**.

7. Midscapular line   This is a vertical line on the posterior aspect of the chest, which runs parallel to the midspinal line and extends through the apices of the scapula.

Different Prominences

1. Sternal angle   This is a transverse bony ridge at the junction of the body of the sternum and the manubrium. This is also known as the *angle of Louis or Ludwig's angle.*

Significance of the sternal angle

i) The second costal cartilage articulates the sternum at this point. Therefore, the rib that corresponds to this point is the second rib. The intercostal space

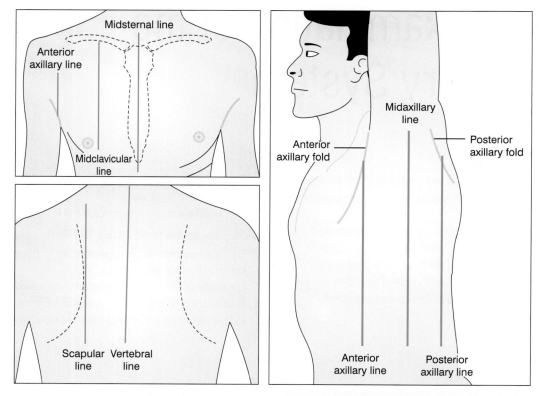

Fig. 52.1   Different lines drawn on the chest for denoting areas of clinical examination of the respiratory system.

below this is the second intercostal space. It helps in identifying all the intercostal spaces.

ii) The trachea bifurcates into two main bronchi at this point.

iv) The level of the upper border of the atria of the heart coincides with this point.

v) The anterior borders of the lungs meet in the midline here.

vi) The disc between the fourth and fifth thoracic vertebrae in the back coincides with this.

2. Suprasternal notch   This is the top of the manubrium.

3. Vertebral prominence   The spinous process of the seventh cervical vertebra is the most prominent on the back and is easily seen and felt.

Lung Fissures and Borders

1. Oblique fissure (major interlobar fissure)   It starts from the second thoracic spine posteriorly and extends obliquely downwards and forwards to the sixth costochondral junction anteriorly.

2. Horizontal fissure (minor interlobar fissure)   It starts from the right fourth costochondral junction and

passes horizontally to meet the oblique fissure in the midaxillary line.

> **Note:** The lower lobe lies below the oblique fissure on either side. Above it, lies the upper lobe on the left side. On the right side, the upper lobe lies above the horizontal fissure. Between the oblique and the horizontal fissures lies the middle lobe of the right lung. The greater part of the back of the chest is occupied by the lower lobe. The anterior aspect of the chest is occupied by the upper lobe in the left and upper and middle lobe in the right.

3. Upper border of lung   It is limited to a level 5 cm above the sternoclavicular joint.

4. Lower border of lung   It lies on the sixth rib on the midclavicular line, on the eighth rib on the midaxillary line and on the tenth rib on the posterior scapular line.

METHODS

Methods of Examination of the Respiratory System

Principle

Examination of the respiratory system is carried out by inspection, palpation, percussion and auscultation of the chest. Inspection shows the configuration, the degree of movement of the chest, and the type and rate of respiration. Palpation confirms the movement of the chest, detects abnormal pulsation, areas of tenderness and the degree of vocal fremitus. Percussion demonstrates the nature of changes (if any) of the lung tissues, bronchi and the pleura, and shows whether the lung tissues contain less or more air than normal and whether the pleura contains less or more fluid than normal. Auscultation detects the type, intensity and nature of breath sounds, and the presence of any other sound.

■ Requirements

1. Measuring tape
2. Stethoscope

■ Procedure

It consists of examination of the chest, which follows observation of a few particular signs in general examination that are relevant to this system. It is best accomplished when the patient is standing or is comfortably seated in an erect position after complete exposure of the chest in good light.

General examination

1. Pallor Presence of anemia is common in patients with chronic hemoptysis.

2. Cyanosis Cyanosis occurs due to the presence of excess deoxygenated hemoglobin (>5 g%). Cyanosis may occur due to inadequate ventilation of perfused lung areas as in pneumonia, or due to the decrease in the total amount of air ventilating the lungs, as seen in poliomyelitis.

3. Clubbing Clubbing is recognised by the bulbousness of the soft, terminal portion of the fingers and by an excessive curvature of the nail in both the longitudinal and lateral planes. It is seen in bronchogenic carcinoma, chronic suppurative diseases of the lung like bronchiectasis, empyema, and lung abscess.

4. Lymph node enlargement The neck and supraclavicular region should be particularly examined to check for enlargement of lymph nodes.

Examination of the chest

Inspection

Inspection of the chest should be done with subject in supine posture on a couch or sitting comfortably on chair, with the chest region fully exposed. As the ribs on both sides of chest extend down to almost middle of the abdomen, the trunk should be exposed up to the umbilicus level (Fig. 52.2).

1. Shape of the chest Examine the shape of the chest. The chest of a normal healthy adult is bilaterally symmetrical. The transverse diameter is greater than the antero-posterior diameter, *the ratio being 7 : 5*. Check for abnormalities of the chest.

2. Symmetry of the chest Look for symmetry of the chest, comparing both sides. The chest may bulge or be depressed either on one or both sides.

3. Movement of the chest Observe whether the chest moves normally and symmetrically equally on both sides with respiration and whether a difference exists in the movement of the chest between the upper and lower parts.

> **Note:** Normally, the movements are equal on both the sides and are more in the base of the lungs than the apex. But one should keep in mind that if lesions are present in both the lungs, the movement may be equally affected on both sides.

4. Respiratory movement Look for the following points while observing the movements of the chest with respiration.

◈ *Rate* The normal rate of respiration in adults is 12–18 per minute. Respiration rate is higher in children. The increased rate of respiration is called tachypnea and the decreased rate of respiration is called bradypnea.

◈ *Rhythm* Determine whether the respiration is regular or irregular.

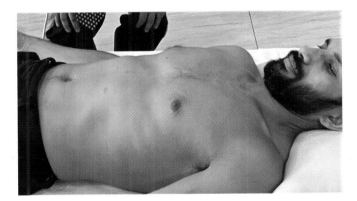

Fig. 52.2 Inspection of the chest. Note that the chest is exposed fully, and trunk is exposed up to the level of umbilicus as the ribs on both sides of the chest extend down to almost the middle of the abdomen.

- ◆ *Depth*   Look for the depth (degree) of respiration. The respiration may be decreased unilaterally or on both sides.
- ◆ *Type*   Note whether the respiration is predominantly thoracic or abdominal. In men, respiration is abdominothoracic and in women, the respiration is thoracoabdominal.

Palpation

1. Expansion of the chest   Expansion of the chest is assessed by placing the two palms firmly on both the sides of the chest and apposing the thumbs in the midline anteriorly (Fig. 52.3A). The subject is asked to take a deep breath and the movement of the thumbs away from the midline is observed (Fig. 52.3B). This indicates the extent of expansion of the chest. Normally, the expansion is more than 5 cm at the base of the lungs in adults, which can be elicited both in the front of the chest (Fig. 52.4A and B) and back of the chest (Fig. 52.5A and B). The expansion is less at the apex

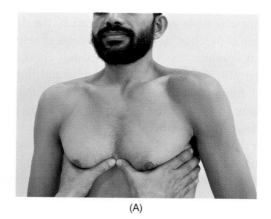

(A)

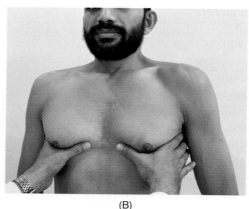

(B)

Fig. 52.4   Demonstration of chest expansion for the base of the lung, anteriorly. (A) Before expansion; (B) After expansion.

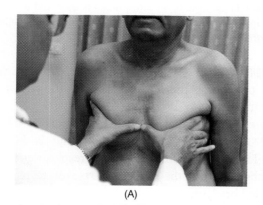

(A)

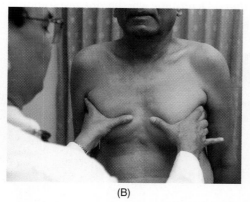

(B)

Fig. 52.3   Demonstration of chest expansion. (A) Chest expansion is performed by firmly holding the chest with both the palms and apposing the thumbs at the centre; (B) The subject is asked to take maximum inspiration possible with which thumbs move apart. The distance between the thumbs is noted as the degree of chest expansion.

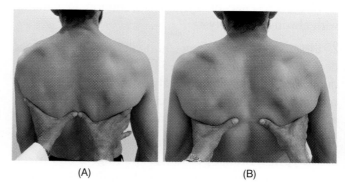

(A)   (B)

Fig. 52.5   Demonstration of chest expansion for the base of the lung, posteriorly. (A) Before expansion; (B) After expansion.

of the lungs, which can be elicited both in front of the chest (Fig. 52.6A and B) and back of the chest (Fig. 52.7A and B). Expansion may be less on the side where the lung is affected by disease.

2. Position of the trachea   The position of the trachea can be detected in three ways.

i)   Place the tip of the index and ring finger of the right hand on the sternoclavicular joints (sternal

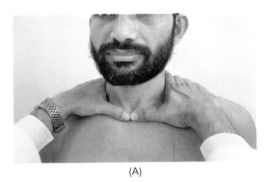

(A)

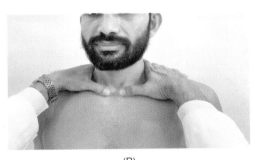

(B)

Fig. 52.6   Demonstration of chest expansion for apex of the lung, anteriorly. (A) Before expansion; (B) After expansion.

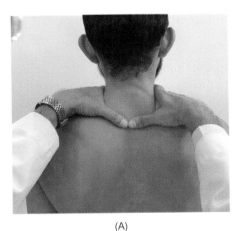

(A)

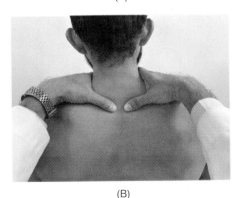

(B)

Fig. 52.7   Demonstration of chest expansion for apex of the lung, posteriorly. (A) Before expansion; (B) After expansion.

ends of the clavicles) on either side, and place the middle finger on the suprasternal notch. Then gently push the middle finger forward to feel the tracheal rings (Fig. 52.8). The position of the trachea is determined by observing the spaces between the finger tips. Normally, the trachea is centrally placed or slightly deviated to the right.

ii) Place the index finger firmly into the suprasternal notch and locate the tracheal rings in relation to the sternum.

iii) Find the space between the anterior border of the sternomastoid muscle and the trachea. If the trachea has deviated to one side, the space becomes narrow on that side.

3. Position of the apex beat   Locate the position of the apex beat (details of the procedure are described in Chapter 53). Displacement of the apex and the trachea to one side indicates the shifting

4. Vocal fremitus (VF)   Ask the subject to repeat 'ninety-nine' or 'one-two-three' and feel the vibration from the surface of the chest by placing the ulnar border of the hand on the surface of the chest, in the intercostal space (Fig. 52.9). To compare both sides (diseased and normal sides), examine the opposite side of the chest in the same intercostal space immediately.

Note: The vibration transmitted to the chest wall from the respiratory passages represents VF. The vibration is conducted from the larynx by the trachea and bronchi to the smaller tubes within the lungs and then through the lung tissues to the chest wall. It should be elicited over symmetrical areas on both the sides of the chest alternately. It may be normal, increased, reduced or absent.

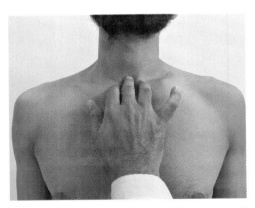

Fig. 52.8   Demonstration of the position of the trachea. Note that the tips of the index and ring finger of the right hand are placed on the sternal ends of the clavicles and the tip of middle finger is placed on the suprasternal notch, which is then gently pushed forward to feel the tracheal rings.

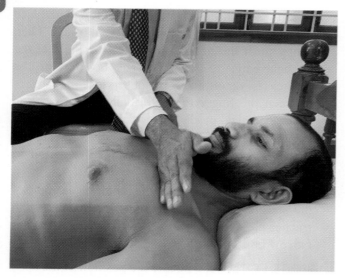

Fig. 52.9   Method of eliciting vocal fremitus (VF). Note that while the subject is uttering '99' or '1-2-3', the examiner feels the vibration from the surface of the chest by placing the ulnar border of the hand firmly in the intercostal space. The opposite side of the chest in the same intercostal space is examined immediately.

5. Tenderness   Palpate all the regions of the chest wall to elicit tenderness if present. Tenderness may be seen in injury to the chest wall, inflammatory conditions of the ribs and intercostal muscles, malignant deposits in the ribs, pleurisy, a painful lung infection and so on.

Percussion

Percuss different areas (supraclavicular, infraclavicular, mammary, inframammary, axillary, infra-axillary, suprascapular, interscapular and infrascapular) on both sides of the chest. While percussing the back of the subject, ask him to cross his arms in front of his chest, the left hand touching the right shoulder and vice versa, and to lean forward. While percussing the axillary region, ask the subject to lift his hands up on to his head. The areas are percussed keeping the pleximeter finger in the intercostal spaces. The clavicle should be percussed directly by the percussing finger without using the pleximeter finger. Percussion of corresponding regions on both sides should be performed and compared simultaneously.

Rules of percussion

1. Apply the pleximeter finger firmly on the surface of the chest (Fig. 52.10).
2. The percussing finger should strike the middle phalanx of the pleximeter finger perpendicularly (vertically).

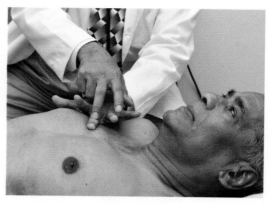

Fig. 52.10   Demonstration of percussion of the anterior aspect of the chest. Note that the pleximeter finger is placed firmly on the anterior surface of the chest in the intercostal space. The percussing finger strokes the pleximeter finger at right angle.

3. The strokes should be delivered from the wrist and finger joints, not from the elbow.
4. The percussing finger should be lifted up immediately after striking the pleximeter finger.
5. The long axis of the pleximeter finger should be parallel to the edge of the organ being percussed.
6. Percussion should be carried out from the more resonant to the less resonant area.

Auscultation

While auscultating, place the chest piece of the stethoscope firmly over the chest and ask the patient to

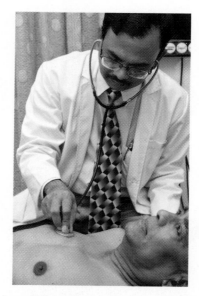

Fig. 52.11   Auscultation of breath sounds. Note that the stethoscope is firmly placed over the chest surface. If the stethoscope is placed loose, chest movement during respiration causes rubbing of the skin against the diaphragm of the stethoscope and produces false adventitious sounds.

breathe regularly and deeply with mouth slightly open (Fig. 52.11).

Auscultate all the areas of the chest in front (supraclavicular, infraclavicular, mammary, and inframammary), all the areas on the side of the chest (axillary and, infra-axillary), and all the areas on the back such as the suprascapular (Fig. 52.12), interscapular (Fig. 52.13) and infrascapular (Fig. 52.14)) regions, and compare both the sides immediately. Usually, breath sounds are clearer and louder on the infrascapular region.

> Note: The purpose of auscultation is to obtain information over and above what the three steps (inspection, palpation, and percussion) of physical examination furnish. Auscultation is done to detect the type of breath sound, the intensity and character of vocal resonance and presence of any adventitious sounds.

Breath sounds Auscultate all the areas over the chest for breath sounds. Use the diaphragm of the stethoscope

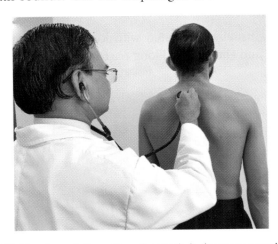

Fig. 52.12   Auscultation of breath sounds in the suprascapular region.

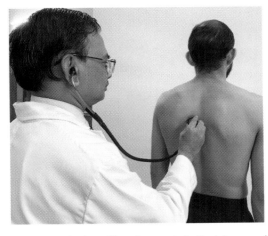

Fig. 52.13   Auscultation of breath sounds in the interscapular region.

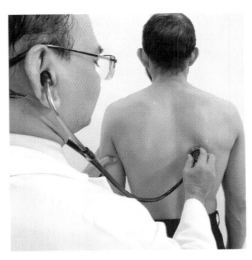

Fig. 52.14   Auscultation of breath sounds in the infrascapular region.

to auscultate breath sounds. Try to note the *intensity* and character of the breath sounds. Also, try to differentiate between the vesicular and bronchial breath sounds. To appreciate the bronchial breath sound, place the diaphragm of the stethoscope on the trachea (Fig. 52.15). The details of differences between vesicular and bronchial breath sounds are detailed in the "Discussion" section.

Vocal resonance Vocal resonance is the auscultatory counterpart of vocal fremitus. Ask the subject to repeat 'one-two-three' or 'ninety-nine' at a constant volume and auscultate the symmetrical areas of both the sides of the chest. The intensity of vocal resonance depends on the loudness and depth of the subject's voice and the

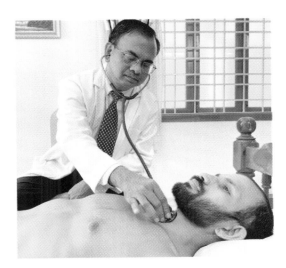

Fig. 52.15   Auscultation of breath sounds on the trachea. Note that normally, tracheal sounds (produced by flow of air through the trachea) resemble bronchial breath sounds.

conductivity of the lungs. It may be normal, decreased or increased. Vocal resonance of normal intensity conveys the impression of being produced just at the chest piece of the stethoscope and is heard as a soft sound.

Adventitious (added) sounds Note the presence of any adventitious sounds.

Precautions

1. The examination should be carried out with the subject standing or seated comfortably with chest fully exposed.
2. General examination should be carried out before examining the chest.
3. Inspection of the chest should be performed without touching the subject.
4. While detecting expansion of the chest, the subject should be instructed to expand his chest as much possible.
5. While detecting the position of the trachea, palpate the tracheal rings gently. If you press hard on the trachea, the subject will feel uncomfortable.
6. Both VF and VR should be elicited on the symmetrical areas on both sides simultaneously and compared.
7. In case of percussion, the rules should be strictly followed, and the maneuver should be carried out on both sides simultaneously to compare the findings.

8. For eliciting VR on different areas of the chest, the subject should be instructed to utter the words at a constant pitch and volume throughout the maneuver.

DISCUSSION

Inspectory Findings

Shape of the Chest

The chest of a normal healthy adult is bilaterally symmetrical and the transverse diameter is greater than the antero-posterior diameter, the ratio being 7 : 5. The following abnormalities should be looked for at inspection (Fig. 52.16).

Flat chest

This is usually associated with long neck, prominent larynx and clavicle, and long narrow chest.

Features
◆ Exaggerated supra- and infraclavicular fossa
◆ Narrow intercostal spaces
◆ Acute subcostal angle

Causes It is seen in healthy persons, but may be associated with:

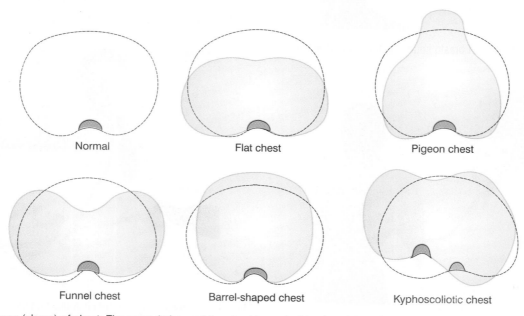

Normal   Flat chest   Pigeon chest

Funnel chest   Barrel-shaped chest   Kyphoscoliotic chest

Fig. 52.16 Types (shape) of chest. The normal shape of the chest is marked by dotted lines. Note that the ratio of transverse to anteroposterior diameter of the normal adult chest is 7 : 5.

- Rickets in childhood
- Chronic nasal obstruction from hypertrophied adenoid
- Bilateral tuberculosis

Pigeon chest

The sternum is unduly prominent and projects beyond the plane of the front of the abdomen. It is seen in:
- Persons with rickets
- Recurrent lung infection in children

Funnel chest

The features are:
- Depression at the lower end of the sternum
- Prominent costochondral junction
- Diminished antero-posterior diameter of the chest
- Causes could be rickets or congenital.

Barrel-shaped chest

The features are:
- Increased anteroposterior diameter of the chest.
- The ribs are wide apart and tend to be horizontal.
- The spine is unduly concave.
- The sternum is more arched.
- Angle of Louis is more prominent.
- Fullness of supraclavicular fossae.

Cause The usual cause is chronic obstructive emphysema.

Kyphosis

This is backward bending of the vertebral column resulting in convexity posteriorly and concavity anteriorly. It causes, shortening of the chest and undue prominence of the vertebrae.

Causes
- Caries spine
- Osteoarthritis
- Secondary osteoporosis
- Chronic obstructive emphysema
- Ankylosing spondylitis

Scoliosis

This consists of lateral bending of the spine and rotation of the vertebrae resulting in undue prominence of the chest and scapula on the side of the convexity, and flattening of the chest.

Kyphoscoliosis

In this, kyphosis is associated with scoliosis.

Harrison's sulcus

This is a transverse groove or constriction in the chest, which begins at the xiphisternum and passes outwards and slightly downwards and may sometimes reach the midaxillary line. It is seen in rickets.

Rickety rosary

This is characterised by the presence of a number of rounded or knob-like projections at the costochondral junctions. It is usually seen in rickets.

Symmetry of the Chest

The chest may bulge or be depressed either on one side or on both the sides.

Localised or unilateral fullness (bulging)
- Pleural effusion
- Pneumothorax
- Intrathoracic tumours

Symmetrical or bilateral fullness
- Emphysema
- Bilateral pleural effusion
- Bilateral pneumothorax

Unilateral depression
- Fibrosis
- Collapse

Bilateral depression
- Bilateral fibrosis
- Bilateral collapse

Respiratory Movements

Rate

The normal rate of respiration in adults is 12–18 per minute. The respiration rate is greater in children than in adults. Increased rate of respiration is called *tachypnea* and decreased rate of respiration is called *bradypnea*.

Causes of tachypnea
A. *Physiological conditions*
   1. Newborns and infants
   2. Children
   3. Gender (rate of respiration is higher in women)
   4. Exercise
   5. Excitement and emotion
   6. Nervousness

B. *Pathological conditions*

Different disease conditions that produce hypoxia; for example, pneumonia causes tachypnea.

Causes of bradypnea

Bradypnea is not seen normally. It is usually seen in conditions of CNS depression, as in narcotic poisoning.

Rhythm

Irregular respiration is commonly seen in intracranial lesions.

Depth

The respiration may be decreased unilaterally or on both sides.

Unilateral restriction of movement

◈ Pleural effusion
◈ Pneumothorax
◈ Fibrosis
◈ Collapse
◈ Consolidation

Bilaterial restriction of movement

◈ Emphysema
◈ Bilateral pleural effusion
◈ Bilateral consolidation

Type

Respiration may be predominantly thoracic or abdominal. In men, respiration is abdominothoracic and in women the respiration is thoracoabdominal.

Types of abnormal respiration

Kussmaul respiration   There is increased rate and depth of respiration (air hunger). It is seen in metabolic acidosis like diabetic ketoacidosis.

Cheyne–Stokes respiration   In this type of respiration, a period of hyperpnea is followed by apnea. It is seen in physiological conditions like sleep (especially in infants), at high altitude, following hyperventilation, and in pathological conditions like cardiac failure, renal failure, brain tumour and narcotic poisoning.

Biot's respiration   The respiration is irregular in depth and rhythm. Irregular pauses with occasional sighs occur. It is seen in meningitis.

Palpatory Findings

Expansion of the Chest

Normally, the expansion is more than 5 cm at the base of the lungs in adults. The expansion is less towards the apex of the lungs. Maximum chest expansion is detected at the fourth intercostal space. It is always less on the side of the chest that is affected by disease of the chest wall or lung.

Position of Apex and Trachea

Displacement of the apex and trachea to one side indicates the shifting of the mediastinum to that side. But, displacement of the apex may occur without displacement of trachea, or the apex and trachea may displace in opposite directions depending on the nature of pathology.

Shifting of mediastinum

i)   The mediastinum shifts to the side of the collapsed and fibrosed lung.
ii) It shifts to the opposite side in pleural effusion, pneumothorax and hydropneumothorax or a mass (for example, tumour) in the thorax.

Vocal Fremitus (VF)

VF may be **normal, increased, reduced or absent**.

VF is increased in:
◈ Consolidation of lungs, for example, lobar pneumonia
◈ Large cavity near the chest surface

VF is diminished in:
◈ Bronchial obstruction
◈ Collapse
◈ Fibrosis
◈ Thickened pleura
◈ Emphysema

VF is absent in:
   VF may be completely absent when the lung is separated from the chest wall by massive pleural effusion or pneumothorax.

Tenderness

Tenderness may be present due to an injury to the chest wall, inflammatory conditions of the ribs and intercostal muscles, malignant deposits in the ribs, pleurisy, or in painful lesions of the lungs.

Percussion Findings

Significance

Percussion is carried out to detect the limit of lung resonance and presence of any pathology in the lungs. Percussion over a normal lung produces a resonant note. 'Resonant' is a relative term as there is no absolute standard. **Cardiac dullness** is noted on the left side between the third and fifth space and **hepatic dullness** is noted on the right side from the fifth rib downwards in the midclavicular line, eighth rib downwards in the midaxillary line and tenth rib downwards in the midscapular line. One should keep in mind that lesions more than 5 cm away from the chest wall or the lesions less than 2–3 cm in diameter will not alter the percussion note. The percussion note is expressed as normal resonance, hyper-resonance, impaired resonance or dullness, and **stony dullness**. When the dullness shifts from one part of the chest to the other, it is called **shifting dullness**.

Hyper-resonance

Hyper-resonance occurs when the amount of air in the lungs or chest cavity is increased. This occurs in:

1. Emphysema
2. Pneumothorax
3. Over an emphysematous bulla
4. Over a large superficial cavity

Dullness or impaired resonance

Dullness or impaired resonance results from any condition that interferes with the production of normal resonant vibrations within the lungs or with the transmission of these vibrations to the chest wall. This is seen in:

1. Consolidation
2. Thickened pleura
3. Fibrosis and collapse
4. Atelectasis

Stony dullness

When the percussion note is very dull, it is called stony dullness. It is seen in pleural effusion.

Shifting dullness

If the dullness shifts when the patient changes position, this is called shifting dullness. It is one of the important tests to detect the presence of air and fluid in the pleural cavity. It is a reliable sign of hydropneumothorax.

Tidal percussion

A dull note obtained above the upper border of liver dullness may be due to liver enlargement or due to a disorder either in the lungs or pleura. Tidal percussion is done to differentiate the pathology. Normally, there is an increase in the area of resonance downwards

by 4–6 cm during full inspiration due to movement of the diaphragm, lungs and liver downwards. In upward enlargement of liver, the increase in the area of resonance in deep inspiration (in tidal percussion) remains within normal limits. In lung pathology, the area of resonance decreases on tidal percussion.

Auscultatory Findings

Auscultation is performed to detect the type of breath sound, the intensity and character of vocal resonance and presence of any adventitious sounds.

Breath Sounds

The breath sounds originate in the large airways due to turbulent airflow during breathing. Sounds produced in the large airways (bronchial breath sounds) are of higher frequencies, above 600 Hz. These sounds are transmitted to the lung tissue, which acts as a low-pass filter, filtering out higher frequency sounds and converting them into low-frequency sounds (vesicular sounds) that are transmitted to the chest wall. Therefore, sounds auscultated from the chest wall in normal persons are vesicular breath sounds though the sounds originate in the large airways (bronchi).

Intensity

The breath sound is produced by the repetitive movement of air into and out of alveoli that are ventilated. The intensity of the sound is directly proportional to the amount of air entering the alveoli. It may be normal, reduced or increased.

Reduced intensity   Breath sounds decrease in intensity if there is a localised airway narrowing, if the lung is extensively damaged by the disease process or if there is interference in the transmission of sound from the lung tissue to the chest wall.

1. Airway narrowing
   - Bronchial obstruction with or without collapse of the lung
   - Consolidation with an obstructed bronchus (obstructive pneumonia)
2. Damage to lung tissue
   - Fibrosis
   - Atelectasis
3. Interference in transmission of sounds
   - Thickened pleura
   - Pleural effusion

- Pneumothorax
- Emphysema

Increased intensity   Breath sounds may be increased in intensity in thin subjects or when the ventilation of lung tissue is increased, as in compensatory emphysema. Loud breath sounds should not be confused with bronchial breath sounds.

Character

On the basis of character, breath sounds are divided into two types: vesicular and bronchial.

A. Vesicular breath sounds   The normal character of breath sounds is vesicular. These sounds originate in large airways, but when transmitted through the lung tissue to the chest wall they become low-pitched vesicular sounds.

These sounds have the ***following characteristics***.

1. Duration of inspiration is more than that of expiration.
2. Intensity of inspiration is greater than that of expiration.
3. There is no gap between inspiration and expiration (Fig. 52.17A).
4. Sounds are rustling in nature.
5. They are low-pitched, with frequencies in the range of 200–600 Hz.

Vesicular breath sound with prolonged expiration   In some diseases, the breath sound is normal in character (vesicular) but the duration of expiration is either equal to or more than that of inspiration. There will be no gap between expiration and inspiration. This is seen when there is partial obstruction of the bronchi as in asthma.

B. Bronchial breath sounds   The bronchial breath sounds originate in the larger airways and are transmitted directly to the chest wall without passing through the alveoli. The sound passing through the lung tissue is not modified and auscultated like bronchial sounds from the chest walls. This sound resembles the sound

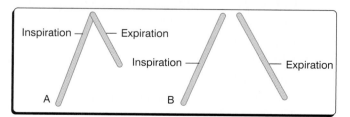

Fig. 52.17   Breath sounds. (A) Vesicular and (B) Bronchial.

obtained by listening over the trachea (directly placing a stethoscope on the trachea).

The following are the **characteristics of bronchial breath sounds** (Table 52.1):

1. Duration of expiration is equal to or longer than that of inspiration.
2. Intensity of expiration is more than that of inspiration.
3. There is a definite gap between inspiration and expiration (Fig. 52.17B).
4. Sounds are harsh or aspirate in nature.
5. They are high-pitched with frequencies above 600 Hz.

Types of bronchial breath sounds   Bronchial breath sounds are of **three types**: tubular, cavernous and amphoric.

The **tubular bronchial breath sound** is a high-pitched sound resulting from the passage of vibrations produced in the small bronchi directly to the chest wall through a solid lung tissue. This is seen when the lung parenchyma becomes a solid mass, as in consolidation.

The **cavernous bronchial breath sound** is a low-pitched bronchial breath sound heard over a cavity, which is situated superficially and communicated to a patent bronchus. The size of the cavity should be more

Table 52.1   Differences between vesicular and bronchial breath sounds.

	Vesicular breath sounds	**Bronchial breath sounds**
Origin	Larger airways, filled with normal air in healthy lung tissues.	Larger airways, but the lung tissue is diseased by infiltration of inflammatory material resulting in consolidation, or there is fibrosis or lung collapse
Location	Heard over the healthy lung fields.	• Normally heard over the trachea (tracheal sound mimics bronchial breath sounds) • In diseases, in which the bronchus is patent but alveoli are not filled with air.
Character	• Low-pitched and soft • No pause between end of inspiration and beginning of expiration	• High-pitched, louder and harsh • Definitive gap between end of inspiration and beginning of expiration
Relative duration	Expiration is less than inspiration	Both inspiration and expiration are equal

than 2 cm in diameter to produce a cavernous breath sound.

The **amphoric bronchial breath sound** is a high-pitched bronchial sound that resembles the sound produced by blowing air into a wide-mouthed bottle. This is heard over a very large cavity communicating pneumothorax. It is also seen in large pulmonary cysts having communication with a patent bronchus.

Vocal Resonance

Vocal resonance is the auscultatory counterpart of vocal fremitus. The intensity of vocal resonance depends on the loudness and depth of the subject's voice and the conductivity of the lungs. It may be normal, decreased or increased.

Increased vocal resonance

When the sounds appear to be nearer to the ear than the chest piece and louder than the normal, the vocal resonance is said to be increased. The **three types** of increased vocal resonance are bronchophony, aegophony and whispering pectoriloquy.

Bronchophony   If the vocal resonance is increased and appears to arise from the earpiece of the stethoscope, it is described as bronchophony. It is seen in consolidation of the lungs as in lobar pneumonia.

Aegophony   When the increased vocal resonance is high-pitched giving a nasal intonation or having a bleating character ('goat voice'), it is called aegophony.

Whispering pectoriloquy   If the vocal resonance is increased to such an extent that the sounds become very clear and seem to be spoken right into the listener's ear, it is whispering pectoriloquy. This is tested by asking the patient to whisper instead of speaking loudly. It is seen in consolidation, and over a large superficial cavity communicating with a patent bronchus.

Diminished vocal resonance

Vocal resonance decreases in:
1. Pleural effusion
2. Pneumothorax
3. Collapse
4. Thickened pleura
5. Emphysema

Adventitious (Added) Sounds

These sounds may arise from the lungs and bronchi or pleura. The sounds that arise from the lungs and bronchi are ronchi, wheeze, stridor and crepitations. The sound that originates from the pleura is the pleural rub.

Ronchi

These are prolonged, uninterrupted musical sounds that occur due to partial obstruction to the flow of air in a narrowed bronchus or bronchiole.

The narrowing of the lumen of the airway may occur due to mucosal swelling, viscid thick secretion, spasm or infiltration of the wall.

Ronchi are of two types. Sibilant and sonorous. *Sibilant ronchi* are high-pitched, and are produced in the smaller bronchi. *Sonorous ronchi* are low-pitched, and are produced in the large bronchi.

Causes
1. Bronchitis
2. Bronchial asthma
3. Obstruction of bronchial tube by a tumour or foreign body

Wheeze

Wheeze is a high-pitched musical sound, which results from partial airway obstruction. This is louder and more persistent during expiration. Sometimes the sound is so loud that it can be heard without the aid of a stethoscope. It is heard during attacks of asthma.

Stridor

This is a jerky, high-pitched and coarse sound usually heard during inspiration. It occurs due to obstruction to inspiratory airflow due to airway obstruction. It is commonly heard in:
- Foreign body impaction
- Tumour (pressing the airway from outside)
- Diphtheria (diphtheric membrane)

Crepitations

These are moist discontinuous crackling or bubbling sounds produced either in the alveoli, bronchi or in cavities. These are produced only in the presence of fluid or secretions.

Crepitations are of **two types**: fine and coarse.

Fine crepitations   These are caused by the opening of collapsed alveoli. It occurs at the end of an inspiration and indicates the presence of exudate in the alveoli. When collapsed alveoli open, the separation of the alveolar wall produces a crackling sound. These are heard in the early stages of pneumonia, localised tuberculosis, and at the base of the lungs in heart failure.

Coarse crepitations   These are heard in any phase of respiration and indicate the presence of secretion in the bronchi or bronchioles. It is heard in:

◆   bronchitis

◆   polycystic diseases of the lungs

◆   resolving stage of pneumonia

◆   bronchiectasis

Pleural rub

This is a rough, harsh crackling sound produced by the rubbing of the visceral and parietal pleura against each other during respiration. It indicates inflammation of the pleura and presence of inflammatory exudates. It can be confused with coarse crepitations. It disappears when the subject is asked to hold his breath and remains unaffected by coughing.

OSPE

I.   Clinically, assess the expansion of the lower part of the chest.

Steps

1.   Give proper instructions to the subject.
2.   Place both the palms on both sides of the lower part of the chest in such a way that the thumbs remain in the front and other fingers on the sides of the chest.
3.   Try to bring the thumbs close to the midline in the front of the chest in such a way that tips of the thumbs just touch each other.
4.   Ask the subject to take a deep breath.
5.   Note the expansion of the chest by observing the movement of the thumbs away from the midline on both sides.

II.   Elicit vocal fremitus from the infraclavicular region of the chest of the given subject and report your findings

Steps

1.   Give proper instructions to the subject.
2.   Place the ulnar border of the hand on the infraclavicular region of one side of the chest.
3.   Ask the subject to say '1-2-3' or '99'.
4.   Feel for the vibration on the chest wall.
5.   Repeat the same on the opposite side and compare.
6.   Report the findings.

III.   Elicit vocal resonance from the infraclavicular region of the chest of the given subject.

Steps

1.   Give proper instructions to the subject.
2.   Place the diaphragm of the stethoscope on the infraclavicular region of one side of the chest.
3.   Ask the subject to say '1-2-3' or '99'.
4.   Hear the sounds on the chest wall.
5.   Repeat the same on the opposite side and compare.
6.   Report the findings.

IV.   Percuss the infraclavicular region of the chest of the given subject and report your findings.

Steps

1.   Give proper instructions to the subject.
2.   Place the pleximeter (middle finger of the left hand) firmly on the intercostal space horizontal to the ribs with the other fingers not touching the chest wall, on one side of the chest.
3.   Strike the pleximeter finger with the percussing finger (middle finger of the right hand) by moving the wrist joint and after each stroke immediately lift the percussing finger.
4.   Percuss all the intercostal spaces and note the resonant sounds.
5.   Percuss the opposite side of the chest and compare.
6.   Report the findings.

V. Assess the position of the mediastinum of the given subject and report your findings.

Steps

1. Stand on the right side of the subject and give proper instructions to him.
2. Place the tip of the index and ring finger of your right hand on the right and left sternal ends of the clavicle, respectively, and the tip of the middle finger on the tracheal rings just above the sternal notch.
3. Palpate the tracheal rings and compare the distance of the middle finger from the index and ring finger to locate the position of the trachea.
4. Place the palm of the right hand on the apical area on the precordium.
5. Localise the apex on the tip of the middle finger.
6. Count the intercostal space and draw the midclavicular line to locate the position of the apex.
7. Compare the tracheal and apical positions to assess the position of the mediastenum.
8. Report your findings.

VIVA

1. *How do you draw the midsternal, midclavicular, anterior-axillary, posterior-axillary, midaxillary, midspinal and midscapular lines?*
2. *How do you locate the sternal angle? What is its significance?*
3. *How do you trace the surface anatomy of major interlobar and horizontal fissures of lungs?*
4. *How do you determine the lower border of the lungs on the chest?*
5. *What is the significance of looking for clubbing and cyanosis before examining the chest?*
6. *What are the common abnormalities of the shape of the chest?*
7. *What are the features of flat chest and in what conditions is it observed?*
8. *What is 'pigeon chest' and in what conditions is it observed?*
9. *What is 'barrel-shaped chest' and in what conditions is it observed?*
10. *What is kyphoscoliosis and in what conditions is it observed?*
11. *What is 'rickety rosary' and in what conditions is it observed?*
12. *What are the causes of unilateral bulging of the chest?*
13. *What are the causes of unilateral depression of the chest?*
14. *What are the causes of tachypnea?*
15. *What are the causes of unilateral restriction of movement of the chest?*
16. *What are the types of abnormal respiration?*
17. *What is Cheyne–Stokes respiration? What are the causes of this abnormal respiration?*
18. *How do you clinically determine the expansion of the chest?*
19. *How do you clinically determine the position of the trachea?*
20. *What are the causes of shifting of mediastinum?*
21. *What are the causes of increased and decreased vocal fremitus?*
22. *What are the rules of percussion?*
23. *What are the causes of hyper-resonance of the lungs?*
24. *What are the causes of dullness of the lungs?*
25. *What is stony dullness and in what conditions does it occur?*
26. *What is shifting dullness and in what conditions does it occur?*
27. *What is tidal percussion and what is its significance?*
28. *What are the types of breath sounds and how do you differentiate between them?*
29. *What are the conditions that decrease the intensity of the breath sound?*
30. *What are the features of bronchial breath sounds?*
31. *What are the types of bronchial breath sounds and how are they produced?*
32. *What do you mean by vocal resonance?*

33. Name the conditions in which vocal resonance is increased and those in which it is decreased.

34. What is bronchophony and in which condition is it seen?

35. What is aegophony and in which condition is it seen?

36. What does whispering pectoriloquy indicate?

37. What are adventitious breath sounds?

38. What is the mechanism of production of ronchi and in what conditions is it seen?

39. What is a wheeze?

40. What are the types and causes of crepitations?

41. What is the mechanism of production of crepitations?

42. What do you mean by pleural rub and in what conditions is it seen?

CHAPTER 53

Clinical Examination of the Cardiovascular System

Learning Objectives

After completing this practical, you will be able to (MUST KNOW):

1. Appreciate the importance of examination of the cardiovascular system (CVS) in clinical physiology.
2. List the parameters to be examined in clinical examination of CVS.
3. Define precordium and apex beat.
4. Draw the midclavicular line on the precordium.
5. Localise the apex of the subject.
6. Locate the different auscultatory areas on the precordium.
7. Auscultate the heart sounds.
8. Examine the neck veins.
9. List the common causes of impalpable apex beat
10. Enumerate the types and causes of heart sounds.

11. Name the waves in JVP and their mechanism of production.

You may also be able to (DESIRABLE TO KNOW):

1. Draw different anatomical lines and borders of the heart.
2. Locate the position of the heart valves and auscultatory areas.
3. Elicit parasternal heave and appreciate the thrill, if present.
4. Percuss to define the border of the heart.
5. List the different conditions in which JVP is raised and prominent 'a', 'c' and 'v' waves are seen in the JVP tracing.
6. Explain the different conditions in which apex is not palpable.
7. List the causes, character and significance of heart sounds.
8. Elucidate the mechanism and causes of split of first and second heart sounds.

INTRODUCTION

The examination of the cardiovascular system (CVS) comprises the **examination of the precordium and blood vessels**. Careful assessment of the arterial and venous pulses should always precede examination of the precordium. Auscultation of the heart should be taken up only after the precordium has been thoroughly examined. Many students do not give enough time to the examination of arterial and venous pulses and the precordium, and directly auscultate the heart to diagnose heart diseases. Beginners especially, become anxious to hear the heart sounds and neglect other aspects of the CVS examination. Before one auscultates the heart, one should have some idea of what abnormalities one expects to detect with the stethoscope. One should also have a minimum knowledge of the physiological basis of production of the heart sounds.

Anatomical Landmarks

The precordium is defined as the anterior aspect of the chest wall, which overlies the heart. Different borders of the heart and the positions of the valves are demarcated on the precordium to make clinical examination of the cardiovascular system convenient.

Different Lines

(*Refer* Fig. 52.1, Chapter 52.)

Midclavicular line This is defined as the vertical line dropped from the centre of the clavicle. The midpoint of the clavicle is determined by taking a point on the clavicle midway between the middle of the suprasternal notch and the tip of the acromion.

Anterior axillary line This is defined as the vertical line descending from the anterior border of the axilla.

Midaxillary line This is defined as the vertical line descending from the centre of the axilla.

Posterior axillary line This is defined as the vertical line descending from the posterior border of the axilla.

Parasternal line This is defined as the vertical line passing through the costochondral junction close to either side of the sternum.

Borders of the Heart

Base of the heart   This is represented by a line joining the right third sternocostal articulation to a point at the level of the left second intercostal space, just internal to the parasternal line.

Right border of the heart   This extends from the right third sternocostal articulation above, to the right seventh intercostal articulation below. It is slightly curved with convexity to the right.

Left border of the heart   This is traced by a line joining the point at the level of the left second intercostal space just internal to the parasternal line above and the apex beat below.

Position of the Heart Valves

Mitral valve   This is obliquely placed behind the inner end of the left fourth costal cartilage and the adjoining part of the sternum.

Tricuspid valve   This is situated obliquely behind the right fifth costal cartilage.

Pulmonary valve   This is placed horizontally at the upper border of the left third costal cartilage.

Aortic valve   This lies obliquely across the left half of the sternum at the level of the lower border of the left third costal cartilage.

Auscultatory Areas

Mitral area   This area corresponds to the apex beat of the heart. The first heart sound is best heard over the mitral area. Normally, this is present in the left fifth intercostal space half an inch medial to the midclavicular line (Fig. 53.1). But in different pathological conditions, the position of the apex changes. Therefore, the auscultatory area of the mitral valve changes with the position of the apex.

Pulmonary area   This area is half an inch in diameter with its centre in the left second intercostal space close to the parasternal line.

Aortic area   This area is half an inch in diameter with its centre in the right second intercostal space close to the parasternal line.

Aortic murmurs are often best heard in the left third intercostal space close to the sternum. Therefore, this area is called second aortic area or **Erb's point**.

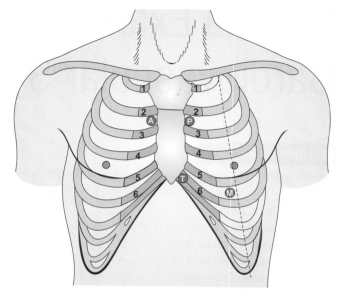

Fig. 53.1   Auscultatory areas on the precordium (A: Aortic area; P: Pulmonary area; T: Tricuspid area; M: Mitral area [apex of the heart]). The vertical dotted line drawn on the left side is the midclavicular line. Note that the second rib is attached to the manubrium sterni.

Tricuspid area   This area is half an inch in diameter with its centre on the left side close to the sternum towards its lower end.

METHODS

Method for Examining the Cardiovascular System

Principle

The process of examination of the cardiovascular system consists of inspection, palpation, percussion and auscultation of the precordium that follows the examination of arterial and venous pulses, recording of blood pressure and a brief general examination of the subject. The functions or any alteration in functions of the CVS are detected by thorough examination of the precordium and blood vessels.

Requirements

1.   **Stethoscope** (an octopus stethoscope should also be available for student's learning)
     Octopus stethoscope   This is a specially designed stethoscope in which the **master stethoscope** (longer and bigger diameter tube, marked with a band at the centre of the tube) originates from the

top of a central cabinet (Fig. 53.2). Another long tube that originates below the cabinet is attached to the chest-piece (diaphragm) of the stethoscope, used for placing the diaphragm on the chest for auscultation. From the peripheral side of the central cabinet, another six tubes originate and branch out to connect to their respective ear-knobs (called **daughter stethoscopes,** which are slightly shorter in length and the tubes having smaller diameter). The Professor (teacher), who demonstrates heart sounds to the students (learners), uses the master stethoscope and learners use the daughter stethoscopes simultaneously. It becomes easy for six learners to follow the demo and identify the types of heart sounds and their qualities, especially of the murmurs, with the help of the octopus stethoscope.

2. **Cardiac bed** or a couch with provision to lift the head end of the bed (Fig. 53.3).

Note: This type of bed used for cardiac patients, which helps in the examination of the jugular venous pulse (JVP) in the neck. With the head of the patient kept at 45° angle to the body, demonstration of JVP becomes easier.

▍ *Procedure*

Examination of the CVS includes: (1) general examination (emphasising a few particular signs) including examination of the radial pulse and blood pressure, (2) examination of the neck veins, and (3) examination of the precordium.

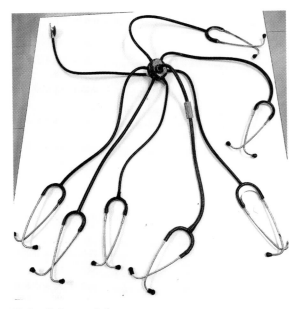

Fig. 53.2   Octopus stethoscope.

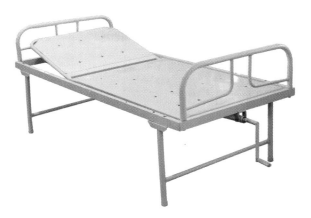

Fig. 53.3   Cardiac bed with provision to raise the head end of the couch, used for cardiac patients. This arrangement to lift the head helps in the examination of jugular venous pulse (JVP) in the neck in the reclined position. With the head of the patient kept at 45° angle to the body, demonstration of JVP becomes easier.

▍ General Examination in Relation to CVS

Anemia

Check for the degree of pallor. The degree of anemia gives a rough idea of the dynamics of circulation, heart rate and blood pressure.

Cyanosis

Check for the presence of cyanosis. This may be present in conditions where there is mixing of arterial blood with venous blood, as seen in Fallot's tetralogy or patent truncus arteriosus.

Edema

Check for the presence of edema in the dependent parts of the body. In cardiac patients, the location of edema depends on the posture of the patient. It is detected by applying pressure over the distal end of the tibia if the patient is mobile. But, if the patient is confined to bed, the sacral area should be examined for the presence of edema.

Clubbing

Nail beds should be examined for the presence of clubbing. If cyanosis is present along with clubbing, this suggests right to left shunt. Clubbing may be present in congenital cyanotic heart disease and in subacute bacterial endocarditis.

Dyspnea

Breathlessness is a feature of heart failure. Dyspnea may be present even at rest.

Abdominal signs

1. Hepatomegaly   A tender hepatomegaly may be present in congestive cardiac failure.

2. Splenomegaly   The spleen may be enlarged in bacterial endocarditis.

3. Ascites   Ascites may be present in heart failure.

4. Epigastric pulsation   Epigastric pulsation may occur due to the following cardiovascular disorders:

- Aortic pulsation usually in thin and nervous patients
- Aneurysm of abdominal aorta
- Hypertrophy of the heart (especially the right ventricle) may give an epigastric systolic thrust

Pulse

Examine the radial pulse for at least one minute. The arterial pulses of both the sides should be examined to check the bilateral symmetry, and the femoral arteries should be examined to detect radiofemoral delay, if present. Brachial, carotid, temporal, popliteal, posterior tibial and dorsalis pedis arteries should also be examined (*also see* Chapter 29).

Blood pressure

Blood pressure (BP) should be detected by sphygmomanometry, preferably by using a mercury manometer. It should be recorded on both sides in cardiac patients. BP should also be recorded by both palpatory and auscultatory methods, especially, if the patient is hypertensive (*see* Chapter 28).

Examination of the Neck Veins

Venous pulses are examined especially in the neck region.

Examine the neck veins in daylight with the patient reclining at an angle of about 45°. If the patient is lying on a cardiac bed or couch (Fig. 53.3), the head end of the bed can be raised to 45° for this purpose. Otherwise, the back of the subject can be supported by the examiner so that the neck muscles are relaxed and the subject reclines at 45° (Fig. 53.4B). Study the level of pressure in the *internal jugular veins* (**jugular venous pressure** (JVP)). The pressure is expressed in terms of centimetres for the vertical distance between the top of the column of blood and the sternal angle, which corresponds to the upper border of the clavicle with the subject reclining at 45° (Fig. 53.4A and B). It may be easier to recognise the pulsation in the external jugular veins, but pulsation in the internal jugular vein is more reliable, because it directly reflects the pressure changes in the right atrium. External jugular veins are not reliable because of the following reasons:

- Venous valves, present in the external jugular veins, prevent the smooth conduction of venous pressure.
- As the external jugular system passes through the fascial planes, they are likely to be affected by external compression.

Why at 45° of neck? The neck of the subject is reclined to 45° because, normally, in this position the sternal

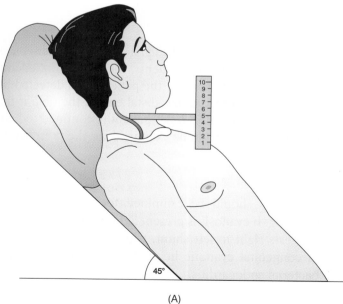

(A)

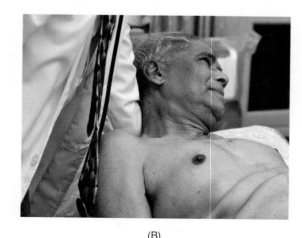

(B)

Fig. 53.4   (A) Method of clinical assessment of jugular vein pressure (JVP). It is measured as the vertical height of JVP above the clavicle with the patient reclining at 45°; (B) Examination of neck veins for JVP. With the support of the examiner, the subject has reclined at 45°.

angle comes to the level of the clavicle. If the person is in good health, the sternal angle corresponds to the middle of the right atrium and approximately represents the normal venous pressure, whatever the position of the subject. When the subject is propped up at an angle of 45°, the venous pressure *appears just at the upper border of the clavicle*, as in this position the sternal angle and clavicle remain at the same level horizontally. Therefore, venous pressure *above the clavicle in this position is considered as raised JVP*.

> Note: In the neck, the arterial pulsation may be confused with venous pulsation. The venous pulses can be differentiated from the arterial pulses by the following parameters.

1. The venous pulse is better seen than felt whereas the arterial pulse is better felt than seen (Table 53.1).
2. The venous pulse has a definite upper level, which falls during inspiration when blood is drawn into the heart.
3. By exerting moderate pressure above the clavicle with a finger, the venous pulse can be obliterated, but not the arterial pulse.
4. If carefully observed, two to three waves can be seen in the venous pulse.

Examination of the Precordium

The process of examination of the precordium consists of inspection, palpation, percussion and auscultation. The subject should lie down on a couch and the examination should be carried out in adequate daylight with the precordium fully exposed (Fig. 53.5).

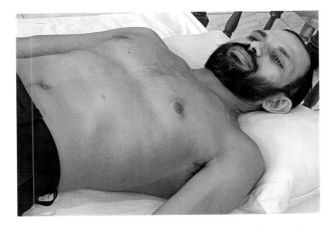

Fig. 53.5 Position of the subject for examination of precordium. The subject should lie down on a couch with the precordium fully exposed, and also the neck part and the upper part of the abdomen (epigastrium) should be exposed.

Inspection

1. **Skeletal deformity** Look for any precordial bulging or depression. The former is usually seen in congenital heart disease.

2. **Dilated and engorged superficial veins** Look for the presence of any dilated and engorged superficial veins over the precordium. This may be seen in superior or inferior venacaval obstruction.

3. **Pulsation**

Apical pulsation Look for pulsation of the apex. Normally, the pulsation of the cardiac apex is visible. Presence of all other pulsations over the precordium is considered abnormal.

Other pulsations Look for pulsation in the other areas of the precordium, especially on the pulmonary and aortic area and in the left parasternal area. Pulsations are seen in the following conditions.
- Pulsation on the pulmonary area is seen in pulmonary hypertension or pulmonary artery dilatation.
- Pulsation on the aortic area may be seen in the aneurysm of the aorta.
- Pulsation on the left parasternal area indicates right ventricular hypertrophy.
- Pulsation over the suprasternal notch indicates aneurysm of the arch of the aorta or coarctation of the aorta.

Palpation

1. **Apex beat** Describe the position and character of the apex.

Position Locate the position of the apex of the heart. This is done by first placing the palm on the precordium to feel the apical impulse (Fig. 53.6A) and then by placing the ulnar border of the palm on the pulsation area horizontally (Fig. 53.6B). Finally, the apex is localised by the tip of the middle or index finger (Fig. 53.6C). If the apex is not palpable in the supine position, ask the subject to sit down and try to locate the apex in the sitting posture. If the apex is still not palpable, ask the subject to lean forward as much as he can in the sitting posture and try to locate the apex in this leaning position. If the apex is still not palpable, palpate the corresponding area of the chest on the right side (in dextrocardia or dextroversion, the apex of the heart may shift to the right). Ideally, the apex should not be palpated in the left lateral position because it shifts the apex laterally, and there is variation in shifting as well.

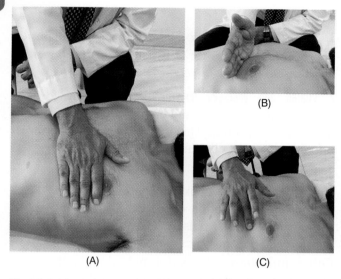

Fig. 53.6   Localisation of the apex of the heart. (A) Palm is gently placed on the precordium to feel the apical impulse; (B) Ulnar border of the palm is placed in the intercostal space to have a better appreciation of the impulse; (C) Finally, the apex is localised by the tip of the middle or index finger.

Note the position of the apex in the intercostal space in relation to the midclavicular line. The intercostal spaces are counted by palpating the manubrium sterni (the most elevated point on the sternum). The second rib joins the manubrium sterni. The space below the second rib is the second intercostal space and accordingly other intercostal spaces are counted.

Note: 1. The apex is defined as the lowermost and outermost definite cardiac impulse. Therefore, if other pulsations are present on the precordium, the apex can be easily identified. 2. The apex beat is normally located in the left fifth intercostal space half an inch medial to the midclavicular line. When students are asked to locate the apex, before they palpate and localise it, they start counting the intercostal spaces and put the tip of the finger medial to the midclavicular line in the fifth space to feel the apex. This is wrong, because the apex may not always be present exactly in that position. Moreover, you do not know if the subject has any pathology in the heart. Therefore, the apex must be first localised as described above and then its position should be demarcated.

Causes of impalpable apex
1. Left-sided pleural effusion
2. Pneumothorax
3. Hydropneumothorax
4. Pericardial effusion
5. Shift of mediastinum to the right (right-sided lung fibrosis and collapse)
6. Obesity (thick chest wall)

7. Apex lying under a rib
8. Dextrocardia (the apex will be palpable on the right side)

Character   Try to describe the character of the apex.

Note: Normally, the apex beat just touches and slightly elevates the examining finger. The common abnormal characters are:
• *Tapping apex*   Seen in advanced mitral stenosis.
• *Forceful and well-sustained apex*   Seen in gross left the ventricular hypertrophy due to chronic systemic hypertension, as it causes pressure overload and increases wall thickness.
• *Forceful but ill-sustained apex*   Seen in right ventricular hypertrophy or mild to moderate left ventricular hypertrophy. In left ventricular hypertrophy due to volume overload (as in aortic regurgitation), there is increase in the ventricular cavity size rather than wall thickness. Therefore, the apex is forceful but ill-sustained.

2. Parasternal heave   Place the ulnar border of the palm firmly on the left parasternal line and feel for any thrust or pulsations and whether the hand is lifted with each pulsation (Fig. 53.7).

Note: Presence of parasternal heave suggests right ventricular hypertrophy.

3. Thrills   Palpate all over the precordium for thrills.

Note: A thrill is a palpable murmur. The thrills are best appreciated when the patient holds his breath in expiration. Thrills may be present in valvular defects or in aneurysm of great vessels.

4. Tender points   Palpate the precordium for presence of any painful points over it.

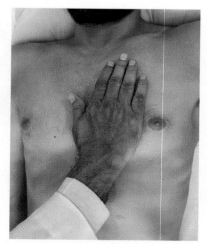

Fig. 53.7   Method of elicitation of parasternal heave. The palm is firmly placed on the left parasternal line to feel the thrust or pulsations, if any, and note if the hand is lifted with each pulsation.

Note: A tender point over the precordium may be due to costochondritis, myalgia, fracture of ribs or pleuritis.

5. Direction of flow in veins

If the veins are dilated and engorged over the precordium, detect the direction of flow in the veins. In superior venacaval obstruction, the direction of blood flow in the veins is from above downwards. In inferior venacaval obstruction, the direction of blood flow in the veins is from below upwards.

Note: The position of the trachea should be checked along with the position of the apex to assess the position of the mediastenum.

Percussion

Percussion is of less significance in the examination of the CVS. But percussion is carried out sometimes to detect the **extent of cardiac dullness** in conditions like pericardial effusion. Cardiac dullness is detected by performing a light percussion. The details of the rules of percussion are discussed in examination of the respiratory system.

Auscultation

With the help of the stethoscope, auscultate the different areas in the following sequence: mitral area, pulmonary area, aortic area and tricuspid area. The diaphragm of the stethoscope should be placed firmly on different areas to hear the heart sounds (Fig. 53.8).

In each area, the following points should be noted during auscultation.

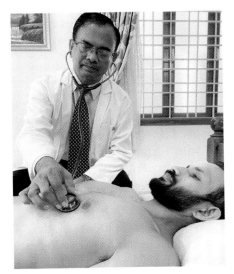

Fig. 53.8 The method of auscultation for heart sounds. Note that the diaphragm of the stethoscope is placed firmly on the apex (mitral area).

1. First (S1) and second (S2) heart sounds

Note their quality, intensity, duration and character. S1 is heard better on the mitral area, and S2 is heard better over the pulmonary and aortic area.

Note: The first and second heart sounds can be differentiated by their pitch and duration. The first heart sound is heard as 'lub' and the second sound as 'dub'. For beginners, it is difficult to differentiate these sounds. They can palpate the carotid artery in the neck while auscultating the heart sounds. The heart sound that coincides with the carotid pulsation is the first heart sound and the sound that follows the pulsation is the second heart sound.

2. Other sounds (if present)

◆ Third heart sound (S3)
◆ Fourth heart sound (S4)
◆ Murmurs
◆ Opening snap
◆ Ejection click

If murmur is present, note the site of origin, timing, character, radiation and its relation with respiration.

DISCUSSION

Clinical Significance

Arterial Pulse

A detailed discussion on arterial pulse is given in Chapter 27.

Venous Pulse

The pulsation of **internal jugular veins** in the neck is examined clinically to determine the atrial pressure activity (Table 53.1). Jugular venous pulse (JVP) has five waves: three positive waves (ascents) and two negative waves (descents). The positive waves are 'a', 'c' and 'v' waves, and negative waves are x and y descents (Fig. 53.9).

a wave : Due to atrial contraction

c wave : Coincides with the onset of ventricular systole and results from the movement (bulging) of the tricuspid valve ring into the right atrium as the right ventricular pressure rises.

v wave : Indicates the passive rise in pressure in the right atrium as venous return continues while the tricuspid valve is closed.

Table 53.1   Differences between jugular venous pulse and carotid arterial pulse.

	Jugular venous pulse	Carotid arterial pulse
Feeling on touching the vessel	Not palpable	Palpable
Height of pulsation in relation to respiration	Varies with respiration	Independent of respiration
Propensity to be occluded	Can be easily occluded	Cannot be occluded, unless substantial pressure is exerted to occlude it
Height of pulsation in relation to abdominal pressure	Height increases with abdominal pressure	Pulse is independent of abdominal pressure
Prominence of pulse in relation to position of the patient	Best observed with neck at 45° angle in relation to body. Prominence of pulsation varies with position of patient	Independent of position of patient
Direction of flow/pulsatility	Rapid inward movement	Rapid outward movement
Peaks in the pulse	Two visible peaks per heart beat	One peak per heart beat (felt but not visible)

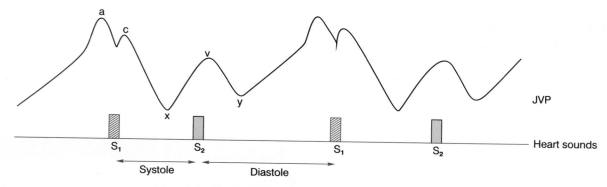

Fig. 53.9   JVP and heart sounds (JVP: Jugular venous pressure; S1: First heart sound; S2: Second heart sound).

x descent : Caused by a fall in right atrial pressure due to relaxation of the right atrium.

y descent : Occurs due to fall in right atrial pressure when blood enters into the right ventricle as the tricuspid valve opens.

Conditions that alter JVP

Raised JVP

1. Right ventricular failure
2. Obstruction of superior vena cava
3. Increase in circulating blood volume
   - Pregnancy
   - Acute nephritis
   - Over-judicious treatment with IV fluids
4. Constrictive pericarditis
5. Tricuspid incompetence

> **Note:** Persistent elevation of JVP is one of the earliest signs of congestive cardiac failure and is probably the most reliable sign of the failure.

Prominent 'a' wave

1. Pulmonary stenosis
2. Pulmonary hypertension
3. Tricuspid stenosis (usually in this condition there is atrial fibrillation, so, the 'a' wave may not be seen).
4. Myxoma of right atrium
5. Distended right atrium in atrial septal defect
6. Cardiomyopathy

Physiological basis   A prominent 'a' wave occurs due to increased force of right atrial contraction associated with right atrial hypertrophy or hypertrophy of right ventricle. When the right atrium contracts against increased resistance, the 'a' wave becomes prominent.

Cannon wave   When the amplitude of the 'a' wave is very high, it is called cannon wave (giant 'a' wave) (Fig. 53.10). It is seen when the right atrium contracts against a closed tricuspid valve. It occurs in:

1. Complete heart block when atrial and ventricular systole coincide.

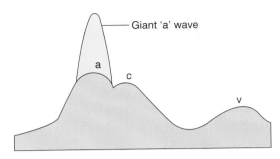

Fig. 53.10   Canon wave. Note the giant 'a' wave in JVP.

2. Nodal rhythm when the atrium and ventricle are activated simultaneously.

Absence of 'a' wave   The 'a' wave disappears in atrial fibrillation.

Prominent 'v' wave   It is seen in tricuspid regurgitation, because when the ventricle contracts during systole, blood enters into the right atrium through the incompetent tricuspid valve. It is also seen in constrictive pericarditis and heart failure.

Precordial Examination

The **two most important parameters** in precordial examination are (1) character and position of the apex of the heart and (2) heart sounds.

Apex of the heart

The position of the apex beat is a valuable physical sign in the examination of the CVS. The apex of the heart is formed by the left ventricle. Therefore, in left ventricular hypertrophy, the apex becomes more forceful. Displacement of the apex occurs due to push or pull from the surrounding viscera. Pushing may be due to pleural effusion and pneumothorax, and pulling may be due to pulmonary fibrosis and collapse. Apical displacement also occurs due to cardiac diseases like enlargement of the left ventricle. It can also occur due to deformity of the thoracic cage like scoliosis.

Heart sounds

Four heart sounds have been described. These are first heart sound (S1), second heart sound (S2), third heart sound (S3) and fourth heart sound (S4). S1 and S2 are heard normally.

First heart sound   The first heart sound represents the beginning of the systole.

Causes   It occurs due to vibration set up by:

◈ Sudden closure of the AV valves.
◈ Rapid increase in tension in the ventricular muscles during isometric contraction acting on full ventricles.
◈ Turbulence created in the blood due to ventricular contraction.

Character   It is a soft sound, heard as 'lub'.
Duration   : about 0.15 seconds
Frequency : 25–45 Hz

Significance   It signifies the beginning of the ventricular systole and AV valve closure.

1. Accentuation of first heart sound
   – Exercise
   – Hyperkinetic circulatory states like anemia and beriberi
   – Hypertension
2. Diminution of first heart sound
   – Shock
   – Acute myocardial infarction
   – Constrictive pericarditis
   – Pericardial effusion
   – Cardiomyopathy (advanced stage)
   – Obesity
   – Emphysema

Splitting   The first heart sound has two components: the mitral and the tricuspid components. The mitral valve closes just before the tricuspid valve. This gives rise to splitting of the first heart sound. But this splitting cannot be detected by auscultation, because both the components are very low-pitched and merge into each other. Therefore, when splitting of the first heart sound is heard, it is always considered as pathological.

Second heart sound

Causes
◈ The second heart sound is primarily caused by the closure of the semilunar valves.
◈ Rushing of blood into the ventricles due to opening of the AV valves also contributes.

Character   This is heard as 'dub'.
Duration   : about 0.12 seconds
Frequency : 50 Hz

Significance   It signifies the end of clinical systole and closure of the semilunar valves.

Loud A2 (increased aortic component) is seen in:
◈ Systemic hypertension

Diminished A2 is seen in:

❖ Aortic stenosis
❖ Aortic incompetence

Loud P2 (increased pulmonary component) is seen in:

❖ Pulmonary hypertension

Diminished P2 is seen in:

❖ Pulmonary stenosis

Splitting   Splitting of the second sound is due to the gap between the aortic and pulmonary components. It is easy to detect because aortic and pulmonary valve closure sounds are high-pitched and can be separated. Aortic valve closure is audible in all areas whereas pulmonary valve closure is audible only in the pulmonary area. Splitting is most easily heard in children and may not be audible in elderly subjects.

Mechanism of splitting   The splitting of the second heart sound is due to the separation between the closure of aortic and pulmonary valves. The closure of pulmonary valve always follows the closure of aortic valve (aortic valve closes first). The splitting is distinctly heard during inspiration. During inspiration, more blood is drawn into the thorax. Therefore, venous return to the right atrium increases and right ventricular stroke volume increases. This increases the duration of right ventricular systole. Thus, P2 is slightly delayed. Also, during inspiration, left ventricular stroke volume decreases, because blood is pooled in the dilated pulmonary vessels and dilated left atrium (this dilatation occurs due to increased negative intrathoracic pressure). Therefore, left ventricular systole is shortened and A2 comes earlier. Therefore, during inspiration, A2 occurs earlier and P2 occurs later. Hence, splitting of the second sound widens during inspiration. Exactly the opposite happens during expiration and splitting narrows.

Reverse splitting   This occurs when the left ventricle takes more time to empty than the right ventricle. It is seen in left bundle branch block (LBBB) and in left ventricular failure.

Third heart sound   Third heart sound is usually not heard in many healthy individuals. Sometimes it may be heard in children and in young adults. It is usually heard in conditions in which the circulation becomes hyperkinetic. The third sound can arise from either side of the heart, but usually it arises in the left ventricle.

Causes

❖ It is caused by the vibration set up in the ventricle during the early period of rapid ventricular filling.

❖ Rebound fencing of the cusp of the valve and chordae of the respective valve due to vigorous elongation of the ventricle caused by rapid inflow of blood also contributes to this.

Character   It is best heard in the mitral area. It follows the aortic component of the second sound and is heard early in the diastole, that is, just after the second sound.

Duration : 0.1 second

Pitch   : low-pitched

Significance

1. This is attributed to rapid ventricular filling. It is found in relatively hyperkinetic circulation, in young persons, and where the mitral diastolic flow is increased as in mitral regurgitation and VSD.

2. It is an important sign of heart failure due to any cause. In heart failure, the atrial pressure is increased and early filling of the ventricle is rapid.

3. It may be heard shortly after myocardial infarction or in diseases where the distensibility of the ventricular muscle is altered. The sound arises from vibration in the atrioventricular valve structures and in the ventricular muscle.

Fourth heart sound   This is also called the atrial sound, because it is produced during atrial contraction. It is not heard in normal individuals. Presence of the fourth heart sound is always considered abnormal.

Causes

❖ It is caused by atrial contraction.

❖ It is produced by the vibration set up within the ventricle due to inflow of blood produced by atrial systole.

Character   It occurs just before the first sound, that is, late in the diastole, and is low-pitched.

Significance

1. It always indicates increased stiffness or non-compliance of the ventricles. Therefore, when a bolus of blood is delivered into the ventricle by atrial contraction, it facilitates a sudden increase of pressure in the ventricle.

2. It is seen in left ventricular hypertrophy due to hypertension, myocardial infarction, pulmonary embolism and pulmonary hypertension.

Triple heart sound   This consists of three heart sounds: the first and second heart sound, and the third one can be either the third or fourth heart sound. The triple rhythm associated with a normal heart may not be a serious one, but if it is present with a definite cardiac pathology, it may signify a serious condition. When the heart rate increases to more than 100 per minute, the triple rhythm is called gallop rhythm, because it produces a typical cadence of the gallop of a horse. The individual sounds cannot be identified separately. If the gallop is due to the third heart sound, it is called a protodiastolic gallop; if it is due to the fourth heart sound, it is called presystolic gallop.

Murmurs Murmurs occur due to **turbulence in the blood flow** at or near a valve, or an abnormal communication within the heart. Murmurs differ from normal heart sounds in the sense that these are of longer duration and higher frequency, whereas heart sounds have shorter duration and lower frequency. When a murmur is present, the following points are carefully noted.

1. **Site of origin**   The area over which the murmur is maximally heard should be noted. The point of maximal intensity usually (but not always) indicates its site of origin.

2. **Timing and duration**   Depending on the timing of the murmur, they are classified into systolic, diastolic or continuous murmurs. Depending on the duration, it may be early diastolic, mid-diastolic, early systolic, pan-systolic, and so on.

3. **Character**   The murmur may be soft, blowing to harsh, rough and rumbling. Loud and rough murmurs are usually associated with organic valvular and congenital lesions, for example, murmur of mitral stenosis is always rough and rumbling in character.

4. **Radiation (conduction)**   From the site of maximum intensity, auscultation is done in different directions to detect whether the murmur is localised or conducted to other parts. Conduction is characteristic of some murmurs, for example, the murmur of mitral stenosis is usually localised whereas the murmur of mitral incompetence selectively propagates towards the axilla.

5. **Relation with respiration**   During inspiration, the stroke volume of the right ventricle increases while that of the left decreases. Therefore, any murmur becoming louder during inspiration is considered to originate from the right ventricle, and any murmur louder during expiration is said to originate from the left side of the heart.

OSPE

I. Locate the apex beat of the subject and report your findings.

Steps

1. Expose the precordium.
2. Inspect for the apex beat.
3. Put the palm on the precordium over the mitral area to feel apical pulsation.
4. Use the ulnar border of the hand to further confirm the pulsation.
5. Use the tip of the middle finger to finally locate the apex, and mark the position.
6. Count the intercostal space and report the exact position of the apex.

II. Examine the neck veins of the given subject and report your findings.

Steps

1. Ask the subject to lie down on the couch and stand on the right side of the subject.
2. Elevate the head end of the bed or support the back of the subject to recline him at an angle of 45°.
3. Turn the subject's head to the opposite side.
4. Ask the subject to relax his neck.
5. Look for the engorgement of the internal jugular vein.
6. If the JVP is raised, look for the upper level of the engorgement and measure the height of the pressure.

III. Auscultate the apex of the given subject and report your findings

Steps

1. Expose the precordium.
2. Localise the apex of the given subject.

3. Lightly place the diaphragm of the stethoscope on the apex to auscultate it.
4. Place fingers gently on the carotid artery to differentiate the first from the second sound.
5. Check for the intensity and character of the sounds and report the findings.

VIVA

1. What are the general physical signs that are specifically looked for before commencing the clinical examination of the cardiovascular system?
2. What is the importance of detecting cyanosis in the examination of the CVS?
3. What are the characteristics of edema seen in cardiac patients?
4. Why should the radial pulse be examined before the examination of the precordium?
5. What is the importance of recording blood pressure in the examination of a patient of CVS?
6. Why are the neck veins usually preferred for the examination of the venous pulse?
7. How do you differentiate venous pulses from arterial pulses in the neck?
8. Why are the internal jugular veins preferred to the external jugulars for examination of the neck veins?
9. What are the waves seen in JVP and how are they produced?
10. In which conditions does an 'a' wave become more prominent?
11. What is a cannon wave and how is it produced?
12. In which pathological conditions can 'a' and 'v' waves be absent?
13. What is the significance of raised JVP and in which clinical conditions is it seen?
14. Define precordium.
15. What are the points one should look for during inspection of the precordium?
16. In what clinical conditions can precordial bulging occur?
17. Define apex beat.
18. What are the procedures to localise the apex if it is not palpable in the supine position?
19. Why should apex beat not be localised in the left lateral position?
20. Name the different conditions in which the apex beat may not be palpable.
21. What are the conditions in which the apex may become forceful and well sustained, and why?
22. What do you mean by 'tapping apex', and in which condition is it seen?
23. What is the importance of examining the position of the trachea along with the location of apex?
24. What is parasternal heave? In what conditions is this seen?
25. What are the different heart sounds normally heard?
26. What are the causes of the first heart sound, and how is it confirmed clinically?
27. What are the conditions in which the first sound becomes louder?
28. What do you mean by splitting of the second sound? Why is splitting better appreciated in inspiration?
29. What is reverse split? In which clinical condition is it seen?
30. What is gallop rhythm, and what is its significance?
31. How are murmurs produced? What are the types of murmurs?

CHAPTER 54

Clinical Examination of the Gastrointestinal System

Learning Objectives

After completing this practical, you will be able to (MUST KNOW):

1. Name the different quadrants of the abdomen.
2. Explain the importance of clinical examination of the GI system.
3. Enumerate the steps of examination of the GI system.
4. Demonstrate the procedures for palpation of the liver and spleen.
5. Percuss the abdomen.
6. Auscultate bowel sounds.

You may also be able to (DESIRABLE TO KNOW):

1. Explain various positive inspectory findings.
2. List the causes of hepatomegaly and splenomegaly.
3. Explain the importance of fluid thrill and shifting dullness.
4. Correlate abnormal bowel sounds with intestinal dysfunctions.

INTRODUCTION

Disorders of the gastrointestinal (GI) system are very common. Dyspepsia, diarrhea, dysentery, indigestion and vomiting are routinely encountered complaints in clinical practice. Many of the causes of these dysfunctions can be easily diagnosed if the physician carries out a thorough and systematic examination of the GI system. **Examination of the abdomen** is the major part of clinical examination of the GI system. While performing abdominal examination, the physician should remember the **anatomical positions of abdominal viscera**. Disorders of abdominal structures can be appropriately diagnosed, as the location of these organs is precise. Therefore, an abnormal sign elicited from a particular region of the abdomen indicates the dysfunction of the viscera underneath.

Anatomical Landmarks

The abdomen is divided into **nine quadrants** by two transverse and two vertical lines (Fig. 54.1). The quadrants are epigastrium, right hypochondrium, left hypochondrium, umbilical, right lumbar, left lumbar, hypogastrium (suprapubic), right ileac and left ileac.

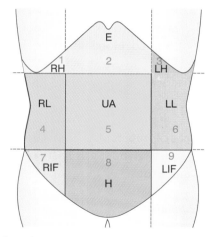

Fig. 54.1 Quadrants of the abdomen (1. Right hypochondrium (RH); 2. Epigastrium (E); 3. Left hypochondrium (LH); 4. Right lumbar (RL); 5. Umbilical (UA); 6. Left lumbar (LL); 7. Right ileac (RIF); 8. Hypogastrium (or suprapubic) (H); 9. Left ileac (LIF)).

METHODS

Method of Examination of GI System

Examination of the GI system proceeds in the following sequence

1. History taking
2. General examination
3. Examination of the oral cavity
4. Abdominal examination

5. Special examinations

History Taking

In a patient with a GI disorder, the following points should be asked (and noted in the examination record) while taking the history. Accurate and relevant present and past histories give the physician important clues to the diagnosis.

1. **Appetite**   Does the patient have a good appetite, or does he have anorexia, nausea or vomiting?
2. Is he able to swallow properly or does he have **dysphagia**?
3. Is there abnormal **flatulence**?
4. Are there frequent acid eructations, retrosternal burning or water brash?
5. **Stool**—Diarrhea, constipation, colour of stools, worms or excess mucus in stools.
6. **Abdominal abnormalities**—Abdominal pain, swelling and distension.
7. Is there a history of **hematemesis** (vomiting out of blood), **melena** (dark tarry stool due to the presence of altered blood in it) or **bleeding per rectum**?
8. Is there a history of jaundice, fever or recent weight loss?
9. Habits—Alcoholism and smoking.
10. Past history of tuberculosis, malaria, kala azar, hemolytic crisis (sudden onset of pallor and dyspnea) and drugs.

General Examination

The following points are particularly noted during general examination.

1. Build and nutrition
2. Examination of nails and conjunctiva for pallor, clubbing, cyanosis and icterus
3. **Signs of liver failure**—Scanty hair, palmar, spider nevi, gynecomastia and testicular atrophy
4. **Vital signs**—Pulse, blood pressure, respiration and temperature

Examination of Oral Cavity

1. Condition of the teeth
2. Health of the tongue and oral mucous membrane
3. Condition of tonsil and oropharynx

Examination of Abdomen

Abdominal examination consists of the following steps:
1. Inspection
2. Palpation
3. Percussion
4. Auscultation

Inspection of abdomen

The subject should lie comfortably on a couch in the supine position with arms by his side. The room should be well lighted. Stand on the right side of the patient. Fully expose the abdomen. Clothing should be drawn up till the xiphisternum and pulled below till the lower margin of the pubic symphysis (sites of hernial orifice should be visible). Closely observe for the following findings (Fig. 54.2).

1. **Shape of abdomen**   Is the abdomen normal in shape, distended or scaphoid?
2. **Umbilicus**   Note the position of umbilicus. Is it central and inverted or everted?
3. **Abdominal movements**   Observe the abdominal movement during inspiration and expiration. Is it free and equal on both sides, markedly diminished or absent?
4. **Pulsations**   Is the pulsation of abdominal aorta visible? Is there any other pulsation?
5. **Dilated veins**   Is there any dilatation of the abdominal vein?
6. **Peristalsis**   Is gastric or intestinal peristalsis visible? Peristalsis is best elicited by patiently observing the abdomen for some time.
7. **Hernial orifices**   Are the hernial orifices bulging with strain or coughing? The hernial sites in the groin should be observed for any swelling. If there

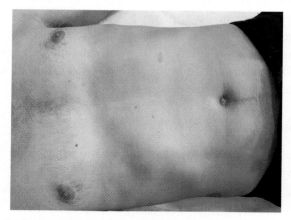

Fig. 54.2   Inspection of abdomen. Abdomen is exposed fully up to the lower level of hypogastrium.

is no swelling, the patient should be asked to stand up, turn his head to one side and cough. The impulse on coughing should be noted if present.

8. **Scars**   Is there any surgical scar mark on the abdomen? Is the scar recent (pink or red) or old (pigmented dark).

9. **Surface and skin of abdomen**   Is the surface smooth? Is the skin shiny? Note any abnormal pigmentation and striae, if present.

Palpation of abdomen

Palpation of the abdomen is an important part of clinical examination of the GI system. The subject should lie on his back, with **legs semi-flexed to relax the abdomen.** Ask him to relax and breathe quietly. Palpation should be done for all areas of the abdomen. Generally, it can start from the left iliac region and then proceed anticlockwise to end in the suprapubic and umbilical regions. If the subject complains of pain in an area, that area should be palpated last.

First, palpation can be performed lightly. Later, deeper palpation can be performed (with both hands if necessary). While palpating, note for **consistency** (softness or rigidity), **tenderness** (can be observed from the facial changes) and guarding of abdomen in any particular region, if present. Then palpate for **liver**, **spleen**, **right** and **left kidneys**, gall bladder, urinary bladder, aorta and para-aortic glands. If a mass is present, note the location, size, surface, borders, consistency and tenderness. If fluid is present, try to confirm the presence of fluid by eliciting fluid thrill and shifting dullness. (This may be learned better in clinical postings. However, a first year medical student should know the procedures for general palpation of the abdomen, and palpation of the liver and spleen).

Palpation of liver   Ask the subject to lie down comfortably on the couch and flex his leg slightly. Give proper instructions. Expose the abdomen (as described above). Sit on the couch beside the right side of the subject. Place both hands side by side flat on the abdomen in the right subcostal region, lateral to the rectus, with the fingers pointing to the ribs. Ask the subject to take a deep breath and at the height of inspiration, press the fingers firmly inwards and upwards. If resistance is encountered, move the hand further down till the resistance disappears. If the liver is palpable, its margin is felt as a sharp regular border that rides beneath the fingers. Note the size of enlargement, surface, consistency and tenderness of liver.

Alternate method of palpation of liver (commonly used)   Sit on a chair to the right side of the subject. Place the right hand lower and parallel to the right subcostal margin in such a way that the index finger remains below it (Fig. 54.3). Ask the subject to breathe deeply and at the height of inspiration, press the index finger slightly inwards. The liver edge is felt against the radial border of the index finger. If resistance is encountered, move the hand further down till the resistance disappears.

> **Note:** The lower limb should be semi-flexed at knee to make the abdomen relaxed, which facilitates palpation of abdominal organs.

Palpation of spleen   From the left subcostal margin, the spleen enlarges downwards towards the right ileac fossa (Fig. 54.4). Therefore, the spleen is palpated

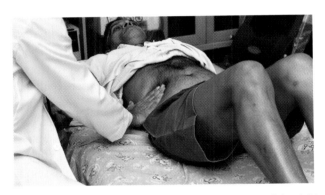

Fig. 54.3   Palpation of liver. Note that the index finger of the right hand is pressed inwards below the right subcostal margin, when the subject takes a deep breath. Also, the legs are semiflexed to relax the abdomen.

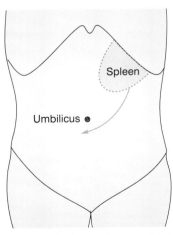

Fig. 54.4   The direction of spleen enlargement. The dotted line below the left subcostal margin depicts the surface marking of an enlarged spleen. The arrow indicates the direction of splenomegaly (towards the right ileac fossa).

along an oblique line, starting from the right ileac fossa towards the left subcostal margin. Place the palm of the right hand on the right ileac fossa lower and to the right of the umbilicus, with fingers close to each other and pointing towards the left subcostal margin (Fig. 54.5). Ask the subject to take a deep breath and press deep with the fingers of the right hand. If the spleen is palpable, it touches the tip of the fingers with each inspiration. Palpate the surface of the spleen and examine for consistency and tenderness.

If the spleen is not palpable, repeat the procedure of palpation 2 cm above in the line of spleen enlargement, and repeat the procedure till you reach the left subcostal margin (Fig. 54.5). If the spleen is still not palpable, place the flat of the right hand beneath the left costal margin and the left hand over the lowermost rib postero-laterally on the left side of the subject. Ask the patient to take a deep breath and press deep with the fingers of the right hand and at the same time exert considerable pressure medially and downward with the left hand. If the spleen is not palpable but suspected to be enlarged, turn the patient halfway on to his right side and ask him to rest/lean on your left hand, and repeat the maneuver.

If the veins are prominently engorged, the direction of flow should be assessed to differentiate between inferior and superior vena caval obstruction (this will be taught in greater detail in the clinical classes). To determine the direction of flow, a section of the vein is emptied using two fingers, and each end of the emptied part is pressed with a finger. One finger is released and the filling of the vein is noted. Similarly, the other finger is released and filling of the vein is noted. Blood enters more rapidly and fills the vein from the direction of the blood flow.

Palpation of kidney   Kidneys are palpated by bimanual technique. Place left hand posteriorly below the lower rib cage and the right hand on the lower part of upper quadrant of abdomen (Fig. 54.6). Push the two hands together firmly, but gently as the patient breathes out. Feel the lower pole as the patient breathes in deeply. Try to trap the palpable kidney between the two hands by delaying application pressure until the end of inspiration. This helps in palpation of kidney as it slides up on expiration. Confirm the structure of kidney by pushing the kidney between two hands (ballotting) and by assessing its degree of movement during respiration. Assess the size, surface and consistency of the kidney. Examine the kidney of the opposite side.

Fluid thrill   Ask the subject to lie on his back. Ask the subject or an assistant to place the ulnar border of his hand firmly on the midline of the abdomen of the patient. Sit on a chair to the right of the subject and place the flat of your left hand on the side of the left lumbar region of the subject. Using your right hand, tap the side of the right lumbar region of the subject (Fig. 54.7). If a large amount of ascites is present, a fluid thrill or a wave is felt as an impulse by the left hand (which is placed on the left lumbar region of the subject).

Percussion of abdomen

Percuss the abdomen lightly following the rules of percussion as described in Chapter 52 (Fig. 54.8). Normally a resonant (tympanitic) note is heard, except on the areas of liver and spleen enlargement and over a tumour, mass or fluid. Absence of dullness over these areas makes the diagnosis of hepatomegaly and

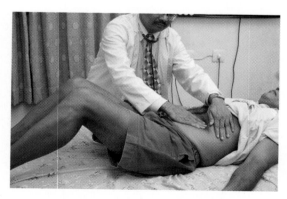

Fig. 54.5   Palpation of the spleen. The palm of the right hand is placed on the right ileac fossa lower and to the right of the umbilicus, with fingers close to each other and pointing towards the left subcostal margin. While the subject takes a deep breath, the examiner presses deep with the fingers of the right hand.

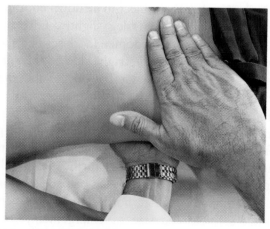

Fig. 54.6   Bimanual palpation of kidney.

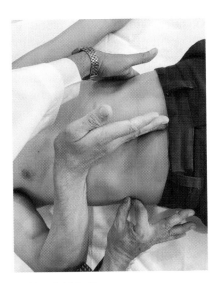

Fig. 54.7 Eliciting fluid thrill.

splenomegaly or an abdominal tumour unlikely. Thus, percussion confirms hepatomegaly and splenomegaly, if present.

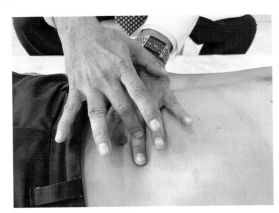

Fig. 54.8 Percussion of the abdomen.

Shifting dullness If presence of fluid is suspected, percussion should be performed first with the patient lying on his back (Fig. 54.9A) and then lying alternately on each side (Fig. 54.9B and C). While lying on one side, the upper flank will be resonant as the fluid is pushed down by gravity to the lower flank. Hence, this is called *shifting dullness*.

Auscultation of abdomen

Auscultation is carried out by placing the diaphragm of the stethoscope on different areas of the abdomen. Auscultation is performed to detect bowel sounds, peristaltic rub and bruit. Note whether bowel sounds are normal, absent or increased. Normal bowel sounds are heard as intermittent low- or medium-pitched gurgles, occasionally interspersed with high-pitched noises.

Special Examinations

The following special investigations are done in some cases.
1. Per rectum (PR) examination
2. Proctoscopy
3. Abdominal ultrasound

DISCUSSION

Inspectory Findings

Shape of Abdomen

The abdomen in a person of normal build is boat-shaped. Abdominal distension occurs due to six factors (the 6 Fs):

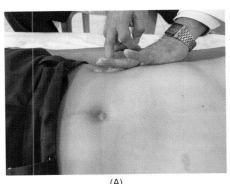
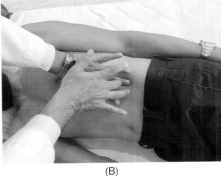
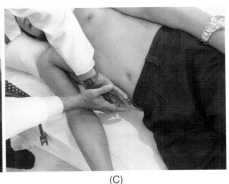

(A)   (B)   (C)

Fig. 54.9 Percussion for demonstration of shifting dullness. (A) With the patient in the supine position, the abdomen is percussed from the central umbilical region to the flank and dullness is noted in the flank if peritoneal effusion is present; (B) Without the examiner changing the position of the hand, the subject is asked to shift his body position to the opposite side, and now on percussion, the dullness is found to be absent as fluid shifts from this upper region to the lower region on the opposite side; (C) The percussion on the other side (the lower side) yields more dullness due to shift of fluid to this lower side.

1. Fat (abdominal obesity)
2. Fluid in excess in peritoneal cavity (ascites)
3. Flatus (excess gas in large intestine)
4. Fetus (pregnant woman)
5. Full urinary bladder
6. Feces (accumulation of excess stool in large intestine as seen in constipation)

Abdominal swelling also occurs in tumours of abdominal organs.

Generalised distension occurs in ascites, obesity and patients with excessive flatus. Localised distension occurs in hepatomegaly (distension in the right hypochondriac region) or splenomegaly (distension in the left hypochondriac region), and in neoplasms. Full bladder and bowel produce distension of the hypogastrium. A scaphoid or sunken abdomen is seen in starvation, and malignancy, especially of the stomach and esophagus.

Umbilicus

Normally, the umbilicus is inverted and situated centrally in the abdomen. The distance between the xiphisternum and the umbilicus is equal to the distance between the umbilicus and the symphysis pubis. In ascites, the distance between the xiphisternum and umbilicus is more than that between umbilicus and symphysis pubis, whereas in ovarian tumours the distance between the xiphisternum and umbilicus is less than that between the umbilicus and symphysis pubis. In ascites, the umbilicus is flattened or everted, whereas in obesity the umbilical cleft is deeper than normal.

Abdominal Movement

Movement of the abdominal wall occurs during respiration. In fact, respiratory rate is counted by observing abdominal movement during respiration. Abdominal movement is absent in peritonitis.

Pulsations

Normally, pulsations are not visible over the abdomen. However, *aortic pulsation* may be visible in the nervous or anemic individual. *Aortic aneurysm* produces expansile pulsations.

Dilated Veins

Presence of dilated veins suggests venous obstruction. In *inferior vena caval obstruction*, there will be dilated veins on the sides with flow of blood from below upwards. This occurs because the blood bypasses the inferior vena cava and travels from the lower limbs to the thorax via the veins of the abdominal wall. In *portal vein obstruction*, the engorged veins are centrally placed and may form a cluster around the umbilicus (caput medusa). The blood in these veins flows in all directions away from the umbilicus. They represent opening of anastomosis between portal and systemic veins.

Peristalsis

Peristaltic wave of the stomach (moving from left to right) is seen in pyloric stenosis in the epigastric and left hypochondriac region. Peristaltic wave of the large intestine (transverse colon) is seen in the same region but moves from right to left. Peristaltic wave of the small intestine is seen as ladder pattern below the centre of the abdomen.

Hernial Sites

The impulse observed at hernial sites on coughing suggests hernia. Femoral or inguinal, and direct or indirect hernia should be differentiated (to be studied in clinical classes).

Skin Over the Abdomen

Smooth and glossy skin indicates abdominal distension whereas wrinkled skin suggests an old distension that has been relieved. Abdominal striae represent the rupture of subepidermal connective tissue as a result of abdominal distension. When formed first, the striae are reddish or pink; when the distension stabilises or regresses, the colour of the striae fades to white. Abdominal striae are seen commonly in obesity, massive ascites and following pregnancy or corticosteroid therapy.

Palpatory Findings

The normal abdomen is soft and no tenderness is elicited on palpation.

Abdominal Tenderness

On applying pressure, the pain felt by the subject is called tenderness. It is commonly found in inflammatory lesions of the viscera and the surrounding peritoneum. The location of tenderness often suggests a specific pathology. Some examples are:

In the epigastrium—peptic ulcer

In the right hyhpochondrium—hepatitis, cholecystitis

In the right iliac fossa—appendicitis

Purely visceral pain such as gastric or intestinal colic may not be associated with tenderness.

Guarding and Rigidity

Abdominal guarding and rigidity are due to contraction of muscles of the abdominal wall; this is often a part of the defence mechanism over a tender region. Abdominal rigidity usually occurs over an inflamed organ as in pancreatitis or cholescystitis. Generalised rigidity occurs in peritonitis.

Fluid Thrill

Presence of fluid thrill indicates accumulation of a large amount of free fluid in the peritoneal cavity (gross ascites).

Hepatomegaly

Hepatomegaly means enlarged liver. Usually, the liver is palpable if enlarged, as normally the lower border of the liver lies at the right subcostal margin. The common causes of hepatomegaly are:

1. Infective hepatitis
2. Chronic amebiasis
3. Malaria
4. Kala azar
5. Congestive heart failure
6. Leukemias
7. Hodgkin's disease
8. Hepatic tumours
9. Portal hypertension
10. Hydatid cyst

Splenomegaly

Splenomegaly is the enlargement of the spleen. To be palpable, the spleen has to enlarge 2.5 times its normal size. Thus, a mildly enlarged spleen is not always palpable and the palpable spleen is considerably enlarged. The common causes of splenomegaly are:

1. Malaria
2. Kala azar
3. Leukemias
4. Lymphomas
5. Hemolytic anemias
6. Portal hypertension
7. Tropical splenomegaly

Percussion Findings

The normal percussion note of the abdomen is resonant (tympanitic). Accumulation of excess gas yields a high tympanitic note and accumulation of fluid yields a dull note. Since fluid first accumulates in the flanks, the areas of dullness on both sides resemble a horseshoe. Hence, it is called *horseshoe dullness,* which is confirmed by eliciting shifting dullness.

In addition to determining the presence of fluid, percussion helps to delineate the border of an enlarged viscera or abdominal tumour. Hepatomegaly, splenomegaly and abdominal lumps or tumours can be confirmed by eliciting the dull note over the respective structures.

Auscultatory Findings

Bowel Sounds

These are intestinal sounds generated by the contractions of the muscular walls of the gut and the resultant vibration of the gut wall produced by the movement of a gas–fluid mixture through the gut. These bowel sounds persist in the fasting state due to the presence of intestinal secretions and swallowed air.

Loud bowel sounds occur due to hyperperistalsis of the intestine (*peristaltic rush*). Exaggerated bowel sounds accompanied by some degree of abdominal distension and cramp-like abdominal pain suggest partial bowel obstruction. Absence of bowel sounds for at least 10 minutes suggests bowel atony or paralytic ileus.

Other Sounds

Arterial bruit These are variable harsh sounds that occur due to turbulence in arterial flow. A loud bruit suggests aortic aneurysm and atherosclerosis or extreme tortuosity of the aorta. Bruit over the kidneys in the flanks suggests renal artery stenosis.

Venous hum Venous hum is a continuous, soft and low-pitched sound. This may be heard over the liver area and umbilicus in portal-systemic shunting of venous flow when portal flow is obstructed.

VIVA

1. Name the various quadrants of the abdomen.
2. What is fluid thrill and what is its importance?
3. What is shifting dullness and what is its importance?
4. What are the types of bowel sounds and how are they produced?
5. What are the common causes of hepatomegaly?
6. What are the common causes of splenomegaly?
7. What is the normal shape of the abdomen and how is the shape altered in different conditions?
8. What is the importance of the position of the umbilicus?
9. What is the importance of abdominal venous engorgement?
10. What is the significance of abdominal guarding?

CHAPTER 55

Clinical Examination of the Nervous System I (Higher Functions and Cranial Nerves)

Learning Objectives

After completing this practical, you will be able to (MUST KNOW):
1. Describe the importance of performing this practical in clinical physiology.
2. List the functions of all the cranial nerves.
3. Perform clinical examination of all the cranial nerves.
4. List the precautions observed while examining each of the cranial nerves.
5. List the parameters to be examined for assessing higher functions and speech.

6. List the common effects of lesions of the cranial nerves.

You may also be able to (DESIRABLE TO NOW):
1. Trace the pathway of all the cranial nerves.
2. Explain the abnormalities observed following lesions of the cranial nerves.
3. List the differences between supra- and infranuclear palsy of the 7th and 12th cranial nerves.
4. List the common problems of higher functions and name the types of aphasias.

Clinical examination of the nervous system is generally performed in the following sequence:
1.   Examination of higher functions and speech
2.   Examination of cranial nerves
3.   Examination of the sensory system
4.   Examination of the motor system

Each examination as listed above requires description in detail. Therefore, the first two examinations are described in this chapter and the third and fourth examinations are described subsequently in separate chapters.

CLINICAL EXAMINATION OF HIGHER FUNCTIONS AND SPEECH

HIGHER FUNCTIONS

Higher mental and intellectual functions are assessed under the following headings.

1. Appearance and behaviour   Is the subject well oriented and well behaved, or is he disturbed and agitated? Note his attention span—whether wandering or experiencing any flight of ideas? Note how he is dressed up, his general hygiene and the condition of nails, hands and hair.

2. Emotional state   Assess the emotional state of the subject. Note, if his mood is elevated or depressed or if there are emotional disturbances. Enquire about the quality and duration of sleep and the quality of dreams.

3. Delusions and hallucinations   Note if the subject is having delusions (false beliefs, which continue to be held despite evidence to the contrary) and hallucinations (false impressions).

4. Level of consciousness and memory   Assess if there is any clouding of consciousness? Also ask questions to assess the evidences of loss of memory, if any.

5. Orientation of place and time   Ask him about the surrounding (whether he is in hospital or at his home), the time, date, month and year. Disorientation if any should be noted.

6. Level of memory   Ask few basic questions to assess his recent and past memory. Loss of recent or remote memory is indicative of brain injury.

7. General orientation and intelligence   Assess this by asking him of his personal history, social history and educational history, especially the nature of his work and habits.

SPEECH (LANGUAGE) FUNCTIONS

Speech is a vital phenomenon to express oneself. The ability to understand and express oneself is the highest quality of the brain and the human being is endowed with this highly developed quality.

Speech has **two components**: the sensory and motor.

1. **The sensory or receptive part** of speech includes vision and hearing of the texts and related sounds.
2. **The motor or expressive part** includes spoken and written speech.

Thus, the disorders of speech may be aphasias or dysarthria.

Assess if the subject is having **aphasias**, i.e., loss of the ability to understand and use symbols, which may be sensory or fluent aphasia that occurs due to lesions in the Wernicke's area or motor (or nonfluent) aphasia that occurs due to lesions in the Broca's area. The patient may also be having global aphasia or **dysarthria**, which is assessed by looking for articulation.

CLINICAL EXAMINATION OF THE CRANIAL NERVES

INTRODUCTION

There are twelve pairs of cranial nerves. Some of them contain only sensory fibres and are thus known as **sensory cranial nerves**. Few cranial nerves are predominantly motor in function and are therefore called **motor cranial nerves**. The remaining cranial nerves contain both sensory and motor fibres and are thus called **mixed cranial nerves**. A systematic and thorough examination of cranial nerves is part of the clinical evaluation of a patient with neurological deficit. The cranial nerves may be affected by a primary disease of the cranial nerve or by a disease of the brain or the meninges, or sometimes secondary to other systemic disorders.

Anatomical and Physiological Considerations

Olfactory or First Cranial Nerve

Anatomy   This nerve arises from the olfactory mucosa. The nasal mucous membrane contains bipolar sensory cells that constitute the first order of neurons. Their central processes pass through the olfactory foramina in the cribiform plate of the ethmoid bone and terminate in the olfactory bulb. From the olfactory bulb, the second order of neurons arises and projects to the olfactory cortex, which consists of the periamygdaloid and prepiriform areas of the piriform lobe.

Function   The olfactory nerve carries the **sensation of smell** from the nasal mucosa to the olfactory cortex of the brain.

Optic or Second Cranial Nerve

Anatomy   This is one of the important cranial nerves as it subserves vision. The fibres of the optic nerve arise in the retina and pass through the optic foramen to form the optic chiasma and then the optic tract. At the chiasma, the fibres from the inner half of each retina decussate while those from the outer half remain on the same side. Thus each optic tract consists of fibres from the outer half of the retina of the same side and from the inner half of the retina of the opposite side (*refer* Fig. 43.1). Most of the fibres of the optic tract pass onto the lateral geniculate body of the thalamus, and some fibres from the optic tract reach the pretectal area, which is involved in regulation of pupillary reflexes and movement of the orbital muscles. The fibres from the lateral geniculate body travel in the optic radiation to reach the visual (calcarine) cortex. The calcarine cortex constitutes the main visual centre and represents the opposite half of the field of **vision**. The area of central or macular vision has extensive cortical representation and has dual blood supply from the middle and posterior cerebral artery.

Function   The optic nerve serves the most important special sensation, vision. Normal vision is dependent on the integrity of the visual pathway, that is, receptors in the retina, optic nerve, optic chiasma, optic tract, lateral geniculate body and visual cortex.

Oculomotor or Third Cranial Nerve

Anatomy   This is predominantly a motor nerve. The third cranial nerve nuclei lie in the midbrain, just anterior to the cerebral aqueduct, at the level of the superior and inferior colliculi. The nerve fibres emerge at the upper border of the pons, pass through the cavernous sinus and superior orbital fissure, and supply the **four extrinsic muscles of the eyeball** (superior rectus, medial rectus, inferior rectus and inferior oblique) (Fig. 55.1). It also supplies the levator palpebrae superioris of the upper eyelid. It carries parasympathetic innervation to the sphincter muscles of the iris (sphincter pupillae) and ciliary muscles (involved in control of accommodation).

Functions

1. It controls all the **movements of the eyeball** except lateral deviation of the eye and depression of the medially deviated eye.
2. It controls the **size of the pupil**.
3. It is involved in the **accommodation** of vision.

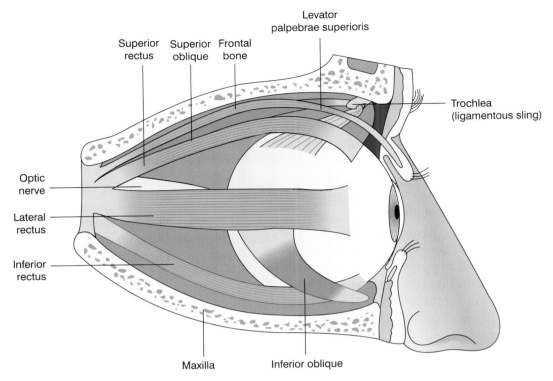

Fig. 55.1 Muscles attached to the left eye.

Trochlear or Fourth Cranial Nerve

Anatomy This is primarily a motor cranial nerve. The nucleus of the fourth cranial nerve is present in the midbrain. The fibres decussate before emerging from the brain and enter the orbit through the superior orbital fissure to supply the superior oblique muscle. It supplies the **superior oblique muscle** of the opposite side of the eyeball. This is a peculiar nerve in the sense that it is the **only cranial nerve that decussates between its nuclei of origin and the point of emergence**.

Function It causes depression of the medially deviated eye.

Trigeminal or Fifth Cranial Nerve

Anatomy This consists of both motor and sensory fibres. It has three subdivisions: **ophthalmic, maxillary and mandibular**. The ophthalmic and maxillary divisions are sensory whereas the mandibular division is both motor and sensory.

Motor component of the fifth nerve The motor fibres originate in the pons and come out of the brain through the foramen ovale to innervate the **muscles of mastication** (masseters and temporalis). Motor fibres

of the fifth nerve are present only in the mandibular division of the nerve.

Sensory component of the fifth nerve Sensory fibres of the fifth nerve are present in all the three divisions of the nerve (Fig. 55.2).

Ophthalmic division The ophthalmic division carries fibres that receive sensation from the skin over the upper eyelid, eyeball, lacrimal glands, nasal cavity, side

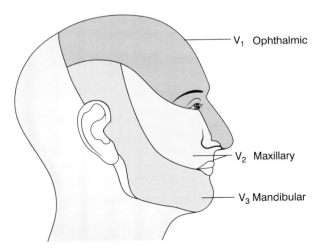

Fig. 55.2 Areas supplied by the three peripheral sensory branches of the trigeminal nerve.

of the nose, the conjunctival surface of the upper but not the lower lid, forehead and the scalp as far as the vertex. These fibres pass through the superior orbital fissure.

Maxillary division   The maxillary division carries sensations from the upper part of the cheek, the lower eyelid and its conjunctival surface, skin and mucous membrane of the nose, the upper lip, the upper teeth, the upper part of the pharynx, the roof of the mouth and soft palate, and the medial inferior quadrant of the cornea. The fibres in the maxillary division enter the brain through the foramen rotundum.

Mandibular division   The sensory fibres in the mandibular division carry sensations from the lower part of the face, the lower lip, the ear, anterior two-thirds of tongue (not taste) and the lower teeth. These fibres pass through the foramen ovale. The sensory fibres from all the three divisions of the trigeminal nerve end in the pons.

Functions   The trigeminal nerve carries general sensation from different parts of the face, and a part of the head and neck. Through its motor functions, it is involved in **mastication** (chewing).

Abducent or Sixth Cranial Nerve

Anatomy   This is primarily a motor nerve. The fibres originate in the nucleus, that is, in the lower part of the pons near the internal genu of the facial canal. After emerging from the pons, it traverses a long intracranial course to enter the orbital cavity through the medial end of the superior orbital fissure **to supply the lateral rectus muscle**. The long intracranial course of this nerve makes it liable to the effects of raised intracranial pressure.

Function   It helps in **lateral deviation** of the eye.

Facial or Seventh Cranial Nerve

Anatomy   The seventh cranial nerve is a mixed nerve. It has motor and sensory components.

Motor component   The motor fibres originate in the pons, pass through the stylomastoid foramen and innervate the muscles of facial expression, scalp and platysma (neck muscle).

Sensory component   Fibres arise from the taste buds present in the anterior two-thirds of the tongue, pass through the stylomastoid foramen and end in the

geniculate ganglion, a nucleus in the pons from where fibres go to the gustatory area in the parietal lobe of the cerebral cortex through the thalamus.

During its course, the facial nerve travels through the **facial canal** in the temporal bone. The chorda tympani nerve, which carries the taste sensation from the anterior two-thirds of the tongue, joins the facial nerve in the facial canal. This part of the nerve is **vulnerable to injury and edema** as it is enclosed in a bony tube.

Functions

1. It supplies all the **muscles of the face and scalp**, (except the levator palpebrae superioris) and platysma. Therefore, it carries out all facial expressions.
2. It carries the taste sensation from the anterior two-thirds of the tongue.

Vestibulocochlear or Eighth Cranial Nerve

Anatomy   It has **two components**, the cochlear and the vestibular.

The cochlear nerve   The auditory (cochlear) fibres arise in the spiral organ (organ of Corti) and form the spiral ganglion. Fibres from the spiral ganglion pass through the internal auditory meatus to reach the nuclei in the medulla, from where the fibres project to the thalamus and from there to the auditory cortex.

The vestibular nerve   The vestibular fibres originate in the semicircular canals, saccule and utricle and form the vestibular ganglion. The fibres from the vestibular ganglion terminate in the vestibular nuclei present in the pons and medulla. A good deal of projection also reaches the cerebellum.

Functions

1. The cochlear fibres convey impulses associated with hearing.
2. The vestibular fibres convey impulses associated with equilibrium.

Glossopharyngeal or Ninth Cranial Nerve

Anatomy   The glossopharyngeal nerve is a mixed nerve. It has motor and sensory components.

The motor fibres   The fibres originate in the nucleus ambiguous in the medulla. It accompanies the tenth and eleventh cranial nerve and comes out of the skull through the jugular foramen to supply the middle constrictor of the pharynx and stylopharyngeous muscle. It also supplies parasympathetic fibres to the parotid gland.

The sensory fibres These fibres arise from the taste buds in the posterior third of the tongue and from baroreceptors in the carotid sinus. They carry general sensation from the nasopharynx and posterior aspect of the soft palate. The fibres terminate in the nucleus tractus solitarius (NTS).

Functions

1. It is involved in the activation of the pharyngeal reflex.
2. It carries the taste sensation from the posterior third of the tongue.
3. It helps in the secretion of saliva.
4. It is involved in the regulation of blood pressure (baroreceptor reflex).

Vagus or Tenth Cranial Nerve

Anatomy The vagus nerve is a mixed nerve. It has motor and sensory components.

The motor fibres The motor fibres originate in the nucleus ambiguous in the medulla. The nerve comes out of the skull through the jugular foramen to supply the structures in the neck, thorax and abdomen. Its function is motor to the soft palate (with the exception of tensor palati), pharynx, larynx, the respiratory passages, esophagus, stomach, small intestine, most parts of the large intestine, gall bladder and heart. Its function is secretomotor to most of these organs.

The sensory fibres It carries sensation from the aortic arch and aortic bodies, which mediate baroreceptor and chemoreceptor reflexes. It also carries the sensation from the structures that it innervates. The fibres pass through the jugular foramen and terminate in the medulla and pons.

Functions

1. It regulates the functions of the cardiovascular system, gastrointestinal tract, respiratory system, urogenital tract and other thoracic and abdominal viscera.
2. It is involved in the elicitation of the **palatal reflex**.
3. It subserves laryngeal and pharyngeal functions.

Accessory or Eleventh Cranial Nerve

Anatomy This is a pure motor nerve, of cranial and spinal origin. The cranial fibres originate in the nucleus ambiguous in the medulla. The spinal fibres emerge from the sixth cervical segment of the spinal cord, ascend through the foramen magnum into the brain and join the cranial fibres. The fibres come out of the skull through the jugular foramen and divide into the cranial and spinal parts. The cranial part supplies a motor nerve to the larynx, pharynx and soft palate. The spinal part supplies the sternomastoid and the trapezius muscle.

Functions

1. The cranial portion mediates swallowing movements.
2. The spinal portion mediates head and shoulder movements.

Hypoglossal or Twelfth Cranial Nerve

Anatomy The twelfth cranial nerve is a pure motor nerve. The fibres originate from its nucleus, which is present in the medulla. It leaves the skull via the hypoglossal canal (anterior condyloid foramen) and joins the ansa hypoglossi in the cervical region. It supplies the muscles of the tongue of the same side. It also supplies the hypoglossus, styloglossus and genioglossus muscles.

Functions

1. It helps in the movement of the tongue and therefore assists in speech and swallowing.
2. It assists in depressing the hyoid bone.

METHODS

Methods to Test Olfactory Nerve

Principle

The olfactory nerve carries the sensation of smell. Therefore, this nerve is tested by various olfactory stimuli.

Requirements

One small bottle each of clove oil, peppermint oil or camphor, and coffee powder (Fig. 55.3).

Procedure

1. Ask the subject to sit comfortably on a stool.

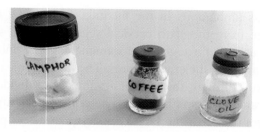

Fig. 55.3   Three types of solutions in bottles for testing sensation of smell.

2. Make sure that both the nostrils are patent and there is no inflammation of the nasal mucosa (no nasal obstruction due to common cold).
3. Ask the subject to close his eyes and one of his nostrils.
4. Remove the cap of the bottle containing clove oil and take the bottle close to the open nostril.
5. Ask the subject if he correctly perceives the smell.
6. Repeat the procedure with peppermint oil.
7. Ask the subject to close this nostril and open the other nostril, and repeat the procedure.
8. Compare the results of both the nostrils.
9. Ask the subject if he has any hallucination of smell.
10. Note your result. Express the result as: Smell—normal, reduced, absent or perverted, separately for each nostril.

Precautions

1. The subject should close his eyes.
2. The subject must be familiar with the odour.
3. Both the nostrils should be examined separately.
4. One nostril should be closed when the other is examined.

Methods to Test Optic Nerve

Principle

The optic nerve carries the sensation of vision. Examination of this nerve reveals intactness of the visual pathway, field of vision and acuity of vision.

Requirements

1. Snellen's chart
2. Lister's or Goldmann's perimeter
3. Ishihara chart

Procedure

The optic nerve is tested for **acuity of vision, field of vision** and **colour vision**.

Tests for acuity of vision, colour vision and field of vision are described in detail in Chapters 43, 44 and 45, respectively.

Clinically, the field of vision is detected by the 'confrontation test' at the bedside of the patient.

Confrontation test

1. Ask the subject to sit on a stool comfortably in an erect position.
2. Sit on a stool in front of the subject in such a way that your eyes and the subject's eyes remain at the same level and at a distance of about 3 feet (Fig. 55.4).
3. Ask the subject to fix his gaze at the tip of your nose.
4. Ask the subject to close one of his eyes and close your opposite eye.
5. Move your finger midway between you and the subject to test the field of vision of four quadrants (upper, lower, nasal and temporal). Bring your finger from the periphery of the four quadrants to the centre of the visual field and ask the subject to say 'yes' when he sees the finger.

Note: If the subject's vision is normal, at the point at which the examiner catches sight of the moving finger, the subject can also see it.

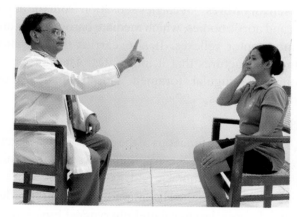

Fig. 55.4   Procedure for testing eyeball movements for assessment of oculomotor nerve function. Note that the eye level of the examiner and the subject is approximately the same. The subject fixes his gaze at the tip of examiner's index finger (with a distance of approximately 25 cm) and follows the movement of the examiner's finger.

6. Compare the patient's field of vision with yours and note your observation.
7. Repeat the procedure with the other eye.

Precautions

1. The distance between the examiner and the subject should be 3 feet.
2. The eye of the examiner should remain level with that of the subject's.
3. The field of vision of the examiner should be normal.
4. The subject should fix his gaze at the centre.
5. The examiner should move his finger midway between him and the subject.
6. While one eye is being examined, the other eye should be closed.
7. The subject should wear glasses during the procedure if he uses them constantly for refractive errors. Restriction of the field of vision due to glasses should be kept in mind.

Method to Test Oculomotor, Trochlear and Abducent Nerves

Principle

The third, fourth and sixth cranial nerves are tested together as they innervate all the external ocular muscles. The eyeball moves in different directions and the movements are named accordingly. Horizontal movement in an outward direction is called **abduction** and in an inward direction is called **adduction,** vertical movement in the upward direction is called **elevation** and in the downward direction is called **depression**. The eye is also capable of rotatory movements. The rolling movement of the eye towards the nose is called **internal rotation** and movement away from the nose is called **external rotation**. The superior and inferior rectus elevate and depress the eye when the eye is in abduction, and the inferior and superior oblique elevate and depress the eye when the eye is in adduction (Fig. 55.5).

Requirements

1. Torch: a pencil torch is preferred (Fig. 55.6)
2. Cardboard

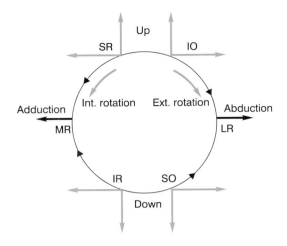

Fig. 55.5 Direction of eyeball movements, based on the mechanism of action of different extraocular muscles. Accordingly, different eye movements are performed for assessing the functions of the 3rd, 4th and 6th cranial nerves (LR: Lateral rectus; MR: Medial rectus; SO: Superior oblique; IO: Inferior oblique; SR: Superior rectus; IR: Inferior rectus).

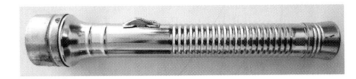

Fig. 55.6 Pencil torch (that sharply focusses light onto the eye).

Procedure

1. Ask the subject to sit comfortably on a stool and you sit in front of the subject.
2. Examine the eyes of the subject for the presence of ptosis (drooping of the eyelid) and nystagmus (rhythmic, involuntary and jerky movement of the eyeball) if any.
3. Give instructions to the subject to follow the direction of the movement of your finger.
4. Bring your index finger to the front of the subject's eyes, keeping a distance of around 25 cm (the normal visual distance) from the subject.
5. Ask the subject to look at and follow the movements of your index finger, and observe the movement of the eyeball of the subject while moving your finger (same instructions as depicted in Fig. 55.4).
6. First, move your finger laterally to the right of the subject (this tests the function of the lateral rectus of the right eye and the medial rectus of the left eye simultaneously). From there, move your finger

vertically upwards (this tests the superior rectus of the right eye and the inferior oblique of the left eye) and downwards (this tests the inferior rectus of the right eye and superior oblique of the left eye) (Fig. 55.5).

7. Then move your finger laterally to the left (this tests the lateral rectus of the left eye and the medial rectus of the right eye). From there, move your finger vertically upward (this tests the superior rectus of the left eye and inferior oblique of the right eye) and downward (this tests the inferior rectus of the left eye and superior oblique of the right eye) (Fig. 55.5).

8. Examine the pupillary reaction to light (**light reflex**). Put a piece of cardboard between the two eyes or place your hand between the eyes (Fig. 55.7A). Switch on the torch and bring the torch from the side of the subject and immediately focus the light onto one of his eyes and look for the reaction of the pupil of that eye (**direct light reflex**) as well the pupil of the other eye (**indirect or consensual light reflex**) (Fig. 55.7B). Repeat the light reflex testing on the opposite eye (Fig. 55.7C).

9. Examine the pupillary reaction to accommodation (*accommodation reflex*). Ask the subject to look at a distant object. Bring the index finger of your hand to a point midway between the two eyes and very close to the eyes of the subject. Ask the subject to look at the tip of your index finger (Fig. 55.8). Examine for medial deviation and pupillary constriction of both the eyes.

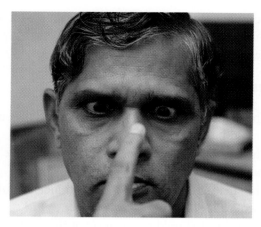

Fig. 55.8   Procedure for assessing accommodation reflex. Note the medial deviation of the eye of the subject and constriction of pupil when he looks at the tip of the examiner's finger kept close to his eyes.

Precautions

1. The examiner's finger should remain about 25 cm (the normal visual distance) from the subject's eyes while testing for eye movement.

2. The light reflexes of both the eyes should be elicited separately by placing a cardboard between both the eyes.

3. For eliciting light reflex, the light should not be projected to the eyes from the front; rather it should be brought from the side of the eye and then immediately focussed on the pupil.

4. For eliciting accommodation, the subject should shift his gaze immediately from a distant object to an object very close to his eyes.

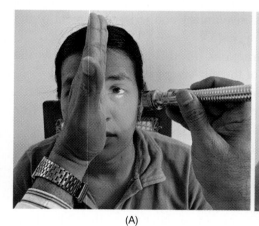 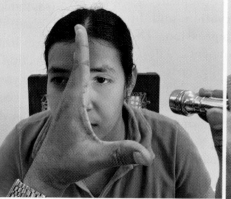 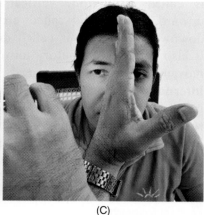

(A)   (B)   (C)

Fig. 55.7   (A) Procedure for assessing light reflex. The examiner, while placing the hand between the eyes, focuses light on the eye by bringing the torch from the side and looks for pupillary constriction; (B) While testing direct light reflex of one eye, also look for the pupillary reaction of the other eye (indirect or consensual light reflex); (C) Testing of light reflex in the opposite eye.

Method to Test Trigeminal Nerve

Principle

The trigeminal nerve supplies the muscle of mastication and carries sensations from the face. Examination of the different sensations on the face and the ability of the subject to chew tests the intactness of the trigeminal nerve.

Requirements

1. Cotton wool
2. Pin
3. Tuning fork, of 128 Hz
4. Glass tubes containing warm and cold water
5. Knee hammer

Procedure

1. Give proper instructions to the subject and explain to him the nature of the examination.
2. Ask the subject to sit comfortably on a stool.
3. Examine all the sensations (as described in Chapter 56) of the face keeping the area supplied by the ophthalmic, maxillary and mandibular division in mind (Fig. 55.2).
4. Examine the motor function. Ask the subject to clench his teeth and palpate the prominence of the temporal and masseter on both sides by palpating the temple and the upper part of the cheek. Ask the subject to open his mouth and look for deviation of the jaw, if present.

Note: If there is paralysis of one side, the muscle on that side will fail to become prominent and on opening the mouth, the jaw deviates towards the paralysed side because it is pushed over by the lateral pterygoid muscle of the healthy side. Normally, the lateral pterygoid muscle pushes the jaw towards the midline.

5. Test the **conjunctival reflex**. Bring a piece of cotton wool from the side of the subject (the subject should not know that you are going to touch his conjunctiva) and immediately touch the conjunctiva (Fig. 55.9A). Look for the response (the subject blinks his eyes).
6. Test the **corneal reflex**. Touch the limbus, that is, the sclerocorneal junction (Fig. 55.9B) of the eye with cotton wool and look for the response (blinking of the eyes).

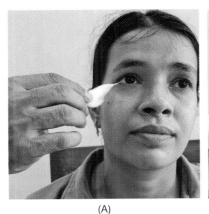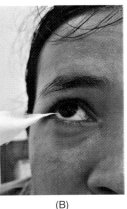

(A)   (B)

Fig. 55.9 (A) Elicitation of conjuctival reflex; (B) Elicitation of corneal reflex. Note that for corneal reflex, the limbus (sclerocorneal junction) is touched but not the cornea, to avoid possible damage to the cornea.

7. Elicit **jaw jerk**. Ask the patient to partially open his mouth. Place your left index finger in the groove under the lower lip and lightly tap on the nail of the finger with the help of the knee hammer (Fig. 55.10). Observe the response (if the jerk is present, the mouth snaps shut).

Precautions

1. The subject should be instructed properly.
2. All the sensations should be elicited from the face according to the distribution of the three subdivisions of the fifth nerve.
3. The masseter and temporalis should be examined on both the sides and compared simultaneously.
4. While eliciting the corneal and conjunctival reflex, the subject should not be aware of the procedure,

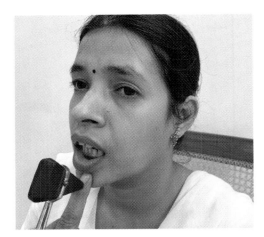

Fig. 55.10 Elicitation of jaw jerk.

otherwise he will close his eyes before the conjunctiva is touched.

Method to Test Facial Nerve

▌ *Principle*

The facial nerve carries the **taste sensation from the anterior two-thirds of the tongue** and supplies the **muscles of facial expression**. Therefore, the examination of the taste sensation of the anterior two-thirds of the tongue and the ability of the subject to perform all facial expressions test the intactness of the facial nerve.

▌ *Requirements*

1. Four small vials containing strong solutions that are sweet (sugar), salty (common salt), bitter (solution of quinine or chloroquine) and sour (lime juice or weak solutions of citric acid) separately.
2. Four glass rods.

▌ *Procedure*

1. Ask the subject to frown or open his eyes wide (Fig. 55.11). Look for the wrinkling of the forehead (to test the frontal belly of the occipitofrontalis).
2. Ask the subject to shut his eyes as tightly as he can. Try to open the eyes while he tries to keep them closed (Fig. 55.12). This is the test for orbicularis oculi.

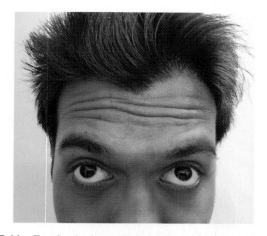

Fig. 55.11   Test for the frontal belly of the occipito-frontalis. Note the wrinkling of the forehead when the subject frowns or open his eyes wide.

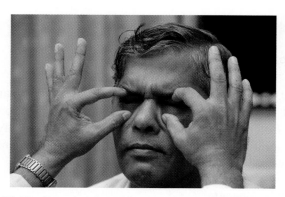

Fig. 55.12   Procedure for testing the orbicularis oculi.

Note: If one side of the nerve is paralysed, the affected eye is either not closed at all, in which case the eyeball rolls upward to make up for the failure of the lid to descend (**Bell's phenomenon**), or if the eye is closed, the eyelashes are not buried. Bell's phenomenon is a normal phenomenon preserved in facial palsies of the lower motor neuron type.

3. Ask the subject to show his teeth. Look for deviation of the angle of the mouth if present (to test for orbicularis oris) (Fig. 55.13).

Note: If the seventh nerve is paralysed, the angle of the mouth on the affected side becomes less prominent and instead of being elevated upwards and laterally, is drawn towards the midline by the unopposed action of the orbicularis oris of the healthy side.

4. Ask the subject to inflate his mouth with air and blow out his cheeks. Tap with the finger on each inflated cheek (test for the buccinator muscle) (Fig. 55.14).

Note: Air escapes from the mouth more easily from the paralysed side.

5. Ask the subject to whistle (test for both orbicularis oris and buccinator) (Fig. 55.15).

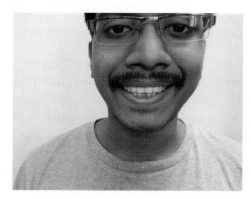

Fig. 55.13   Test for orbicularis oris. Deviation of the angle of the mouth is noted when the subject shows his teeth.

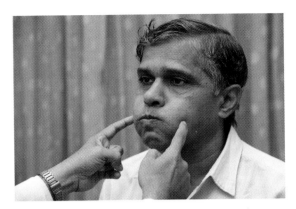

Fig. 55.14 Procedure for testing of buccinator muscle.

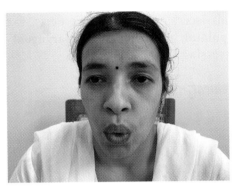

Fig. 55.15 Test for both orbicularis oris and buccinator. Ability to whistle is assessed.

6. Ask the subject to clench his teeth and observe the prominence of the platysma muscle in the neck (Fig. 55.16).
7. Test the taste sensations from the anterior two-thirds of the tongue. Ask him to protrude his tongue. Dip one glass rod in the sweet solution and touch different parts of the tongue of the subject with the tip of the rod. Ask him what taste

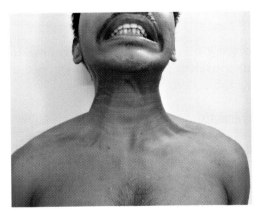

Fig. 55.16 Procedure for testing the platysma. Note the prominence of platysma in the neck, while the subject clenches his teeth.

he senses. Similarly repeat the procedure with the salty, sour and bitter solutions by using separate glass rods for each solution.

> **Note:** While testing for different taste sensations, the relative distribution of taste buds in the tongue for different modalities of taste should be kept in mind. The taste buds for sweet are more concentrated at the tip, bitter at the back and salt and sour on the sides of the tongue.

Precautions

1. The subject should be properly instructed.
2. Functions of both sides of facial muscles should be tested simultaneously and compared.
3. Separate rods should be used for testing different taste solutions.
4. Sensation for bitterness should be tested last.
5. Rinse the mouth after testing with each solution.

Method to Test Vestibulocochlear Nerve

Principle

The eighth nerve has two components, vestibular and cochlear. The cochlear nerve is involved in hearing and the vestibular in balance and equilibrium. Therefore, eighth nerve functions are tested by performing hearing and vestibular tests. The tests of hearing are described in Chapter 51.

Requirements

No special requirement.

Procedure

1. Ask the subject whether he has giddiness, dizziness and vertigo (external objects seem to move around him).
2. Examine the subject's eye for the presence of **nystagmus** (involuntary rhythmic jerky movement of the eyeball).

> **Note:** Nystagmus is observed by asking the subject to look in a different direction, if not found. Nystagmus can be elicited clinically by hyperextending the neck and rapidly moving the head from side to side.

3. Elicit nystagmus by performing caloric test or rotation test (not usually done in physiology).

Caloric test

Irrigate the ear with warm water or with cold water. This produces nystagmus. Irrigation with warm or cold water sets up convection currents in the endolymph of the semicircular canals and produces nystagmus.

Rotation test

Rotate the subject in a special rotating chair. Rotation induces nystagmus.

Method to Test Glossopharyngeal Nerve

▊ Principle

The ninth cranial nerve carries general as well as taste sensations from the posterior third of the tongue and mucous membrane of the pharynx, and supplies motor fibres to the middle constrictor of the pharynx and the stylopharyngeous muscle. It also carries sensation from the carotid sinus. Therefore, functions of the ninth nerve are tested by eliciting **taste sensations from the posterior third of the tongue, pharyngeal reflex**, and by testing the heart rate and blood pressure response to standing.

▊ Requirements

1. Different taste solutions, as described for the seventh nerve
2. Swab stick
3. Sphygmomanometer

▊ Procedure

1. Ask the subject to sit comfortably on a stool and elicit all the taste sensations in the posterior third of the tongue as described for the seventh nerve.
2. Ask the subject to open his mouth wide. Tickle the back of the pharynx with the help of a swab stick, and observe the contraction of the posterior pharyngeal wall (pharyngeal reflex).
3. Ask the subject to lie down and record his blood pressure. Then ask him to stand up and immediately record his blood pressure.

Note: A fall in blood pressure of more than 20 mm Hg is considered as **orthostatic hypotension**, and may indicate dysfunction of the ninth nerve.

▊ Precautions

1. Precautions are similar to the ones followed for testing the taste sensations of the seventh nerve.

2. Swab sticks should not be placed for a longer duration in the pharynx to elicit pharyngeal reflex.
3. The blood pressure should be recorded immediately (preferably within 15 seconds) after standing.

Method to Test Vagus Nerve

▊ Principle

The vagus nerve supplies motor fibres to the soft palate, pharynx and larynx. It also innervates the respiratory passage and most of the thoracic and abdominal viscera. Therefore, this nerve is tested by eliciting **palatal, pharyngeal and laryngeal reflexes**, and by assessing visceral function.

▊ Requirement

1. Swab stick

▊ Procedure

1. Ask the subject to open his mouth wide and say 'aaah'. Observe the arch of the palate and whether the arch is formed equally on both the sides or is flat on one side or both sides.
2. Elicit the pharyngeal reflex as described for the ninth nerve.
3. The laryngeal reflex is tested by laryngoscopy.
4. Visceral functions of the tenth nerve can be tested separately.

Method to Test Accessory Nerve

▊ Principle

The accessory nerve supplies the **sternomastoid and trapezius muscles**. Therefore, its functions are tested by testing the actions of these muscles.

▊ Requirements

No special requirements.

▊ Procedure

1. Stand behind the subject and press his shoulder. Ask the subject to shrug his shoulders against the passive resistance (Fig. 55.17).

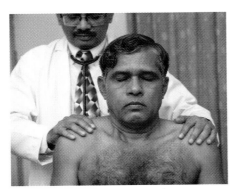

Fig. 55.17   Testing the function of the 11th cranial nerve (trapezius muscle).

> **Note:** This test is done to assess the function of the trapezius.

2.   Ask the subject to move his chin to one side. Try to prevent it by opposing the movement (Fig. 55.18). Note the prominence of the sternomastoid muscle of the opposite side. Repeat the procedure by asking the subject to move his chin against resistance to the opposite side (Fig. 55.19). Ask the subject to depress his chin against the resistance of your hand (Fig. 55.20).

> **Note:** Movement of chin to one side against resistance assesses the power of the sternomastoid of the opposite side. Depressing the chin against resistance assesses the power of the sternomastoid of both sides simultaneously.

Precautions

1.   The examiner should stand behind the subject for testing the trapezius.
2.   While testing for trapezius, press moderately on the shoulders.

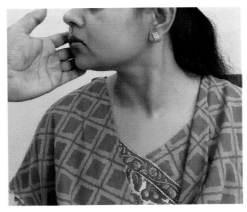

Fig. 55.18   Testing the function of the 11th cranial nerve (sternocleidomastoid muscle of one side).

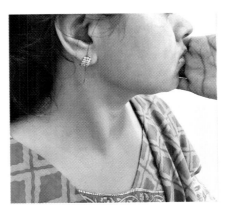

Fig. 55.19   Testing the function of the accessory nerve of the other side.

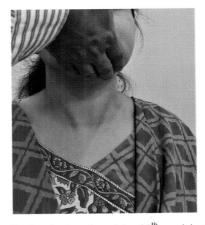

Fig. 55.20   Testing the function of the 11th cranial nerve (sternocleidomastoid muscle of both the sides). Note the prominence of both sternocleidomastoid muscles, while the subject depresses her chin against resistance.

3.   While testing for the sternomastoid, offer gentle resistance against the movement of the chin.

Method to Test Hypoglossal Nerve

Principle

The hypoglossal nerve is a pure motor nerve that supplies the muscles of the tongue and the depressors of the hyoid bone. Therefore, this nerve is tested by testing the movement of the tongue and hyoid bone.

Requirements

No special requirements.

Procedure

1.   Ask the subject to protrude his tongue and note if the median raphe of the tongue is concave towards

one side. Also observe atrophy, fasciculation or tremor if present.

2. Ask the subject to move his tongue from side to side and push his cheek laterally from inside. Resist the tongue movements by pressing it from the outside of the cheek (Fig. 55.21).

DISCUSSION

The cranial nerves are examined thoroughly to detect the abnormalities of these nerves and to localise the lesions at various levels of the brainstem. The lesions of the cranial nerve may occur either in the supranuclear pathway (in the corticonuclear fibres), in the nucleus, or in the infranuclear pathway, that is, in the nerves. The nuclear and infranuclear palsies of the cranial nerves, whether unilateral or bilateral, manifest with definite clinical features, but the unilateral supranuclear palsies of most of the cranial nerves do not manifest with physical signs because of their bilateral cortical representation. The bilateral supranuclear lesions of the cranial nerves manifest with specific features, especially the lesions of facial and hypoglossal nerves.

Olfactory Nerve

A lesion of the olfactory nerve manifests as various disorders of smell like anosmia, parosmia and olfactory hallucinations.

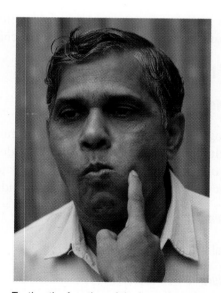

Fig. 55.21   Testing the function of the hypoglossal nerve (strength of the tongue muscle). The subject pushes his cheek with the tongue from inside and the examiner resists it from outside.

Anosmia

Definition   Complete abolition of sense of smell is called anosmia.

Causes   Unilateral and bilateral anosmia could have different causes.

Unilateral anosmia
* Tumour of olfactory bulb
* Tumour of frontal lobe
* Meningiomas pressing on the olfactory bulb or olfactory tract

Bilateral anosmia
* Common cold
* Head injuries in which the cribiform plate of the ethmoid bone is fractured
* Atrophic rhinitis

Hyposmia

Definition   Decreased sensation of smell is called hyposmia.

Causes   Same as anosmia.

Parosmia

Definition   When the sensation of smell is perverted, it is known as parosmia. The offensive smell may seem like a pleasant odour or vice versa. This is also called cacosmia.

Causes   It could be due to
* Mental disorders
* Can occur as an aura in epilepsy
* Sometimes in head injury

Olfactory Hallucination

Definition   When the sensation of smell is perceived without actual presence of any odour.

Cause   It is typically seen as an aura of temporal lobe epilepsy.

Optic Nerve

A lesion of the optic nerve results in defects in the acuity of vision, field of vision and colour vision. These defects are discussed separately under 'Perimetry', 'Acuity of Vision' and 'Colour Vision' (Chapters 43–45).

Oculomotor Nerve

The lesion of the oculomotor nerve results in ptosis, nystagmus, abnormal reaction of pupil to light and accommodation, diplopia and defects in eye movement.

Ptosis

Definition Drooping of the eyelid is called ptosis.

Causes
- Impairment of the functions of the third cranial nerve
- Horner syndrome (sympathetic lesion)
- Myasthenia gravis (disorder of neuromuscular junction)

The **ptosis of Horner syndrome** is always minimal. Therefore, presence of gross ptosis excludes sympathetic lesions. In sympathetic lesions, the pupil of the affected side is smaller (constricted). In third nerve palsy, ptosis is complete and the pupil of the affected side is larger (dilated). In myasthenia, ptosis is usually bilateral and the pupil remains unaffected.

Nystagmus

Definition This is the involuntary, rhythmic and jerky movement of the eyeball. The nystagmus may be horizontal, vertical or rotatory.

Causes
- Vestibular lesion
- Cerebellar lesion
- Lesion of third cranial nerve
- Congenital

Nystagmus of visual origin is mostly pendular and often rotatory on central fixation of the eyes.

Pupillary Reactions

The pupils constrict in response to light (**light reflex**).

The pathway for both direct and indirect light reflexes are summarised in Fig. 55.22.

In **accommodation reflex**, there is convergence of the eyeballs, constriction of pupils and increased convexity of the lens. The pathway for accommodation reflex is depicted in Fig. 55.23.

There are **different abnormalities** in which pupillary reactions are altered.

1. Argyll Robertson pupil

Definition Absence of the reaction of pupils to light with preservation of the reaction to accommodation is called Argyll Robertson pupil (ARP, mnemonic for accommodation reflex present).

Causes It is usually seen in neurosyphilis. Neurosyphilis is very rare in recent times after the advent of modern antibiotics.

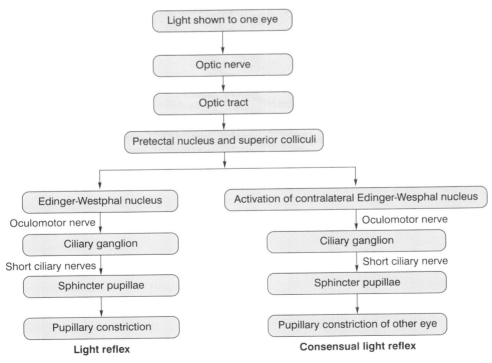

Fig. 55.22 Schematic diagram for the reflex pathway for direct and consensual light reflexes.

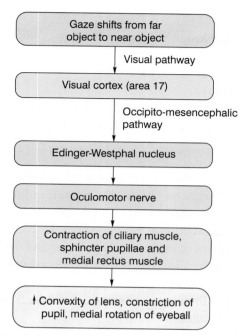

Fig. 55.23   Schematic diagram for the reflex pathway for accommodation reflex.

2. Adie's pupil

Definition   The extremely decreased reaction of the pupil to light and darkness is called Adie's pupil. In light, the pupil constricts very slowly, and in darkness, it dilates very slowly. It also reacts sluggishly to accommodation.

Causes
- Holmes-Adie syndrome (decreased tendon reflexes)
- Sometimes seen in young girls

3. Unilateral dilated and fixed pupil

Cause   Unilateral third nerve palsy. It is associated with ptosis and laterally deviated eye.

4. Hippus

Definition   Alternate rhythmic dilatation and constriction of pupil in response to light is called hippus.

Cause   Usually seen in retrobulbar neuritis.

Abnormalities of Ocular Movement

Normally, the movement of the two eyes are symmetrical, so that the visual axes meet at the point at which the eyes are directed. This is called conjugate movement of the eyes. In third nerve palsy, the ability of the eye to move medially, to move upward in the adducted position and to move upward and downward

in the abducted position is lost. The eye deviates laterally due to unopposed action of the lateral rectus, which is supplied by the sixth cranial nerve.

Strabismus

Definition   Deviation of the eyeball is called strabismus or squint. The visual axes do not meet at the point of fixation.

There are **two types of strabismus**: paralytic and non-paralytic. ***Paralytic strabismus*** occurs due to weakness of extraocular muscles. Paralytic strabismus causes diplopia (double vision) because defective movement of one eye results in images formed by the two eyes falling upon non-identical points of two retinas. Therefore, binocular fusion cannot occur in the visual cortex and two separate images are perceived.

Diplopia

Definition   The occurrence of double vision is called diplopia.

Physiologic basis   Diplopia occurs only over that part of the field of vision towards which the affected muscles move the eye. If both the eyes are functional, and one deviates, binocular diplopia results. Monocular diplopia results from lens opacities and astigmatism.

Causes   Diplopia can occur in third, fourth and sixth nerve palsy.

Trochlear Nerve

The trochlear nerve innervates the superior oblique muscle. Therefore, a lesion of the trochlear nerve results in impaired downward movement of the eye. The eyeball rotates outward by the unopposed action of the inferior rectus when the subject attempts to look downward. Usually, there is no squint, but diplopia may occur below the horizontal plane.

Abducent Nerve

The abducent nerve innervates the lateral rectus muscle. Therefore, lesions of the sixth nerve result in the inability to move the eye outwards and diplopia occurs when the subject looks in that direction. A convergent squint may occur because of unopposed action of the medial rectus.

Trigeminal Nerve

A lesion of the trigeminal nerve results in sensory and motor deficits.

Sensory Deficits

1. There is loss of general sensation from different parts of the face depending on the division of the fifth nerve affected.
2. Though the fifth nerve does not carry the taste sensation, in the suspected lesion of the fifth nerve, the sensation of taste should be examined as the seventh nerve runs in close association with the fifth nerve in the brain.

Motor Deficits

1. Paralysis of the fifth nerve of one side causes the muscles of mastication on that side to fail to become prominent. On opening the mouth, the jaw deviates towards the paralysed side, being pushed over by the healthy lateral pterygoid muscle.
2. Jaw jerk is diminished in infranuclear fifth nerve palsy. The jaw jerk is exaggerated in supranuclear fifth nerve palsy (upper motor neuron lesion above the nucleus of the fifth nerve).

Reflex Deficits

Corneal and conjunctival reflexes are abolished in fifth nerve lesions.

Trigeminal neuralgia

Neuralgia (nerve pain) of one or more branches of the trigeminal nerve is called the trigeminal neuralgia (tic douloureux). It may be associated with sensory loss and muscle weakness in the area of its distribution.

Facial Nerve

A lesion of the facial nerve is the commonest of the cranial nerve lesions. Bell's palsy is the most common cranial nerve disorder.

Effects of Paralysis

1. The affected side of the face loses its expression.
2. The nasolabial fold is less pronounced.
3. The eye on the affected side is more widely open than on the other side, and does not close totally even during sleep.
4. The mouth is drawn to the healthy side.
5. The food is collected between the lips and gum on the affected side.
6. The fluid and saliva escape from the affected angle of the mouth.
7. There is loss of taste sensation from the anterior two-thirds of the tongue. However, if the lesion is below the joining of the chorda tympani nerve that is distal to the stylomastoid foramen, taste will not be affected.

Types of Paralysis

Facial nerve lesion may be infranuclear or supranuclear.

Infranuclear facial palsy

This is the commonest of all lesions of cranial nerves. Idiopathic infranuclear facial palsy is called **Bell's palsy**. It usually occurs due to viral infection, or may be idiopathic. The common features are:

1. Both upper and lower parts of the face are equally affected.
2. Taste sensation may be lost depending on the site of lesion.
3. No involvement of emotional components of facial expression.

Supranuclear facial palsy

Facial palsy due to a lesion above the nucleus involving the corticonuclear fibres is called supranuclear facial palsy. The common features are:

1. The lower part of the face is mainly affected whereas the upper part of the face is either totally spared or affected minimally. This is because the frontal belly of occipitofrontalis has bilateral cortical innervation.
2. Taste sensation may not be altered.
3. Muscles of the voluntary movement of the face are paralysed, but muscles involved in emotional expressions of the face, for example, crying, remain intact or exaggerated (mimic paralysis). This occurs because the emotional movements are not dependent on the same cortical innervation as voluntary movements.

Vestibulocochlear Nerve

The effect of cochlear nerve lesion is discussed separately in Chapter 53.

Effect of Lesion of Vestibular Nerve

1. Patient complains of vertigo, dizziness and giddiness. Vertigo is the sensation of rotation in the absence of actual rotation (hallucination of movement).
2. Patient may vomit and nystagmus may be present.
3. Orientation in space may be lost.

Glossopharyngeal Nerve

Effects of Paralysis

1. Loss of taste and general sensation from the posterior third of the tongue.
2. Absence of pharyngeal reflex and difficulty during swallowing.
3. Decreased secretion of saliva.
4. Orthostatic hypotension may occur.

Vagus Nerve

Effects of Paralysis

1. Loss of the pharyngeal and palatal reflex. Swallowing becomes difficult.
2. Nasal regurgitation of fluid may occur.
3. Uvula deviates to the healthy side.
4. Paralysis of vocal cord causes aphonia.
5. Paralysis of larynx (all the muscles of the larynx except the cricothyroid are supplied by the recurrent laryngeal nerve, a branch of the vagus nerve) results in hoarseness of voice.
6. Impairment of sensation from many organs.
7. Increase in heart rate and impairment in regulation of blood pressure.

Accessory Nerve

A lesion of the accessory nerve causes inability to raise the shoulders and difficulty in turning the head. There may be drooping of shoulders.

Hypoglossal Nerve

The features of hypoglossal nerve lesion depend on the type of paralysis.

Lower Motor Neuron Paralysis

Unilateral paralysis

The common features are:
1. Tongue is pushed to the paralysed side.
2. Median raphe becomes concave towards paralysed side.
3. Atrophy (with flaccidity) of tongue occurs on the affected side.
4. Fasciculation may be seen on the affected side.

Bilateral paralysis

The common features are:
1. Marked wasting with fasciculation on both sides.
2. Protrusion of tongue becomes impossible.
3. Dysarthria and difficulty in pronouncing 'T' and 'D' may be seen.

Upper Motor Neuron Paralysis

Unilateral paralysis   The common features are:
1. Usually asymptomatic.
2. Tongue may be pushed to the opposite side.

Bilateral paralysis   The common features are:
1. Tongue is spastic.
2. Dysarthria may be associated with emotional disturbances.
3. Dysphagia may be present. This is due to the inability to swallow because the tongue cannot manipulate food properly.

OSPE

I. Check the acuity of vision of the subject by the confrontation test.
    Steps
    1. Give proper instructions to the subject.
    2. Make the subject sit comfortably on a stool.
    3. Sit at a distance of about 3 feet from the subject taking care that your eye level remains at the eye level of the subject.

4. Ask the subject to fix his gaze at the tip of his nose and instruct the subject to say 'yes' when he sees the tip of his finger in the field of vision.

5. Ask the subject to close one of his eyes and close your opposite eye.

6. Move your finger midway between you and the subject from the periphery to the centre of four quadrants to check the field of vision.

7. Compare the field of vision of the subject with your own field of vision.

8. Repeat the procedure with the other eye.

II. Examine the III, IV and VI cranial nerves of the subject and report your findings.

Steps

1. Instruct the subject to look at the tip of the finger and follow the movement of the finger.

2. Bring the tip of your index finger to the eye level of the subject keeping a distance of 25 cm from the subject's eye.

3. Examine the functions of different extrinsic muscles of the eye by making appropriate movements of the finger.

4. Ask the subject to look straight at a distant object and then ask him to look immediately at the fingertip brought close to his eyes.

5. Examine the pupillary reflex (both direct and consensual) by focusing light to the eye of the subject. For this, focus the light by bringing the light from the side of the head of the subject and by placing a cardboard between both eyes.

III. Examine the VII cranial nerve of the subject and report your findings.

Steps

1. Give proper instructions to the subject.

2. Ask the subject to frown.

3. Ask the subject to shut his eyes against (examiner's) resistance.

4. Ask the subject to show his teeth, smile and whistle.

5. Ask the subject to inflate his mouth and blow out his cheeks.

6. Ask the subject to clench his teeth. Look for the prominence of the platysma muscle.

7. Ask for testing taste sensations from anterior two-thirds of the tongue (need not perform).

IV. Examine the IX cranial nerve of the subject and report your findings.

Steps

1. Give proper instructions to the subject and ask him to sit comfortably on a stool.

2. Ask the subject to open his mouth wide, and with the help of a swab stick, tickle the back of the pharynx and observe the contraction of the posterior pharyngeal wall.

3. Ask the subject to lie down and record his blood pressure, and then record the blood pressure immediately after asking the subject to stand.

V. Examine the XI cranial nerve of the subject and report your findings.

Steps

1. Give proper instructions to the subject and ask him to sit comfortably on a stool.

2. Stand behind the subject and place your hands on both the shoulders.

3. Ask the subject to elevate his shoulders. Try to prevent this.

4. Ask the subject to move his chin to one side. Try to prevent it by opposing his chin movement, and look for the prominence of the sternocleidomastoid muscle of the opposite side of the neck.

5. Repeat the procedure to check the action of the sternocleidomastoid muscle of the opposite side.

VI. Examine the XII cranial nerves of the subject and report your findings.

Steps

1. Give proper instructions to the subject.

2. Ask the subject to protrude his tongue and observe for the presence of fasciculation, tremor or atrophy; and also check the position of the median raphe of the tongue.

3. Ask the subject to move his tongue to one side and to push the cheek of that side from inside. While the subject does this, try to assess the strength of the tongue by offering resistance from outside the cheek.

4. Repeat the procedure by asking the subject to push the cheek of the opposite side.

VIVA

1. Which cranial nerves are sensory in function, motor in function, or mixed?
2. What is the pathway for olfactory nerves?
3. What is anosmia? What are its causes?
4. What is parosmia?
5. Why should a distance of 3 feet be maintained between the subject and the examiner for performing confrontation test and for detecting acuity of vision?
6. What are the functions of the third cranial nerve?
7. Why should a distance of 25 cm be maintained between the eye of the subject and the finger of the examiner for assessing eye movements?
8. What are the effects of a lesion of the third cranial nerve?
9. What is diplopia and what are its causes?
10. What is ptosis and what are its causes?
11. What is nystagmus?
12. What are the causes of unilateral and bilateral dilated pupils?
13. What are the divisions of the fifth cranial nerve and what are their functions?
14. How do you test for the motor function of the fifth cranial nerve?
15. Why is the fourth cranial nerve more liable to be affected by raised intracranial pressure?
16. What is the course of the seventh cranial nerve?
17. How do you test for the motor functions of the seventh cranial nerve?
18. Why is the facial nerve more prone to injury in the facial canal?
19. What is Bell's palsy?
20. Differentiate between supranuclear and infranuclear palsy of the seventh nerve?
21. Why does the upper part of the face escape in supranuclear seventh nerve palsy?
22. How do you assess the functions of the vestibular division of the eight nerve?
23. What are the functions of the ninth cranial nerve?
24. What are the effects of a lesion of the ninth cranial nerve?
25. What are the functions of the vagus nerve?
26. What are the effects of a lesion of the vagus nerve?
27. How do you assess the functions of the eleventh cranial nerve?
28. What are the effects of a lesion of the eleventh cranial nerve?
29. How do you assess the functions of the twelfth cranial nerve?
30. What are the effects of a lesion of the twelfth cranial nerve?
31. What are the differences between upper motor and lower motor neuron paralysis of the twelfth cranial nerve?

CHAPTER 56

Clinical Examination of the Nervous System II (Sensory System)

Learning Objectives

After completing this practical, you will be able to (MUST KNOW):

1. Describe the importance of performing this practical in clinical physiology.
2. Classify different sensations and receptors.
3. Draw the sensory map of the body.
4. Elicit all the sensations.
5. List the precautions taken during elicitation of sensations.

6. Trace the pathway of all sensations.
7. Name the common abnormalities of alteration in sensations.

You may also be able to (DESIRABLE TO KNOW):

1. Explain the abnormalities of alterations of sensations.
2. Correlate the clinical findings with abnormalities if present.
3. Localise the diseases affecting different parts of the sensory system.
4. Explain the effects of lesions at various levels in the sensory pathways.

CLINICAL EXAMINATION OF THE SENSORY SYSTEM

INTRODUCTION

Anatomical and Physiological Considerations

The sensory information conveyed to the central nervous system by the peripheral nerves originates in the special structures that are distributed in the skin, subcutaneous tissues, muscles, tendons and joints. These special structures are known as receptors, which are modified nerve endings. From the peripheral nerves, the sensations enter the spinal cord through the posterior nerve roots. In the spinal cord, the sensations ascend in different sensory tracts to finally reach the sensory cortex via the thalamus. Some of the sensory inputs also reach the cerebellum, and these inputs are mainly the unconscious proprioceptive and kinesthetic sensations that are involved in the modulation of motor activities. Lesions at different levels of the sensory system produce specific sensory deficits.

Sensory Modalities

Sensations are broadly classified into **general sensations, special sensations and visceral sensations**.

General Sensations

◆ The different types of general sensations are:
◆ Touch and pressure
◆ Warmth
◆ Cold
◆ Pain
◆ Vibration
◆ Movement and position of joints (proprioception)

Special Sensations

The sensations that originate in the special sensory receptors present in the structures like the eye and ear are called special sensations. Different types of special sensations are:
◆ Vision
◆ Hearing
◆ Smell
◆ Taste
◆ Acceleration (rotational and linear)

Visceral Sensations

Sensations that originate in the visceral structures are referred to as visceral sensations. Some of the examples of visceral sensations are lung inflation, distension of the stomach and change in arterial blood pressure.

Receptors

Receptors are transducers that convert various forms of energy in the environment into the action potentials in the neurons. They may be a part of the neuron or a specialised cell that generates action potential in the neurons. Very often, the receptors are associated with non-neural cells that surround them to form a sense organ.

Types of Receptors

The receptors are divided into **four categories:**

1. Exteroceptors   These receptors are concerned with the changes in the external environment close to the body. Exteroceptors are distributed on the surface of the body, in the skin and subcutaneous tissues. These cutaneous sense organs are broadly divided into expanded endings and encapsulated endings.

The **expanded endings** are:
- Merkel's discs and
- Ruffini endings

Merkel's discs and Ruffini endings are slow-adapting touch receptors.

The **encapsulated endings** are:
- Pacinian corpuscles,
- Meissner's corpuscles and
- Krause's end-bulbs

Meissner's and Pacinian corpuscles are rapidly adapting touch receptors. Most of these sensory endings are present around the hair follicles, therefore, the slightest movement of hair, elicits the sensation of touch. Some of the endings, especially Ruffini endings and Pacinian corpuscles, are also found in deep fibrous tissues. It appears that none of these endings are needed for elicitation of sensations, because sensory modalities can be elicited from the areas that contain only free nerve endings.

2. Interoceptors   These are concerned with the changes in the internal environment of the body, like osmoreceptors that respond to change in osmolality of body fluids.

3. Proprioceptors   These provide information about the position of the body in space at any given time. The conscious component of proprioception comes from the receptors in the joints, and from the cutaneous touch and pressure receptors.

4. Teleceptors   These are concerned with the events that occur at a distance from the body.

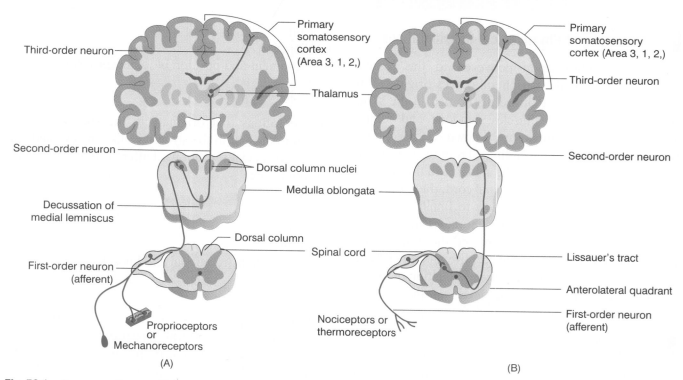

Fig. 56.1   Sensory pathways. (A) Dorsal column (lemniscal) pathway; (B) Anterolateral (spinothalamic) pathway.

Sensory Pathways

The sensory pathways are divided in the **two systems**. The pathways that ascend in the posterior column of the spinal cord are frequently called the **lemniscal system** and the pathways that ascend in the anterior and lateral quadrant of the spinal cord are referred to as the **anterolateral system** (Fig. 56.1). The neurons in the sensory pathways are placed in sequential order and accordingly they are called first, second and third order of neurons. The first order of neurons sends the encoded information from the receptors to the spinal cord and medulla. The second order of neurons transmits the impulse from the spinal cord and medulla to the thalamus from where the third order of neurons conveys the information to the cortex.

Fine Touch

Touch receptors are present in large numbers in the skin of the fingers and lips and in fewer numbers in the skin of the trunk. The first order of neurons carrying fine touch sensation enter the spinal cord via the posterior root and then ascend up in the dorsal column of the spinal cord of the same side. They terminate in the nucleus gracilis and cuneatus of the medulla. The second order of neurons arises from these nuclei, crosses to the opposite side in the medulla and ascends in the contralateral medial lemniscus, to terminate in the ventral posterior nucleus and related specific sensory nuclei of the thalamus. The third order of neurons arises from the thalamus and reaches the sensory cortex via thalamic radiation. The **sensations that are carried in the posterior column** of the spinal cord are:

◆ Fine touch
◆ Proprioception (joint sensation and sense of position)
◆ Sense of vibration
◆ Tactile localisation
◆ Two-point discrimination
◆ Stereognosis

Crude Touch

The first order of neurons after entering the spinal cord synapse on the second order of neurons in the dorsal horn of the cord. The second order of neurons crosses to the opposite side at that spinal segment and ascends in the contralateral ventral spinothalamic tract to terminate in the specific sensory relay nuclei of the thalamus. The third order of neurons arises from the thalamus and terminates in the sensory cortex through thalamic radiation.

Proprioception

The pathway for proprioceptive inputs is the same as that of fine touch. A large part of proprioceptive input goes to the cerebellum in addition to its projection to the sensory cortex, which is involved in modulation of motor activities.

Pain

The sense organs for pain are free nerve endings. The sensation of pain is transmitted to the central nervous system by a two-fibre system. The Aδ fibres carry fast pain whereas the C fibres carry slow pain. The Aδ fibres terminate mainly on the neurons in the laminas I and V, and the C fibres terminate on the neurons in the laminas I and II. The second order of neurons crosses to the opposite side of the spinal cord, at the same segmental level and then ascends in the contralateral lateral spinothalamic tract to terminate in the specific sensory relay nuclei in the thalamus. From the thalamus, the third order of neurons arises and projects to the sensory cortex. Many fibres activated by pain terminate in the reticular system from where they project to the midline and intralaminar (non-specific projection) nuclei of the thalamus and from there to many different parts of the cortex. Many pain fibres also terminate in the periaqueductal gray in the midbrain.

Temperature

There are two types of sense organs for temperature sensation; one type for eliciting cold and the other one for eliciting warmth. The afferents for cold are Aδ fibres and C fibres, and for warmth, only C fibres. The first order of neurons terminates in the same segmental level of the spinal cord. The second order of neurons crosses to the opposite side and ascends in the contralateral lateral spinothalamic tract to terminate in the thalamus from where the third order of neurons arises and terminates in the sensory cortex.

The receptors and pathways for various sensations are summarised in Table 56.1.

Table 56.1 Testing primary sensation.

Sensations	Testing method/object	Receptors		Afferent Fiber Size	Pathway
Pain	Pinprick	Cutaneous nociceptors		Small	Spinothalamic also D
Temperature, heat	Warm metal object	Cutaneous thermoreceptors for hot		Small	Spinothalamic
Temperature, cold	Cold metal object	Cutaneous thermoreceptors for cold		Small	Spinothalamic
Touch	Cotton wisp, fine brush	Cutaneous mechanoreceptors, also naked endings		Large and small	Lemniscal (fine touch), also D and Spinothalamic (crude touch)
Vibration	Tuning fork, 128 Hz	Mechanoreceptors, especially pacinian corpuscles		Large	Lemniscal, also D
Joint Position	Passive movement of specific joints	Joint capsule and tendon endings, muscle spindles		Large	Lemniscal, also D

D: Diffuse ascending projections in ipsilateral and contralateral anterolateral columns; Lemniscal: Posterior column and lemniscal projection, ipsilateral; Spinothalamic: Spinothalamic projection, contralateral

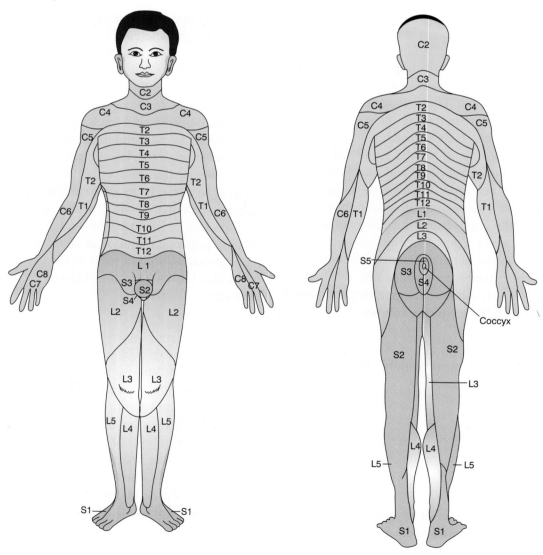

Fig. 56.2 Sensory map of the body.

Sensory Map

The spinal cord is made up of different segments. From each segment, a pair of motor and sensory nerve roots arise. The sensory fibres from each segment innervate a specific dermatome of the body. This dermatomal innervation by sensory fibres constitutes the sensory map of the body (Fig. 56.2). Sensations are elicited from the skin of different dermatomes to check the intactness of a particular segment of the spinal cord.

METHODS

Method of Examination of Sensory System

Principle

Different sensory modalities are elicited from different dermatomes of both sides and compared.

Requirements

1. Cotton
2. Von Frey's hair aesthesiometer (Fig. 56.3)
3. Compass aesthesiometer (Fig. 56.4)
4. Tuning fork (128 Hz)

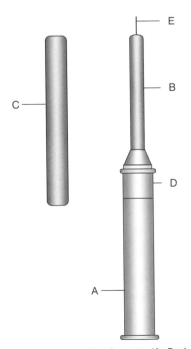

Fig. 56.3   Von Frey's hair aesthesiometer (A: Body; B: Sliding graduated tube; C: Protective cap; D: Body tube; E: Protruding horse hair).

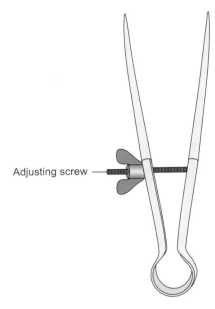

Fig. 56.4   Compass aesthesiometer.

5. Pin
6. Algometer
7. Test tubes containing warm and cold water
8. Ballpoint pens

Procedure

The following different forms of sensation are tested.
1. Tactile sensibility which includes:
   – Fine touch
   – Pressure (crude touch)
   – Tactile localisation (ability to localise a point on the surface of the body being touched)
   – Two-point discrimination (ability to discriminate between two points when the two points are touched simultaneously)
   – Stereognosis (ability to feel and recognise the familiar objects by their size, shape and form)
2. Position sense, and the appreciation of passive movement (proprioception)
3. Vibration
4. Pain
5. Temperature

Tactile sensibility

Fine touch

Steps

1. Give proper instructions to the subject (to raise his finger or say 'yes' when he feels the sensation of touch).

2. Ask the subject to close his eyes.

3. With the help of cotton wool (Fig. 56.5A), or Von Frey's hair aesthesiometer (Fig. 56.5B) lightly touch the skin of the different parts of the subject.

4. If the subject raises his finger or says 'yes' enquire whether the feeling is normal or different. If the subject does not feel the sensation, compare carefully with the corresponding area on the opposite part of the body.

5. Elicit the sensation dermatome-wise on both sides of the body.

> **Note:** Areas of hypoaesthesia, paraesthesia, or hyperaesthesia, if present, should be properly delineated.

6. Note down your observation.

Precautions

1. Give proper instructions to the subject to gain maximum cooperation.

2. The subject should close his eyes throughout the entire procedure.

3. Sensations should be elicited according to different dermatomes of the body.

4. Sensation of the corresponding area of the opposite side of the body should also be elicited simultaneously and compared.

5. If the sensation is altered in a particular part of the body, the area of alteration of sensation should be properly delineated.

Pressure (Crude Touch)

Steps

1. Give proper instructions to the subject.

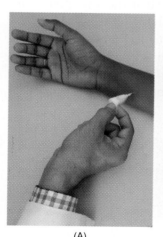 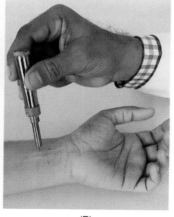

(A)   (B)

Fig. 56.5   Elicitation of fine touch. (A) Using cotton wool; (B) Using hair aesthesiometer.

2. Ask the subject to close his eyes.

3. Elicit the pressure sensation by pressing with your finger tip on the skin of different dermatomes.

4. Record your observation.

Precautions   Same as are described for 'Fine touch'.

Tactile localisation

Steps

1. Give instructions to the subject to localise (with the help of a ballpoint pen) the part of the body, which is touched by the tip of a pen.

2. Ask the subject to hold a pen and close his eyes.

3. Touch the skin of one area of the body with the help of a ball pen and ask the subject to immediately localise that point by touching with the pen that he is holding.

4. Measure the distance between the two points (this is called the localisation distance).

> **Note:** This distance varies greatly in different parts of the body. It corresponds with the concentration of touch spots which are numerous on the tips of the fingers and palms and fewer on the back. The localisation distance is less if the concentration of touch spots is more.

5. Likewise, determine the localisation distance on different parts of the body on both sides.

Precautions

1. The subject should be instructed properly regarding his role in the experiment.

2. The subject should close his eyes throughout the procedure.

3. Sensations should be elicited according to different dermatomes of the body.

4. The localisation distance of the corresponding area of the opposite side of the body should also be elicited simultaneously and compared.

Two-point discrimination

Steps

1. Give instructions to the subject to say whether he feels the touch of one point or two points when he is touched by a compass aesthesiometer. Use smaller aesthesiometer for fingers, hand and forearm and big aesthesiometer for trunk of the body (Fig. 56.6).

2. Ask the subject to close his eyes.

3. Separate the two limbs of the compass aesthesiometer a little and touch the skin of the subject lightly with the two points of the aesthesiometer simultaneously.

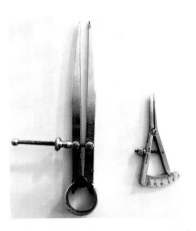

Fig. 56.6 Big and small Weber's compass aesthesiometers.

Ask the subject to say whether he is being touched at one or two points.

4. If the subject says one point, increase the distance between two points a little more and repeat the test till two separate points are appreciated by the subject (the distance between two points when the subject feels it as two points is called the minimum separable distance).

Note: This distance varies greatly in different parts of the body with the richness of touch spots. Normally, it is about 2 mm on finger tips, 5 mm on the hands and more on other parts of the body.

5. Record the minimum separable distance on different parts of the body on both the sides.

Precautions

1. Proper instruction should be given to the subject to gain maximum cooperation.
2. The subject should close his eyes throughout the procedure.
3. The sensation should be elicited by starting from the minimum distance between the two limbs of the aesthesiometer, and the distance should be increased little by little till the minimum separable distance is obtained.
4. The two points of the aesthesiometer should be touched simultaneously.
5. The sensation of the corresponding part of the opposite side of the body should be elicited and compared simultaneously.

Stereognosis

Steps

1. Give instructions to the subject to identify the object when asked to handle it.

2. Ask the subject to close his eyes.
3. Place a familiar object in one hand of the subject and ask him to recognise it by palpating the object.
4. Repeat the procedure with four to five familiar objects.
5. Repeat the procedure in the opposite hand.

Precautions

1. The subject should be instructed properly.
2. The subject should close his eyes during the experiment.
3. The sensation should be elicited by giving objects that are familiar to the subject.
4. The test should be repeated with at least three different objects.
5. The sensation should be elicited in one hand at a time and should be repeated in the other hand.

Sense of position and joint movement

This is tested by passively moving the limbs of the subject to a particular position with the eyes closed and asking him to recognise the position of the limb. The perception of movement is closely related to the sense of position; therefore, both the senses are tested together.

Steps

1. Give proper instructions to the subject (to recognise the particular position of the limb when the limb is moved).
2. Ask him to close his eyes.
3. Move his finger or hand, up or down and ask the subject to recognise the movement by calling out the position of the finger/limb or by imitating the same movement in the other limb.
4. Repeat the procedure by changing the position of all the limbs.
5. Make movement at all the joints (all small and big joints) and ask the subject to recognise the joint movement (Fig. 56.7A and B).

Note: Note the angle through which the limb was moved. If the sense of movement is decreased, this angle is greater than that in the normal limb. Movements of less than 10° are appreciated at all the normal joints.

6. Make a particular movement (flexion or extension at a joint) and ask the subject to recognise the direction of movement.

Note: The patient can sometimes recognise the occurrence of a movement but not its direction. **Romberg test** for assessing body position is described in Chapter 57, under "Coordination of Movement."

Precautions

1. The subject should be properly instructed to cooperate fully in the experiment.
2. The subject should close his eyes during the experiment.
3. Movement at different joints and position of different parts of the limbs should be performed.
4. The sensation should be elicited on both the sides and compared simultaneously.

Sense of vibration

Steps

1. Give proper instructions to the subject.
2. Make the tuning fork vibrate by hitting the blades of the fork against the hypothenar eminence of the palm or against the thigh.
3. Place the foot of the vibrating tuning fork on the surface of the body, especially on a bony prominence like the lower end of the tibia, styloid process of the ulnar (Fig. 56.8A), and medial or lateral malleolus (Fig. 56.8B), and ask the subject whether he feels the vibration.
4. Ask the subject to raise his finger when he ceases to feel the vibration.
5. Immediately place the tuning fork on the corresponding bony prominence of your body and note whether you can still perceive the vibration.

> **Note:** If the examiner perceives the vibration after the subject ceases to perceive it, the sense of vibration is impaired in the subject.

6. Elicit vibration sense on all the bony prominences of the body.

Precautions

1. The subject should be instructed properly.

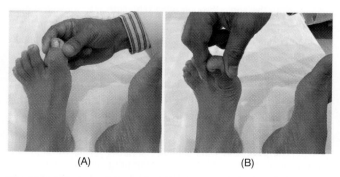

Fig. 56.7 Demonstration of joint movement by bending the great toe. (A) By forward bending; (B) By backward bending.

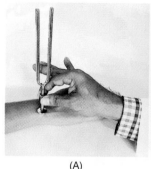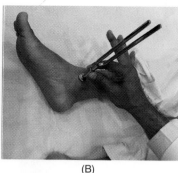

Fig. 56.8 Testing for sense of vibration. (A) In upper limb (on styloid process of ulna); (B) In lower limb (on medial malleolus).

2. The tuning fork should be allowed to vibrate by hitting the blades of the fork against the hypothenar eminence of the palm or against the thigh, not against any hard surface.
3. The examiner should hold the tuning fork by holding the stem of the fork close to the base without touching the blades.
4. The vibrating fork should be placed only on the bony prominence.
5. After the subject ceases to feel the vibration, the examiner should place the fork immediately on the corresponding point on his own body to check if the vibration has actually ceased.
6. The sensation should be elicited on the corresponding bony prominence of the opposite side of the body.

Pain

Superficial pain

Steps

1. Give proper instructions to the subject.
2. Explain properly that you will be eliciting pain.
3. With the help of a pin (not a needle), lightly prick the skin of different parts of the body and ask the subject to indicate whether he feels pain.
4. Elicit pain from all the dermatomes of both sides of the body.
5. Delineate the area of analgesia, hypoalgesia or hyperalgesia, if present.

Precautions   Same as described for 'Fine Touch'

Pressure pain

Steps

1. Give proper instructions to the subject.
2. With an algometer (Fig. 56.9), carefully press on the surface of the body and note the minimum pressure required to produce pain.

3. Repeat the procedure on the identical points of the body on the opposite side and compare the results.

Note: Clinically pressure pain is elicited by squeezing the muscle or tendon (Achilles tendon) till pain is produced.

Temperature

Steps

1. Give proper instructions to the subject (to say whether he feels cold or warm when touched with different glass tubes).
2. Take two test tubes containing warm and cold water separately (Fig. 56.10).
3. Place the test tubes on the skin of the subject, each in turn or randomly and ask the subject to say whether he feels warm or cold.
4. Examine warm and cold sensation on all the dermatomes of both sides of the body and note your observation.

Precautions Same as described for 'Fine Touch'

DISCUSSION

Abnormalities of Sensation

Tactile Sensation

Anesthesia

Anesthesia means loss of all sensation. Anesthesia is graded as hypoesthesia when the sensation is decreased

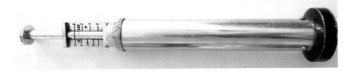

Fig. 56.9 Algometer, for eliciting deep or pressure pain.

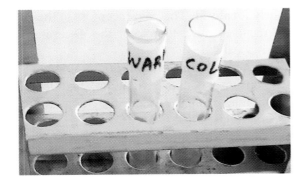

Fig. 56.10 Warm and cold solutions, for eliciting temperature sensation.

or complete anaesthesia when the sensation is totally lost.

Causes of hypoesthesia It is seen in lesions of the central sensory structures, like lesions of the thalamus, internal capsule or cortex. Usually it affects the distal parts of the limbs more than the proximal parts.

Causes of complete anaesthesia

◈ Usually occurs in peripheral nerve lesions. The common causes are leprosy and complicated diabetes mellitus. Lesions of peripheral nerves result in anaesthesia corresponding to the distribution of sensory fibres.
◈ Complete anaesthesia also occurs in **complete transection of the spinal cord** where anaesthesia is seen in the limbs and trunk below the level of the lesion.

Dissociated anaesthesia

When the **sensation of pain and temperature is lost with the preservation of the touch sensation**, the condition is known as dissociated anaesthesia.

Physiologic basis Dissociated anaesthesia occurs in conditions where the grey matter of the spinal cord near the central canal is damaged. The fibres carrying the touch sensation ascend in the dorsal column of the spinal cord and are therefore spared. The fibres carrying pain and temperature cross to the opposite side of the spinal cord at the same segmental level of the cord. While crossing to the opposite side, the fibres travel very close to the central canal, therefore they are damaged in the disease process involving the grey matter of the spinal cord.

Causes

◈ Syringomyelia
◈ Intramedullary tumours
◈ Brainstem lesions (syringobulbia)
◈ Thrombosis of the posterior inferior cerebellar artery.

Hemianaesthesia

This is loss of sensation that affects the face, arm and leg of one side (usually opposite side) of the body.

Causes Usually seen in lesions of the thalamus, internal capsule or cortex.

Hyperaesthesia

When the response to a sensory stimulation is exaggerated, the condition is called hyperaesthesia.

Cause   Thalamic lesions

Paraesthesia

When the touch **sensation is perverted** (touch may produce an unpleasant sensation almost amounting to pain) is called paraesthesia. This consists of sensations like pricking, numbness or band-like sensations around the trunk.

Causes

◆ *Nerve compression*   This is the commonest cause of paraesthesia. It occurs when peripheral nerves are stretched or subjected to pressure. The commonest example is paraesthesia (numbness and pricking) after sitting for a longer time with legs crossed.

◆ Spinal tumours

◆ Subacute combined degeneration of spinal cord (Vitamin B12 deficiency)

◆ Disseminated sclerosis

◆ Thalamic lesions

Proprioceptive Sensation

The proprioceptive sensation is that of joint movement, sense of the position of different parts of the body and the sense of vibration. The loss of proprioceptive sensation can occur without loss of other sensations. It is characteristic of the lesions of the posterior column or lesion of the fibres ascending in the posterior column to the medulla. **Romberg test** to describe abnormalities of sense of position is described in Chapter 57.

Loss of proprioception is seen in:

1. Tabes dorsalis
2. Subacute combined degeneration of spinal cord

Pain

Analgesia

Loss of pain sensation is called analgesia.

Causes   Analgesia occurs with anaesthesia, and usually seen in peripheral nerve lesion. Analgesia can also occur without anaesthesia. A hereditary analgesia syndrome has been described, in which the pain receptors are totally absent in the body.

Hypoalgesia

Partial loss of pain sensibility is called hypoalgesia.

Cause   Nerve compression

Hyperalgesia

This is a condition of exaggerated sensibility to pain. In this condition, a mild stimulus, which ordinarily does not produce pain, causes severe pain. It may occur in response to a mild cutaneous stimulus or sometimes as an intractable spontaneous activity (without stimulus).

Causes

◆ Spinal cord disease, for example, tabes dorsalis

◆ Thalamic lesions

◆ Deep-seated lesions in the parietal lobe

Common Clinical Conditions

Peripheral Nerve Pain

This occurs due to injury to the nerve, neuritis and neuropathy. It may be associated with other sensory loss with or without motor changes. Sometimes only nerve pain may occur without other sensory or motor loss. Then it is called neuralgia; for example, trigeminal neuralgia.

Root Pain

Pain is seen in the area of distribution of a particular root that is affected. The most common examples are cervical and lumbar root pain distributed to the appropriate limb, as in cervical spondylosis or lumbar disc prolapse. It is characteristic of extramedullary cord compression.

Causalgia

This is an abnormal type of burning sensation usually seen after limb injuries. It occurs when the nerve injury is mild.

Visceral Pain

This occurs due to diseases of the viscera. For example, inflammation of abdominal viscera produces pain. Visceral pain differs from somatic pain in various ways. These are:

1. **Poorly localised.** The pain receptors in the viscera are relatively few, therefore, the visceral pain is poorly localised.

2. **Associated with autonomic changes** like hypotension, nausea, vomiting and sweating. Autonomic changes occur due to activation of visceral reflexes.

3. **Associated with muscle guarding** (spasm of the abdominal wall). Muscle guarding occurs due to reflex contraction of the skeletal muscle in the abdominal wall. This is a protective reflex as it prevents further injury to the viscera.

4. Often **radiates or is referred to other areas**. Usually visceral pain is referred to a somatic structure that is developed from the same dermatome of the visceral structure in which the pain originates. The most common example is pain of myocardial infarction radiating to the ulnar border of the left hand or the pain of cholecystitis radiating to the tip of the shoulder.

Brown–Sequard Syndrome

This occurs in a **hemisection of the spinal cord**. It is usually seen in injury to the spinal cord or in tumours that affect one half of the cord. ***On the side of the lesion***, the dorsal column sensations (the fine touch sensation, proprioceptive sensations and the tactile localisation and discrimination) are lost. ***On the opposite side*** of the lesion pain, temperature and crude touch sensations are lost. This occurs because the sensation for fine touch, proprioception, and two-point discrimination ascend the dorsal column of the same side, whereas the sensation for pain, temperature and crude touch ascend the anterolateral system of the opposite side of the spinal cord.

Syringomyelia

In this condition there is a lesion around the central canal of the spinal cord. The lesion interrupts the pain and temperature fibres passing to the opposite side of the spinal cord. Therefore, there is **loss of pain and temperature with preservation of touch** and postural sensibility.

Physiological Significance

Examination of sensory system is performed to localise disease processes that affect any part of the neuraxis of the sensory system. This is called localisation of lesion of the sensory system. Localisation of lesion partly depends on the distribution of the sensory loss and partly on the type of sensory loss. The disease may affect the nerve, the nerve root, the spinal cord, the brainstem, the thalamus or the cortex.

Nerve Lesion

Lesion of a peripheral nerve results in anaesthesia corresponding to the distribution of that particular nerve (Figs. 56.11 and 56.12).

Nerve Root Lesion

There is **segmental anaesthesia** in root lesions corresponding to the involvement of the segment of the spinal cord from where the nerve root arises.

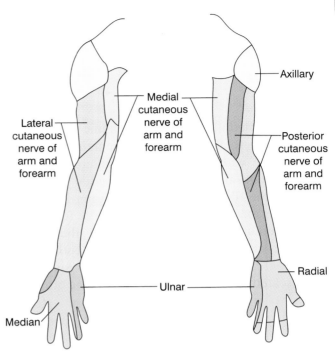

Fig. 56.11   Peripheral nerve lesions in the upper limbs.

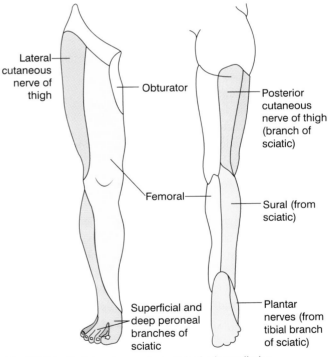

Fig. 56.12   Peripheral nerve lesions in the lower limbs.

Spinal Cord Lesion

Complete section of spinal cord causes anaesthesia in the limbs and trunks below the level of lesion. **Hemisection** of the spinal cord results in **dissociation of anaesthesia** (dissociated sensory loss as seen in

Brown–Sequard syndrome). A lesion around the central canal of the spinal cord results in loss of pain and temperature on both the sides below the level of the lesion with preservation of other sensations.

Brainstem Lesion

Above the medulla, the spinothalamic tract (fibres of the anterolateral system) remains in close association with the trigeminothalamic tract in the tegmentum, whereas the medial lemniscus carrying the fibres of posterior column lies medial to it. A lesion of the lateral part of the tegmentum causes hemianalgesia and thermoanaesthesia in the opposite side of the body without affecting other sensations (as the medial lemniscus is spared). A deep-seated lesion in the upper part of the brainstem may involve the medial lemniscus without affecting the spinothalamic fibres. This results in loss of posterior column sensations with preservation of pain and temperature.

Thalamic Lesion

Severe and extensive lesion of the thalamus results in gross impairment of sensory modalities on the opposite side of the body. The threshold for pain may be raised, but a less painful stimulus may cause an exaggerated response (hyperalgesia). The touch sensation may induce an unpleasant sensation (paraesthesia). This is called the **thalamic syndrome**, which occurs in the lesions of the lateral and ventral nucleus.

Cortical Lesion

The cortex is primarily involved in processing the finer aspect of sensations, especially the spatial and discriminatory sensibility. Tactile localisation, two-point discrimination and stereognosis are therefore called cortical sensations. The cortical lesion results in impairment of tactile localisation, two-point discrimination and stereognosis. Other sensations may remain intact.

OSPE

I. Elicit touch (fine touch) sensation of anterior aspect of the forearms of the subject and report your findings.
   Steps
   1. Give proper instructions to the subject.
   2. Ask the subject to close his eyes.
   3. With cotton wool, lightly touch the skin of anterior aspect of one forearm (according to the different dermatomes).
   4. Elicit touch sensation on the other forearm and compare the finding.
   5. Report your findings.

II. Elicit crude touch sensation of the anterior aspect of the forearms of the subject and report your findings.
   Steps
   1. Give proper instructions to the subject.
   2. Ask the subject to close his eyes.
   3. With the help of his fingertips, lightly press the skin of the anterior aspect of one forearm (according to the different dermatomes).
   4. Elicit crude touch sensation on the other forearm and compare the finding.
   5. Report your findings.

III. Elicit two-point discrimination of the anterior aspect of the right forearm of the subject and report your findings.
   Steps
   1. Give proper instructions to the subject.
   2. Ask him to close his eyes.
   3. Separate the two limbs of the compass aesthesiometer a little and touch the skin of the subject lightly with the two points of the aesthesiometer simultaneously. Ask the subject to say whether he is being touched at one or two points.
   4. If the subject says one point, increase the distance between the two points a little more and repeat the test till two separate points are appreciated by the subject as two points.
   5. Repeat the procedure in the other forearm of the subject and compare.

6. Report your findings.

IV. Elicit pain sensation of the anterior aspect of the right forearm of the given subject and report your findings.

Steps

1. Give proper instructions to the subject.
2. Explain properly that you will be eliciting pain.
3. With the help of a pin (not a needle) lightly prick the skin of the right forearm and ask the subject to say whether he/she feels pain.
4. Repeat the procedure on the opposite side of the body.
5. Delineate the area of analgesia, hypoalgesia or hyperalgesia, if present.
6. Report your findings.

V. Perform tactile localisation in the anterior aspect of the forearms of the given subject and report your findings.

Steps

1. Give proper instructions to the subject and ask him to hold a ballpen.
2. Ask the subject to close his eyes.
3. With the help of a pen, touch the right forearm at a particular point and ask the subject to touch the same point with his pen.
4. Repeat the procedure on the other side of the body and compare.
5. Report your findings.

VI. Test the vibration sense in the upper limbs of the given subject and report your findings.

Steps

1. Select a tuning fork of 128 Hz or less.
2. Instruct the subject.
3. Make the tuning fork vibrate by striking it against the hypothenar eminence of your hand or against the thigh.
4. Hold the tuning fork by holding the stem of the fork close to the base without touching the blades.
5. Immediately place the vibrating tuning fork on the bony prominence of the upper limb and ask the subject to report when the vibration ceases.
6. When the subject gives indication of the cessation of vibration, immediately place the tuning fork on the same point on yourself to feel if the vibration has actually ceased.
7. Repeat on the other limb.
8. Report your findings.

VII. Test the sensation of joint movement and position in the lower limbs of the given subject and report your findings.

Steps

1. Give proper instructions to the subject (to recognise the particular position of the limb when the limb is moved).
2. Ask him to close his eyes.
3. Move his toes or foot, up or down and ask the subject to recognise the movement by saying the position of the toes/foot or ask him to imitate the same movement in the other limb.
4. Repeat the procedure by changing position of the limb at different joints.
5. Make a particular movement (flexion or extension at a joint) and ask the subject to recognise the directions of the movement.
6. Repeat the procedure in the other limb.
7. Report your findings.

VIVA

1. *How do you classify sensations?*
2. *Define a receptor.*
3. *What are the types of receptors?*
4. *What are the sensations carried in the dorsal column?*

5. What are the sensations carried in the anterolateral system of the spinal cord?
6. Trace the pathway for fine touch.
7. Trace the pathway for proprioception.
8. Trace the pathway for pain and temperature.
9. What is a sensory map? What is its physiologic significance?
10. What are the precautions to be observed during elicitation of fine touch sensation?
11. What are the precautions to be observed during elicitation of tactile localisation and two-point discrimination?
12. Why is the tuning fork placed on the bony prominence for eliciting vibration sensibility?
13. What are the precautions to be taken during elicitation of vibration sensibility?
14. What is dissociated anaesthesia?
15. What are the causes of dissociated anaesthesia and what is its physiological?
16. What is hyperaesthesia and what are its causes?
17. Define paraesthesia. Give two causes of paraesthesia.
18. What is hyperalgesia? What are its causes? What is causalgia?
19. How does visceral pain differ from somatic pain?
20. What is the Brown–Sequard syndrome? What are its features?
21. What are the sensory changes seen in syringomyelia?
22. What is the physiological significance of examination of the sensory system?
23. What are the sensory features of brainstem lesion?
24. What is the effect of a lesion of the thalamus on sensory functions?
25. What is the effect of a lesion of the cortex on sensory functions?

CHAPTER 57

Clinical Examination of the Nervous System III (Motor System)

Learning Objectives

After completing this practical, you will be able to (MUST KNOW):

1. Describe the importance of performing this practical in clinical physiology.
2. Measure the bulk of the muscles.
3. Estimate and grade the strength of various individual and groups of muscles.
4. Assess the tone of flexors and extensors at various joints.
5. Elicit superficial and deep reflexes.
6. Test the coordination of movement in the upper and lower limbs.
7. Name the descending motor pathways.
8. Trace the pathway of corticospinal tracts.
9. List the differences between upper and lower motor neuron paralysis.

You may also be able to (DESIRABLE TO KNOW):

1. Trace the pathway of all descending motor tracts.
2. List the functions of motor pathways, basal ganglia, cerebellum and motor cortex.
3. Explain briefly the role of alpha and gamma motor neurons in regulation of muscle tone.
4. Name the common conditions associated with alteration in bulk, tone and strength of the muscles and reflexes.
5. Explain the changes in motor function in upper and lower motor neuron paralysis.
6. List the differences in coordination of movement in cerebellar, sensory and corticospinal pathway disorders.
7. Describe the different types of abnormal gaits and involuntary movement.

CLINICAL EXAMINATION OF THE MOTOR SYSTEM

INTRODUCTION

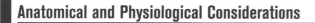

Anatomical and Physiological Considerations

The motor system consists of **motor areas in the brain, the upper motor neurons, the lower motor neurons and the muscles**. The motor system deals with the body functions related to movement of different parts of the body. Movement occurs due to contraction and relaxation of the agonists and antagonists. **Agonists** are muscles that facilitate movement by their contraction, whereas **antagonists** facilitate movement by their relaxation. Movement depends on the maintenance of posture and balance. A balanced posture provides a stable background for movement.

Muscles

Muscles can be classified in various ways. But, to understand motor physiology, the muscles can be best classified as the **medial (proximal)** and the **lateral (distal)** group.

The proximal group of muscles

The proximal groups of muscles are the muscles of the trunk, girdles and proximal parts of the limbs. These muscles are primarily involved in the **maintenance of posture** and equilibrium.

The distal group of muscles

The distal groups of muscles are the intrinsic muscles of the digits and the muscles of the distal parts of the extremities. They are not required for postural activities, but are primarily involved in the **control of skilled voluntary movement**, that is, manipulatory activities.

Lower Motor Neuron

The lower motor neurons are the final common pathway for the output of the motor system. The cell bodies of the lower motor neurons are present in the anterior horn of the spinal cord. The lower motor neurons consist of the **anterior horn cells and the homologous cells in the brainstem, their efferent nerve fibres** that pass via the anterior spinal nerve roots and peripheral nerves to the muscles, and the terminal axonal branches that innervate the muscle fibres. In the ventral horn, the most medially situated motor neurons innervate the proximal groups of muscles (the axial muscles and the proximal limb muscles) and the most laterally situated motor neurons innervate the distal groups of muscles of the body. Therefore, the **medial groups of motor neurons are involved in postural control**, whereas the **lateral groups of motor neurons are involved in manipulatory (skilled) activities**.

Upper Motor Neuron

The upper motor neurons originate in the motor cortex and other areas in the brain that are involved in the regulation of motor activities, and terminate on the anterior horn cells. The upper motor neurons are classically divided into **two types**: (i) pyramidal fibres (corticospinal tract) and (ii) extrapyramidal fibres. The **pyramidal fibres** are the motor neurons that pass through the pyramid in the medulla, regardless of their cells of origin. The **extrapyramidal fibres** are the neurons that do not pass through the pyramid of the medulla. The **corticospinal tract** is synonymous with the pyramidal tract for all clinical purposes. The extrapyramidal tracts are rubrospinal, vestibulospinal, reticulospinal and tectospinal tracts. Strictly speaking, some of the fibres of the pyramidal system do not pass through the pyramid and some of the fibres of the extrapyramidal system pass through the pyramids. Therefore, from the physiological point of view, the upper motor neurons are better divided into the **medial system pathways** and **the lateral system pathways**.

The lateral system

The upper motor neurons of the lateral system descend in the lateral funiculus of the spinal cord and terminate directly or indirectly on the laterally placed motor neurons in the anterior horns. This includes **two major pathways**: the **lateral corticospinal tract** and the **rubrospinal tract**. As the lateral system fibres terminate on the lateral group of motor neurons (in the anterior horn) that innervate the distal group of muscles of the body, they are primarily involved in **regulation of skilled voluntary activities**.

The medial system

The upper motor neurons of the medial system descend in the ventral funiculus of the spinal cord and terminate mostly indirectly on the medially placed motor neurons in the anterior horns. This includes the **vestibulospinal** (lateral and medial), **reticulospinal** (medullary and pontine), **tectospinal** and **interstitiospinal** tracts. As the medial system fibres terminate on the medial group of motor neurons in the anterior horn cells that innervate the proximal group of muscles of the body, they are primarily involved in **regulation of posture and equilibrium**.

Corticospinal tracts

Origin, course and termination   The fibres of the corticospinal tract originate in the fifth layer of the motor cortex. Fibres pass through the posterior limb of the internal capsule (Fig. 57.1) where all the fibres coming from different areas of the motor cortex converge into a narrow space (therefore a *lesion in the internal capsule causes maximum motor deficit*). Then the fibres descend down through the midbrain and pons into the medulla where they form the pyramid. In the medulla, 80–90 per cent of the fibres after passing through the pyramid, cross over (decussate) to the opposite side and then enter the contralateral spinal cord to form the **lateral corticospinal tract**. These upper motor neurons enter the anterior grey horn of the spinal cord and project directly onto the lower motor neurons. Fibres of this tract have monosynaptic connections with the motor neurons that **innervate the distal groups of muscles**. The remaining 10–20 per cent of the fibres in the medulla do not cross over to the opposite side. They descend down ipsilaterally in the same side of the spinal cord as the **anterior corticospinal tract** and cross over to the opposite side only at the segmental level (at the segments in the spinal cord where they innervate the muscles through the lower motor neurons). These fibres project onto the lower motor neurons (mostly indirectly) through interneurons that *supply the proximal groups of muscles*.

Functions

1. The lateral corticospinal tract conveys the information from the motor cortex to the distal group of skeletal muscles on the opposite side of the body, which coordinates and regulates skilled voluntary movement.

2. The anterior corticospinal tract conveys the information from the motor cortex to the proximal group of skeletal muscles on the opposite side of the body, which coordinates and regulates the movement of the axial skeleton (that is involved in the control of posture).

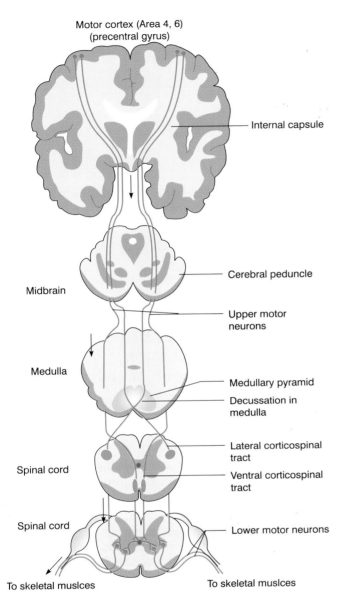

Motor cortex (Area 4, 6)
(precentral gyrus)

Internal capsule

Midbrain

Cerebral peduncle

Upper motor
neurons

Medulla

Medullary pyramid

Decussation in
medulla

Lateral corticospinal
tract

Spinal cord

Ventral corticospinal
tract

Spinal cord

Lower motor neurons

To skeletal musices

To skeletal musices

Fig. 57.1 Pyramidal (corticospinal) tract.

Rubrospinal tract

Origin, course and termination This tract originates from the red nucleus in the midbrain, which receives input from the motor cortex, basal ganglia and cerebellum. The fibres cross over to the opposite side in the midbrain and descend down in the contralateral spinal cord to terminate on the lower motor neurons in the anterior horn, which innervate the distal groups of muscles.

Functions This tract conveys motor impulses from the red nucleus to the skeletal muscles on the opposite side of the body, which govern precise, discrete movements of the hands and feet (skilled voluntary movements).

Vestibulospinal tracts The vestibulospinal tract conveys motor impulses from the vestibular nuclei, which receive inputs regarding head movement from the vestibular apparatus in the inner ear, to the skeletal muscles on the same side of the body, which are involved in maintenance of balance and posture. The **lateral vestibulospinal tract** (LVST) originates from the Deiter's nucleus that receives input from the utricles and saccules and traverses the length of the spinal cord. The LVST is involved in the adjustment of body posture in relation to linear acceleration. The **medial vestibulospinal tract** (MVST) originates from the medial and the descending vestibular nuclei, which receive input from the semicircular canals, and traverses up to the midthoracic level. This tract adjusts body posture (head, neck and trunk movement) in relation to angular or rotational acceleration.

Reticulospinal tracts The reticulospinal tracts originate from the reticular formation, traverse through the entire length of the spinal cord and convey information to the proximal group of muscles. Therefore, these tracts are involved in the regulation of posture. The **medullary reticulospinal tract** facilitates flexor reflexes, inhibits extensor reflexes and decreases muscle tone. The **pontine reticulospinal tract** inhibits flexor reflexes, facilitates extensor reflexes and increases the tone of antigravity muscles. Therefore, pontine RST is the most important tract involved in the **control of posture**.

Tectospinal tract

Origin, course and termination The fibres in the tectospinal tract originate from the superior colliculus and immediately cross over to the opposite side. This tract descends down only up to the midcervical segments in the spinal cord and innervates the muscles of the head and neck.

Function The tectospinal tract conveys impulses from the superior colliculus to the skeletal muscles on the opposite side of the body, which are involved in the movement of the head and neck in response to visual stimuli. Therefore, it controls **visually guided head movements**.

The Motor Areas in the Brain

The motor areas in the brain include the **cortical motor areas** and the other areas that are involved in regulation of motor activities. Corticospinal tracts (the pyramidal tract) arise from cortical motor areas. The other descending motor pathways, especially extrapyramidal tracts, do not directly arise from the cortical motor areas, rather they originate from the brainstem areas that receive inputs from the basal ganglia, cerebellum and motor cortex. Therefore, apart from the cortical motor areas, the important motor areas in the brain are the **basal ganglia** and **cerebellum**.

The cortical motor areas

The cortical motor areas in the brain include the areas in the cortex that on stimulation produce motor activities. This includes the **primary motor cortex** (area 4), **premotor cortex** (lateral portion of the area 6), the **supplementary motor cortex** (medial portion of the area 6), the **somatosensory cortex** (areas 3, 1, 2), and the **posterior parietal cortex** (areas 5, 7). About 60 per cent of the fibres in the corticospinal tract come from motor areas (primary motor cortex, premotor cortex and supplementary motor cortex) whereas the remaining 40 per cent originate from the sensory areas in the cortex.

Basal ganglia

The basal ganglia are subcortical structures that consist of several groups of nuclei in each cerebral hemisphere, which include the neostriatum (caudate nucleus and putamen), globus pallidus, subthalamic nucleus and substantia nigra. The basal ganglia receive inputs from the cortex and thalamus and project back to the cortex via the thalamus. They are involved in the control of posture and movement, especially in the initiation, planning, programming and smoothening of movement.

Cerebellum

The cerebellum receives inputs from the vestibular apparatus, the spinal cord and the cortex. It influences the lower motor neuron activities indirectly via its projection to the vestibular nuclei, the brainstem areas and the cortex. The **vestibulocerebellum** (archicerebellum) is involved in the maintenance of equilibrium and balance, the **spinocerebellum** (paleocerebellum) is involved in smoothening and coordination of movement, and the **corticocerebellum** (neocerebellum) is involved in the planning and programming of movement.

METHODS

Methods of Examination of Motor Functions

Principle

The integrity of the motor system is assessed by examining the size, tone and strength of the muscles, and by evaluating the reflex response of the muscle to stretch, and coordination of movement.

Requirements

1. Measuring tape (Fig. 57.2)
2. Knee hammer (Fig. 57.3)

Procedure

The following aspects of motor functions are assessed while examining the motor system:
1. Bulk of muscles
2. Tone of muscles
3. Strength of muscles
4. Reflexes
5. Coordination of movement
6. Gait
7. Involuntary movement (if present)

Bulk of muscles

The bulk of the muscles can be easily estimated by **inspection and palpation**.
1. Ask the subject to sit on a stool or lie down on a couch comfortably and remove all his clothing.
2. **Inspect the muscle mass** of all parts of the body and note if there is any wasting (atrophy) or hypertrophy of any particular group of muscles.
3. **Palpate the muscle** to assess the consistency.

> **Note:** Wasted or **atrophic muscles** are not only smaller, but also softer and flabbier than normal muscles, especially when they are contracted. **Hypertrophic muscles** are usually firm in consistency. If muscle wasting is associated with fibrosis as is in polymyositis, the muscles are hard to palpate and inelastic.

4. Compare the bulk of the muscles of both sides of the body.

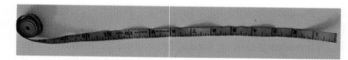

Fig. 57.2   Measuring tape.

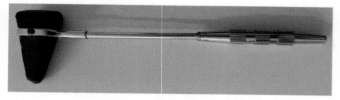

Fig. 57.3   Knee hammer.

5. Measure the **midarm** (Fig. 57.4A) and **midforearm** (Fig. 57.4B) circumference in the upper limbs, and **midthigh** (Fig. 57.4C) and **midcalf** (Fig. 57.4D) circumference in the lower limbs of both sides with a measuring tape.

> **Note:** Measurement of the girth of the muscles is the best way of estimating the bulk of the muscle.

Tone of muscles

Tone is a **state of partial contraction** of muscles. Clinically, tone means the **resistance of the muscle to passive stretching**. It is estimated by handling and passively moving the parts of the body.

1. Ask the subject to relax completely.
2. Passively move different parts of the body at various joints and try to feel the **degree of resistance encountered** during each passive movement (Fig. 57.5).

> **Note:** The degree of resistance offered by the muscle during passive movement indicates the state of tone. This is perceived by **feeling the resistance to movement**, not by palpating the muscle. For example, passive flexion of the forearm stretches the triceps muscle and passive extension of the forearm stretches the biceps muscle. Therefore flexion assesses the tone of the triceps and extension assesses the tone of the biceps muscle. The tone may be normal, decreased (**hypotonia**) or increased (**hypertonia**). **Do not palpate muscle** while making passive flexion movement for eliciting tone, as handling of muscle could stimulate muscle sensory receptors and alter muscle tone due to interference.

3. Assess and compare the tone of muscles of both sides of the body simultaneously.

Strength of muscles

The strength of muscles is better estimated by **active movement against resistance**.

1. Ask the subject to perform a movement of any part of the body (say flexion of the forearm)

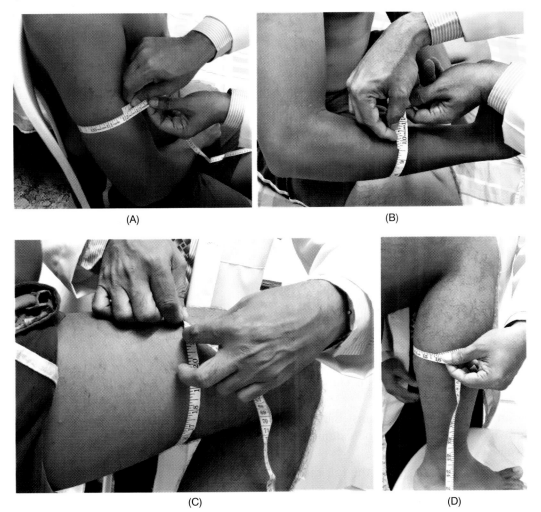

(A)　　　　　　　　　　　　　(B)

(C)　　　　　　　　　　　　　(D)

Fig. 57.4　Measurement of the circumference of the various parts of the limbs. A: Midarm; B: Midforearm; C: Midthigh; D: Midcalf.

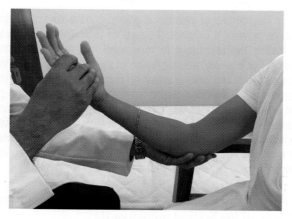

Fig. 57.5   Eliciting the tone of biceps muscle by passively extending at the elbow joint. Note that the examiner appreciates the feeling of resistance offered to passive extension movement, not by actively palpating the muscle. The limb is supported to ensure and facilitate passive movement.

and you oppose the movement actively (oppose flexion of the forearm by placing your palm on his forearm and giving maximum resistance to stop flexion).

> **Note:** The strength of the subject is assessed by comparing with the strength of the examiner. Age, sex and build of the person should be kept in mind while comparing the strength.

2. Compare strength of the same group of muscles of the other side simultaneously.
3. Test the strength of muscles of the lower limbs, upper limbs and the trunk of the body.

Grading of the strength of the muscles

Strength or weakness of muscles is graded into six degrees by the Indian Medical Research Council Scale.

Grade 0 : Complete paralysis (no contraction)

Grade 1 : A flicker of contraction only (without any resultant movement of any limb or joint)

Grade 2 : The muscle can make movement only when the opposing force of gravity is eliminated by appropriate positioning

Grade 3 : The limb can be moved against the force of gravity, but not against the examiner's resistance

Grade 4 : The muscle is able to make the full range of normal movement, but can be overcome (by resistance) to a variable extent

Grade 5 : Normal power

Testing the strength of muscles of the upper limbs

Interossei and lumbricals

First dorsal interosseous   Ask the patient to abduct his index finger against resistance; while doing so, this muscle becomes prominent and the contraction of the muscle can be felt (Fig. 57.6).

Dorsal interossei   These are abductors of the fingers. Therefore, their power can be tested by asking the patient to abduct the fingers against resistance.

Palmar interossei   These are the adductors of the fingers. These are tested by placing a paper or card between the fingers and trying to pull out the paper/card (Fig. 57.7).

Lumbricals   These are tested by asking the patient to flex his metacarpophalangeal joints and to extend his distal interphalangeal joints. This can be done by asking him to hold a pen. While the terminal phalanx of the thumb is being apposed against the terminal

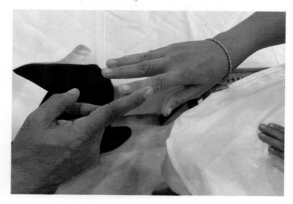

Fig. 57.6   Procedure of testing the strength of the first dorsal interosseous.

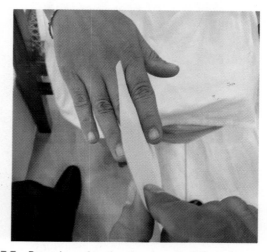

Fig. 57.7   Procedure of testing the strength of the palmar interossei.

phalanx of any other finger, the examiner may try to dislodge the pen by force. This gives a combined test for opponens pollicis and lumbricals (Fig. 57.8).

Flexors of the fingers   Flexors of the fingers are flexor pollicis longus, flexor pollicis brevis, flexor digitorum superficialis and flexor digitorum profundus. These are tested by asking the subject to squeeze your index and middle finger (Fig. 57.9).

Flexors of the wrist   Flexors of the wrist are flexor carpi radialis, flexor pollicis brevis, and palmaris longus. Ask the subject to bring the tips of his fingers towards the front of the forearm so as to touch the crease on the front of the wrist joint (Fig. 57.10).

Extensors of the wrist   These are extensor carpi radialis and extensor carpi ulnaris. Ask the subject to flex the fingers in the form of a fist and the hand is held with the palm downwards. Then hold the wrist joint firmly

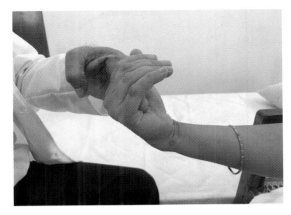

Fig. 57.10   Procedure of testing the strength of the flexors of the wrist.

and ask the subject to extend the wrist joint against resistance (Fig. 57.11).

Brachioradialis   Place the arm midway between the prone and the supine position. Then ask the subject to bend the forearm upwards. Oppose the movement by grasping the hand. The brachioradialis becomes prominent (Fig. 57.12).

Biceps   Ask the subject to lift up the forearm against resistance offered by grasping the hand or wrist with the forearm in full supination. The biceps becomes prominent as it contracts (Fig. 57.13).

Triceps   Ask the subject to straighten out his forearm while the examiner tries to keep it flexed by passive resistance (Fig. 57.14).

Supraspinatus   Ask the subject to keep his arm by the side of the body and then direct the subject to lift it straight outward at right angles to his side. The first 30° angle

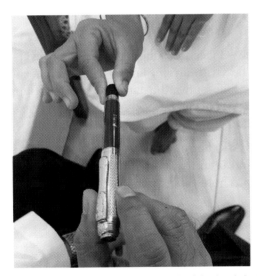

Fig. 57.8   Procedure of testing the strength of the lumbricals.

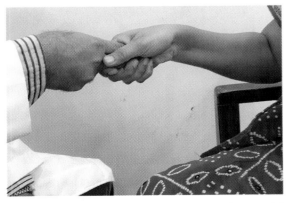

Fig. 57.9   Procedure of testing the strength of the flexors of the fingers.

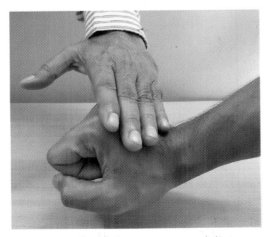

Fig. 57.11   Procedure of testing the strength of the extensors of the wrist.

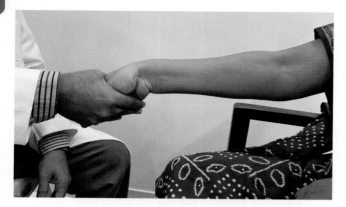

Fig. 57.12   Procedure of testing the strength of the brachioradialis. Note the prominence of the brachioradialis.

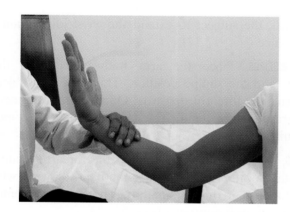

Fig. 57.13   Procedure of testing the strength of the biceps. Note the prominence of the biceps.

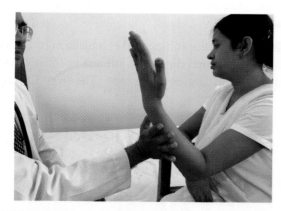

Fig. 57.14   Procedure of testing the strength of the triceps. Note the prominence of the triceps.

of movement is carried out by the supraspinatus (Fig. 57.15). The remaining 60° angle is produced by the deltoid.

Deltoid   It can be tested along with the supraspinatus. The subject is asked to make forward and backward movements of the abducted arm at a 45° angle against

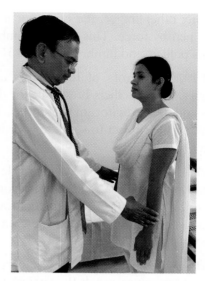

Fig. 57.15   Procedure of testing the strength of the supraspinatus.

resistance (the anterior and posterior fibres of the deltoid help to draw the abducted arm forward and backward, respectively) (Fig. 57.16).

Infraspinatus   Place the subject's elbow by his side with a forearm flexed to a right angle, then ask the subject to rotate the limb outward against the resistance applied to the middle of the outer aspect of the forearm (Fig. 57.17). Contraction of the muscle can be seen and felt.

Pectorals   Ask the subject to stretch his arm out in front of him and then to clap his hands while the examiner attempts to hold them apart (Fig. 57.18).

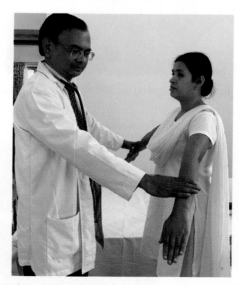

Fig. 57.16   Procedure of testing the strength of the deltoid. Note the prominence of the triceps. Note also that when arms are abducted at a 45° angle, resistance is given for forward and backward movements, and also for lifting them.

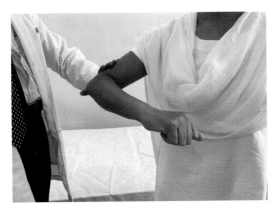

Fig. 57.17   Procedure of testing the strength of the infraspinatus.

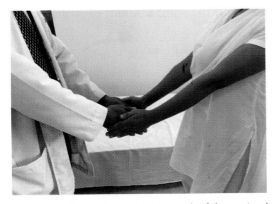

Fig. 57.18   Procedure of testing the strength of the pectorals.

Serratus anterior   If the muscle is paralysed, the subject will be unable to elevate his arm above a right angle when asked to do so. Paralysis of this muscle causes winging of the scapula. Therefore, look for 'winged scapula'. The deformity becomes more prominent

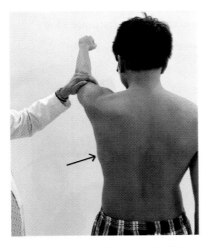

Fig. 57.19   Procedure of testing the strength of the serratus anterior. Note that elevating the arm above right angle makes the serratus anterior prominent (the tip of the black arrow points to the prominence of the serratus anterior).

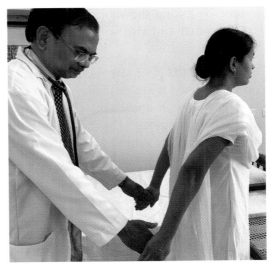

Fig. 57.20   Procedure of testing the strength of the latissimus dorsi.

when the patient is asked to push forward against the wall with both hands (Fig. 57.19).

Latissimus dorsi   The subject is asked to clap his hands behind his back while the examiner (standing behind the subject), offers passive resistance to the downward and backward movement (Fig. 57.20).

Testing the strength of muscles of the trunk

Abdominal muscles   The weakness of the muscles of the abdomen is detected by observing the subject's inability to raise himself in bed without the aid of his arms. Babinski's rising-up sign is also checked.

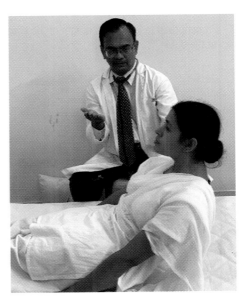

Fig. 57.21   Procedure of testing the strength of the abdominal muscles. Note that the subject rises without using the hand.

This is done by asking the subject to lie on his back with legs extended and rise without using his hands (Fig. 57.21).

Erector spinae and muscles of the back   Ask the subject to lie down on his face and try to raise his head from the bed by extending the neck and back. The examiner may provide passive resistance (Fig. 57.22). If the back muscles are healthy, the subject will be able to raise her head and muscles will stand out prominently during this effort.

Testing the strength of muscles of the lower limb

Intrinsic muscles of the foot   It is difficult to examine the strength of intrinsic muscles of the foot (lumbricals and interossei). If the interossei are weakened or paralysed, claw-foot develops.

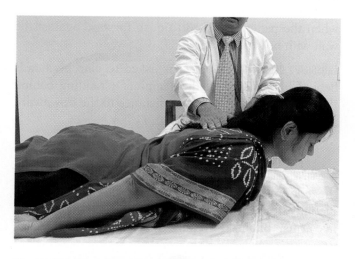

Fig. 57.22   Procedure of testing the strength of the erector spinae and muscles of the back.

Dorsiflexor and plantar flexors of the feet and toes   Dorsiflexors are peronei, and plantar flexors are tibialis posterior, gastrocnemius and soleus. These are tested by asking the patient to to dorsiflex (Fig. 57.23A) or plantarflex (Fig. 57.23B) the part against resistance. The observer should try to fix the ankle or apply resistance against the patient's movement.

Evertors and invertors of the foot   Evertors (Fig. 57.24A) are peronei, and invertors (Fig. 57.24B) are tibialis anterior and tibialis posterior.

Extensors of the knee   Quadriceps are the extensors of the knee. Bend the patient's knee and then pressing with your hand on the shin, ask him to straighten his limb (Fig. 57.25).

Flexors of the knee   These are biceps femoris, semitendinosus and semimembranosus. Raise the straightened lower limb, supporting the thigh with your left hand and holding the ankle with your right hand. Then ask the subject to bend his knees (Fig. 57.26).

Extensors of the thigh   Gluteus maximus is the extensor of the thigh. Lift the subject's foot off the bed when the knee is extended and ask him to depress the limb against resistance (Fig. 57.27A).

Flexors of the thigh   These are the iliopsoas and the tensor fascia lata. In the extended leg, ask the subject to raise his lower limb against resistance, without bending the limb at knee joints (Fig. 57.27B).

Adductors of the thigh   These are the adductor longus, adductor brevis, adductor magnus and gracilis. Abduct the lower limb and then ask the subject to bring it back to the midline against resistance (Fig. 57.28A).

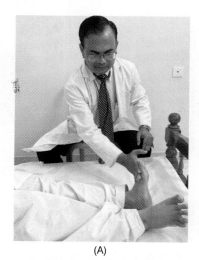
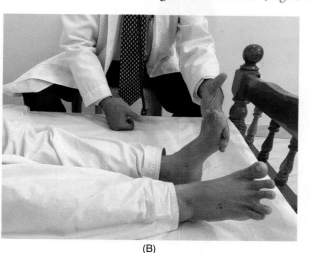

(A)   (B)

Fig. 57.23   Procedure of testing the strength of muscles of the feet and toes. (A) Dorsiflexors; (B) Plantar flexors.

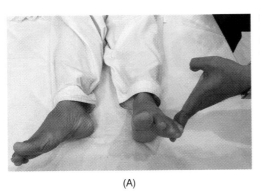
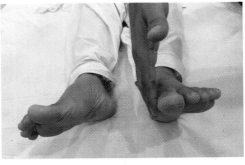

Fig. 57.24   Procedure of testing the strength of the muscles of the feet. (A) Evertors; (B) Invertors.

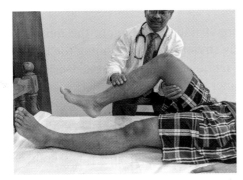

Fig. 57.25   Procedure of testing the strength of extensors of the knee. Note that the subject straightens the leg against resistance from the bent position of the knee.

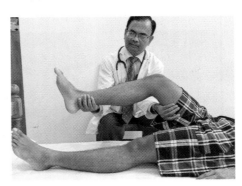

Fig. 57.26   Procedure of testing the strength of flexors of the knee. Note that the subject bends his knees of the lifted and straightened limb against resistance given at the ankle.

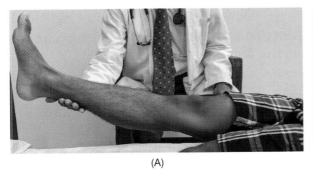
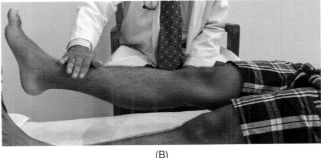

Fig. 57.27   Demonstration of the strength of extensors and flexors of the thigh. (A) For extensors of the thigh, the fully extended limb with extension at the knee joint is brought down from a little height by the subject against resistance given at the ankle from below by the examiner; (B) For flexors of the thigh, the fully extended limb is raised by the subject against resistance given at the ankle from above by the examiner.

Abductors of the thigh   These are the gluteus medius and gluteus minimus. Bring the lower limb to the midline and then ask the subject to move it outward against resistance (Fig. 57.28B).

Rotators of the thigh or hip   These are the gluteus medius, gluteus minimus, obturator externus and obturator internus. With the subject's lower limb extended on the bed, ask the subject to rotate the limb outwards (Fig. 57.29A) and inwards (Fig. 57.29B) against resistance.

Reflexes

Clinically, reflexes are of **three types**: tendon or deep reflexes, superficial reflexes, and visceral or sphincteric reflexes.

Tendon or deep reflexes

The **contraction of the muscle in response to a sudden stretch** produced by striking the tendon (with a knee hammer) is called a tendon reflex. Tendon reflexes are **stretch reflexes** because they are elicited by stretching

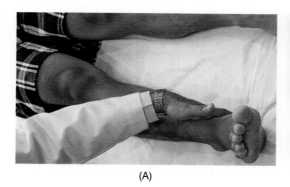
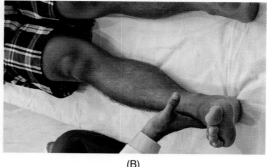

(A)   (B)

Fig. 57.28   (A) Demonstration of the strength of adductors; (B) Demonstration of the strength of abductors of the thigh. Note that in the fully extended limb, the subject adducts and abducts the whole limb against resistance given at the ankle from the side by the examiner.

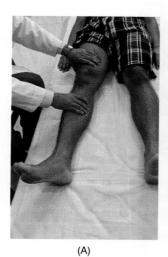
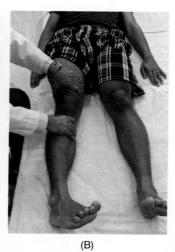

(A)   (B)

Fig. 57.29   Demonstration of the strength of the rotators of the thigh and hip. (A) For outward rotators, the subject rotates the entire limb in the outward direction in the fully extended position of the limb against resistance given by the examiner to prevent this outward rotation; (B) For inward rotators, the subject rotates the entire limb in the inward direction in the fully extended position of the limb against resistance given by the examiner to prevent this inward rotation.

the muscle. These stretch reflexes are **monosynaptic reflexes**. The tendon reflexes assess the integrity of the afferent and efferent pathways and excitability of the anterior horn cells in the spinal segment of the stretched muscle.

The following **precautions** should be observed for eliciting tendon reflexes:

1. The subject should be completely relaxed.
2. Reassure the subject that the knee hammer is not a harmful instrument and will not cause pain while eliciting reflexes.
3. The subject's limb should be appropriately positioned.

4. Before striking the tendon, the muscle should be lightly stretched by positioning the limb.
5. The tendon should be stroked briskly by a knee hammer making a sudden jerky movement at the wrist joint.
6. The knee hammer should be appropriately held between the thumb and the index finger, so that it swings freely in an arc, yet is controlled in its direction.
7. The homologous reflex on the opposite side should always be tested immediately for comparison.
8. If the reflexes are not elicited, the reinforcement technique (Jendrassik's maneuver) should be used.

Grading of the tendon reflexes   Tendon reflexes can be graded into **five degrees** as given below.

Grade 0 : Absent (no response)
Grade 1 : Present but diminished (as a normal supinator jerk)
Grade 2 : Brisk (as a normal knee jerk)
Grade 3 : Very brisk (hyperactive)
Grade 4 : Clonus

Note: Normal supinator jerk is less than average and normal knee jerk is brisker than average reflexes.

Biceps jerk (C5,6)

1. Ask the subject to relax.
2. Flex the elbow of the subject and place his forearm in a semi-pronated position and support with your hand (Fig. 57.30), with subject in sitting position (Fig. 57.31) or in supine position (Fig. 57.32) or by placing his elbow on his abdomen, with the subject in the lying position on the bed (Fig. 57.33).
3. Place your thumb firmly on the biceps tendon.

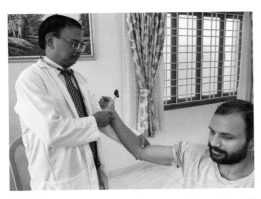

Fig. 57.30 Procedure to hold the forearm of the subject for eliciting biceps reflex. Note that the elbow of the subject has to be flexed and his forearm to be placed in a semi-pronated position, and you support him with your hand. Ensure that the subject's upper limb is fully relaxed with your support.

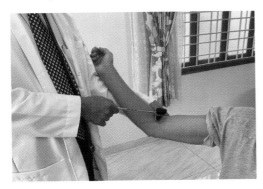

Fig. 57.31 Demonstration of biceps jerk in sitting or standing posture. Note that the subject rests his forearm on the forearm of the examiner with elbow joint flexed. The examiner strikes the biceps tendon by striking his own thumb (placed and pressed on the tendon), using the narrow end of the knee hammer.

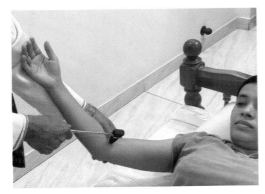

Fig. 57.32 Elicitation of biceps jerk with subject in the lying position with limb outstretched and supported.

4. Strike your thumb with the help of the pointed end of the knee hammer so that the biceps tendon stretches by striking the thumb.

5. Observe the contraction of the biceps muscle and the flexion at the elbow.

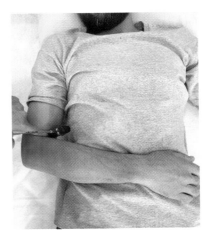

Fig. 57.33 Demonstration of biceps jerk in supine posture. Note that the subject rests his forearm on his abdomen with elbow flexed at an angle of 90°. The examiner strikes the biceps tendon by striking his own thumb (placed and pressed on the tendon), using the narrow end of the knee hammer.

6. Elicit biceps jerk of the other limb (Fig. 57.34) and compare.

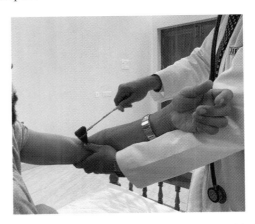

Fig. 57.34 Elicitation of biceps reflex of the opposite side (left side).

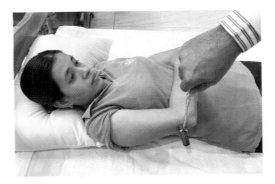

Fig. 57.35 Demonstration of triceps jerk in supine posture. Note that the subject rests his forearm on his abdomen with elbow flexed at an angle of 90°. The examiner strikes the triceps tendon by using the broad end of the knee hammer.

Triceps jerk (C6,7)

1. Flex the subject's arm at the elbow and allow the forearm to rest on his abdomen (Fig. 57.35) or be supported by your hand (Fig. 57.36).
2. Tap the triceps tendon directly above the olecranon.

> **Note:** Take care not to strike the belly of the triceps muscle.

3. Observe the contraction of the triceps muscle and extension at the elbow.
4. Elicit the triceps jerk of the other side and compare (Fig. 57.37).

Supinator or brachioradialis jerk (C5,6)

1. Hold the hand of the subject in sitting position (Fig. 57.38), supine position (Fig. 57.39) or allow the forearm of the subject to rest on his abdomen in supine position (Fig. 57.40) and slightly stretch the brachioradialis muscle by laterally bending the hand in the opposite direction.

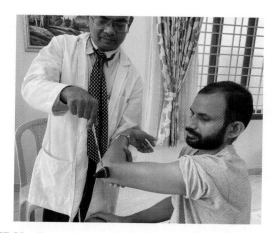

Fig. 57.36 Demonstration of triceps jerk in sitting or standing posture. Note that the forearm of the subject rests on the forearm of the examiner with his elbow joint flexed at 90°. The examiner strikes the triceps tendon by using the broad end of the knee hammer.

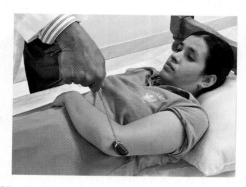

Fig. 57.37 Elicitation of triceps jerk of the opposite side (left side of the subject).

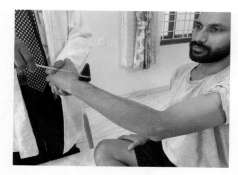

Fig. 57.38 Demonstration of supinator jerk in the sitting or standing posture. Note that the examiner holds the hand of the subject and slightly dorsiflexes it and then strikes the brachioradialis tendon at the wrist by using the broad end of the knee hammer.

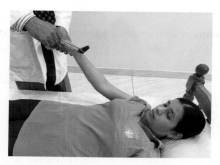

Fig. 57.39 Elicitation of supinator jerk with subject in supine position.

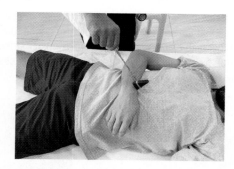

Fig. 57.40 Demonstration of supinator jerk in the supine posture. Note that the subject rests his forearm on his abdomen and the examiner strikes the brachioradialis tendon at the wrist by using the broad end of the knee hammer.

2. With the help of a knee hammer, strike the radius 1–2 inches above the wrist over its styloid process.
3. Observe the flexion at the elbow and supination of the forearm.
4. Elicit the supinator jerk of the other side (Fig. 57.41) and compare.

Knee jerk (L2, 3, 4)

It can be tested with the subject either in the supine or sitting position.

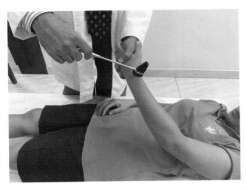

Fig. 57.41   Elicitation of supinator jerk of the opposite side (left side of the subject).

In the supine position (Figs. 57.42, 57.43 and 57.44)

1. Expose the part (up to the upper thigh)
2. Pass your forearm under the knee to be tested and place your hand on the opposite knee (the knee to be tested should rest on the dorsum of your wrist and forearm).
3. Semiflex the knee and lift your hand slightly so that the weight of the knee rests on your hand.

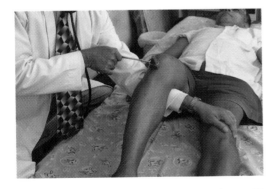

Fig. 57.42   Demonstration of knee jerk in the supine position. Note that the examiner supports the leg to be examined by placing his hand below the leg in such a way that he lifts it with the help of the other leg.

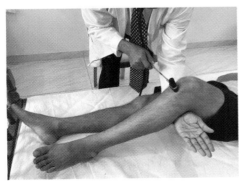

Fig. 57.43   Elicitation of knee jerk of the left side, in supine position, the examiner lifting the leg using his forearm as shown.

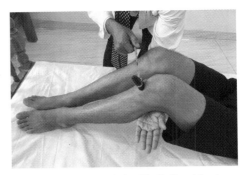

Fig. 57.44   Elicitation of knee jerk of both the sides in one lifting, in supine position.

4. Strike the patellar tendon directly with the help of a knee hammer (by using the narrow end of the hammer).
5. Observe the contraction of the quadriceps and the brief extension at the knee.
6. Elicit the knee jerk of the opposite side and compare.

In the sitting position (Figs. 57.45 and 57.46)

1. Ask the subject to sit over the edge of the bed or a stool in such a way that his legs dangle freely from the edge, or ask the subject to keep one knee (the knee to be tested) on the other knee.
2. Ask him to relax completely.
3. Strike the patellar tendon.
4. Observe the contraction of the quadriceps and the extension at the knee joint.

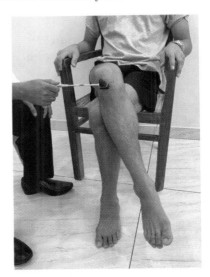

Fig. 57.45   Demonstration of knee jerk in the sitting position. Note that the subject sits on a stool or chair crossing the leg to be examined over the other leg. The examiner strikes the patellar tendon. The legs of the subject should hang freely (should not touch the ground).

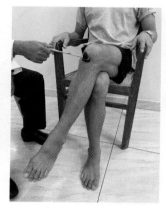

Fig. 57.46 Elicitation of knee jerk of the opposite side (left side of the subject) in sitting position.

Ankle jerk (S1,2)   The ankle jerk can be tested with the subject in the supine, kneeling or prone position.

In the supine position

1. Place the lower limb (to be examined) of the subject on the bed in such a way that it is everted and slightly flexed.
2. With one hand, slightly dorsiflex the foot so as to stretch the Achilles tendon (Fig. 57.47).
3. With the other hand, strike the tendon on its posterior surface (by using the broad end of the knee hammer).
4. Observe for any contraction of calf muscles and plantar flexion of the foot.
5. Elicit the ankle jerk of the other side (Fig. 57.48) and compare.

In the kneeling and prone position

1. Ask the subject to kneel on a chair with feet projecting out (Fig. 57.49A).

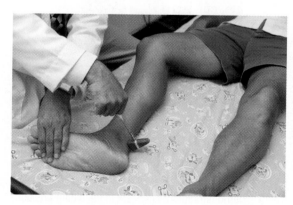

Fig. 57.47 Demonstration of elicitation of ankle jerk in the supine posture. Note that the examiner strikes the Achilles tendon after slightly dorsiflexing the foot. Also note that the knee of the examined leg is flexed to an angle of 120°.

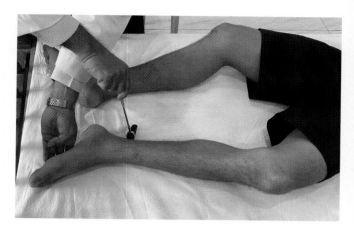

Fig. 57.48 Elicitation of ankle jerk of the opposite side (left side of the subject) in supine position.

2. With the subject in prone position, keep the ankle at right angle and slightly dorsiflex the foot (Fig. 57.49B).
3. Strike the Achilles tendon.
4. Observe for contraction of calf muscles and plantar flexion of the foot.

Jaw jerk

1. Ask the subject to partially open his mouth.
2. Place a finger firmly on his chin (Fig. 57.50).
3. Strike the finger with the help of a knee hammer (using the narrow end of the hammer).
4. Observe for immediate closure of the mouth (due to contraction of the elevators of the jaw).

Jendrassik's maneuver

This is performed by asking the subject to make a strong voluntary muscular effort using following methods:

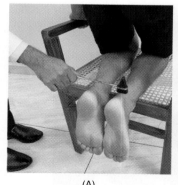
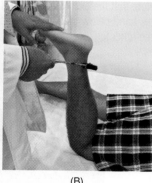

(A)   (B)

Fig. 57.49 Demonstration of ankle jerk. (A) In kneeling posture; (B) In prone posture. Note that the subject kneels on a chair or lies down on the bed in prone posture with knee bent at right angle and the examiner strikes the Achilles tendon. Slight dorsiflexion of the foot may be needed if ankle is not at right angle.

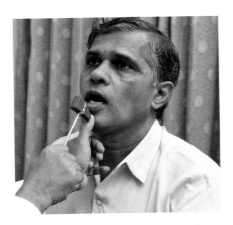

Fig. 57.50 Demonstration of jaw jerk. Note that the examiner strikes the thumb placed on the chin of the subject (subject partially opens his mouth).

1. While testing the reflexes of the lower limb, ask the subject to hook the fingers of two hands together and then pull them apart (against one another) as hard as possible (Fig. 57.51).
2. While testing the reflexes of the upper limb, ask the subject to clench his teeth or to make a fist in the other hand (Fig. 57.52).

> **Note:** Jendrassik's maneuver works by increasing the excitability of the anterior horn cells and by increasing the sensitivity of the muscle spindle primary sensory endings to stretch by increasing the gamma fusimotor discharge.

Superficial reflexes

The superficial reflexes are elicited by stimulating the cutaneous receptors. The stimulation of an area of the skin by scratching results in contraction of certain

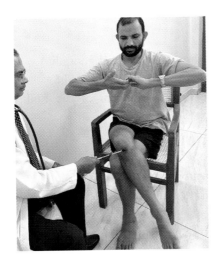

Fig. 57.51 Demonstration of Jendrassik's maneuver. Note that the subject pulls apart the fingers of both the hands hooked against each other, during which the examiner elicits the jerk.

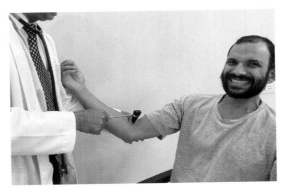

Fig. 57.52 Jendrassik's maneuver for upper limbs. Note that subject clenches his teeth firmly while the examiner elicits the reflex.

muscles supplied by the same spinal segment. These reflexes are polysynaptic reflexes. Superficial reflexes are of two types, spinally mediated and cranially mediated. The *chief superficial reflexes of spinal origin* are:

1. Plantar reflex
2. Cremasteric reflex
3. Bulbocavernosus reflex
4. Anal reflex
5. Abdominal reflex
6. Scapular reflex

Superficial reflexes of cranial origin are:

1. Conjunctival reflex (*refer* Fig. 55.9A)
2. Corneal reflex (*refer* Fig. 55.9B)
3. Pupillary reflexes (light and accommodation reflex)
4. Palatal reflex (described under 10th Cranial Nerve in Chapter 55). *Refer* Fig. 55.7 and Fig. 55.8.

Plantar reflex (L5 S1)

1. Ask the subject to lie down on the couch.
2. Partially flex the lower limb and rotate it externally.
3. With one (left) hand, grasp the leg just above the ankle joint.
4. Ask the subject to relax completely.
5. In the other hand, with the help of a pointed object (pointed metallic portion of the knee hammer or a pointed key) gently scratch the outer edge of the sole of the foot from the heel towards the little toe and then medially across the metatarsus towards the ball of the great toe (Fig. 57.53).
6. Observe for the plantar response.

> **Note:** The plantar response may be a flexor plantar response or an extensor plantar response. The **flexor plantar response** is characterised by inversion and dorsiflexion of the ankle with flexion of all the toes at the metatarsus. This is normally present in healthy subjects. The **extensor plantar response** is

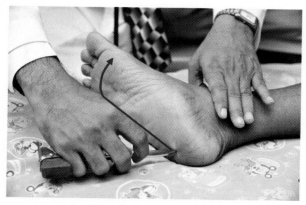

Fig. 57.53   Demonstration of plantar reflex. Note that a pointed object is used to stroke or scratch on the lateral aspect of the sole in the direction of the arrow depicted in the figure.

characterised by dorsiflexion of the great toe and abduction or fanning of other toes with dorsiflexion of the ankle. It is found in patients with corticospinal tract lesions and is a pathognomonic feature of upper motor neuron paralysis. This abnormal response is also called **Babinski's sign** as it was first described by Babinski. It is also normally seen in newborns and infants.

Cremasteric reflex (L1,2)   This is elicited only in male subjects.

1. Expose the part (genitalia and upper thigh).
2. Lightly scratch the inner aspect of the upper part of the thigh.
3. Observe the elevation of the testicle on that side and the contraction of the dartos muscle as evidenced by increase in wrinkling of the skin of the scrotum.
4. Elicit the cremasteric reflex of the opposite side.

Abdominal reflex (T7–12)

1. Ask the subject to lie down in the supine position.
2. Expose the abdomen fully.
3. Ask him to relax completely.
4. Stroke lightly but briskly each side of the abdomen above and below the umbilicus, with a key or a pencil or the pointed metallic end of the knee hammer (Fig. 57.54), from the outer aspect towards the midline (Fig. 57.55).
5. Observe the contraction of the abdominal muscles after every stroke as evidenced by the deviation of the umbilicus towards the stimulus.

Note: It is often impossible to elicit abdominal reflexes in obese, elderly and anxious patients and in multiparous women.

Bulbocavernosus reflex (S3,4)

This is elicited only in male subjects.

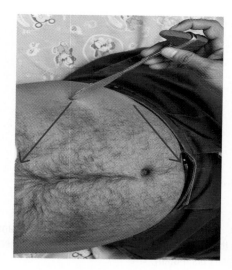

Fig. 57.54   Note that with the pointed metallic end of the knee hammer, the surface of the abdomen is scratched from the outer aspect towards the midline in the direction of the arrow.

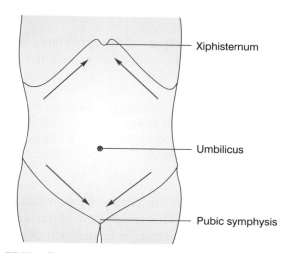

Fig. 57.55   Site and direction of stimulation for elicitation of abdominal reflex.

1. Expose the part (external genitalia).
2. Pinch the dorsum of glans penis.
3. Observe the contraction of the bulbocavernosus muscle.

Anal reflex (S3,4)

1. Expose the anal region.
2. Ask the subject to relax completely.
3. Stroke or scratch the skin near the anus.
4. Observe the contraction of the anal sphincter.

Scapular reflex (C5–8, T1)

1. Expose the upper portion of the back.
2. Stroke the skin in the interscapular region.
3. Observe the contraction of the scapular muscles.

Sphincteric reflexes

These reflexes are concerned with swallowing, defecation and micturition. They depend upon complex muscular movement excited by increased tension in the wall of the viscera concerned.

Swallowing   Ask the subject whether he has any difficulty in swallowing (dysphagia). Also ask whether there is any regurgitation of food through the nose. If dysphagia is present, ascertain whether it is predominantly for liquids or solids or both.

Defecation   Ask the subject if he has any problem in passing stools. The subject should also be questioned regarding the presence of normal or abnormal anorectal sensation.

Micturition   The subject should always be asked regarding his bladder habits, and whether he has any problem in controlling or initiating micturition. Retention of urine, incontinence or urgency of micturition should be noted.

Coordination of movement

Coordination of movement means smooth recruitment, interaction and cooperation of muscles or groups of muscles to carry out a precise and definite motor act. Coordination of movement should be tested both in the upper and lower limbs.

In the upper limbs

Finger-nose test

1. Give proper instructions to the subject regarding the test.
2. Ask the subject to touch the tip of his nose with the tip of his index finger from the maximally outstretched hand (Fig. 57.56A), rapidly and repeatedly, first with the eyes open (Fig. 57.56B), and then with the eyes closed (Fig. 57.56C).
3. Observe whether the subject is able to touch his nose every time, especially when done at a little faster speed.
4. Ask him to repeat the test with the other hand (Fig. 57.56D and E).

Finger-finger-nose test   In addition to the procedure of finger-nose test, the subject from the outstretched hand (Fig. 57.57A) first touches the finger of the examiner (Fig. 57.57B) and then the tip of his/her nose (Fig. 57.5C), and does it rapidly and repeatedly. Then repeats the procedure in the other hand (Fig. 57.57D).

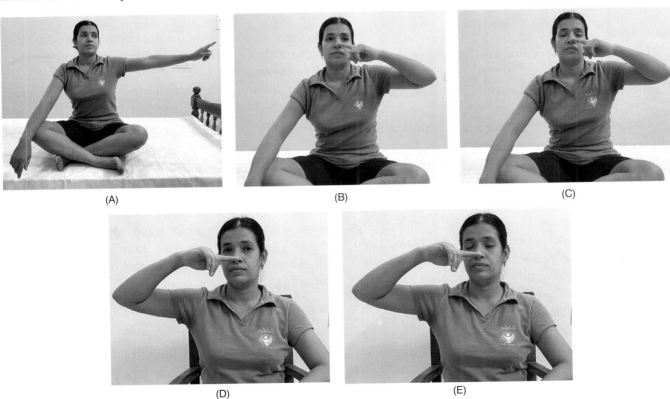

(A)   (B)   (C)

(D)   (E)

Fig. 57.56   Procedure for finger-nose test. (A) The subject is asked to touch the tip of her nose with the tip of her index finger with her maximally outstretched hand; (B) Then she repeats the same rapidly, first with the eyes open;(C) Then she repeats the same with the eyes closed; (D and E) Then she repeats the entire procedure in the other hand.

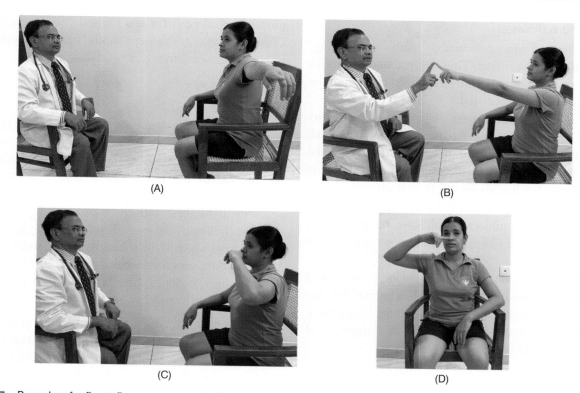

Fig. 57.57   Procedure for finger-finger-nose test. (A) The subject stretches the hand out; (B) With outstretched hand she touches the finger of the examiner; (C) She then touches the tip of her nose. She does it repeatedly in quick succession, with eyes open. (D) Then she repeats the procedure using the other hand.

Making a circle

1. Give proper instructions to the subject regarding the test.
2. Ask the subject to draw a circle in the air with his forefinger.
3. Observe whether the subject is able to draw a circle.
4. Ask him to repeat with the other hand.

Dysdiadokokinesis

Dysdiadokokinesia is the inability to execute rapidly repeated alternate movements. Diadokokinesis can be tested in different ways.

1. Ask the subject to flex his elbow to a right angle and then ask him to perform supination and pronation of his forearm as rapidly as possible, or
2. Ask him to tap the palm with the tips of his fingers as fast as possible in an arhythmic manner, or
3. Ask the subject to clap over the dorsum of one hand with the palm of another hand as quickly as possible. He may be asked to perform this movement alternately on either hand.

Romberg test   Romberg test is the test for body's sense of positioning and proprioception, which requires intactness of dorsal column. But it is used to investigate the cause of loss of motor coordination (ataxia). It is performed to differentiate between incoordination of movement due to cerebellar disease, and sensory system disease. The patient is asked to stand fully erect with both the feet close together and then instructed to close the eyes (Fig. 57.58). If the patient has loss of balance after closing the eyes, Romberg test is positive, which indicates that ataxia is due to sensory deficit (loss of proprioception and sense of body position). If the Romberg test is not positive (patient does not lose balance with eye closure) but the patient loses balance as soon as he is made to stand with eyes open, the ataxia is cerebellar in nature. Romberg test is mainly for assessing coordination of the trunk of the body including the neck and head.

In the lower limbs

Knee-heel test

1. Ask the subject to lie down in the supine position.
2. With the eyes open, ask him to place one heel (Fig. 57.59A) on the opposite knee and then to slide the heel down the shin of his leg towards the ankle (Fig. 57.59B).
3. Ask him to repeat the procedure in quick succession.

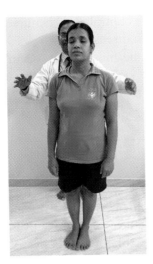

Fig. 57.58 Procedure for Romberg test. The patient is asked to stand with the feet close together. Then he/she is instructed to close the eyes. If the patient has loss of balance after closing the eyes, Romberg test is positive. Note that the examiner stands close to the subject, to support immediately if the patient falls after closing the eyes.

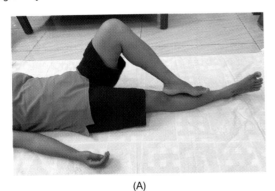

(A)

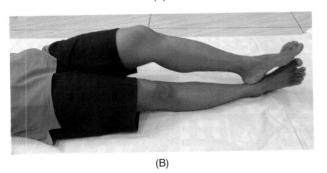

(B)

Fig. 57.59 Procedure for knee-heel test. (A) With eyes open, the subject is asked to place one heel on the opposite knee; (B) Then the subject slides the heel down the shin of his/her leg towards the ankle. He/she repeats the procedure in quick succession, and perform it in the other limb.

4. Observe whether he performs the action properly.
5. Ask him to repeat the procedure with the other limb.

Making a circle

1. Ask the subject to draw a circle in the air with his toes.
2. Observe whether he is able to draw a circle.

Walking

1. Ask the subject to walk on a straight line.
2. Observe whether he is able to walk on a straight line.

Gait

Gait is defined as the **attitude of walking**. It is tested by asking the subject to walk with bare feet on a straight line. Ask him to walk a distance and then to turn round and come back. While the subject is walking observe the following points:

1. Whether he walks at all.
2. If he walks, does he walk in a straight line or does he tend to deviate to one side.
3. If he tends to fall, in what direction?

Involuntary movement

Involuntary movements are not seen normally. In some diseases of the nervous system there are involuntary, unintended movements. Observe whether there is any involuntary movement of any part of the body. If involuntary movements are present, note the type of movement.

DISCUSSION

Bulk of the Muscle

The bulk of the muscle may be normal, decreased (atrophy) or increased (hypertrophy).

Muscle Atrophy

Muscle atrophy is seen in neurological disorders, especially in lower motor neuron disease. Generalised wasting of the muscle occurs in non-neurological conditions like malignancy, diabetes, thyrotoxicosis and tuberculosis. Localised wasting is seen in arthritis or myopathy.

Muscle Hypertrophy

Hypertrophy occurs due to excessive use of muscles as in athletes and gymnasts. It can also occur in some myotonic disorders.

Tone of the Muscle

The tone of the muscle is the state of partial contraction of the muscle. Healthy muscles always exhibit certain degrees of tone. In some diseases, the tone of the muscles increases (hypertonia) and in others the tone of the muscles decreases (hypotonia).

Hypertonia

Hypertonia is a feature of upper motor neuron lesion. Hypertonia manifests as spasticity or rigidity.

Spasticity

Spasticity is a term used to describe a state of increased tone of muscle, which is of the **'clasp-knife' type**. The tone is much more increased in the antigravity muscles, that is, in the flexors of the upper limbs, and extensors and adductors of the lower limbs. Clasp-knife rigidity is seen in pyramidal tract lesion.

Rigidity

Rigidity is seen in all muscles, without any relation to gravity. There are two types of rigidity: lead pipe and cogwheel. This is seen in lesions of extrapyramidal tracts.

Lead pipe rigidity   The resistance to passive movement is uniform throughout the range of movement. It is seen in catatonic states, dementia and Parkinsonism.

Cogwheel rigidity   The resistance to passive movement is seen alternately, that is, there is alternate resistance and relaxation. This is typically seen in diseases of the basal ganglia, particularly in the involvement of the substantia nigra.

Strength of Muscles

If muscle strength is decreased, there is paresis and if there is no strength, there is paralysis.

Hemiplegia means paralysis of one side of the body, especially of the arms and legs, **paraplegia** means paralysis of both legs, **monoplegia** means paralysis of one limb and **quadriplegia** means paralysis of all four limbs.

Hemiplegia is usually seen in *lesions of the corticospinal tract at the level of the internal capsule.* **Paraplegia** is seen in spinal cord lesions below the midthoracic level and **quadriplegia** is seen in spinal cord lesion above the upper thoracic level. **Monoplegia** usually occurs due to lesions of a nerve plexus. **Crossed paralysis** refers to paralysis of the ipsilateral cranial musculature with contralateral hemiplegia. It is usually seen in brainstem disease.

Weakness of the muscle may occur in the absence of paralysis. It occurs due to myasthenia gravis, myopathies and myotonic dystrophy.

Reflexes

Tendon Reflexes

Tendon reflexes are stretch reflexes that are activated in response to a **sudden stretch of the muscle**. These are **monosynaptic reflexes** that are activated by stretching of the muscle spindle, which conveys information via **Ia fibres** directly to the motor neurons in the spinal cord (Fig. 57.60). Stimulation of the a motor neuron causes contraction of the muscle that was stretched. The presence of the tendon reflexes indicates the **integrity of the afferent and efferent pathways**, and of the **excitability of the anterior horn cells** in the spinal segment of the stretched muscles. The tendon reflexes are continuously affected by the activities in the descending (from supraspinal centres) pathways. The higher centres usually inhibit the spinal reflexes. Therefore, the *tendon reflexes are exaggerated in upper motor neuron lesions.* The tendon reflexes are **diminished or absent in lower motor neuron lesions** as there is disruption in the final common pathway.

Gamma motor neurons increase the sensitivity of the muscle spindle to stretch. Therefore, *increased g motor neuron discharge increases the reflex activity.* The γ

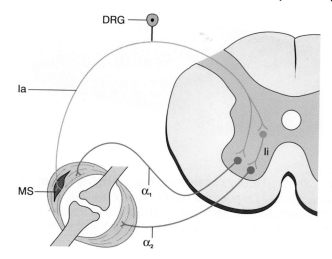

Fig. 57.60   The stretch reflex (DRG: Dorsal root ganglion; MS: Muscle spindle; Ii: Inhibitory interneuron; α_1 and α_2: Motor neurons to agonist and antagonist muscle respectively; Ia: Ia afferents).

motor neurons are usually under the inhibitory influence of supraspinal inputs. Therefore, a lesion of the upper motor neuron results in exaggeration of deep reflexes.

Superficial Reflexes

The superficial reflexes are polysynaptic and involve many centres in the neuraxis. These are elicited by stimulating the cutaneous receptors that carry information to higher centres by sensory pathways. The higher centres then convey information to the concerned muscles by motor pathways. Therefore, superficial reflexes are lost in both upper and lower motor neuron paralysis.

Coordination of Movement

Normal movement is dependent on the ability of the agonist muscles to contract to the degree needed and the simultaneous relaxation of the antagonist muscles. Impairment in these abilities produces incoordination of movement. This incoordination may be due to a disease of the cerebellum, the corticospinal tract or the sensory system. Lack of proper coordination is known as **ataxia**.

Cerebellar Disease

In cerebellar ataxia, the errors of movement tend to occur at right angles to the intended direction of movement. A useful sign of **cerebellar ataxia** is dysdiadokokinesia which is the impaired ability to execute rapidly repeated alternate movements. All the aspects of movement (initiation, rate, range, direction and termination) are affected.

Corticospinal Tract Disease

The incoordination is characterised by **slowness and clumsiness in finger movements**. This is tested by asking the patient to rapidly approximate each finger to the thumb. Corticospinal tract disease does not cause incoordination of movement at the more proximal joints, that is, knee, hip, elbow and so on; it also does not cause incoordination of movement in the leg. However, if it is associated with muscle weakness, impairment in walking occurs.

Sensory System Disease

Incoordination of movement can be produced in the arms or legs by impaired sensation. This is called **sensory ataxia**. It is tested by the Romberg sign. The patient is asked to stand with his feet close together

and if he can do so, he is asked to close his eyes. If the subject sways or falls, the Romberg sign is positive. It is an important physical sign of impaired position and joint sense in the lower limb.

Gait

Gait is the posture of the subject while walking. The character of the gait is often important in the diagnosis of neurological diseases. Normally, when a person walks, he partially flexes the hip and knee joint of one lower limb and dorsiflexes his foot. As he does so, his foot is lifted above the ground and the other lower limb supports the whole weight of the body. As the first lower limb is moved forward and takes up his weight, the other lower limb is flexed and the whole cycle is repeated. If the smooth manner in which the whole movement is performed is disturbed, the gait becomes abnormal. The common **abnormal gaits** are:

* Spastic gait
* Ataxic gait
* Festinant gait
* Waddling gait
* High-stepping gait
* Limping gait

Spastic Gait

Spastic gait is probably the commonest abnormal type. The patient walks on a narrow base, has difficulty in bending his knees and drags his feet along as if they are glued to the ground. The movement is slow and the flexion of the knee and hip joints is either absent or imperfectly performed. The affected leg tends to remain adducted. The foot is raised from the ground by tilting the pelvis and the leg is then swung forwards so that the foot tends to describe an arc (circumduction), the toe scraping along the floor. It is characteristically seen in **corticospinal tract lesions**. There are two types of spastic gaits: (i) hemiplegic and (ii) scissor.

Hemiplegic gait   In this type of gait only one leg is affected. It is seen in hemiplegia.

Scissor gait   The spasticity is present on both sides. The patient walks in a typical criss-cross fashion. It is typically seen in congenital spastic paraplegia.

Ataxic Gait

This occurs due to ataxia. Ataxic gaits are of **two types**, stamping and drunken.

Stamping gait It is a high-stepping ataxic gait in which the movements in the lower limbs are not coordinated. The patient raises his feet suddenly and often abnormally to a higher level and then jerks them forward, bringing them to the ground again with a stamp, and often heel first. Ataxia increases in darkness or if the eyes are closed. It is best seen in **tabes dorsalis and severe peripheral neuritis**.

Drunken gait The patient walks on a broad and irregular base, the feet being planted widely apart. The ataxia is equally severe whether the eyes are opened or closed. It is typically seen in **cerebellar disorders**.

Festinant Gait

The patient walks with an attitude of generalised flexion (bent forward) so that the centre of gravity of the body lies outside in front of him. To bring the centre of gravity to its proper place, the patient takes rapid, short and shuffling steps. But, the centre of gravity moves forward and continues to elude him. Thus, he attempts to catch the centre of gravity. His arms do not swing. It is typically seen in **Parkinsonism**.

Waddling Gait

This is like the gait of a duck. The patient sways from side to side, the body is tilted backwards with an increase of lumbar lordosis and with a protruberant abdomen. The feet are planted widely apart, and the heels and toes tend to be brought down simultaneously. It occurs in proximal muscular weakness, which is seen in **myopathies and muscular dystrophies**. It is also seen in **advanced pregnancy**.

High-Stepping Gait

The patient walks taking high steps. It is typically seen in foot drop, as in **peripheral neuritis or peroneal muscular dystrophy**.

Limping Gait

The patient limps with short steps, keeping the painful limb semiflexed and dropping the pelvis towards the painful side. It is seen in tuberculosis of the knee and hip joints and in sciatica.

Involuntary Movement

Involuntary movements can occur either at rest or during voluntary movement. Involuntary movements are classified into two types, localised and generalised

Localised involuntary movement
1. Fibrillation
2. Fasciculation
3. Myoclonus
4. Tremor

Generalised involuntary movement
A. Extrapyramidal abnormalities
   - Athetosis
   - Chorea
   - Choreoathetosis
   - Hemiballism
   - Torsion dystonia
B. Spasms
   - Tonic spasm
   - Clonic spasm

Fibrillation

This occurs due to contraction of a single muscle fibre. Usually it cannot be seen. Clinically, fibrillation, if present, can be observed in the tongue but it can be recorded electromyographically.

Fasciculation

This occurs due to contraction of a bundle of muscle fibre. It can be seen as well as recorded electromyographically. It occurs due to irritation of the anterior horn cells or nerve roots during inflammation or degeneration.

Causes
- Motor neuron disease
- Cervical spondylosis
- Syringomyelia
- Peroneal muscular dystrophy

Myoclonus

Sudden shock-like contraction of a single muscle or group of muscles is called myoclonus. It is involuntary and arrhythmic. There are different varieties of myoclonus. When myoclonus occurs in the face, it is called facial myoclonus, when it occurs during muscular activity it is called action myoclonus, and when it occurs in different parts of the body and disappears during sleep it is called myoclonus simplex.

Tremor

Tremor is a regular, rhythmic, purpose-less, to and fro movement of a part of the body (usually limbs) due to contraction of a group of muscles and their antagonists. It usually involves the distal parts of the limbs, tongue, and rarely the trunk. It is divided into resting or static tremor (when it occurs at rest) and intention or kinetic tremor (when it occurs during a purposeful movement of limbs). **Resting tremor** is typically seen in Parkinsonism and **intention tremor** in cerebellar disorder. Tremor is also divided into **fine and coarse tremors**. Fine tremor is seen in anxiety, hyperthyroidism and so on. Coarse tremor is seen in Parkinsonism (pin-rolling tremor).

Causes of tremor

I. **Physiological**
1. Anxiety
2. Exposure to cold
3. Old age (senile tremor)
4. Congenital

II. **Pathological**
A. Neurological
1. Parkinsonism
2. Cerebellar disorder
3. Disseminated sclerosis
4. Benign essential tremor
B. Metabolic
1. Thyrotoxicosis
2. Hypoglycemia
3. Hepatic coma
4. Uremia
C. Toxic
1. Alcoholism
2. Barbiturate poisoning
3. Opium poisoning
4. Heavy metal poisoning

Chorea

This is a rapid involuntary dancing type of movement. It occurs in lesions of the caudate nucleus. It is seen in Huntington's disease (Huntington's chorea) and chronic rheumatic disease (Sydenham's chorea).

Athetosis

This is characterised by continuous, slow or writhing movements. It occurs due to a **lesion in the globus pallidus**.

Choreoathetosis

When chorea and athetosis are present together, the condition is called choreoathetosis.

Ballism

This is an involuntary movement, which is sudden, flailing, intense and violent. It occurs in the **lesion of the subthalamic nucleus**. When it occurs in one side of the body, it is called hemiballism.

Torsion Dystonia

The torsion of the limbs and vertebral column causes distorted posture of the limbs and trunk. Persistent increase in muscle tone occurs. The dystonia disappears during sleep.

Tonic Spasm

Tonic spasm of the muscle is seen in tetanus and strychnine poisoning.

Clonic Spasm

Clonic spasm of the muscle is seen in epilepsy.

Tics

These are sudden rapid, repeated, coordinated and purposeless movements that occur usually in the same region intermittently. Usually tics occur in the form of blinking of the eyes or wriggling of the shoulders.

Upper Motor Neuron (UMN) Paralysis

Features

- Muscles are affected in groups (individual muscles are never affected)
- No muscle atrophy (disuse atrophy may occur in chronic patients)
- Spasticity (hypertonia)
- Exaggeration of tendon reflexes
- Loss of superficial reflexes
- Positive Babinski sign (extensor plantar response)
- No fascicular twitches
- No denervation potential in EMG
- Normal nerve conduction studies

Causes

The corticospinal pathways can be interrupted by lesions at any level, starting from the cerebral cortex, subcortical white matter, internal capsule, brainstem, to the spinal cord. The most common site of lesion of the corticospinal tract is the internal capsule that is usually involved in cerebral hemorrhage due to damage to

Charcot's artery (the artery of cereberal hemorrhage), a branch of the middle cerebral artery. Corticothalamic, corticostriate, corticorubral, corticopontaine, cortico-olivary, and corticoreticular fibres also pass through the internal capsule. Therefore, a lesion in the internal capsule not only affects the pyramidal (corticospinal) tract but also the extrapyramidal and other fibres. Therefore, the paralysis is called upper motor neuron paralysis, instead of pyramidal paralysis.

The extrapyramidal motor system includes the basal ganglia and the cerebellum. These two structures influence the extrapyramidal tracts by projecting directly or indirectly to the brainstem. Extrapyramidal lesions do not cause paralysis (Table 57.1).

Table 57.1   Differences between pyramidal (corticospinal) and extrapyramidal lesions.

		Pyramidal	Extrapyramidal
1.	Muscle tone	Spasticity (clasp-knife rigidity)	Plastic (cogwheel rigidity)
2.	Distribution of hypertonus	Flexors of arm and extensors of leg	Generalised
3.	Shortening and lengthening reaction	Present	Absent
4.	Involuntary movement	Absent	Present
5.	Tendon reflexes	Exaggerated	Normal
6.	Babinski's sign	Positive	Negative
7.	Paralysis	Of voluntary movement	No paralysis

Physiological basis

In upper motor neuron (UMN) paralysis, there occurs not only lesions of the corticospinal tract (the so-called pyramidal tract), but a few extrapyramidal fibres (especially corticoreticular fibres that project onto the reticulospinal tract) are also disrupted. This occurs in UMN paralysis due to a lesion at the internal capsule (the commonest site of UMN lesion). The pontine reticulospinal tract is excitatory to the muscles involved in postural control, that is, the **antigravity muscle**, and this reticulospinal tract is under the inhibitory control of corticoreticular fibres.

◆ In UMN lesions, disruption of corticoreticular fibres facilitates the excitatory output of the pontine reticulospinal pathway. Therefore, **hypertonia and spasticity** occur in a UMN lesion.

◆ Deep reflexes are exaggerated because of the **increased discharge and sensitivity of the gamma motor neurons**. Excitability of the gamma motor neurons regulates spinal reflex activity. Gamma motor neurons are usually inhibited by many supraspinal influences. In UMN lesions, loss of inhibitory influence increases gamma motor neuron discharge and therefore increases the reflex activity.

◆ The corticospinal tract excites flexor motor neurons and inhibits the extensor motor neurons of the digits of the limbs. Therefore, normally stroking of the sole elicits plantar flexion. In UMN paralysis, disruption of corticospinal influence on the lumbosacral motor neurons causes dorsiflexion of the big toe and fanning of other toes (**Babinski's sign or extensor plantar response**).

Lower Motor Neuron (LMN) Paralysis

Lower motor neurons may be injured or diseased in the cranial nerve nuclei or spinal anterior horn cells, in the anterior nerve roots, or in the nerves themselves. The most common acute lesion of the anterior horn cell is poliomyelitis. The chronic degeneration of anterior horn cells occurs in motor neuron disease (progressive muscular atrophy). The anterior nerve roots may be damaged by trauma, especially in association with cervical spondylosis or by an inflammatory or neoplastic lesion. The peripheral nerves are mainly affected by injury, inflammation and toxic or metabolic disorders (neuropathies). As the nerves carry both motor and sensory information, pure motor deficit rarely occurs. Usually muscular paralysis is associated with sensory changes.

Features

◆ Usually individual muscles are affected
◆ Muscle atrophy is pronounced (Table 57.2)
◆ Flaccidity
◆ Hypotonia is seen in the affected muscles
◆ Tendon reflexes and superficial reflexes are diminished or absent
◆ Babinski's sign is negative (plantar flexion)
◆ Fascicular twitches may be present
◆ Denervation potentials (fibrillation, fasciculation, positive sharp waves) are observed in the EMG
◆ Nerve conduction studies reveal abnormalities

Table 57.2 Comparison of upper motor neuron and lower motor neuron paralyses.

		UMN paralysis	LMN paralysis
1.	Muscles affected	Muscles are affected in groups	Individual muscles are affected
2.	Size of the muscles	Atrophy not seen (slight atrophy may occur due to disuse)	Pronounced atrophy (may be up to 80 per cent of the total bulk) of muscles
3.	Type of paralysis	Spastic paralysis	Flaccid paralysis
4.	Tone of the muscles	Hypertonia	Hypotonia
5.	Power of the muscles	Paralysis occurs (no voluntary movement)	Paralysis occurs
6.	Tendon reflexes	Exaggerated	Diminished or absent
7.	Superficial reflexes	Absent	Absent
8.	Babinski's sign	Positive (extensor plantar reflex)	Negative (flexor plantar reflex)
9.	Involuntary movement	Absent	Fascicular twitches may be present
10.	EMG changes	No denervation potentials seen in EMG	Denervation potentials (fibrillations, fasciculations, and sharp waves) are seen in EMG
11.	Nerve conduction	No abnormalities in nerve conduction	Abnormal nerve conduction (decreased studies conduction)

OSPE

I. **Measure the bulk of the muscles of the right arm of the subject.**

Steps
   1. Give proper instructions to the subject.
   2. Detect the midpoint of the right arm of the subject by measuring (with the help of a measuring tape) the distance between the median olecranon process and the tip of the humerus
   3. Ask him to relax completely.
   4. Measure the midarm circumference with a measuring tape.
   5. Measure the midarm circumference of the other (left) side and compare.

II. **Assess the tone of the flexors and extensors of the right elbow of the subject.**

Steps
   1. Give proper instructions to the subject.
   2. Ask him to relax completely.
   3. Make passive movements (flexion and extension) of the forearm at the elbow joint.
   4. Feel (can also palpate the muscles) the tone of the extensors and flexors.
   5. Repeat the procedure in the other elbow joint and compare.

III. **Assess the strength of the biceps muscle of the right side of the subject.**

Steps
   1. Give proper instructions to the subject.
   2. Ask the subject to bend his right forearm against resistance (the examiner prevents flexion of the forearm by applying resistance).
   3. Look for the prominence of the biceps muscle and assess the strength (in terms of grade) of the biceps.
   4. Repeat the procedure in the opposite side and compare.

IV. **Elicit biceps jerk of the right side of the subject.**

Steps
   1. Give proper instructions to the subject.
   2. Flex the right elbow of the subject and make the forearm semipronated by resting it on the abdomen or on your (examiner's) left forearm.

3. Expose the front of the arm.
4. Ask the subject to relax completely.
5. Place your thumb on the biceps tendon firmly to stretch the muscle.
6. Strike with the narrower end of the hammer on his thumb.
7. Observe the contraction of the biceps and flexion of the forearm.
8. Elicit the biceps jerk of the opposite side and compare.

V. Elicit triceps jerk of the right side of the subject.

Steps

1. Give proper instructions to the subject.
2. Flex the right elbow of the subject and rest the forearm on his (the subject's) chest or on your own (examiner's) forearm.
3. Expose the back of the arm.
4. Ask the subject to relax completely.
5. Tap the triceps tendon with the broader end of the hammer with movements at the wrist joint.
6. Look for contraction of the triceps and extension of the forearm.
7. Elicit the triceps jerk on the opposite side and compare.

VI. Elicit right side supinator jerk of the subject.

Steps

1. Give proper instructions to the subject.
2. Slightly flex the right forearm of the subject and support the forearm by holding the hand.
3. Ask the subject to relax completely.
4. Tap the radius about 1–2 inches above the wrist over its styloid process.
5. Look for flexion at the elbow and supination of the forearm.
6. Elicit supinator jerks of the opposite side and compare.

VII. Elicit knee jerk of the right side of the subject in the supine position.

Steps

1. Give proper instructions to the subject.
2. Pass your hand under the knee to be tested; and place it upon the opposite knee in such a way that the tested knee rests on the dorsum of your wrist.
3. Ask the subject to relax completely.
4. Strike the patellar tendon with the broader end of the hammer with movement at the wrist joint.
5. Observe the contraction of the quadriceps and extension at the knee joint.
6. Elicit knee jerk of the opposite side and compare.

VII. Elicit ankle jerk of the right side of the subject in the supine position.

Steps

1. Give proper instructions to the subject.
2. Place the right lower limb of the subject on the bed so that it lies everted and slightly flexed.
3. Slightly dorsiflex the foot so as to stretch the Achilles tendon.
4. Strike the tendon on its posterior surface with the broader end of the hammer, with movement at the wrist joint.
5. Observe the contraction of the calf muscles and plantar flexion at the ankle joint.
6. Elicit ankle jerk of the other side and compare.

IX. Elicit plantar reflex of the subject.

Steps

1. Ask the subject to lie down in the supine position.
2. Fix the foot by placing the left hand on the medial malleolus.
3. Ask the subject to relax completely.
4. Gently scratch with a key or the pointed metallic end of the knee hammer on the outer edge of the sole of the foot, from the heel towards the little toe and then medially across the metatarsus.
5. Observe the response.

6.   Elicit the plantar reflex of the opposite side and compare.

X. Elicit the abdominal reflex of the subject in the supine position.

Steps
1.   Give proper instructions to the subject.
2.   Expose the abdomen.
3.   With the help of a key or the pointed metallic end of the knee hammer, scratch lightly but briskly from the outer aspect of the abdomen towards the midline in all four quadrants.
4.   Look for contraction of the muscle and deviation of the umbilicus.

XI. Elicit the cremasteric reflex of the subject.

Steps
1.   Give proper instructions to the subject.
2.   Expose the part (external genitalia and upper portion of the thigh).
3.   With the help of a key, scratch the upper and inner aspect of the thigh lightly and briskly.
4.   Look for contraction of the dartus muscle and lifting of the testicle.
5.   Elicit the cremasteric reflex of the other side and compare the findings.

XII. Perform the finger-nose test of the subject.

Steps
1.   Give proper instructions to the subject.
2.   Ask the subject to touch the tip of the nose with the tip of one of his index fingers rapidly and repeatedly, first with the eyes open and then with the eyes closed.
3.   Ask him to repeat the same with the opposite index finger; compare the findings.

XIII. Perform the knee-heel test of the subject in the supine position.

Steps
1.   Give proper instructions to the subject.
2.   Ask the subject to place one of his heels on the opposite knee and then to slide the heel down his shin towards the ankle.
3.   Ask him to repeat the same rapidly 4–5 times.
4.   Ask him to do the same on the other side; compare the findings.

VIVA

1.   *What are the different aspects of motor functions that are assessed while examining the motor system?*
2.   *How do you measure the bulk of the muscles in the upper and lower limbs?*
3.   *What is the tone of the muscle and how is it assessed?*
4.   *How do you grade the strength of muscles?*
5.   *How do you estimate the strength of intrinsic muscles of the hands?*
6.   *How do you assess the strength of the flexors and extensors of the wrist?*
7.   *How do you assess the strength of the biceps, triceps and brachioradialis?*
8.   *How do you assess the strength of the abdominal muscles?*
9.   *How do you assess the strength of the intrinsic muscles of the foot?*
10. *How do you assess the strength of extensors and flexors of the knee and those of the thigh?*
11. *What are the precautions observed for eliciting deep reflexes?*
12. *How do you grade tendon reflexes?*
13. *What is the root value of different important tendon jerks?*
     Ans: Biceps jerk (C5,6), triceps jerk (C6,7), supinator or brachioradialis jerk (C5,6), knee jerk (L2,3,4), ankle jerk (S1, 2), plantar reflex (L5, S1), abdominal reflex (T7-12), jaw jerk (fifth cranial nerve, mandibular division), cremasteric reflex (L1,2), anal reflex (S3,4).

14. Name the superficial reflexes.
15. What are the tests for coordination of movement in the upper and lower limbs?
16. What is dysdiadokokinesis?
17. Define gait.
18. In what conditions are atrophy and hypertrophy of muscles observed? Why?
19. What is the cause of spasticity in upper motor neuron paralysis?
20. What is the cause of flaccidity in lower motor neuron paralysis?
21. What are the differences between pyramidal and extrapyramidal tract lesions?
22. What are the differences between upper motor neuron and lower motor neuron paralysis?
23. How do you classify muscles clinically?
24. What do you mean by lower and upper motor neurons?
25. What are the descending motor tracts?
26. Name the extrapyramidal systems.
27. Trace the pathway of corticospinal tracts.
28. What are the functions of corticospinal tracts?
29. What are the functions of extrapyramidal systems?
30. What are the areas in the brain involved in regulation of motor activities?
31. What are the functions of the motor cortex?
32. What are the functions of the basal ganglia?
33. What are the functions of the cerebellum?

CHAPTER 58

Introduction to Animal Experiments and Appliances

INTRODUCTION TO ANIMAL EXPERIMENTS

A student of physiology should be familiar with the apparatus that he uses in experimental physiology. He should know the basic principle of the working of the instruments, the uses of the apparatus and the instructions for the safe use of the apparatus. As electric current is used as the stimulus to perform most of the experiments, proper earthing (grounding) and insulation of the wires must be ensured before starting an experiment.

In most experimental work, especially that dealing with the study of the response of tissues to various stimuli, **four set-ups are needed**: (i) the source of stimulation, (ii) a stimulating device, (iii) tissue preparation and (iv) a recording device.

Source of Stimulation

The stimulus may be mechanical, chemical, thermal or electrical. But, in most experimental procedures, **electrical stimulus is usually preferred** because of its many advantages:

1. The electrical stimulus is easy to deliver. The operator can handle it conveniently.
2. The apparatus for delivering the stimulus is tidy.
3. The stimulus is easily controlled by the break or make of a key.
4. It is possible to stimulate the tissue with the desired strength, frequency and duration, accurately and easily.
5. The stimulus can be accurately localised on the tissue.
6. The stimulus can be controlled from a long distance.
7. This is the least injurious type of stimulus to the tissue.

Stimulating Device

The stimulating device is the inductorium, which is described in detail later in this chapter.

Tissue Preparation

For amphibian nerve muscle experiments, the sciatic nerve and the gastrocnemius muscle of the frog are usually used.

Advantages of Using Frog

- It is easily available.
- It is easy to handle.
- It is harmless.
- It is less expensive.
- To maintain the tissue preparation of frogs, no extra supply of oxygen is needed as the frog muscles can directly imbibe oxygen from the environment.

* The tissue preparation of a frog can be maintained for a long duration if handled properly.
* It is easy to dissect the frog.

The **advantages of using a gastrocnemius-sciatic preparation** are:

1. The sciatic nerve and gastrocnemius muscle are easy to locate and dissect.
2. The sciatic nerve is the longest nerve and is therefore easy to place on the electrodes that are kept a short distance away from the muscle.
3. The gastrocnemius muscle is a big muscle (has more cross-sectional area) and therefore on contraction, produces more force to lift the lever and records a good magnitude of contraction.
4. The gastrocnemius muscle cannot be easily fatigued.

Recording Device

Recording of muscle contractions is done by using a writing lever that inscribes on the smoked surface of a moving drum fitted to a kymograph.

DESCRIPTION AND USES OF APPLIANCES

Source of Current

Electrical stimulation can be given either with a **direct current** (DC) source and a pair of stimulating electrodes (**galvanic current**) or by using an induction coil and the electrodes (**faradic current** or **induced current**). In most experiments, direct current is used. Direct current (6 volts) is available at the battery terminals of all experimental tables. To obtain an induced current, a constant current (galvanic) of low voltage is fed into the primary coil of the inductorium. To supply low-voltage direct current, a central low-voltage unit is installed in most laboratories. The output terminals feed a direct current of 3–15 volts to all the working seats in the table. This direct current is a rectified current, which comes from the central eliminator. Direct current can also be obtained from dry cells connected in series.

Wires

Usually **copper or aluminium wires** are used in laboratories to carry electric current. A single thick wire is used to supply direct current. The wires are insulated by cotton, silk or enamel. For the connection or to supply current, the insulation from the tip of the wires

is removed and polished with the help of fine sandpaper to give a good contact. **Copper wires are usually used**. The wire should not be damaged or have cracks. The wires are usually rolled on glass rods into spirals.

Keys

The key is a device used for completing or interrupting a circuit. Two types of keys are used, the simple or tap key, and the short-circuiting key.

The tap key   This key (Fig. 58.1A) is connected in the primary circuit in series with the DC source. The key is pressed gently and released to make and break the circuit.

The short-circuiting key   This key (Fig 58.1B) is connected in the secondary circuit in parallel to prevent accidental leakage of current into the tissue. This also prevents unipolar induction. The key is kept closed to check unnecessary stimulation of the tissue, and when stimulation is required, it is left open. Different types of short-circuiting keys are available, but the Du Bois-Reymond key (Fig. 58.1C) is usually used in the laboratory.

The reversing key   This key (Fig. 58.1D) is also used in the laboratory when two electrodes are required for shunting the current from one electrode to the other.

Inductorium

The inductorium (induction coil) (Fig. 58.2) is a device from which a faradic (alternate) current is obtained by feeding a galvanic current. The inductorium used is known as the **Du Bois-Reymond inductorium** (introduced by Du Bois-Reymond in 1849). This is a simple device for transforming direct current into induced current. This is basically a step-up transformer used to obtain a high-voltage stimulus from a low-voltage direct current source, by using the principle of Faraday's electromagnetic induction. It consists of two separate coils: the primary coil and the secondary coil. The primary coil is fixed on a frame and the secondary coil is movable and covers the primary coil, but has no connection with it.

The primary coil   The primary coil consists of 300 turns of insulated thick copper wire wound around a soft iron core. The primary coil, the direct current source and the tap key are connected in series and this constitutes the primary circuit.

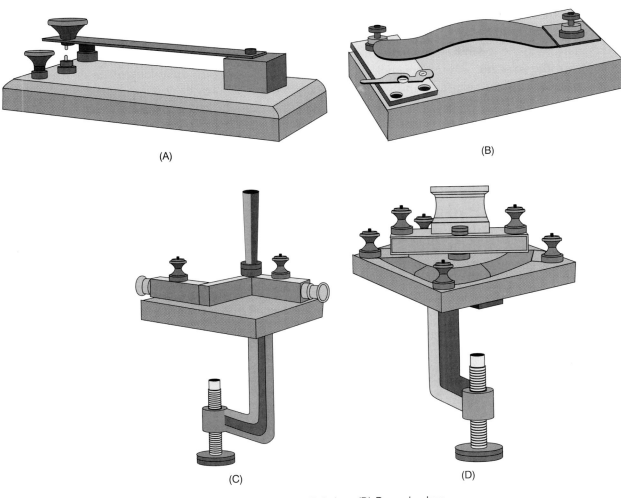

Fig. 58.1   Keys. (A) Tap key; (B) Short-circuiting key; (C) Du Bois key; (D) Reversing key.

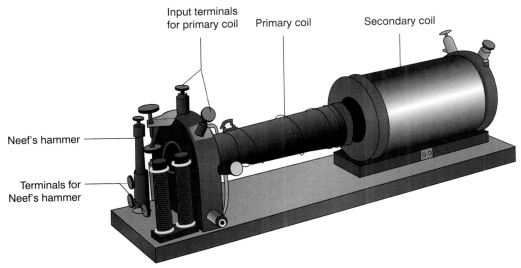

Fig. 58.2   Du Bois-Reymond inductorium.

The secondary coil   The secondary coil is made of 5000 turns of very fine copper wire. The secondary coil can slide on two horizontal metal slide rods. On one of the slide rods, a scale is marked (in cm) by which the distance between the coils can be measured. The two terminals of the secondary coil are connected to the stimulating electrodes. The secondary coil and the stimulating electrodes form the secondary circuit.

A current is induced in the secondary coil only when there is a change in the strength of the magnetic field of the primary coil. When the strength of the current passing through the primary coil is constant, changes in the strength of the magnetic field occur only at commencement (make) and termination (break) of the current. Therefore, a current is induced in the secondary coil at 'make' or 'break' of the current in the primary coil. No current is induced in the secondary coil when the current passing through the primary coil is constant. The induced current is always of short duration.

The time taken by the current in the primary circuit at 'make' to develop from zero to maximum voltage is longer than that taken by it to fall from maximum to zero at 'break'. This is due to the development of Faraday's extra current at 'make'. Therefore, the *induced current in the secondary coil is stronger at 'break' than at 'make'*. The break stimulus is always stronger than the make stimulus. The strength of the stimulating current can be increased or decreased by changing the distance or the angle between the primary and the secondary coils. Other factors also determine the strength of the induced current.

The inductorium also has a built-in interruptor (**Neef's hammer**) which works on the same principle as that of an electric bell. When the Neef's hammer is introduced in the primary circuit, the alternate make and break stimuli are rapidly repeated (40/s); this produces repeated induced current in the secondary circuit.

Factors That Affect the Strength of the Induced Current

1. **The distance between the two coils**—when the distance between the two coils increases, the strength of the stimulating current decreases and when the distance decreases, the strength of the current increases.
2. **The angle between the coils**—when the two coils are placed straight, the strength of the current is maximum. The strength of the current reduces by turning the secondary coil away from the primary coil. When the secondary coil is placed at right angles to the primary coil, there is no induction of current.
3. **Number of turns in the coils**—usually fixed.
4. The **strength of the direct current** fed into the primary coil.

Stimulating Electrodes

Electrodes used in biological experiments differ depending on their manufacture and use. They are designed to provide low resistance between the preparation and the amplifier input. Stimulating electrodes (Fig. 58.3) are used for delivering the electrical stimulus to the tissues. A stimulating electrode consists of two copper wires held together by a piece of perspex.

Signal Marker

It is always better to indicate the point of application of stimulus, below the tracings. A signal marker marks (Fig. 58.4A) the moment of stimulation below the recording of the muscle contractions. It has two electromagnets and a writing lever. The lever marks the point of stimulation on the smoked paper. It is always included in the primary circuit.

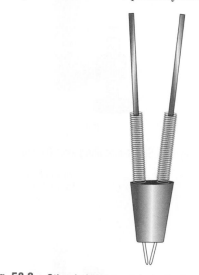

Fig. 58.3   Stimulating (simple) electrode.

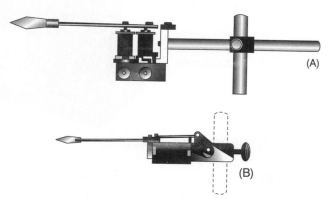

Fig. 58.4   (A) Signal marker; (B) Simple time-marker.

This simple time-marker (Fig. 58.4B) with a single magnet can also be used for this purpose.

Power Shaft and Pulleys

A horizontal power shaft driven by an electric motor is provided on the table. Cone pulleys with four grooves are fixed to the power shaft at each seat.

Kymograph

Kymograph (Fig. 58.5) is the name given to any instrument that records movements on a moving surface. It consists of a metal gear box to which a vertical rotating shaft is connected. The shaft is powered by a horizontal axis running through the metal case. To this axis, on one side, a series of pulleys are attached. A belt connects one of these pulleys to one of the pulleys in the power shaft. A cylinder (6″ × 6″), also called drum, is fixed to the shaft. The drum rotates with the shaft. A gear switch on the left side of the kymograph provides high and low gears. In each gear, the drum can be made to turn at different speeds by connecting different-sized pulleys of the kymograph and the power shaft. The drum can be started or stopped by turning a clutch on the left side of the metal gear box.

There are two horizontal **contact arms** that project from the lower end of the vertical shaft. These contact arms can be separated and fixed with various angles

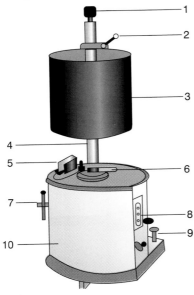

Fig. 58.5   The kymograph (1: Screw lift for cylinder; 2: Cylinder fixing lever; 3: Cylinder; 4: Spindle; 5: Contact block; 6: Contact arm; 7: Clutch lever; 8: Speed regulator; 9: Levelling screw; 10: Body of kymograph).

between them. The tips of the arms, when they revolve, make contact with a spring at the left side of the top of the kymograph. The insulated carrier of the spring is adjustable and is clamped by a screw. There are two terminals for electrical connection: one is attached to the insulated spring and the other to the metal case of the gear box. By means of these connecting terminals, the insulated carrier along with the spring can be made to act as a key in the primary circuit. The circuit is 'made' or 'broken' when the tip of the contact arm makes and breaks contact with the insulated spring.

Muscle Trough

The muscle trough (Fig. 58.6) is a perspex or plastic chamber used to keep the muscle moist and viable in Ringer's solution. A block carrying the stimulating electrodes is fixed on the side walls of the trough. The writing lever is fixed on the other side wall of the trough. From the base of the muscle trough, a drainage pipe is provided with a clamp that helps to drain the Ringer's solution from the trough whenever required.

Levers

Different types of levers are used in experimental physiology for various purposes. The commonly used levers are the writing simple lever, the starling heart lever, the isometric lever, the afterload lever (Fig. 58.7) and the frontal lever (Fig. 58.8).

The Writing Lever

This is used to magnify and record the muscle contraction on the drum. The lever consists of a horizontal arm, which bears holes and notches for hanging the weights (Fig. 58.9). The lever is fixed to the side wall of the muscle trough. The writing point of the lever is made up of a triangular piece of photographic film.

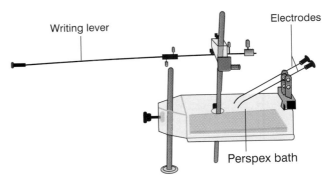

Fig. 58.6   Muscle trough.

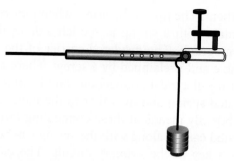

Fig. 58.7 Afterload lever.

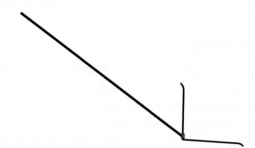

Fig. 58.8 Frontal lever.

An ink writing stylus can be fitted into the writing lever, which can write on a white glazed paper instead of on a smoked drum. There is a screw (afterload screw) near the fulcrum of the lever, which limits the downward movement of the lever.

The Starling Heart Lever

This is used for recording the cardiogram of a frog's heart. This lever is more sensitive than the writing lever, as it records the contractions of the heart, which are weaker than the contractions of the gastrocnemius muscle. It consists of a frame with a light steel lever, with holes and notches, supported by a fine adjustable nickel silver spring (Fig. 58.10).

Isometric Lever

This consists of a holder that carries a steel tension spring and a flat writing lever (Fig. 58.11). It is used for recording isometric contractions.

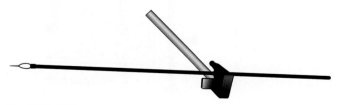

Fig. 58.9 Simple lever.

Myograph Stand

This is a vertical rod fixed to a heavy and triangular base (Fig. 58.12). The muscle trough can be fitted to the rod and can be moved up and down with the help of a fitted screw. The rod can be turned on its axis so that the writing point of the muscle lever can be made to touch or be removed from the drum without disturbing other adjustments.

Tuning Fork

A tuning fork (Fig. 58.13) with a frequency of 100 vibrations per second (100 Hz) is used for measuring different time intervals. To the end of one arm of the tuning fork, a writing point is attached. The tuning fork is set to vibrate and is then made to write on the fast rotating drum to obtain a tracing. This tracing consists of different waves. Each wave of the tracing (from crest to crest) measures 0.01 seconds (10 ms).

Pohl's Commutator

This is used to change the direction of current. It consists of a vulcanite base on which a rocking metallic cradle is mounted (Fig. 58.14). There are six cup-like depressions filled with mercury, and six terminals are attached to these cups. Two narrow copper strips connect the diagonally opposite corner cups.

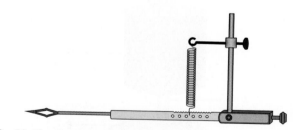

Fig. 58.10 Starling heart lever.

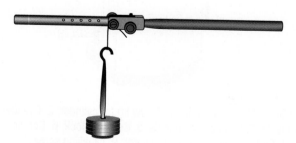

Fig. 58.11 Isometric lever.

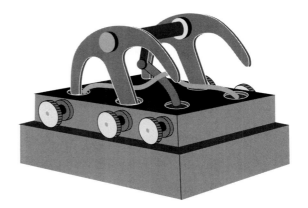

Fig. 58.14 Pohl's commutator.

1. To check the primary circuit, connect a short piece of wire to one of the low volts terminals and strike the other terminal with its free end. A spark indicates the presence of current. Check the simple key and the contact block on the kymograph. Each time the striker makes contact, a spark is produced.
2. To check the secondary circuit, place the tissue on the wires connected to the secondary coil terminals. If twitchings occur in the tissue with each revolution of the spindle, the connection is correct. If the muscle does not contract, place the electrodes directly on the muscle. If the muscle contracts due to direct stimulation, check if the nerve is damaged during the dissection.

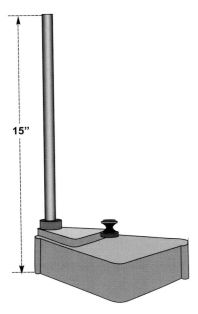

15"

Fig. 58.12 Myograph stand.

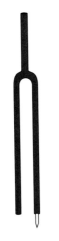

Fig. 58.13 Tuning fork.

Student's Stimulator

This is an electronic stimulator with a DC output of 0–15 volts. The strength (volts), frequency and duration of the stimulus are indicated on the apparatus. More advanced stimulators, which are required for special experiments and research, are also available.

EXERCISES

Making Electrical Connections

Make the **primary and secondary circuits** as depicted in Figs. 58.15A and B. Check whether the primary and secondary circuits are made correctly.

Smoking

Before smoking the drum, a piece of a glazed paper is properly pasted on the drum. Then the drum is placed on the horizontal arm of the smoking stand (Fig. 58.16). The burner is put on and the drum is smoked uniformly by rotating manually on the flame. A thin and uniformly black smoking is aimed at.

Varnishing

Varnishing is done to fix the recording on the smoked paper. Labelling of the recording is done before varnishing. The paper is cut at the jointed portion and taken out of the drum and dipped in the 2 per cent solution of resin or methylated spirit. Then the paper is clipped and hung till it is completely dry.

Precautions

1. The primary and secondary circuits should be made perfectly.

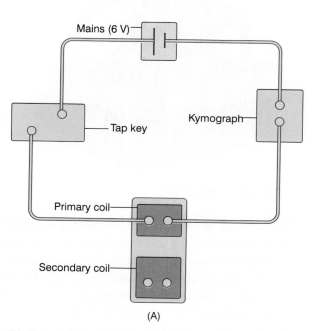

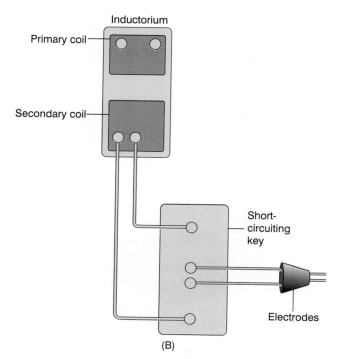

Fig. 58.15 (A) Primary circuit; (B) Secondary circuit.

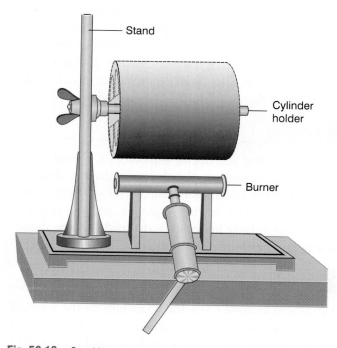

Fig. 58.16 Smoking stand.

2. Loose connections in the circuits should be detected and dealt with.
3. The wires used for making the circuit should be as short as possible. Long wires can be shortened by winding them around a glass rod or a pencil.
4. The kymograph should be properly levelled by using the levelling screws at its base.
5. The drum should be tightly fixed to the vertical shaft.
6. The drum should always be rotated clockwise.
7. The writing lever should always be arranged on the right side of the drum.
8. The writing lever should be tangential with the recording surface.
9. The tip of the writing lever should touch the smoked surface evenly and lightly.
10. The initial and resting positions of the writing lever should always be horizontal.
11. The tracing should be taken at least one inch above the lower edge of the drum.
12. The contact arm should be tightly fixed.

VIVA

1. What are the different types of stimuli and why is the electrical stimulus usually preferred?
2. Why is the frog selected for amphibian practicals?
3. What are the advantages of using the gastrocnemius-sciatic preparation for frog experiments?
4. What are the types of keys used in amphibian experiments and what are their uses?
5. What is the principle of working of the inductorium?
6. What are the factors that determine the strength of induced current?
7. Why is the 'break' stimulus stronger than the 'make' stimulus?
8. What is the use of the short-circuiting key?
9. What is the use of a signal marker?
10. What is the principle used in the working of a kymograph?
11. How is the speed of the kymograph regulated?
12. What is the use of the contact arm of the kymograph?
13. How is the time tracing obtained in the recording?
14. What are the precautions taken for making electrical circuits?
15. How are the recordings fixed?

CHAPTER 59

Nerve-Muscle Preparation

Learning Objectives

After completing this practical, you will be able to:
1. Hold a living frog.
2. Pith the frog.
3. Dissect the frog to isolate the sciatic nerve and gastrocnemius muscle.
4. List the precautions taken during pithing and making the nerve-muscle preparation.
5. List the reasons why the gastrocnemius muscle and sciatic nerve of frogs are preferred for amphibian nerve muscle experiments.
6. State the composition of Ringer's solution.

INTRODUCTION

For any amphibian nerve-muscle experiment, the sciatic nerve and the gastrocnemius muscle of the frog are used for of the following reasons:
1. The sciatic nerve is a long nerve, and is therefore easy to mount in the muscle trough.
2. The gastrocnemius muscle is a bulky muscle and therefore it gives good amplitude of contraction on stimulation. It cannot be fatigued easily.

Before making the nerve-muscle preparation, the frog should be pithed by destroying the brain and spinal cord.

Methods

Nerve-Muscle Preparation

Principle

A pithed frog is dissected to isolate the intact sciatic nerve and gastrocnemius muscle. This nerve-muscle preparation is mounted on the muscle trough to perform various experiments.

Requirements

1. Frog (living)
2. Pithing needle
3. Dissecting set
   • Dissection board

• A pair of scissors with blunt ends (8″)
• A pair of scissors with sharp ends (6″)
• A pair of pointed forceps
• A glass rod
4. Ringer's solution

Procedure

There are two broad steps in nerve-muscle preparation: pithing of the frog and dissection to make the nerve-muscle preparation.

Pithing

1. Hold the frog gently but firmly with the help of cloth or cotton.

Note: The skin of the frog is slippery. Therefore, the animal should be held with a dry cloth or cotton.

2. Hit a blow on its head to make the animal unconscious.

Note: This procedure is called stunning.

3. Hold the unconscious frog in your hand and ventroflex its head.
4. Feel the depression at the junction of the skull and vertebral column.

Note: This corresponds to a point in the middle of the line joining the posterior borders of the tympanic membranes.

5. Insert a pithing needle firmly through the skin, muscle and bone tissue into the spinal cord.

6. Manipulate the needle anteriorly into the skull and rotate it to destroy the brain.
7. Withdraw the needle and direct it backwards into the spinal cord and rotate the needle to destroy the cord.

Note: Immediately after the needle is directed into the spinal cord, the muscles of the lower limb and trunk become spastic. They become flaccid after destruction of the spinal cord. This procedure is called pithing. After pithing, the animal loses its voluntary and reflex movements, but is still alive and can be used for experiments.

Dissection

1. Cut the skin of the frog around the middle of the trunk and strip off the skin from the trunk and hind limbs.
2. Place the frog on the frog board on its abdomen.
3. Pick up the tip of the urostyle with the forceps and lift it carefully. Cut the pelvic girdle on its sides taking care not to injure the underlying sciatic nerve.
4. Identify the sciatic plexus.
5. Isolate a 2 cm long piece of vertebral column from where the sciatic plexus originates by cutting the vertebral column above and below the exit of the sciatic nerve with scissors.
6. Bisect the vertebral column vertically into two halves with the help of the bone cutting scissors.
7. Expose the sciatic nerve in the thigh between the muscle mass posteriorly by separating the muscle with the help of the blunt glass probe (Fig. 59.1).
8. Clean the nerve from its surrounding fascial attachments.

Note: Do not pull the nerve; do not touch it with any metal object. Use only a glass rod for handling the nerve.

9. Identify, separate and cut the gastrocnemius tendon from its attachment and tie a long thread around the tendon.
10. Free the muscle from the tibia and cut the tibia close to the knee joint, then cut the femur close to the knee joint. The knee joint should be kept intact.
11. Remove all redundant muscles (other than the gastrocnemius).
12. Lift the nerve-muscle preparation (Fig. 59.2) carefully and transfer it to a container filled with Ringer's solution.
13. Keep the nerve-muscle preparation immersed in Ringer's solution until it is used for the experiment.

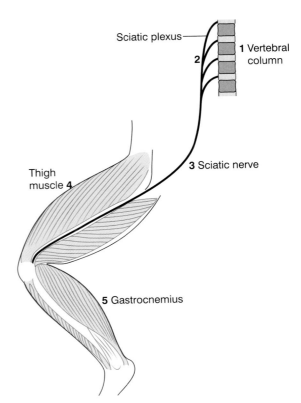

Fig. 59.1 Anatomical position of the sciatic nerve and gastrocnemius muscle of frog.

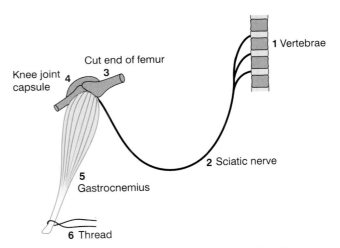

Fig. 59.2 The sciatic-gastrocnemius preparation. Note that a thread is tied to the tip of the tendon and that a portion of the vertebral column is kept intact with the nerve.

Note: If required, a nerve-muscle preparation from the other side can be obtained.

Precautions

1. The frog should be stunned before pithing (pithing of a conscious frog is painful for the frog).

2. The frog should be held by wrapping it with a cloth piece or cotton as the skin is slippery.

3. During pithing, the whole of the spinal cord should be destroyed.

4. Care should be taken not to injure the sciatic nerve plexus while cutting the pelvic girdle.

5. The knee joint should be kept intact with the preparation as it becomes easy to fix the muscle through the knee joint in the muscle trough.

6. A piece of vertebral column should be kept intact with the nerve (the nerve should not be cut from its origin). It becomes easy to place the nerve on the electrodes if the vertebral column is intact with the nerve.

7. The nerves should be identified, traced and exposed with the help of a glass rod. The nerve should not be handled with metallic objects, as metals may stimulate the nerve.

8. While dissecting, to obtain the preparation, the nerve and the muscle should not be strained.

9. The nerve-muscle preparation should be immediately transferred into Ringer's solution as soon as the dissection is over. The preparation should not be allowed to dry.

10. Once the preparation is ready, mount in the muscle trough to start the experiment. Otherwise, the muscle may be fatigued.

DISCUSSION

Once the nerve-muscle preparation is made, it should be immediately immersed in Ringer's solution. The preparation should be mounted in the muscle trough as early as possible and the experiment should be started.

Composition of Ringer's Solution

$NaCl$: 0.6% (isotonic with frog plasma)
KCl : 0.014% (maintains membrane potential)
$CaCl_2$: 0.012% (maintains muscle excitability)
$NaHCO_3$: 0.02% (maintains pH)
NaH_2PO_4 : 0.001% (maintains pH)
Dextrose : 0.1% (provides nutrition)

VIVA

1. Why is the frog chosen for amphibian experiments?
2. Why are the gastrocnemius muscle and sciatic nerve selected for nerve-muscle experiments?
3. Why is the animal stunned before pithing?
4. What are the precautions to be followed during dissection for the nerve-muscle preparation?
5. How can you assess that a frog is properly pithed?
6. Why is the knee joint kept intact with the muscle for making the preparation?
7. Why is the nerve not handled with any metallic objects?
8. Why is the preparation immersed in Ringer's solution immediately after dissection?
9. What is the composition of Ringer's solution?
10. What are the uses of Ringer's solution?

CHAPTER 60

Simple Muscle Twitch

Learning Objectives

After completing this practical, you will be able to:

1. Dissect and make a sciatic nerve and gastrocnemius muscle preparation.
2. Make primary and secondary circuits.
3. Record the response of the muscle in response to a single electrical stimulus to the nerve.
4. Record the time-tracing below the recording of the simple muscle curve.
5. Calculate the latent period, contraction period and relaxation period from the recording.

INTRODUCTION

When a muscle is stimulated with a single induction shock, it exhibits a momentary twitch like a contraction. This momentary contraction of the muscle in response to electrical stimulation is called simple muscle twitch. The contraction recorded on a moving kymograph is known as a simple muscle curve. The simple muscle curve is recorded to study the latent period, contraction period and relaxation period of the skeletal muscles (Fig. 60.1).

The latent period is the period from the point of stimulus to the point of onset of contraction. The contraction period is the period between the point of onset of contraction to the point that corresponds to the peak of contraction. The relaxation period is the period from the peak of contraction to the end of relaxation.

Methods

Method to Study Simple Muscle Twitch

Principle

When a muscle is stimulated with a single induction shock, the muscle contracts. This lifts the lever to record a curve on a revolving smoked drum.

Requirements

1. Dissection instruments
2. Kymograph
3. Muscle trough
4. Inductorium
5. Short-circuiting key
6. Tap key
7. Ringer's solution
8. Smoked drum
9. Low-resistance wires
10. Electrodes
11. Tuning fork (100 Hz)
12. Thread
13. Hook and weights (Fig. 60.2)

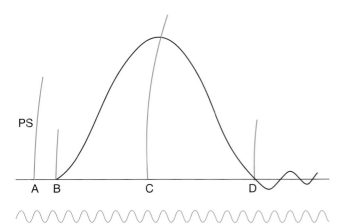

Fig. 60.1   Simple muscle twitch with time-trace below the curve (PS: Point of stimulation; AB: Latent period; BC: Contraction period; CD: Relaxation period).

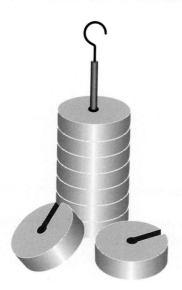

Fig. 60.2   Hook with weights.

Procedure

1. Arrange the primary and secondary circuits for recording a muscle twitch (*Refer* Fig. 58.15).
2. Include the kymograph in the primary circuit.
3. Select the fastest speed of the kymograph (first gear; pulleys 4 : 1).
4. Dissect a frog to obtain a sciatic nerve-gastrocnemius preparation.
5. Fix the nerve-muscle preparation in the muscle trough.
6. Pour Ringer's solution into the trough.
7. Hang a 10 g weight from the writing lever and keep the muscle in the afterloaded position.
8. Adjust the writing lever in such a way that the lever touches the drum lightly in the horizontal position.
9. Adjust the secondary coil to obtain a contraction at break stimulus only.
10. Set the drum in motion and record a baseline.
11. Press the tap key and release it as soon as you record the first contraction.
12. Vibrate the tuning fork by hitting against the thigh or against the hypothenar eminence of the hand and record a time-tracing below the simple muscle curve.
13. Stop the drum and close the short-circuiting key.
14. Rotate the drum manually so that the contact arms touch the kymograph key.

Note: This marks the instant when the primary circuit will be complete if the tap key is closed, which results in a stimulus from the secondary coil.

15. Mark the point of stimulation by moving the writing lever over the smoked drum.
16. Mark the beginning of contraction, peak of contraction and end of relaxation by moving the lever vertically on the drum manually on the corresponding points in the curve.
17. Calculate and record the duration of latent period (LP), contraction period (CP) and relaxation period (RP).

Precautions

In addition to the precautions described for 'nerve-muscle preparation' in Chapter 59, the following precautions should be observed:

1. The stimulus should be given briefly for a single induction shock.
2. The point of stimulus should be accurately marked.
3. While marking for latent period, contraction period and relaxation period, the lever should be placed exactly on the points.
4. Time-tracing should be taken just below the recording.

Observations and Results

Observe and study the simple muscle curve (Fig. 60.1). Express the duration of LP, CP and RP in ms; and also calculate the CP and RP as a percentage of the total muscle curve (CP + RP) duration.

DISCUSSION

The latent period, contraction period and relaxation period vary according to the type of muscle.

The latent period is due to:
- Time taken for the stimulus to travel along the nerve to the neuromuscular junction.
- Time taken for the impulse to cross the neuromuscular junction, to stimulate the muscle.
- Time taken for the excitation–contraction coupling to occur.
- Time taken by the lever to overcome the inertia of rest.
- Time taken to overcome the viscous resistance of the muscle.

The latent period is normally about 10 ms. The contraction period represents the duration of mechanical contraction. It normally ranges between 20 and 40 ms.

The relaxation period represents the time taken by the muscles to relax. It is normally more than the contraction period and ranges between 30 and 50 ms.

VIVA

1. *What are the causes of the latent period?*
2. *What is isometric contraction and how does it differ from isotonic contraction?*
3. *Give examples of isometric and isotonic contractions.*
4. *What is the normal duration of the contraction and relaxation periods of the frog skeletal muscle and what do they represent?*
5. *Can you determine the duration of LP, CP and RP without obtaining the time-tracing below the curve?*
    Ans: Yes, it can be derived from the speed of the drum.
6. *Why is induced current used for recording a simple muscle twitch?*
    Ans: Induced current gives a stimulus of short duration of desired intensity.
7. *Why is a 10 g weight placed on the lever?*
    Ans: The weight placed on the lever checks the amplitude of the contraction, overcomes the inertia of the lever, and keeps the lever horizontal.

CHAPTER 61

Effect of Temperature on Simple Muscle Twitch

Learning Objectives

After completing this practical, you WILL be able to:

1. Demonstrate the effect of temperature on muscle contraction.

2. State the precautions taken for recording the effects of temperature on muscle contraction.

3. Explain the effect of temperature on muscle contraction.

INTRODUCTION

A change in temperature in Ringer's solution causes a change in muscle contraction. With a change in temperature, there is a change in amplitude and the duration of different periods of contraction (latent, contraction and relaxation periods). The changes are mainly due to change in the rate of conduction velocity in the nerve, enzymatic and chemical activities in the muscle and a change in the viscosity of the muscle.

METHODS

Method to Study Effect of Temperature on Muscle Contraction

Principle

A change in the temperature of the environment affects muscle contraction. The effects of temperature on muscle contraction are studied by changing the temperature of Ringer's solution. The effects are studied on the same point of stimulus and same baseline. The change in amplitude of contraction, the duration of latent period, contraction period and relaxation period are noted.

Requirements

1. Same as that for 'simple muscle twitch'
2. Cold Ringer's solution (10°C)
3. Warm Ringer's solution (40°C)
4. Centigrade thermometer

Procedure

1. Pith and dissect the frog to make the nerve-muscle preparation.

2. Set up the nerve-muscle preparation for recording the simple muscle curve.

3. Record a simple muscle curve on the revolving drum with Ringer's solution in the muscle trough at room temperature.

4. Drain the Ringer's solution from the muscle trough and replace with warm Ringer's solution and wait for 1–3 minutes to allow the muscle to warm up.

5. Using the same baseline, same point of stimulation and same strength of stimulus, record the effect of warm Ringer's solution on the simple muscle curve.

6. Note the temperature of the Ringer's solution and drain the solution from the muscle trough.

7. Pour the normal Ringer's solution and wait for some time for the preparation to come back to normal temperature. Pour cold Ringer's solution into the muscle trough and wait for 2–5 minutes to allow the muscle to cool.

8. Using the same baseline, point of stimulation and strength of stimulus, record the effect of cold Ringer's on muscle contraction.

9. Record a time-tracing below the recordings with the help of a tuning fork.

10. Calculate the latent period, contraction period and relaxation period of the muscle contraction with different temperatures.

11. Record your observations in a tabular form (Table 61.1).

Table 61.1 Tabulation of experimental recordings.

Temperature of Ringer's soln.	L P (ms)	C P (ms)	R P (ms)	Height of contraction (cm)
1. Normal (25°C)				
2. Warm (40°C)				
3. Cold (10°C)				

Observation

Compare the recordings of the three muscle curves recorded at three different temperatures of Ringer's solution. Study the height and slope of contraction, and the duration of latent period, contraction period and relaxation period of each curve (Fig. 61.1).

Precautions

The precautions are the same as that for 'simple muscle twitch'. In addition to these, the following precautions are also to be kept in mind:

1. The point of stimulation, the baseline and the strength of stimulation for all the recordings should be kept constant.
2. The temperature of Ringer's solution should not exceed 42°C.

Note: When the temperature of the solution is 43°C or more, the muscle proteins are denatured. Muscles remain in a state of sustained contraction. This phenomenon is known as heat rigor.

3. The temperature of the cold solution should not be less than 4°C.

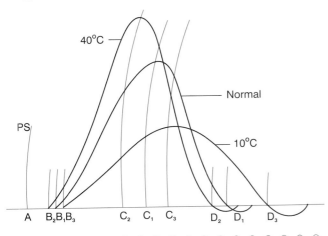

Fig. 61.1 Effect of temperature on simple muscle twitch. AB_1, AB_2 and AB_3 are the latent periods; B_1C_1, B_2C_2 and B_3C_3 are the contraction periods; C_1D_1, C_2D_2 and C_3D_3 are the relaxation periods of normal, high (40°C) and low (10°C) temperatures respectively.

Note: When the temperature of the solution is very low, the muscle proteins are coagulated. This prevents muscle contraction.

4. The temperature of the solution should be recorded just prior to or immediately after muscle contraction.
5. The effects of the warm solution should be recorded before recording the effects of cold Ringer's, because cold Ringer's inhibits all enzymatic and metabolic activities of the muscle. It may be difficult to revive muscle activities from the effects of cold Ringer's.

DISCUSSION

When muscle contraction is recorded with **higher temperature** of Ringer's solution, the *latent period, contraction period and relaxation period decrease, and the height of contraction increases*. The decrease in latent period is due to:

◈ Increase in conduction velocity in the nerve
◈ Increased rate of neuromuscular transmission
◈ Inertia of the lever being overcome faster

The shortening of the contraction and relaxation periods is due to faster contraction and relaxation. This occurs due to **activation of myosin ATPase activity** and **decreased resistance** of the muscle to contractions as the viscosity of the muscle decreases with increased temperature. The amplitude of contraction increases due to *increased enzymatic and chemical activities* in the muscle.

When muscle contraction is recorded with **low temperature of Ringer's solution**, the *opposite effects* are observed. They are due to **decreased rate of conduction** of impulse in the nerve and through the neuromuscular junction, **increased viscosity of the muscle, decreased enzymatic and chemical activities** in the muscle.

The change in the muscular activities of **human beings** due to change in environmental temperature, though similar, may be different from these experimental observations. This is because physical efficiency depends on various factors like **training, motivation, state of nutrition**, environmental temperature, humidity and so on. However, the body temperature never rises to the extent of causing heat rigor. But, if a person is exposed to a high temperature for a long duration, a phenomenon akin to heat rigor occurs; if a person is exposed to very low temperatures, muscle contraction is inhibited.

VIVA

1. What are the precautions taken when recording the effects of temperature on muscle contraction?
2. What are the changes in muscle contraction, which occur in response to warm Ringer's solution? What are the causes of these changes?
3. What are the changes in muscle contraction, which occur in response to cold Ringer's solution? What are the causes of these changes?
4. What is heat rigor?
5. Why is the effect of warm Ringer's recorded before recording the effect of cold Ringer's?
6. What is the effect of temperature on performance in human beings?

CHAPTER 62

Effect of Increasing Strength of Stimuli on Muscle Contraction

Learning Objectives

After completing this practical, you will be able to:

1. Define subthreshold, threshold and supra-maximal stimuli.
2. Differentiate between make and break stimuli.
3. Demonstrate the effect of increase in strength of stimuli on muscle contraction.
4. Explain the physiological basis of these changes.

INTRODUCTION

The amplitude of contraction increases with increase in the strength of the stimuli. There are different types of stimuli:

1. A **subminimal stimulus** or subthreshold stimulus is a stimulus that does not evoke a response.
2. A **threshold stimulus** is the minimum strength of stimulus that is just sufficient to evoke a response. This is also called minimal or liminal stimulus.
3. A **maximal stimulus** produces maximum response.
4. A **supramaximal stimulus** is stronger than a maximal stimulus, but does not change the magnitude of contraction after reaching a peak level.

When a muscle is stimulated with increasing strength of stimuli, more and more motor units are recruited. This results in an increase in the amplitude of contraction. A *motor unit* is defined as a single motor neuron (together with its branches) and the muscle fibres that it supplies.

Factors that affect the magnitude of contraction:

1. Number of motor units activated by the stimulus
2. The strength of the stimulus
3. The frequency of the stimulus

METHODS

Method to Study Effects of Strength of Stimuli on Muscle Contraction

Principle

The amplitude of contraction increases with increase in the strength of the stimuli. Increasing the strength of single 'make' and 'break' stimuli are applied to the muscle by stimulating the nerve starting from the subthreshold to supra-maximal levels. The muscle contractions are recorded on a stationary drum.

Requirements

1. Electrical connections for single induction shock (with a spring key in the primary circuit and a short-circuiting key in the secondary circuit)
2. Kymograph
3. Muscle trough and lever
4. Nerve-muscle preparation (freshly dissected)

Procedure

1. Set up the myograph and the nerve-muscle preparation for recording a simple muscle twitch.
2. Exclude the drum from the primary circuit and engage the gear in the neutral position.
3. Move the secondary coil of the inductorium far away from the primary coil.
4. Keep the writing point of the lever away from the drum and press and release the spring key. Observe for the contraction at 'make' and 'break'.
5. If there is no contraction, move the secondary coil 1 cm closer to the primary coil and press and release the key, and look for contraction at 'make' and 'break'.
6. Repeat the procedure till the break shock gives a contraction and record the contraction on the smoked drum. Measure and note the distance (in cm) between the primary and secondary coils.
7. Move the secondary coil 1 cm closer to the primary

coil, rotate the drum manually and record the contraction at both 'make' and 'break'. Record each pair of 'make' and 'break' contractions close to each other, as given in Fig. 62.1.

8. Repeat this procedure by moving the secondary coil closer to the primary coil till there is no further increase in the amplitude of contraction, by increasing the intensity of the stimulus. Measure the distance between the primary and secondary coils for each stimulus.

9. Label the response as M for make stimulus and B for break stimulus below each pair of recordings.

Summation of subminimal stimuli

1. Set up the apparatus for a simple muscle twitch with a spring key in the primary circuit.
2. Reduce the strength of induction shock to just below the minimum.
3. Give a single induction shock and note that no contraction occurs.
4. Stimulate repeatedly by tapping the key repeatedly and rapidly and observe the contraction, which usually occurs on the fifth or sixth stimulus.

Observation

Observe and study the recording (Fig. 62.1). Observe that there was no contraction at subminimal stimuli. The contraction was recorded only with the break stimulus at minimal strength. With further increase in the strength of the stimuli, the contractions were recorded with both make and break stimuli and the amplitudes of the contractions increased in a graded manner. In all recordings, the height of the contractions of the break stimuli is more than the height of the contractions of the make stimuli, when the stimuli were submaximal. At maximal stimulus, the height of the contraction is maximum, but there is no difference between the recordings of the make and break stimuli. After reaching the maximal level, there was no further increase in the height of contractions following application of supramaximal stimuli. In the case of supramaximal stimuli, the height of make and break stimuli also remain the same and are unchanged.

Precautions

1. The drum should be excluded from the primary circuit.
2. Contractions of both make and break stimuli should be recorded.
3. The recording should start from the subminimal level and should continue to the supra-maximal stimuli.
4. Each pair of recordings should be labelled to indicate the make and break stimuli.
5. The writing point should be brought in contact with the drum with the same friction for all the recordings.

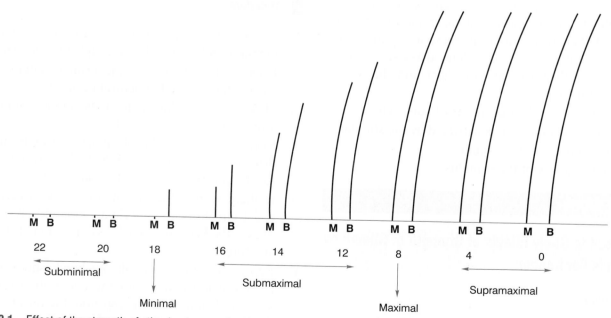

Fig. 62.1 Effect of the strength of stimulus on muscle contraction (M: Make stimulus; B: Break stimulus). The numbers below the stimuli indicate the distance (in cm) between the primary and secondary coils.

6. A minimum of 15 seconds should be allowed between application of the make and break shocks to avoid the beneficial effects on muscle contraction.

DISCUSSION

At subminimal (subthreshold) stimulus, the muscle does not contract since the current supplied does not have enough strength to excite muscle fibres to result in a muscle contraction. A threshold stimulus excites few motor units and gives a weak contraction. Minimal stimuli contraction is recorded only with the break stimulus, because the break stimulus is stronger than the make stimulus. As the strength of stimuli increases, **more and more motor units are recruited**, which results in increased magnitude of contraction. When the strength of the stimulus reaches maximal level, there is no increase in the magnitude of contraction with further increase in the strength of stimuli (supra-maximal stimuli) because the maximum number of motor units have already been utilised.

VIVA

1. Define subminimal, threshold and supra-maximal stimuli.
2. Why does the contraction occur only with the break stimulus at the threshold level?
3. Why does the magnitude of contraction increase with increase in the strength of stimuli?
4. Why is no change observed in the magnitude of the contraction with an increase in the strength of the contraction after reaching the maximal level?
5. Define a motor unit.
6. Why does only the break stimulus evoke a response with application of minimal stimuli?
7. Why is 15 seconds allowed between the application of the make and break stimuli?

CHAPTER 63

Effect of Two Successive Stimuli on Muscle Contraction

Learning Objectives

After completing this practical, you will be able to:

1. Define absolute and relative refractory period.
2. Describe the physiological basis of the beneficial effect.
3. Demonstrate the effect of two successive stimuli on muscle contraction.
4. Explain the mechanisms of these effects.

INTRODUCTION

When two successive stimuli are paired, the response of the muscle to the paired stimuli depends on the timing of the second stimulus. If the second stimulus is applied in the absolute refractory period of the previous stimulation, it does not evoke any response.

If it falls in the relative refractory period, a response may be obtained. The muscle and nerve are unresponsive during the refractory period of the action potential. However, the mechanical response (the contractile machinery) has no refractoriness. Therefore, the two successive stimuli can be added up.

Absolute refractory period

This is the period during which a second stimulus does not produce any response, no matter how strong the stimulus is or how long the duration of the application of the stimulus is.

Relative refractory period

This is the period during which a stimulus of greater strength may evoke a response.

The beneficial effect

When a muscle is stimulated by two successive stimuli, the magnitude of the contraction of the second stimulus is greater than the first. This occurs because the first stimulus becomes beneficial for the second one. The calcium ions released from the terminal cisterns during muscle contraction are pumped back into the cisterns during relaxation. Therefore, when the second stimulus falls in the relaxation period or immediately following the relaxation period of the first one, some amount of calcium is left in the sarcoplasm due to incomplete relaxation. This increases the calcium concentration for the second stimulus, as it adds to the calcium that has been left in the sarcoplasm from the first stimulus. Therefore, the height of the contraction increases with the second stimulus. The increase in temperature and the decrease in viscosity of the muscle by first contraction also contribute to the beneficial effect.

METHODS

Method to Study Effect of Two Successive Stimuli on Muscle Contraction

Principle

When two successive stimuli are paired and applied to the muscle, the magnitude of contraction changes depending on the timing of the second stimulus. This is recorded by separating the contact arms of the kymograph and recording the contractions at different angles between the arms.

Requirements

The requirements are the same as that for simple muscle twitch.

Procedure

1. Set up the nerve-muscle preparation for recording a simple muscle twitch.
2. Arrange the induction coil to obtain maximal or supra-maximal stimuli.

3. Separate the two contact arms attached to the spindle of the drum by an angle such that the second twitch immediately follows the first twitch.

4. Stimulate the nerve and record the muscle contraction. Mark the two points of stimulation.

5. Reduce the angle between the two contact arms to such an extent that the second stimulus falls during the relaxation period of the first twitch. Record the contraction and mark the point of stimulation.

6. Continue to record by reducing the angle between the two contact arms so that the second stimulus falls during the contraction period, and during the first half and second half of the latent period of the first contraction.

Observation

Study your observations. Note that there is no effect of the second stimulus on muscle contraction if the stimulus falls in the first half of the latent period of the first muscle twitch. But if the second stimulus falls in the second half of the latent period or in the contraction period, the magnitude of the contraction increases. When the second stimulus falls in the relaxation period of the first contraction, a conjoint second contraction (two peaks of the contraction) appears, which obscures the relaxation period of the first contraction. The second peak is bigger than the first one. When the

second stimulus falls immediately after the relaxation period of the first contraction, the second contraction is bigger than the first one (Fig. 63.1).

Precautions

1. The distance between the contact arms should be gradually decreased so as to apply the second stimulus on different phases of contraction of the first stimulus.

2. The point of stimulus of both the twitches should be marked.

3. The beneficial effect should be demonstrated.

4. The stimuli should be of maximal or supra-maximal strength as these stimuli activate all motor units and give maximum response.

DISCUSSION

When the second stimulus falls in the **first half of the latent period** of the first contraction, it *does not evoke any response* as it falls in the absolute refractory period of the first stimulus.

❖ When the second stimulus falls in the **second half of the latent period or in the contraction period**, there is *summation of contraction and the magnitude of the contraction increases*.

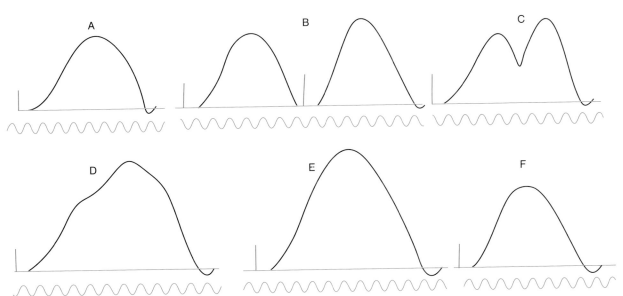

Fig. 63.1   Effect of two successive stimuli on muscle contraction. (A) Simple muscle twitch; (B) Second stimulus given immediately following the relaxation period of the first one; (C) Second stimulus applied during the relaxation period of the first one; (D) Second stimulus applied during the contraction of the first one; (E) Second stimulus applied during the second half of the latent period of the first stimulus; (F) Second stimulus applied in the first half of the latent period of the first stimulus.

- When the second stimulus **falls in the relaxation period** of the first, the *relaxation is arrested and the second contraction occurs*. In this case, the height of the second contraction is more than the first one because of the beneficial effect.

- When the second stimulus falls **immediately following the relaxation** of the first contraction, a *second twitch is recorded*, which is of *higher magnitude* than the first one. The increase in magnitude of the second twitch is also due to the beneficial effect. The increased magnitude of contraction is actually due *to the summation of the responses* (contractions) rather than the summation of stimuli.

VIVA

1. Why is the supra-maximal stimulus used in this experiment?
2. What is the beneficial effect and what is its physiological basis?
3. Define absolute and relative refractory periods.
4. Explain why the second stimulus does not evoke any response if it falls in the first half of the latent period of the first twitch.
5. Why is the magnitude of a contraction more when the second stimulus falls in the second half of the latent period or the contraction period of the first twitch?
6. Why is the magnitude of a contraction of the second stimulus more than the first one when the second stimulus falls in or following the relaxation period of the first one?

CHAPTER 64

Genesis of Tetanus

Learning Objectives

After completing this practical, you will be able to:

1. Define treppe, clonus and tetanus.
2. Demonstrate the effects of increasing frequency of stimulation on muscle contraction.
3. List the precautions taken during genesis of tetanus in this experiment.
4. Calculate the minimal tetanisable frequency (MTF).
5. List the factors that affect MTF.
6. Explain the physiological basis of treppe, clonus and tetanus.
7. Differentiate between experimental and clinical tetanus.
8. List the causes, features and prevention of tetanus (the disease).

INTRODUCTION

Tetanus refers to a state of sustained tonic contraction of the muscle (without relaxation) due to rapidly repeated stimulation. It does not occur if the muscle is stimulated at a lower rate (lower frequency). If the rate of stimulation increases (higher frequency), tetanus ensues. When the muscle is stimulated below the tetanising frequency, incomplete tetanus (clonus) occurs.

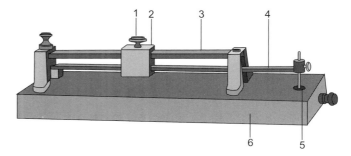

Fig. 64.1 Vibrating reed (1: Clamping plate; 2: Thumb screw; 3: Vibration scale; 4: Metal guide; 5: Mercury cup; 6: Base board).

METHODS

Method to Study Genesis of Tetanus

Principle

If a muscle is stimulated at higher frequencies, there is sustained tonic contraction of the muscle (tetanus). The nerve-muscle preparation is stimulated at different frequencies using a vibrating interrupter till tetanus ensues.

Requirements

1. Same as that for 'simple muscle twitch'.
2. Vibrating variable interrupter (Fig. 64.1). The reed is calibrated to vibrate at a frequency of 5, 7, 10, 20, 30 and 40 vibrations per sec. This is achieved by sliding the clamping plate along the metal guides fixed to the base board.

3. Signal marker.

Procedure

1. Arrange an electrical circuit for single induced shocks, including vibrating interrupter and signal marker in the primary circuit. Exclude kymograph from the circuit.
2. Set up the kymograph and nerve-muscle preparation as for the recording of the simple muscle curve.
3. Adjust the inductorium for weak break shocks.
4. Adjust the length of vibrating reed of the interrupter to provide five interruptions (stimuli) per second.
5. Start the kymograph using slow speed (fast gear; pulley 1:4) and set the reed vibrating. Open the short-circuiting key to stimulate the muscle and close it after recording 5–7 contractions on the drum.

6. Now increase the rate of interruptions (stimulation) to 10, 15, 20, 30 and 40 per second and take a record of each stimulation, using fresh space on the smoked paper. Avoid unnecessary stimulation.

Note: If high frequency for obtaining tetanus is not available, use Neef's hammer by including it in the primary circuit.

7. Note the frequency of stimulation, which produced complete tetanus in your experiment.
8. Above each set of recordings, indicate the rate of stimulation as given in the figure.
9. Fix the recording by varnishing the paper.

Observation

Observe and study the graph (Fig. 64.2). Observe the staircase phenomenon (treppe) of the first initial stimuli. At the low frequency of stimulation, single contractions occur; with increasing frequency, first clonus (partial tetanus) and then tetanus occur.

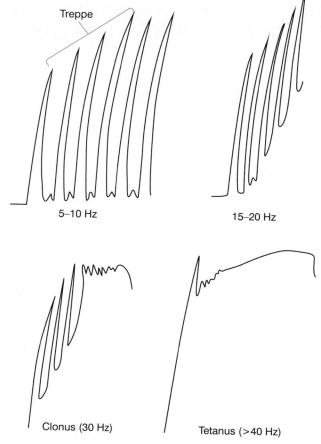

Fig. 64.2   Genesis of tetanus.

Precautions

1. The kymograph should be excluded from the circuit.
2. The inductorium should be adjusted for weak break shocks.
3. The preparation should be stimulated from lower frequency to higher frequency.
4. Unnecessary stimulation should be avoided.
5. If tetanising frequency in not obtained, Neef's hammer should be included in the primary circuit.

DISCUSSION

Minimal Tetanisable Frequency

The minimal tetanisable frequency (MTF) of a muscle can be calculated from the simple muscle curve (measuring the contraction period) by using the following formula:

$$MTF = \frac{1}{Contraction\ period}$$

For example, if the contraction period is 0.04 seconds, the MTF = 1/0.04 = 25 Hz.

Factors That Affect MTF

1. Type of muscle   In slow muscles, the MTF is low because they produce slow, sustained contractions (longer contraction period). In fast muscles, the MTF is greater because the contraction period is less. An example of a slow muscle is soleus, and examples of fast muscles are the muscles of the eye.

2. Temperature of the environment   Tetanisable frequency is lower in a hot environment and higher in a cold environment.

3. Load acting on the muscle   If the load acting on the muscle is greater, the tetanisable frequency decreases.

Treppe

Treppe is also known as the **staircase phenomenon**; it is the *progressive increase in the force of contraction for the first two to three contractions* when a muscle is stimulated repeatedly. This occurs due to the accumulation of calcium in the sarcoplasm due to application of repeated stimuli. Treppe is also seen in cardiac muscles. However, the cardiac muscle cannot be tetanised because of a longer refractory period.

Clonus

Clonus is a state of **partial tetanus** observed in experimental conditions (experimental clonus). This should not be confused with the clinical clonus, for example, ankle clonus, seen in upper motor neuron type of paralysis. In experimental clonus, relaxation is incomplete.

Tetanus

Tetanus is a **state of sustained contraction**. The muscle remains in a state of tonic contraction without relaxation. This occurs when a nerve-muscle preparation is stimulated at a higher frequency. Rapid and repeated stimulation leads the stimuli to fall during the contraction phase so that the contractile processes are repeatedly activated. The muscle does not get time to relax. Therefore, with each stimulation, the *muscle contracts without relaxation. Individual responses fuse* to give a state of sustained contraction (tetanus). The muscles of our body, which are involved in the maintenance of posture exhibit tetanic contraction (sustained contraction). An erect posture is maintained due to sustained contraction of the antigravity muscles. Tetanic contraction of the skeletal muscles is also observed during an isometric exercise.

Tetanus is also seen clinically when a person is infected by a group of bacteria called *Clostridium tetani*. Tetanus usually occurs following an injury (cut, wound) through which the bacteria enter the body. The tetanus toxin released by the bacteria stimulates the motor neurons repeatedly at a higher frequency and results in tetanus. The facial muscles are commonly affected. In severe cases, all the skeletal muscles of the body may be affected. The disease can be prevented by prior immunisation with the tetanus vaccine or receiving the vaccine within twelve hours of injury.

VIVA

1. *Define treppe, clonus and tetanus.*
2. *What is the mechanism of the staircase phenomenon?*
3. *How is tetanus produced experimentally?*
4. *What is minimal tetanisable frequency (MTF)? How is the MTF calculated and what are the factors that affect MTF?*
5. *Explain why the cardiac muscle cannot be tetanised.*
6. *Give an example of tetanic contractions in our body.*
7. *Why is the tension developed by a tetanically contracting muscle more than the tension developed by the muscle during a single twitch?*
   Ans: During a single contraction of the muscle, any calcium released into the sarcoplasm is quickly taken back into the cisterns during relaxation. But if the muscle is stimulated repeatedly, there is accumulation of calcium in the sarcoplasm as calcium cannot be pumped back fully into the cisterns. This increases the tension in the muscle.
8. *What is the cause of tetanus (disease) and how is the disease prevented?*
9. *What is tetany?*
   Ans: Tetany occurs due to hypocalcemia, for example, hypoparathyroidism. It is not connected with tetanus.

CHAPTER 65

Genesis of Fatigue

Learning Objectives

After completing this practical, you will be able to:
1. Define fatigue.
2. Demonstrate the site of fatigue in the nerve-muscle preparation.
3. List the precautions taken during the recording of the genesis of fatigue.
4. Name the site of fatigue in isolated and intact preparations.
5. Explain the causes of fatigue in isolated preparations.
6. Explain how recovery can be expedited.

INTRODUCTION

Fatigue is defined as *decrease in performance due to continuous and prolonged activity*. It can occur in the whole organism or in isolated preparations. The mechanism of fatigue is different in an intact organism and in an isolated preparation. Fatigue is a **reversible phenomenon** and there is no permanent functional or structural damage to the tissues. **In humans**, fatigue first occurs **in the central nervous system** whereas **in isolated preparations**, the *neuromuscular junction* is the first site of fatigue.

METHODS

Method to Study Genesis of Fatigue

Principle

A muscle is fatigued when it is stimulated repeatedly and continuously. The phenomenon of fatigue is recorded by stimulating the preparation without changing the baseline, the point of stimulation and the strength of the stimulus.

Requirements

The requirements are the same as that for 'simple muscle twitch'.

Procedure

1. Dissect the frog to make the nerve-muscle preparation.
2. Mount the preparation in the muscle trough and set it up for recording a simple muscle curve. Mark the point of stimulation.
3. Repeatedly stimulate the nerve and record the first, second and third contractions on a fast-moving drum without changing the point of stimulation. Note the beneficial effect.
4. Move the writing lever away from the drum.
5. Without changing the point of stimulation, stimulate the nerve repeatedly by keeping the tap key pressed and record every tenth contraction by applying the writing lever to the drum.

Note: The drum rotates without recording the muscle contraction. Only the tenth contraction is recorded on the drum. This is done to avoid overlapping recordings. Recording can be made with each stimulation, but overlapping of the recordings will make it difficult to study the graph.

6. Continue to record every tenth contraction till the contractions are too feeble to be recorded.
7. Change the point of stimulus to record a muscle contraction at a different place adjacent to the fatigue curve and on the same baseline.
8. Stimulate the muscle directly and record the contraction on the changed point of stimulus.

9. Drain the Ringer's solution and replace with fresh solution.

10. Allow the nerve-muscle preparation to rest for five minutes.

11. Again change the point of stimulus on the same baseline in such a way that the next recording will be adjacent to the previous recording.

12. Stimulate the nerve to record the muscle contractions.

Observation

Record the amplitude and duration of the phases of the first three contractions and the subsequent contractions. Note that with the onset of fatigue, the relaxation period of the muscle twitches is prolonged and the baseline goes up (Fig. 65.1A). Muscle contraction occurs by direct stimulation of the muscle (Fig. 65.1B) following fatigue. Muscle contraction also occurs in response to nerve stimulation following recovery (Fig. 65.1C).

Precautions

1. All the precautions described for the recording of simple muscle twitch should be taken (Chapter 60).

2. All the contractions should be recorded on the same point of stimulus and on the same baseline for the fatigue curve (fatigue produced by stimulation of nerve).

3. The muscle should be directly stimulated immediately after recording the fatigue by stimulating the nerve, and the contraction should be recorded on a different point of stimulus but on the same baseline.

4. The preparation should be allowed a minimum of five minutes for recovery before stimulating the nerve, to record the effect of recovery.

5. To facilitate recovery, the old Ringer's solution should be removed and replaced by the fresh solution.

DISCUSSION

In isolated preparations, fatigue can occur at **three sites**: the *muscle, the neuromuscular junction and the nerve*. The *nerve is theoretically unfatiguable*, therefore the possible sites may be either the muscle or the neuromuscular junction. But the muscle contraction recorded by directly stimulating the muscle following the genesis of fatigue indicates that the muscle is not fatigued. Therefore, it can be inferred that the *first site of fatigue is the neuromuscular junction*.

The *cause of this fatigue is the depletion of acetylcholine*, the neurotransmitter from the myoneural junction. If the preparation is allowed to rest for some time and fresh Ringer's solution is supplied to the preparation, the muscle contracts in response to the stimulation of the nerve (following the period of recovery). This again proves that the site of fatigue was the neuromuscular junction, as recovery allows re-synthesis of neurotransmitters at the nerve endings. The Ringer's solution supplies nutrition and facilitates recovery.

If the *muscle is directly stimulated continuously*, it can also be *fatigued due to exhaustion of glycogen storage*. But in this condition, there will be no recovery, as the utilised glycogen cannot be replaced.

An **early sign of fatigue** is the *prolongation of the relaxation period*. When a muscle is fatigued, the relaxation becomes incomplete and then it remains in a state of partial contraction. This is called **contraction remainder**. It occurs due to a decrease in the ATP content and accumulation of the metabolites in the muscle. The baseline increases due to contraction remainder.

In human beings, the first site of fatigue *is the CNS*, not the neuromuscular junction.

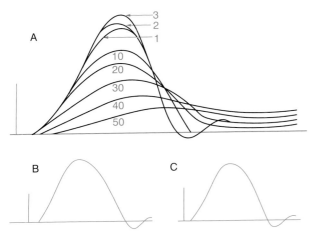

Fig. 65.1 Demonstration of the phenomenon and site of fatigue. (A) Genesis of fatigue following repeated stimulation of the nerve. Numbers depicted with the curves indicate the number of stimuli. Note the beneficial effects with the first three contractions. Also, note the decrease in amplitude, prolongation of relaxation period and rise in baseline with the onset of fatigue; (B) Recording of the curve by directly stimulating the muscle immediately following onset of fatigue; (C) Recording of the curve by stimulating the nerve following recovery.

VIVA

1. Define fatigue.
2. What is the difference between the fatigue of an intact animal and that of an isolated preparation?
3. What is the site of fatigue in an isolated preparation and how do you demonstrate it?
4. What is the mechanism of fatigue in an isolated preparation?
5. How can the recovery be facilitated?
6. What is contraction remainder?
7. What is the early sign of fatigue in an isolated preparation?

CHAPTER 66

Conduction Velocity of Nerves in Frogs

Learning Objectives

After completing this practical, you will be able to:

1. State the importance of the determination of nerve conduction in clinical physiology.

2. Demonstrate the recording of the conduction velocity of nerves in frog.
3. List the factors that affect nerve conduction velocity.

INTRODUCTION

The detection of the velocity of nerve conduction is one of the important tests in clinical neurophysiology. In human beings, the velocity of conduction is determined by using nerve conduction apparatus (*see* Chapter 31). But the recording of conduction velocity in frogs is a simple experiment. Conduction velocity mainly depends on the diameter and myelination of the nerve.

METHODS

Method to Determine Conduction Velocity of Nerves in Frogs

Principle

The velocity of conduction is determined by dividing the distance between the two points of stimuli (proximal and distal) by the difference in the latent period of both the recordings.

Requirements

1. Same as that for simple muscle twitch
2. Scale

Procedure

1. Make a gastrocnemius-sciatic nerve preparation and set up to record a simple muscle twitch.

2. Stimulate at the vertebral end of the sciatic nerve and record a simple muscle twitch. Mark the point of placement of the electrodes on the nerve.
3. Mark the point of stimulus and the point of onset of the contraction to record the latent period.
4. Stimulate at the muscular end of the sciatic nerve and record a simple muscle twitch on the same baseline and on the same point of the stimulus, and calculate the latent period. Mark the point of placement of the electrodes on the nerve.
5. Deduct the latent period of the second recording (recording of the stimulation of the muscular end) from the latent period of the first recording (recording of the stimulation at the vertebral end).
6. Measure the distance between the points of stimulation of the vertebral end and the muscular end of the nerve in centimetres.
7. Calculate conduction velocity by dividing the distance by time.

Note: The distance is the length of the nerve (in cm) between the two points of stimuli and the time is the difference in the latent period of the two recordings (in ms).

Observation

Observe the difference in the latent period of the two recordings (Fig. 66.1) and calculate the conduction velocity from the given recordings. Express your result in m/s.

Note: The normal value of the conduction velocity of the sciatic nerve of a frog is 40–60 m/s.

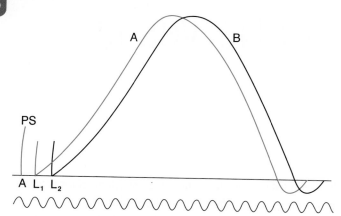

Fig. 66.1   Determination of nerve conduction velocity in frog. (A: Simple muscle curve following stimulation of the nerve close to the muscle; B: Simple muscle curve following stimulation of the nerve close to the vertebra; PS: Point of stimulation; AL_1: Latent period of the curve A; AL_2: Latent period of the curve B).

▋ *Precautions*

1. The point of stimulus of both the ends of the sciatic nerve should be marked at the time of stimulation.

2. The distance between the two points should be accurately measured.

3. The difference in the latent periods should be accurately measured.

DISCUSSION

The sciatic nerve is a mixed nerve and a thick nerve. The conduction velocity of a nerve is determined mainly by the fibre diameter and the degree of myelination of the nerve. As the fibre diameter increases, the velocity of conduction increases. The velocity of conduction is higher in myelinated than in unmyelinated fibres. The velocity of conduction of a somatic nerve (like the sciatic nerve) having a fibre diameter of 12–20 µm ranges between 60 and 120 m/s. The decrease in conduction velocity indicates injury to the nerve or some defect in the nerve.

Other factors that affect nerve conduction are temperature, height of action potential and stimulating and recording systems.

VIVA

1. What is the clinical significance of determining the conduction velocity of nerves?
2. What is the normal velocity of conduction of the sciatic nerve of the frog?
3. What are the factors that affect the velocity of conduction in the nerve?
4. In which condition does the velocity of conduction decrease?

CHAPTER 67

Normal Cardiogram of Frog

INTRODUCTION

The normal cardiogram of a frog is the recording of the mechanical activities of the heart of the frog on a smoked drum. Since the cardiogram is the **recording of the mechanical activities**, it records the systole and diastole of the different chambers of the heart. In a frog, the atria are called **auricles**, the **ventricles are single-chambered**, and the electrical rhythm for generating an impulse is located in the **sinus venosus** instead of the SA node as seen in the mammalian heart (Table 67.1). Therefore, in an ideal tracing, the mechanical activities of the sinus venosus, auricles and ventricles are recorded. A white crescentic line is present between the auricles and the sinus venosus(Fig. 67.1). The normal heart rate of a frog is 40–50 beats per minute.

METHODS

Method of Recording Normal Cardiogram of Frog

▌ Principle

The mechanical activities of the amphibian heart are directly recorded by connecting the heart to the writing lever with a thread which transmits the waves of contraction and relaxation from the heart to the lever. The cardiac activities are recorded on a moving drum.

▌ Requirements

1. Kymograph with Sherrington–Starling drum
2. Frog board

Table 67.1   Differences between amphibian and mammalian heart.

		Amphibian heart	Mammalian heart
1.	Heart chambers	Three-chambered heart; two auricles and a ventricle	Four-chambered heart; two atria and two ventricles
2.	Sinus venosus	Present; receives venous blood	Absent; venous blood directly drains to right atrium
3.	Coronary arteries	Not well developed	Well developed
4.	Blood in ventricle	Mixed (arterial and venous)	Not mixed
5.	Myocardial perfusion	Directly from the blood present in the ventricle	Through coronaries
6.	Pacemaker	Pacemaker is present in sinus venosus	SA node is the pacemaker, which is present in the right atrium
7.	White crescentic line	Present; works as parasympathetic ganglion	Absent

3. Myograph stand
4. Starling's heart lever or simple heart lever
5. Frog Ringer's solution
6. Pins (also one hooked pin)
7. Thread

▌ Procedure

1. Pith the frog (destroy only the spinal cord).
2. Lay the pithed frog on its back on the frog board.

3. Make a median incision through the skin over the sternum.

4. Raise the xiphisternum with blunt forceps and separate it from the underlying tissue using a pair of blunt scissors, taking care not to injure the heart.

5. Insert one of the blades of the scissors under the pectoral girdle and cut on both sides so that the anterior wall of the thorax can be removed.

6. Pull the forelimbs laterally and fix them on to the board with pins so as to keep the chest wide open.

7. Identify the heart, beating inside the thin membrane (pericardium).

8. Observe that at the apex of the heart, there is a small clear space between the heart and pericardial membrane. With the help of forceps, pinch and lift the pericardium at the apex at this clear space, taking care not to touch the heart.

9. Make a slit in the pericardium with the help of a pair of fine scissors and then cut the pericardium up to the base of the heart, taking care not to injure the heart.

10. Study the different parts of the heart (Fig. 67.1).

Note: On the ventral aspect of the heart, the initial dilated portion of the aorta, which is known as bulbus arteriosus, divides into two aortae. On the dorsal aspect (lift the ventricle), identify the sinus venosus separated from the auricles by a white crescentic line. Note that two superior vena cavae and the inferior vena cava enter the sinus venosus. Observe the change in the colour of the chambers during systole (contraction) and diastole (relaxation).

11. Fix the pericardium through the base of the heart to the frog board with a pin.

12. Hook a bent pin through the apex of the heart taking care not to puncture the chambers of the ventricle.

13. Tie one end of the thread to the pin and lift the ventricle by the thread. Tie the other end of the thread to the heart lever.

Note: Keep the thread vertical and taut enough to transmit the contraction of the heart to the writing point of the lever.

14. Keep the writing arm of the lever horizontal.

15. Touch the writing point of the heart lever lightly to the smoked paper on the drum in the lower third (about 5 cm from the lower margin) of the drum.

16. Set the drum to rotate at a slow speed (1.2 mm/s) and record the cardiogram starting from just after the joint of the paper on the drum.

17. Take a time-tracing below the recording.

18. Repeat the recording of the cardiogram at a higher speed (2.5 mm/s).

Note: Recording at a faster speed will clearly show the different components of the cardiogram.

Observation

Identify the different components of the cardiogram recorded at slow and fast speeds as given in Fig. 67.2.

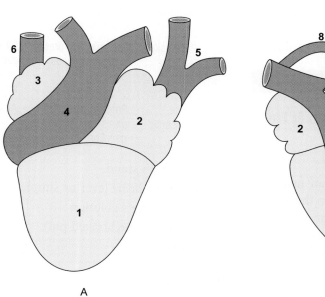
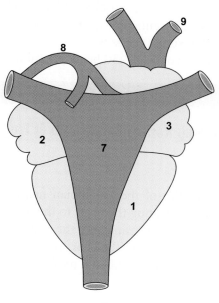

Fig. 67.1   Frog's, heart. (A) Dorsal view; (B) Ventral view (1: Ventricle; 2: Left auricle; 3: Right auricle; 4: Truncus arteriosus; 5: Left anterior caval vein; 6: Right anterior caval vein; 7: Sinus venosus; 8: Pulmonary vein; 9: Right systemic arch; 10: Posterior caval vein).

Observe the rhythmicity (whether regular or irregular) and calculate the heart rate.

Precautions

1. While cutting the sternum of the frog with a median incision, care should be taken not to damage the heart.
2. The heart should be exposed by cutting the pericardium.
3. While cutting the pericardium, take care not to damage the heart.
4. The hooked pin should be introduced at the apex of the heart through the wall of the ventricle. While introducing the hooked pin, care should be taken not to puncture the ventricle (the pin should not enter the ventricular cavity).
5. The thread connecting the heart and the lever should be placed vertically.
6. The lever should be placed horizontally.

7. The base of the heart should be fixed. It increases the amplitude of recording as the force of contraction is directly transmitted to the lever due to the pulling of the apex towards the fixed base during each systole.
8. Frog Ringer's solution should be poured on the heart at regular intervals to prevent it from drying.

DISCUSSION

The properties of the heart, which are studied in this experiment, are **automaticity, rhythmicity, conductivity and contractility**. Automaticity is studied by observing the automatic beating of the heart, which occurs due to the impulse generated automatically in the heart; rhythmicity is studied by the rhythmical beating of the heart; conductivity is studied by conduction of impulse from the sinus venosus to the ventricles (better *demonstrated by Stannius ligatures*); and contractility is recorded by observing the contraction of the heart and recording the systole and diastole in the tracings.

In the heart of a frog, the cardiac impulse is generated in the sinus venosus. Impulse is transmitted from the sinus venosus to the auricles and then to the ventricles. A slight pause is seen between auricular and ventricular contraction and this is due to the delay (partial conduction block) in conduction of the impulse from the auricles to the ventricles. In a frog, the rate of impulse generation is maximum in the sinus venosus. Therefore, the *sinus venosus is the natural pacemaker* of the heart.

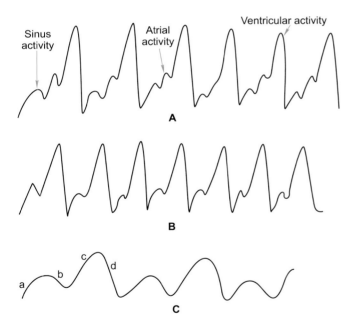

Fig. 67.2 Normal cardiogram of frog. (A) Ideal recording (at slow speed; 1.2 mm/s); (B) Usual recording (at slow speed; 1.2 mm/s); (C) Usual recording at fast speed (a: atrial systole; b: atrial relaxation; c: ventricular contraction; d: ventricular relaxation).

The Cardiogram

Different waves in the cardiogram represent the activities of different chambers of the heart. Usually only two **types of waves** are seen. The **'a' wave** represents auricular systole (upgoing) and diastole (downgoing), and the **'v' wave** represents ventricular systole and diastole. In an ideal recording, the **'s' wave** is that which appears before the **'a' wave** is seen. The **'s' wave** represents the systole and diastole of the sinus venosus.

VIVA

1. What is the difference between the cardiogram (recorded in this experiment) and the electrocardiogram?
2. What is the normal heart rate in a frog?
3. What are the properties of the cardiac muscle? What properties of the cardiac muscle are demonstrated in this experiment?
4. What are the differences between the amphibian and mammalian hearts?
5. Where is the pacemaker of a frog's heart situated?
6. What does the crescentic line represent?
7. What are the different waves recorded in a normal cardiogram of a frog's heart? How are these waves produced?
8. What are the precautions taken during dissection to expose the heart?
9. Why is the base of the heart fixed?
10. Why should only the spinal cord be destroyed during pithing?

   Ans: Cardiovascular centres are present in the brain. Therefore, if the brain is destroyed with pithing, there may be an alteration in heart function.

CHAPTER 68

Effect of Temperature on Frog's Heart

Learning Objectives

After completing this practical, you will be able to:

1. State the physiological importance of performing this practical.
2. Demonstrate the effect of cold and warm Ringer's solution on the sinus venosus and the ventricle.
3. List the precautions taken for studying the effect of cold and warm Ringer's solution on the sinus venosus and the ventricle.
4. Explain the changes in cardiac activities following the application of cold and warm Ringer's solution on the sinus venosus and the ventricle.

INTRODUCTION

The application of cold and warm Ringer's solution on the sinus venosus changes the heart rate by changing the pacemaker activity, which is present in the sinus venosus in frogs. The application of cold and warm Ringer's solution on the ventricle changes the force of contraction by directly affecting the contractile machinery of the myocardium.

This experiment is carried out to study the effect of temperature on the sinus venosus and the ventricle, and to know the site of impulse generation in the frog's heart.

METHODS

Method to Study Effect of Temperature on Frog's Heart

Principle

The application of cold and warm Ringer's solution on the sinus venosus changes the heart rate and that on the ventricle changes the force of contraction. These changes are observed by applying cold and warm Ringer's solution separately on the sinus venosus and on the ventricle, and recording the effect on a moving drum.

Requirements

1. Same as that for Chapter 67.
2. Cold Ringer's solution (15°C)
3. Warm Ringer's solution (35°C)
4. Dropper
5. Blotting paper

Procedure

Expose the heart of a pithed frog and record a normal cardiogram as described in Chapter 67. Then carry out the experiment separately on the sinus venosus and on the ventricle as described below.

On the sinus venosus

1. Record a normal cardiogram (about 10 beats).
2. Apply cold (15°C) Ringer's solution to the sinus venosus with the help of a dropper and record its effect on the cardiogram (about 10 beats).
3. Apply Ringer's solution at normal room temperature and record a normal cardiogram (about 10 beats).
4. Apply warm Ringer's (35°C) to the sinus venosus with the help of a dropper and record its effect on the cardiogram (about 10 beats).
5. Apply Ringer's solution at normal room temperature and record a normal cardiogram (about 10 beats).

On the ventricle

1. Record a normal cardiogram (about 10 beats) at room temperature.
2. Apply cold (15°C) Ringer's solution to the ventricle with a piece of blotting paper and record its effect on the ventricle.

Note: The small piece of blotting paper is soaked in cold Ringer's solution and the paper is then placed on the ventricle with the help of forceps, taking care not to allow the solution to trickle down to the sinus venosus.

3. Apply Ringer's solution at normal room temperature and record a normal cardiogram (about 10 beats).

4. Apply warm Ringer's (35 °C) to the ventricle with blotting paper and record its effect on the ventricle.

Note: The blotting paper is soaked in warm Ringer's solution and then placed on the ventricle with forceps, taking care not to allow the solution to trickle down to the sinus venosus.

5. Apply Ringer's solution at normal room temperature and record a normal cardiogram (about 10 beats).

Tabulate the effects of temperature on the sinus venosus and on the ventricle with reference to heart rate and force of contraction.

Observation

Study the effect of temperature on the sinus venosus and the ventricle. Note that cold Ringer's decreases the heart rate but increases the force of contraction, and warm Ringer's increases the heart rate but decreases the amplitude of contraction when applied to the sinus venosus. Cold Ringer's decreases the amplitude of contraction without changing the heart rate and warm Ringer's increases amplitude of contraction without changing the heart rate when applied to the ventricle (Fig. 68.1).

Precautions

1. The normal cardiogram should be recorded prior to the recording of the effects of cold and warm Ringer's solution on the sinus venosus and the ventricle.

2. The temperature of cold Ringer's should be 15°C and the temperature of warm Ringer's should be 35°C. If the solution is very cold or very hot, the heart may be damaged.

3. The temperature of the solutions should be recorded just before their application.

4. Care should be taken to apply the solution only on the sinus venosus when the effect of cold and warm Ringer's solution is carried out.

5. Care must be taken to prevent the trickling down of the solution to the sinus venosus from the ventricle, when the effect of cold and warm Ringer's is carried out. For recording the cardiogram, the ventricle is placed above the sinus venosus, blotting paper (not the dropper) is used to pour cold and warm Ringer's solution on the ventricle so that the solution does not trickle down to the sinus venosus.

6. The heart should be moistened with normal Ringer's solution frequently to prevent drying.

7. When not recording, the lever of the heart should be lowered to prevent deterioration of the function of the heart.

DISCUSSION

Cold Ringer's on the Sinus Venosus

The application of cold Ringer's solution on the sinus venosus *decreases the heart rate and increases the amplitude of contraction*. The heart rate decreases because cold Ringer's *directly inhibits the pacemaker activity* of the heart. This is **the primary effect**. The

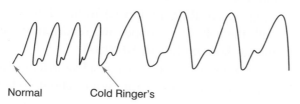

Normal   Cold Ringer's

A. On sinus venosus

Normal   Warm Ringer's

Normal   Cold Ringer's

B. On ventricle

Normal   Warm Ringer's

Fig. 68.1   Effect of temperature on frog's heart.

increase in amplitude of contraction is *due to the Frank–Starling law*. When the heart rate decreases, the ventricular end diastolic volume increases as the ventricle gets more time to fill. The increased ventricular filling increases the length of the ventricular muscle fibre prior to the onset of systole. Therefore, the force of the contraction increases. This is the **secondary effect**.

Warm Ringer's on the Sinus Venosus

The application of warm Ringer's solution on the sinus venosus *increases the heart rate and decreases the force of contraction*. The increase in heart rate is the **primary effect** and the decrease in the force of contraction is the **secondary effect**. The heart rate increases due to stimulation of the pacemaker activity in the sinus venosus by the warm solution. The force of contraction decreases due to less filling of heart (decreased end diastolic volume) as the heart gets less time to fill.

Cold Ringer's on the Ventricle

The application of cold Ringer's solution to the ventricle **decreases the force of contraction** due to the *inhibition of myocardial contractility* by the cold solution. The heart rate does not change as the pacemaker of the heart is present in the sinus venosus, which remains unaffected in this experiment. The myocardial activity is depressed by the cold Ringer's solution because at the low temperature, the *enzymatic activity of the myocardium decreases and the viscosity of the myocardial tissue increases*.

Warm Ringer's on the Ventricle

The application of warm Ringer's solution to the ventricle *increases the force of contraction* due to the accentuation of myocardial activity by the direct action of warm solution on it. The heart rate remains unchanged as the pacemaker is present in the sinus venosus. Warm Ringer's stimulates myocardial contractility by **increasing the enzymatic activity and decreasing the viscosity** of the myocardial tissue.

These experiments prove that the sinus venosus is the pacemaker of the frog heart.

VIVA

1. *What is the effect of cold Ringer's on the sinus venosus and the ventricle? What is the physiological basis?*
2. *What is the Frank–Starling law of the heart?*
3. *What is the effect of warm Ringer's solution on the sinus venosus and the ventricle? What is the physiological basis?*
4. *What are the precautions taken for demonstrating the effect of cold and warm Ringer's on the sinus venosus and the ventricle?*
5. *What is the physiological basis of the difference between the effect of cold and warm Ringer's on the sinus venosus and the ventricle?*

CHAPTER 69

Effect of Stannius Ligatures on Frog's Heart

Learning Objectives

After completing this practical, you will be able to:

1. Explain the clinical implication of this practical.
2. Demonstrate the effect of Stannius ligature on the frog heart.
3. Explain the effect of Stannius ligatures.
4. State the rate of discharge of different potential pacemakers of the heart.
5. Classify heart blocks.

INTRODUCTION

In humans, the cardiac impulse is generated in the SA node and conducted to all parts of the heart. Therefore, the SA node is the pacemaker of the heart. In a **frog's heart**, the **pacemaker is present in the sinus venosus**. The cardiac muscle has the property of automaticity, that is, it has the power to generate its own impulse. Though normally an impulse is generated in the SA node (primary pacemaker), automaticity is not limited to the SA node alone. When the SA node is diseased, the other potential pacemakers of the heart take over the responsibility to generate the impulse. The first to take over the work of the SA node is the AV node. The next in the hierarchy are bundle of His, the Purkinje system and the ventricular muscle. In humans, the *rate of discharge is maximum in the SA node as it is the natural pacemaker of the heart*. The rate of discharge gradually *decreases in the hierarchy of the pacemakers*.

In humans, the **rate of discharge of the different pacemakers** is as follows:

SA node	: 60–100/min
AV node	: 50–70/min
His bundle	: 40–60/min
Purkinje system	: 30–50/min
Ventricular muscle	: 15–40/min

This practical demonstrates the hierarchy of pacemaking activity of the different tissues of the heart.

METHODS

Method to Study Effect of Stannius Ligatures on Frog's Heart

Principle

The rate of discharge of impulses is different in different potential pacemakers of the heart. Their rhythms are demonstrated by separating (appropriately placing ligatures) them from each other.

Requirements

1. Same as that for Chapter 67
2. Aneurysm needle
3. Thread

Procedure

1. Set up the experiment as for recording a normal cardiogram.
2. Pass a threaded aneurysm needle between the truncus arteriosus and the atria.
3. Hook up the heart and record the normal cardiogram on a slow-moving drum.
4. Bring forward the thread under the truncus arteriosus and tie it at the junction of the sinus venosus and the atria (on the white crescentic line).

Note: This is the first Stannius ligature (Fig. 69.1). It records the atrial rhythm.

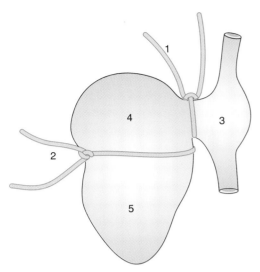

Fig. 69.1 Position of Stannius ligatures as seen in the side view of the heart (1: First Stannius ligature; 2: Second Stannius ligature; 3: Sinus venosus; 4: Auricles; 5: Ventricle).

5. Record the effect of ligation on the cardiogram.
6. Apply the ligature at the atrioventricular junction and record the effect of ligation on the cardiogram.

Note: This is the second Stannius ligature. It records the ventricular rhythm. Note that the ventricle starts beating after a pause, and at a much slower rate (idioventricular rhythm).

Observation

Note that the frequency of heart beat after placing the first Stannius ligature is significantly less than the normal rhythm. The frequency of heart beat is much lower after placing the second Stannius ligature (Fig. 69.2).

Precautions

1. The first Stannius ligature should be tied between the truncus arteriosus and the atria.

2. The second Stannius ligature should be tied between the atria and ventricle.
3. Recording should be done immediately after placing the ligatures.

DISCUSSION

The **sinus venosus (SA node in humans)** is the **primary pacemaker** of the heart. Therefore, the **first Stannius ligature**, which prevents transmission of impulses from the sinus venosus to atria, decreases the heart rate as the impulse is now generated by the atria (**atrial rhythm**). After placing the **second Stannius ligature**, which prevents transmission of impulse from the atria to the ventricle, the heart rate decreases further as the impulse is now generated by the ventricle (**ventricular rhythm**). This indicates that the primary pacemaker in the frog heart is present in the sinus venosus.

Clinical Significance

Heart Blocks

As already noted, the SA node normally controls the heart rate. Interruption of impulse transmission from the atria to the ventricle is called heart block. There are three degrees of heart blocks: first, second and third. In **first degree and second degree heart blocks**, impulse transmission is not completely interrupted between the atria and the ventricle, therefore these are called **incomplete heart blocks**. However, impulse transmission is completely blocked between the atria and the ventricle in the **third degree heart block**, and therefore it is called **complete heart block**.

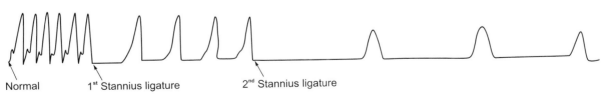

Normal   1ˢᵗ Stannius ligature   2ⁿᵈ Stannius ligature

Fig. 69.2 Recording of the effects of Stannius ligature on frog's heart.

VIVA

1.   *What is the effect of the first Stannius ligature on the heart?*
2.   *What is the effect of the second Stannius ligature on the heart?*
3.   *What is the rate of discharge of the different potential pacemakers of the heart?*
4.   *What is heart block? What are the different types of heart blocks?*

CHAPTER 70

Properties of the Cardiac Muscle

Learning Objectives

After completing this practical, you will be able to:

1. Explain the importance of studying the properties of the cardiac muscle.
2. List the properties of the cardiac muscle.
3. Define extrasystole, compensatory pause, refractory period, all or none law and the staircase phenomenon.
4. Elaborate on the physiological basis of the different properties of the cardiac muscle.
5. Explain why the cardiac muscle cannot be tetanised.
6. Explain the physiological basis of the staircase phenomenon.

INTRODUCTION

The properties of the cardiac muscle can be divided into two groups: **properties** that can be studied in a beating heart and those studied in a quiescent heart.

Properties that can be studied in a beating heart

◆ Automaticity   ◆ Rhythmicity
◆ Contractility   ◆ Conductivity
◆ Excitability   ◆ Long refractory period
◆ Extrasystole and compensatory pause

Properties that can be studied in a quiescent heart

◆ All or none law
◆ The staircase phenomenon
◆ Length–tension relationship
◆ Summation of subminimal stimuli

In this practical, the properties that you will study are extrasystole, compensatory pause, refractory period, all or none law, the staircase phenomenon and the summation of subminimal stimuli. The last three properties can be studied in a quiescent heart.

METHODS

Method to Study Properties of the Cardiac Muscle

▍ *Principle*

The properties of the cardiac muscle are studied in a beating heart and in a quiescent heart.

▍ *Requirements*

1. Same as that for recording of a normal cardiogram
2. Electrical circuit for cardiac stimulation
3. Signal marker
4. Aneurysm needle

▍ *Procedure*

▍ I. Recording of Extrasystole, Compensatory Pause and Refractory Period

A. In a beating heart

1. Set up the experiment as would be done for recording a normal cardiogram.
2. Apply electrodes to the base of the ventricle for stimulating it with single induction shocks.
3. Adjust a signal marker close to the heart lever to record the movement of stimulation.
4. Record normal heart beats on a slow-moving drum.
5. Stimulate the ventricle during different phases of the cardiac cycle.

Note: While stimulating the ventricle, it should be observed that the stimuli during the systole are ineffective, but the stimuli during diastole elicit a premature contraction (extrasystole) which is followed by a compensatory pause. The contraction following the compensatory pause is higher in magnitude than the previous one (Fig. 70.1A).

6. Label your record to show the systole and diastole in a normal heart beat, point of application of the extra stimulus, extrasystole and compensatory pause.

B. In a quiescent heart

1. Make electrical connections for delivering single induced shocks with the drum in circuit.
2. Apply the first Stannius ligature by tying the heart with a thread at the white crescentic line to make the heart quiescent.
3. Place the electrodes at the base of the ventricle.
4. Stimulate the ventricle by adjusting the angle between the contact arms so that the stimuli fall during different phases of the cardiac cycle.
5. Record the effect of the stimuli on the drum running at medium speed.
6. Mark the point of stimulation for each graph before changing the angle of the contact arms and the position of the cylinder.
7. Obtain at least three sets of graphs as mentioned below:
   i. The second stimulus is applied when the ventricle is completely relaxed after the first contraction.
   ii. The second stimulus is applied during the diastole of the first heart beat (relative refractory period).
   iii. The second stimulus is applied during the systole of the first heart beat (absolute refractory period).

II. All or None Law

1. Make electrical connections to stimulate the ventricle with single induced shocks.
2. Apply the first Stannius ligature to make the heart quiescent.
3. Apply electrodes to the base of the ventricle.
4. Adjust the writing lever to record on a stationary drum.
5. Stimulate the ventricle with subthreshold stimuli and observe the effect.
6. Increase the strength of the stimulus till a contraction is recorded.
7. Increase the strength of the stimulus every thirty seconds; rotate the drum through 1 cm each time and record the contraction.

Note: Observe that the height of the contraction remains the same irrespective of the strength of the stimulus, that is, the amplitude of contraction of the threshold stimulus is the same as the amplitude of contraction recorded with the stimuli of higher strength. No recording occurs with subthreshold stimuli (Fig. 70.1B).

III. Staircase Phenomenon

1. Adjust the inductorium for a single effective shock.
2. Make the heart quiescent by applying the first Stannius ligature.
3. Stimulate the ventricle repeatedly at intervals of two seconds and record each contraction at 1 cm intervals on a stationary drum.

Note: Observe that the first few contractions show a successive increase in amplitude, which is known as the staircase phenomenon (Fig. 70.1C).

IV. Summation of Subminimal Stimuli

1. Make the heart quiescent by putting the first Stannius ligature.
2. Find a stimulus by adjusting the position of the inductorium, which just fails to produce a contraction.

Note: The stimulus is a subthreshold stimulus.

3. Repeatedly stimulate the ventricle at intervals of one second till the ventricle gives a full contraction.

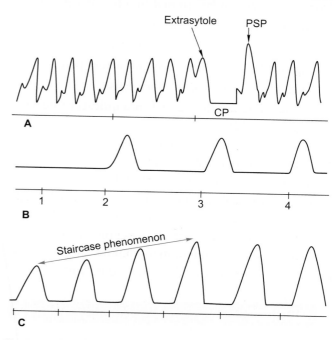

Fig. 70.1   Demonstration of the properties of the cardiac muscle. (A) Extrasystole (1: Stimulus applied during systole produces no extrasystole; 2: Stimulus applied during diastole produces an extrasystole which is followed by a compensatory pause; PSP: Postextrasystolic potentiation); (B) All or none law (1: Subthreshold stimulus; 2: Threshold stimulus; 3 and 4: Suprathreshold stimuli); (C) Staircase phenomenon (stimuli applied every 2 seconds).

Note: Usually between the tenth and twentieth stimulus the ventricle contracts.

Observation

Observe and study the properties of the cardiac muscle recorded in a beating heart and in a quiescent heart.

Precautions

1. For recording of the extrasystole and compensatory pause, the stimulus should be applied in the diastole of the heart.
2. To study the refractory period, one stimulus should be applied in the systole and another in the diastole of the heart.
3. The all or none law, staircase phenomenon and summation of subminimal stimuli should be studied in a quiescent heart.
4. To study the all or none law, stimuli should be given in different strengths starting from the subthreshold to the suprathreshold level.
5. To study the staircase phenomenon, the ventricle should be stimulated repeatedly at intervals of 2 seconds.
6. To study the effect of the summation of subminimal stimuli, the subthreshold (that just fails to evoke a response) stimuli should be given repeatedly at intervals of 0.5–1 second.

DISCUSSION

Extrasystole and Compensatory Pause

When the ventricle is **stimulated in the relaxation period** (relative refractory period), the heart muscle may contract. This *contraction comes earlier* than the normally expected contraction. Therefore, it is called an **extrasystole**. The next impulse arrives in the refractory period of the extrasystole, hence fails to evoke a response. This results in **a pause (silence),** following the extrasystole, which is known as a **compensatory pause**. The response following the compensatory pause is greater than the previous one due to the accumulation of calcium ions during the pause.

Refractory Period

The cardiac muscle has a **long refractory period**. The **absolute refractory period** is about 250 ms and the **relative refractory period** is around 50 ms (Fig. 70.2). During the absolute refractory period, a stimulus cannot re-excite the tissue, no matter how strong the stimulus is. The duration of the action potential of the cardiac muscle is almost the same as the duration of the mechanical activity. A fresh action potential should be accompanied by a mechanical response. The mechanical responses of the cardiac muscle cannot be merged. Therefore, contraction and relaxation of the cardiac muscle to a stimulus must be over before the muscle responds to another stimulus. Therefore, the **cardiac muscle cannot be tetanised.**

The All or None Law

The **threshold stimulus** is the *weakest stimulus that evokes a response*. If the heart muscle is stimulated with subthreshold stimuli, no response is seen. The **amplitude of contraction** in response to the suprathreshold stimuli *remains the same* as that with the threshold stimuli. This is known as the all or none law. This is due to two reasons: (a) the heart muscle being an excitable tissue

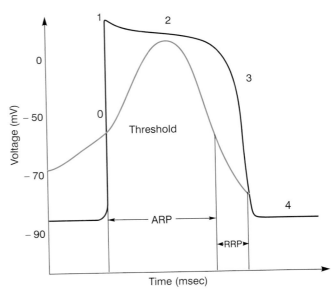

—— Slow fibres, present in the SA and AV nodes. Resting membrane potential is –50 to –70 mV and the conduction velocity is 2–10 cm/sec. Note the spontaneous diastolic depolarisation in phase 4 and slow phase 0.

—— Fast fibres (atrial and ventricular myocardial cells and cells in specialised conduction tissues). Resting membrane potential is –90 mV and the conduction velocity 30–100 cm/sec,

ARP: absolute refractory period, i.e., an interval in which no stimulus, however strong, can initiate an action potential

RRP: relative refractory period, i.e., an interval during which a supranormal stimulus can initiate an action potential

Fig. 70.2 Action potential of cardiac muscle showing five phases.

follows the all or none law and (b) the heart muscle behaves as the functional syncytium. Therefore the whole heart contracts with the same force.

Staircase Phenomenon

If the heart is stimulated repeatedly with the interval between the consecutive stimuli not less than 10 seconds, the **first 2–5 contractions progressively increase in amplitude**. This is called the staircase phenomenon. This is due to the *accumulation of calcium ions* in the sarcoplasm. With each stimulus, calcium ion is released into the sarcoplasm and if the next stimulus reaches within 10 seconds, the calcium ions may not be totally pumped back into the sarcotubular system. Therefore, the next contraction is accentuated due to an increase in the concentration of calcium ions (calcium released by the stimulus plus the extra calcium left by the previous stimulus). The staircase phenomenon also occurs *due to increased temperature* in the muscle during the previous contraction.

Summation of Subminimal Stimuli

When subminimal stimuli are applied repeatedly, with the interval between the consecutive stimuli being less than one second, the *stimuli summate and produce a response*.

VIVA

1. What is extrasystole? Why is extrasystole followed by a compensatory pause?
2. Explain why the cardiac muscle cannot be tetanised.
3. Define and explain the absolute and relative refractory periods.
4. What is the all or none law? Why does the cardiac muscle exhibit the all or none law?
5. Why should the intervals between the stimuli be less than 10 ms to demonstrate the all or none law?
6. What is the staircase phenomenon? What is its physiological basis?
7. What is the mechanism of summation of the subminimal effects?

CHAPTER 71

Effect of Stimulation of Vagosympathetic Trunk on Frog's Heart

Learning Objectives

After completing this practical, you will be able to:

1. Explain the clinical implications of performing this practical.
2. Explain the differences between vagal and sympathetic innervation of the frog and human heart.
3. Identify the vagosympathetic trunk in the frog.
4. Demonstrate the effect of vagal stimulation on the heart.
5. Understand the phenomenon of vagal inhibition and vagal escape.
6. Explain the physiological basis of vagal inhibition and vagal escape.
7. Explain the effect of vagal stimulation in humans.

INTRODUCTION

The vagal and sympathetic fibres to the heart in a frog cannot be stimulated separately, as these fibres are mixed to form a single nerve, the vagosympathetic trunk (VST). **Stimulation of VST results in cardiac inhibition** as the vagal effect is dominant over the sympathetic effect. But if VST is stimulated for a long period, the facilitatory effect of the sympathetic may become dominant. The **white crescentic line** is the parasympathetic ganglion (**Remak's ganglion**) in the frog's heart and its stimulation causes cardiac inhibition.

The postganglionic parasympathetic neurons that are embedded in the heart muscle at the junction of atria and ventricle form the white crescentic line.

METHODS

Method to Study Effect of Stimulation of Vagosympathetic Trunk on Frog's Heart

Principle

Stimulation of the vagosympathetic trunk results in cardiac inhibition. However, if the stimulation continues, the heart recovers from this inhibitory effect.

This is demonstrated by effect of vagosympathetic stimulation of the heart recorded on a moving drum.

Requirements

1. Same as that for the recording of a normal cardiogram
2. Electrical circuit for stimulating the heart
3. Frog

Procedure

1. Pith the frog.
2. Expose the chest of the frog by making an incision on the sternum.
3. Extend the incision upwards to the lower jaw.
4. Cut the platysma.
5. Remove the tissue running from the angle of the jaw to expose the petrohyoid muscle (a thin muscle that runs from the base of the skull to the posterior corner of the hyoid bone).

Note: The petrohyoid muscle is identified by its shining colour. The glossopharyngeal and the hypoglossal nerves are seen superficial to the petrohyoid. Along the lower border of the petrohyoid, a neurovascular bundle is seen. This neurovascular bundle is formed by the laryngeal nerve, the carotid artery and the vagosympathetic trunk. The vagosympathetic trunk is identified by its close association with the artery (Fig. 71.1).

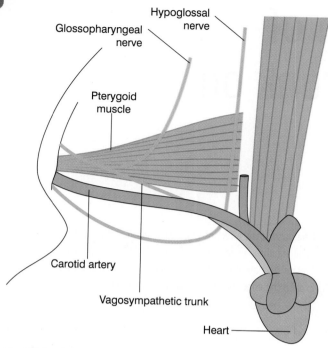

Fig. 71.1   Anatomy of the vagosympathetic trunk.

6. Isolate the vagosympathetic trunk carefully with a thin glass rod and pass a thread below the nerve.

7. Confirm the vagosympathetic trunk by observing the cardiac inhibition (slowing of the heart) by stimulating the nerve.

8. Record a normal cardiogram.

9. Stimulate the vagosympathetic trunk with a stimulus of lower strength and record the effect of stimulation.

10. Repeat the procedure by gradually increasing the strength of the stimuli till the heart stops.

Note: For studying the effect of different strengths of the stimulus, record the cardiogram before, during and after the stimulation of the vagosympathetic trunk. The slowing and final stopping of the heart due to vagosympathetic stimulation is known as vagal inhibition.

11. After the heart stops, continue stimulating the vagosympathetic trunk till the heart starts beating.

Note: The recovery of the heart from the inhibitory influence of the vagus when the vagosympathetic trunk is stimulated for a longer duration is known as vagal escape.

12. Indicate the beginning and termination of vagal stimulation on the recording, and label the vagal inhibition and vagal escape.

Observation

Study the effect of stimulation (of different strengths) of the vagosympathetic trunk on the cardiac activities (Fig. 71.2). Note that at a lower strength of stimulation, there is a slowing down of the heart, but the heart stops with a higher strength of stimulus. Also note that the heart beat reappears when stimulation is continued for a longer duration. The heart rate of the vagal escape is significantly less than the heart rate prior to the vagal stimulation (normal heart rate).

Precautions

1. The vagosympathetic trunk should be identified by its anatomical landmark.

2. Before carrying out the experiment, the vagosympathetic trunk should be confirmed by stimulating the trunk and observing the slowness of the heart.

3. The effect of vagal stimulation on the heart should be studied from a stimuli of lower strength to one of higher strength.

4. After recording vagal inhibition, the stimulation should be continued to study the phenomenon of vagal escape.

5. The cardiogram should be recorded before, during and after stimulation of the vagosympathetic trunk.

6. The recording should be labelled properly to mark the start and termination of stimulation.

DISCUSSION

Effect of Stimulation of the Vagus Nerve

A. In Frog

Vagal inhibition

When the vagus nerve (vagosympathetic trunk) is stimulated in a frog, there is inhibition of the heart. The *heart rate and the force of contraction decrease*. This is called vagal inhibition. If the stimulus is strong, the heart stops. Cardiac inhibition occurs due to the **release of acetylcholine** at the nerve endings. This increases the potassium conductance in the nodal tissues by *opening a special set of potassium channels*. Acetylcholine also decreases the concentration of cyclic

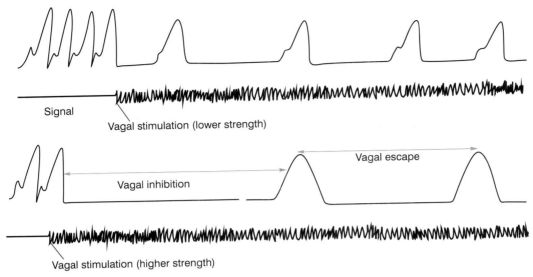

Fig. 71.2   Effect of vagal (vagosympathetic trunk) stimulation on frog's heart.

AMP in the cells. The decrease in cyclic AMP slows the opening of the calcium channels, which decreases the firing rate. A decrease in calcium concentration in the myocardial cells decreases the force of contraction.

Vagal escape

A **strong vagal stimulation** may abolish the spontaneous discharge of the heart for some time and the heart stops temporarily. But the **heart recovers automatically** even after the continuation of vagal stimulation. This is called **vagal escape**. The heart rate following vagal escape is significantly lower than the normal heart rate because the escape rhythm is the ventricular rhythm.

Causes of vagal escape

1. ***Idioventricular rhythm*** When the heart stops due to vagal stimulation, the ventricle starts generating the impulse, which is known as idioventricular rhythm. It is so called because the cardiac rhythm is due to the pacemaker activity of the ventricular muscle, and the exact cause of the ventricular pacemaking activity was not known (idiopathic). As the discharge rate of the ventricle is much less, the idioventricular rhythm is significantly lower than the normal heart rate.

2. ***Depletion of acetylcholine*** When the vagus nerve is stimulated continuously, the acetylcholine released at the nerve ending is depleted after some time. Acetylcholine is degraded rapidly by the enzyme cholinesterase. Therefore, the effect of vagal stimulation on the heart is temporary.

3. ***Sympathetic stimulation*** It is believed that when the vagosympathetic trunk is continuously stimulated, the sympathetic fibres are also activated and stimulate the heart.

B. in Humans

In mammals including human beings, the vagal and sympathetic fibres innervating the heart are present separately in separate nerves. Therefore, *stimulation of the vagus shows the effect of only parasympathetic activation.* However, continuous stimulation of the vagus nerve results in **vagal escape,** which is predominantly due to idioventricular rhythm.

Vasovagal attack

Stimulation of the vagus nerve causes sudden and transient loss of consciousness. This is known as **vasovagal syncope** or vasovagal attack. It occurs due to inadequate cerebral blood flow which results from abrupt vasodilation and decreased cardiac output.

Vagal tone

The normal heart rate in humans is about 70/mm (range: 60–100) which is significantly less than the **intrinsic heart rate** (100–120/mm). Intrinsic heart rate is the heart rate when the heart is denervated (devoid of parasympathetic and sympathetic innervation). This reduced heart rate (in comparison to intrinsic heart rate) is **due to vagal tone.** Therefore, vagal tone is the tonic inhibitory influence of the vagus nerve on the heart. There is also the **sympathetic tone**, which stimulates the heart. But normally, the vagal tone is dominant over the sympathetic tone. This is the reason why the heart rate is normally less than the intrinsic rate. The balance between the vagal and sympathetic drives is known as **sympathovagal balance.**

VIVA

1. What is the difference between vagal and sympathetic innervation of the heart in frogs and humans?
2. What is vagal inhibition? What is the mechanism involved in vagal inhibition?
3. What is vagal escape? What are the causes of vagal escape?
4. Why is the heart rate following vagal escape significantly less than the normal heart rate?
5. What is a vasovagal attack?
6. What is vagal tone?

CHAPTER 72

Perfusion of Frog's Heart and Effect of Drugs and Ions

Learning Objectives

After completing this practical, you will be able to:

1. Explain the importance of performing this practical in cardiovascular physiology.

2. List the effects of drugs and chemicals on the normal cardiogram.

3. Explain the effect of various chemicals on the heart.

INTRODUCTION

The activities of the heart depend primarily on the concentration of intracellular and extracellular ions. Different drugs and chemicals change cardiac function by changing the ionic concentration of the nodal tissues and myocardial cells by either acting directly on the ion channels or by acting on different receptors that affect the ion channels. Usually, various chemicals **alter heart function by changing the cyclic AMP and calcium** concentration in the cardiac cells. Many of the drugs used in clinical practice for cardiac ailments act by modulating the ionic concentration of cardiac cells.

METHODS

Method to Study Perfusion of Frog's Heart and Effect of Drugs and Ions

Principle

Different drugs and ions change the rate and force of contraction of the heart. The effects of these chemicals are observed on the cardiogram of a frog and recorded on a moving drum.

Requirements

1. Same as that for recording a normal cardiogram
2. Different chemicals (1% $CaCl_2$, 1% KCl, 1% NaCl, 1 in 100,000 adrenaline, and 1 in 10,00,000 acetylcholine)

3. Syme's cannula
4. Mariotte's bottle

Procedure

1. Pith the frog.
2. Expose the thorax of the frog.
3. Remove the pericardium.
4. Pass a fine thread around the sinus venosus.
5. With a pair of sharp scissors make a small slit in the sinus venosus and introduce Syme's cannula.
6. Tie the thread around the neck of the cannula and cut the heart out of the frog.
7. Connect the cannula with Mariotte's perfusion bottle containing frog's Ringer's solution.
8. Perfuse the heart with Ringer's solution and record the heart beat on a slow-moving drum (Fig. 72.1).
9. Record the effect of the following drugs and ions by applying each chemical separately with the help of separate droppers:
   i) 1 ml of 1% $CaCl_2$
   ii) 1 ml of 1% KCl
   iii) 2 ml of 1% NaCl
   iv) 0.5 ml of 1 in 100,000 solution of adrenaline hydrochloride
   v) 0.5 ml of 1 in 10,00,000 acetylcholine

Note: Normal cardiogram should be taken before and after recording the effect of each chemical.

Observation

Observe the changes in the cardiogram following application of different chemicals. Note that calcium

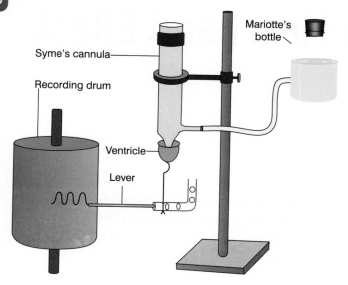

Fig. 72.1   Perfusion of a frog's heart.

2. While introducing the cannula into the sinus venosus, care should be taken not to puncture other heart chambers (Fig. 72.1).

3. The thread should be tied tightly so that it does not loosen during the experiment.

4. The concentration and amount of the chemicals should be appropriate.

5. Separate droppers should be used for applying different chemicals.

6. The normal cardiogram should be recorded prior to the application of the chemicals.

7. The heart should be washed with frog's Ringer's solution each time before the application of each chemical.

8. The effect of stimulatory chemicals should be recorded before the recording of inhibitory chemicals.

chloride and adrenaline stimulate the heart whereas potassium chloride and acetylcholine depress the heart. Sodium chloride increases the heart rate but decreases the force of contraction (Fig. 72.2).

Observe the effect of different chemicals on the recording (Fig. 72.2).

Precautions

1. Same as that for the recording of a cardiogram.

DISCUSSION

Adrenaline

Adrenaline **increases the inotropic, chronotropic, dromotropic** and **bathmotropic** actions of the heart. It exerts its effect on the heart by acting **on β₂ adrenergic receptors** that *increase intracellular cyclic AMP concentration*. Increased intracellular cyclic AMP in the nodal cells facilitates the *opening of longstanding*

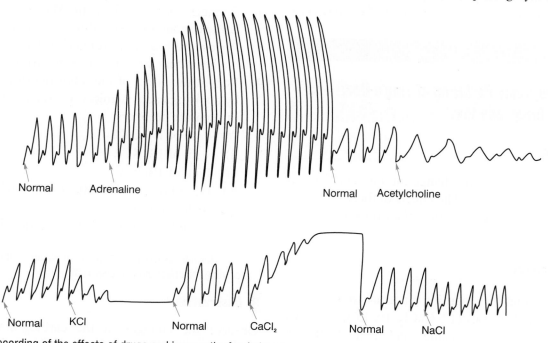

Fig. 72.2   Recording of the effects of drugs and ions on the frog's heart.

calcium channels, which increases the depolarisation phase of the impulse, thereby increasing the heart rate. Adrenaline also increases intracellular calcium in the myocardial cells by **acting on β_1 receptors** present on the cardiac muscles and thereby increases the force of contraction.

Acetylcholine

Acetylcholine **decreases the heart rate and the force of contraction**. The heart rate decreases because the membrane becomes hyperpolarised and the slope of prepotentials is decreased due to the action of acetylcholine on **muscarinic receptors and K^+ channels**. Acetylcholine increases the K^+ conductance in the nodal tissue by directly opening the K^+ channels. By acting on **M_2 receptors** on the nodal cells, acetylcholine decreases the concentration of intracellular cyclic AMP that slows down the opening of calcium channels. This decreases the firing rate of the nodal tissue. Therefore, the heart rate decreases. Acetylcholine also decreases cyclic AMP in the myocardial cells, and therefore decreases the magnitude of contraction.

Potassium Chloride

Potassium chloride **decreases the resting membrane potential**. Therefore, the fibres become inexcitable. The heart stops in diastole.

Calcium Chloride

Calcium chloride **increases the force of contraction and decreases the relaxation time**. Therefore, the heart stops in systole (tonic contraction). This is called **calcium rigor**. It may not affect the heart rate.

Sodium Chloride

Sodium chloride **facilitates depolarisation**, and hence *increases the heart rate*. But it competes with calcium ions, and therefore decreases the force of contraction.

VIVA

1. What are the effects of various drugs and chemicals on the heart? State the physiological basis for each.
2. What is calcium rigor?

CHAPTER 73

Effect of Drugs and Ions on Isolated Mammalian Intestine

Learning Objectives

After completing this practical, you will be able to:
1. Classify smooth muscles.
2. List the properties of smooth muscles.
3. Name the steps of contraction of smooth muscles.
4. Describe the effect of various drugs and chemicals on intestinal movement.
5. Explain the mechanism of action of these drugs and chemicals.

INTRODUCTION

Intestinal movements are possible due to the activities of smooth muscles present in the walls of the intestine, which generate their own impulse.

Smooth Muscles

Smooth muscles are broadly classified into **two types**: (a) visceral or single unit smooth muscles and (b) multiunit smooth muscles. **Visceral smooth muscles** are found in the stomach, intestines, uterus, urinary bladder and the walls of the small arteries and veins. **Multiunit smooth muscles** are found in the walls of the large arteries, in the large airways (bronchioles), in the erector pili (muscles in the hair follicles) and radial and circular muscles of the eye.

Properties of Visceral Smooth Muscles

1. They are **involuntary**, innervated by **autonomic fibres**.
2. They show continuous, irregular contractions independent of their nerve supply. This helps them maintain a state of partial sustained contraction called **tonus or tone**. The sustained contraction occurs due to the **latch-bridge mechanism** in which dephosphorylated myosin cross-bridges remain attached to the actin for some time after the cytoplasmic calcium concentration falls.

3. Visceral smooth muscle is unique in that it **contracts in response to a stretch** in the absence of any extrinsic innervation. The stretch causes the decline in membrane potential, increased spike frequency and increased tone.
4. There is **no true resting membrane potential**. But, during the period of quiescence, the RMP is about -50 mV.
5. Spikes (slow **sine wave-like fluctuations**) of a few millivolts appear on the resting potential.
6. They exhibit **autorhythmicity**. Pacemaker potentials appear at multiple foci.
7. The **excitation contraction coupling is very slow**. The muscle contracts about 200 ms after the start of the spikes and 150 ms after the spike is over. The peak contraction reaches about 500 ms after the spike.
8. The thick and thin filaments are **not arranged in an orderly fashion**. Therefore, there are no A and I bands. Smooth muscles do not exhibit cross striations. Therefore, they are named smooth muscles. They also contain intermediate filaments.
9. They **lack transverse tubules and contain very few sarcoplasmic reticulum** for storage of calcium. For contraction, they receive calcium mainly from ECF.
10. Intermediate filaments attached to the **dense bodies** play a role during contraction. During contraction, intermediate filaments pull the dense bodies attached to the sarcolemma, which causes lengthwise shortening of the muscle fibre.

11. Muscles exhibit **plasticity**, which is the variability of the tension that it exerts at any given length. This allows the smooth muscle to undergo great changes in length while still retaining the ability to contract effectively.

12. **Calmodulin** and myosin light chain kinase are the regulator proteins for contraction.

Major Steps of Contraction of Visceral Smooth Muscle

1. Acetylcholine binds to the muscarinic receptors.
2. Calcium influx of the cell increases.
3. Calcium binds with calmodulin-dependent myosin kinase.
4. Phosphorylation of myosin occurs.
5. Myosin binds with actin, which increases myosin ATPase activity.
6. This causes contraction of the muscle.
7. Dephosphorylation of myosin occurs by various phosphatases.
8. Sustained contraction or relaxation occurs due to the latch-bridge mechanism.

METHODS

Method to Study Effect of Drugs and Ions on Isolated Mammalian Intestine

Principle

Segments of the small intestine continue to contract and respond to various stimuli if kept in a suitable medium at optimum temperature with the provision for oxygen supply.

Requirements

1. **Dale's apparatus** This consists of a large perspex rectangular bath meant for keeping water at appropriate temperature (37°C) with the help of a heating element and thermostat. There is a central organ bath of 20 ml capacity, which is provided with an outlet. There is a hollow bent glass tube curved at the lower end for fixing intestine and other tissues. This tube can be inserted in the centre of the organ bath and is also used for supplying oxygen through the solution. A frontal lever can be attached to the assembly for recording movement on a moving kymograph (Fig. 73.1).

2. **Tyrode's solution** The composition of the Tyrode's solution (for preparing 10 litres of stock solution) is as follows:

NaCl	: 80 g
KCl (10%)	: 20 ml
$MgSO_4$ (10%)	: 26 ml
NaH_2PO_4 (5%)	: 13 ml
Glucose	: 10 g
$NaHCO_3$	: 10 g
$CaCl_2$ (molar)	: 18 ml
Aerating gas	: Oxygen or air

3. Petri dish
4. Thread and needle
5. Oxygen supply
6. Frontal lever
7. Kymograph and smoked drum
8. Pipette/syringe
9. A living rabbit
10. Drugs and chemicals

Procedure

1. Keep the rabbit fasting overnight.

> Note: The intestine of a fasting rabbit shows good contraction.

2. Fill the organ bath with the Tyrode's solution and the outer bath with water.
3. Heat the water of the outer bath to keep the temperature constant at about 37°C.
4. Keep the petri dish containing the Tyrode's solution ready.
5. Stun (kill) the rabbit and open the abdomen.
6. Take out a small part (about 5 cm) of the jejunum close to the duodenum and place the intestine in a petri dish containing Tyrode's solution.
7. Rinse the intestinal lumen with Tyrode's solution with the help of a pipette or by pushing the solution gently through the lumen with the help of a syringe.
8. Pass the threaded needle through the wall of one of the cut ends of the segment and make a loop from the thread.
9. To the other end of the intestinal segment, tie a long thread for attaching to the lever.
10. Mount the segment in the organ bath filled with Tyrode's solution by securing the threaded loop to the curved end of the glass tube.
11. Allow oxygen to pass through the solution at a rate of 2–3 bubbles per second.

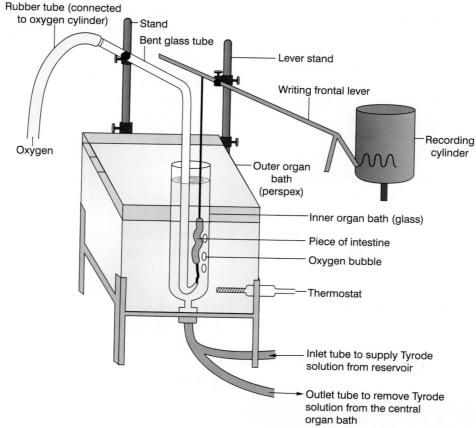

Fig. 73.1   Dale's apparatus.

12. Keep the temperature of the water bath at 37°C. Check the temperature frequently.
13. Attach the intestine to the frontal lever.
14. Record the normal movements of the intestine on a slow-moving drum.
15. Study the effect of the following drugs/chemicals by taking 1 ml of each solution in a pipette and mixing the solution in the central organ bath.

Acetylcholine	: 1 in 10,00,000
Adrenaline	: 1 in 1,00,000
Atropine	: 0.01%
Histamine	: 50 mg
KCl solution	: 1%
CaCl$_2$ solution	: 1%
Barium chloride	: 2%

Note: After recording the effect of each drug, the Tyrode's solution should be drained and replaced with fresh Tyrode's solution. The effect of the next drug should be recorded only after the intestine shows the normal movement.

16. By placing arrow marks below the recordings, indicate the drugs used for the recordings.

Observation

Observe the rate and amplitude of movement of intestinal contraction following application of each chemical (Fig. 73.2).

Precautions

1. The animal should not be fed the previous night, to get good intestinal contraction.
2. The temperature of the outer organ bath should be maintained at 37°C throughout the experiment.
3. The apparatus should be kept ready before killing the animal and dissecting the intestine.
4. The lumen of the intestine should be rinsed quickly and placed in the Tyrode's solution immediately after separating from the GI tract of the animal.
5. Oxygen should be supplied throughout the experiment.
6. Separate pipettes should be used to put the chemicals into the organ bath, or if one pipette is used, the pipette must be thoroughly cleaned before taking the chemical.

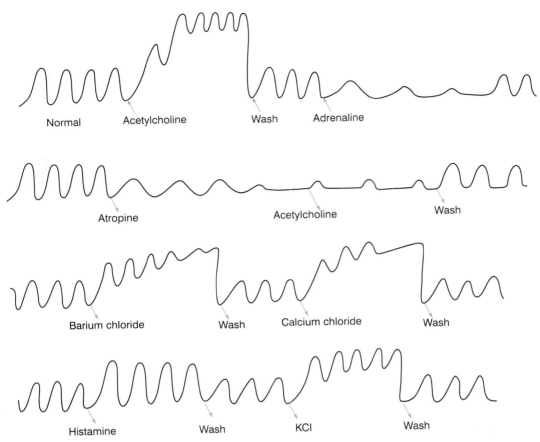

Fig. 73.2   Recording of effects of drugs and ions on rabbit intestine.

7. Between applications of chemicals into the organ bath, the Tyrode's solution should be replaced with fresh solution every time.

8. Normal recordings should be taken before and after the recording of the effect of each chemical.

9. The effect of acetylcholine should be studied before the application of atropine.

10. The effect of acetylcholine should also be studied immediately after the application of atropine.

DISCUSSION

Adrenaline

When adrenaline is added to the preparation, the membrane potential becomes larger, **the frequency of contraction decreases, the muscle relaxes and the amplitude of contraction decreases.** Adrenaline exerts its inhibitory effect by acting on both α and β receptors present on the muscle. The action on the β receptor is mediated by a **decrease in cyclic AMP** in the cells and increased intracellular binding of calcium so that less calcium is available in the cell. This decreases the muscle tension in response to excitation. The action on the α receptor is mediated by **increased calcium efflux** from the cells so that *less calcium is available* in the cell. This also decreases the magnitude of contraction.

Acetylcholine

Acetylcholine decreases the membrane potential and the muscle becomes more active. The **rate and height of contraction increase.** There is an increase in tonic tension in the muscle. Acetylcholine exerts its effect by **activating the phospholipase C**, which in turn forms ionositol triphosphate (IP3). IP3 increases the intracellular calcium concentration by mobilising calcium from the intracellular stores and by facilitating calcium entry into the cell. This increases the activity of the muscle.

Atropine

Atropine is a cholinergic **muscarinic blocker**. It prevents the action of acetylcholine on the smooth muscle of the intestine. It *decreases muscle activity*. If acetylcholine is applied to the preparation following application of atropine, the effect of acetylcholine is abolished.

Histamine

Histamine *increases the tone* of the smooth muscle. It increases the amplitude of contraction. It acts by activating the H_1 and H_2 receptors. By acting on **H_1 receptors**, it *activates phospholipase C* that in turn *increases intracellular calcium* concentration and by acting on H_2 receptors, it increases cyclic AMP concentration in the cells.

Potassium Chloride

Just like acetylcholine, this **stimulates** intestinal movements.

Calcium Chloride

$CaCl_2$ when applied increases calcium entry into the cell and **stimulates contraction** of the intestine. Calcium causes tonic contraction of the muscle.

Barium Chloride

Barium chloride mimics the action of acetylcholine. The intestine contracts strongly due to direct action of barium ions on the intestinal smooth muscle.

VIVA

1. What are the types of intestinal movement?
2. What are the types of smooth muscles?
3. What are the special properties of smooth muscles?
4. What are the steps of contraction of smooth muscles?
5. What are the effects of different chemicals on intestinal movement? What are their mechanisms of action?

CHAPTER 74

Effect of Drugs on Mammalian Uterine Contraction

INTRODUCTION

The **myometrium** of the uterus is made up of **smooth muscles**. Uterine smooth muscles respond to various hormones in different phases of the menstrual cycle and pregnancy. The ovarian hormones especially **estrogen, progesterone and relaxin, and oxytocin** secreted from the posterior pituitary, modify the activities of the uterus by acting on the myometrial and epithelial cells. These hormones alter the activities of the myometrial cells of the uterus in different phases of gestation to facilitate smooth continuation and termination of pregnancy. This practical is designed to study the effect of some of these drugs on uterine contraction.

METHODS

Method to Study Effect of Drugs on Mammalian Uterine Contraction

Principle

An estrogen-primed uterus is sensitive to different drugs. The effect of different drugs is studied on an isolated uterus in Dale's apparatus.

Requirements

1. Dale's apparatus (a detailed description is given in Chapter 73).
2. Dale's solution
3. Gas mixture (95% O_2 and 5% CO_2)
4. Frontal lever
5. Petri dish
6. Needle and thread
7. Kymograph with smoked drum
8. Living adult female rat primed with estrogen
9. Drugs: oxytocin, estrogen, progesterone, acetylcholine and adrenaline.

Procedure

1. Take a female rat in the estrous phase or prime it with estrogen.

Note: Estrogen-priming is done by injecting estrogen into the animal, 24 hours prior to commencement of the experiment. The primed uterus increases the sensitivity of the uterine tissue to different drugs.

2. Stun (kill) the animal and open the abdomen.
3. Locate the two cornu (horns) of the uterus.
4. Cut the upper end of each horn to separate it from the ovary and the surrounding fat.
5. Split the lower end of the uterus and separate each horn.
6. Divide each horn into two pieces so that four segments are available from each rat.
7. With the help of the needle, make a loop of thread at one cut end and attach a long thread to the other end.
8. Mount the segment in Dale's solution by placing the hook in the curved glass rod in Dale's organ bath and connect the other end to the frontal lever.
9. Maintain the temperature of the solution at 37°C.

10. Allow the bubble of gas mixture to pass through the solution continuously.
11. Record the normal contraction of the uterus.
12. Study the effect of oxytocin, estrogen, progesterone, acetylcholine and adrenaline on uterine contraction. Wash the tissue with fresh Dale's solution before and after application of each drug. Record normal uterine contractions before studying the effect of each drug.
13. Indicate on the recording by placing arrow marks below the point of application of drugs.

Observation

Observe the normal uterine contraction and the effect of different drugs on uterine contraction (Fig. 74.1).

Precautions

1. The animal should be in the estrous phase or should be primed with estrogen.
2. Each uterus should be cut into two separate segments.

3. The temperature of the organ bath should be maintained at about 37°C.
4. The tissue should be washed with fresh Dale's solution before recording the effect of each drug.
5. Normal uterine contraction should be recorded before recording the effect of each drug.

DISCUSSION

Effect of Different Drugs

Oxytocin

Oxytocin *increases the frequency and amplitude of uterine contraction*, and **the tone of the muscle**. Oxytocin acts on the receptors present on the myometrium. It *increases intracellular calcium concentration* and therefore stimulates contraction.

Estrogen

Estrogen **stimulates uterine contraction** by acting on the receptors in the myometrial cells. It combines with

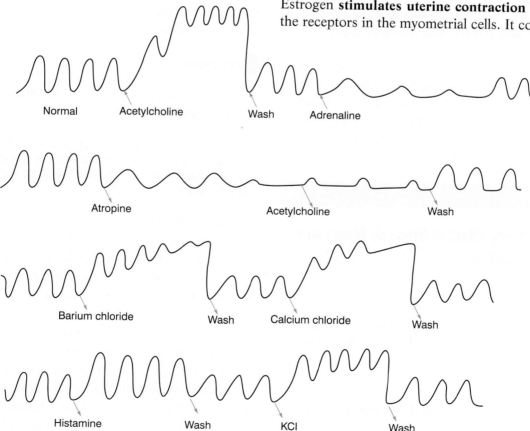

Fig. 74.1 Effect of drugs on uterine contraction. Note that oxytocin, estrogen and acetylcholine are stimulatory whereas progesterone and adrenaline are inhibitory. Oxytocin and acetylcholine increase the tone of uterine muscle.

the intracellular protein receptors, and the hormone receptor complex binds to the DNA that **promotes the formation of mRNA**. mRNA in turn regulates the formation of new proteins that facilitate cell function.

Progesterone

Progesterone **inhibits uterine contraction and decreases the tone** of the muscle. It inhibits myometrial cells, decreases the excitability of the myometrium and decreases the sensitivity of the myometrium to oxytocin. It also decreases the number of estrogen receptors in the myometrial cells. Progesterone acts by acting on the receptors inside the cell, which regulates DNA that in turn controls new mRNA synthesis.

Acetylcholine

Acetylcholine **increases tone, frequency and amplitude** of the uterine contraction, probably by similar mechanisms imparted on intestinal smooth muscle.

Adrenaline

Adrenaline **decreases uterine contraction**, probably by similar mechanisms that take place in intestinal smooth muscle.

Clinical Significance

Oxytocin

The number of oxytocin receptors in the myometrium increases 100 times in late pregnancy and reaches a peak at term. *Estrogen increases the number of oxytocin receptors* on the myometrial cells. At term, the distension of the uterus and dilatation of the cervix gives **feedback information** to the posterior pituitary to release more oxytocin. It also increases the sensitivity of the myometrium to the normal oxytocin concentration in the blood. Oxytocin facilitates uterine contraction which finally leads to **parturition**.

Estrogen

Estrogen increases the amount of uterine muscle and its content of contractile proteins. The myometrial cells become more excitable and active. The **estrogen-dominated uterus is more sensitive to oxytocin**. During the early part of pregnancy, the estrogen concentration in plasma is low. Therefore, there are no uterine contractions, which prevents abortion. Close to term, the estrogen concentration increases in plasma, which along with oxytocin facilitates parturition.

Progesterone

Progesterone has antiestrogenic activity. It **decreases uterine excitability and contraction**, decreases the estrogen receptors on the myometrial cells and decreases the sensitivity of the uterus to estrogen. Progesterone concentration increases during pregnancy; it is the main hormone that **maintains pregnancy**.

VIVA

1. *What are the hormones of the ovary that act on the uterine myometrium?*
2. *What are the actions of oxytocin, estrogen, progesterone, acetylcholine and adrenaline on uterine contraction? What is their mechanism of action?*
3. *What is the mechanism of initiation of labour?*
4. *What is the role of oxytocin in parturition?*
5. *What is the role of estrogen in parturition?*
6. *What is the role of progesterone in pregnancy?*

CHAPTER 75

Estrus Cycle in Rat

Learning Objectives

After completing this practical, you will be able to:
1. Describe the different phases of the estrus cycle in rats.
2. Identify different phases by microscopic examination of vaginal smears.
3. Correlate these changes with the phases of the menstrual cycle in humans.

INTRODUCTION

Under the influence of hormones, cyclical changes occur in the reproductive organs in females during their reproductive life. The regular cyclic changes in females are meant for their preparation for fertilisation and pregnancy. In primates, the cycle is referred to as menstrual cycle and periodic vaginal bleeding (menstruation) is an important feature of the cycle. In **non-primate mammals** like rats that do not menstruate, sexual cycles are referred to as **estrus cycles**. The cyclical changes in vaginal smears in rats are relatively well-marked, whereas similar vaginal changes in humans and other species though present are not so specific. In humans, specific changes occur in the uterus and the ovaries during the cycles, but it is not easy to study the changes in these organs.

METHODS

Method to Study Estrus Cycle in Rat

Principle

The vaginal epithelium undergoes cyclical changes during the estrus cycle under the influence of ovarian hormones. These changes are identified by examining the vaginal smears under microscope.

Requirements

1. Microscope
2. Pipette
3. Methylene blue
4. Slides and coverslips
5. Adult non-pregnant female rats

Procedure

1. Place a drop of methylene blue stain on a slide.
2. With the help of a pipette, aspirate vaginal fluid from the rat.
3. Mix the vaginal fluid with the stain and put a coverslip on the mixture.
4. Make similar smears from five different rats (in different phases of the cycle).
5. Observe the cellular pattern under the high-power microscope.

Observation

The presence of vaginal cells and leucocytes helps in the identification of different phases of the cycle (Fig. 75.1).

1. Proestrus : Predominance of vesicular (nucleated) cells
2. Estrus   : Predominance of non-nucleated, cornified or keratinised cells
3. Metestrus : Presence of leucocytes and cornified cells
4. Diestrus : Mainly leucocytes and few other cells

Precautions

1. Adult non-pregnant female rats should be used for the experiment.
2. Smears should be prepared by collecting vaginal fluid from different rats.

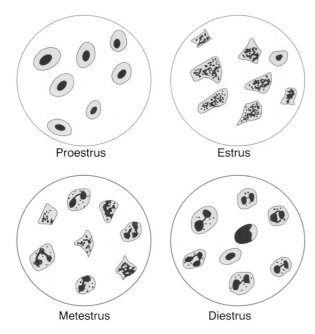

Proestrus   **Estrus**

Metestrus   **Diestrus**

Fig. 75.1   Microscopic appearance of vaginal smear of different phases of the estrus cycle in rats.

3. Vaginal fluid should be collected by introducing the tip of the pipette into the vagina and then by aspirating the fluid.
4. Vaginal smears should be examined under the high-power microscope.

DISCUSSION

The **estrus cycle in rat is 4–5 days**. The proestrus phase persists for few hours only. The estrus phase is the heat phase which marks the first day of the cycle and denotes ovulation in rats. The estrus phase corresponds to the ovulation phase in humans. In humans, the menstrual cycle is divided into two phases, proliferative and secretory. In the first half of the cycle (proliferative or follicular phase), the ovarian follicle matures. In the middle of the cycle, ovulation occurs which is followed by the secretory or luteal phase, the second half of the cycle. Menstrual bleeding occurs at the end of the secretory phase.

VIVA

1. Why are non-pregnant adult female rats selected for this experiment?
2. What are the different phases of the estrus cycle in rats and how do you identify these phases by studying the vaginal smear?
3. In which phase of the estrus cycle does ovulation occur in rats?
4. What are the phases of the menstrual cycle in humans?
5. What are the uterine changes observed in different phases of the menstrual cycle?
6. What is the mechanism of ovulation? What are the indicators of ovulation?
7. Why is it important to know the date of ovulation?

Index of Normal Values

A. Blood

1. Hemogram

Total RBC count	
Men	4.5–6 million/mm^3
Women	4–5.5 million/mm^3
Hemoglobin	
Men	14–18 g/dl
Women	12–16 g/dl
Packed cell volume (Hematocrit)	
Men	40–50%
Women	37–47%
Mean corpuscular volume (MCV)	78–96 fl
Mean corpuscular hemoglobin (MCH)	27–33 pg
Mean corpuscular Hb conc (MCHC)	30–37%
Colour index	0.85 0 1.10
Total leucocyte count	4000–11,000/mm^3
Differential count	
Neutrophils	50–70%
Eosinophils	1–4%
Lymphocyte	20–40%
Monocyte	2–8%
Basophils	0–1%
Total platelet count	150,000–400,000/mm^3
Reticulocyte count	0.5–1% of red cells
ESR	
Westergren method	
Men	3–5 mm at the end of 1 h
Women	5–12 mm at the end of 1 h
Wintrobe method)	
Men	0–9 mm at the end of 1 h
Women	0–20 mm at the end of 1 h
Osmotic fragility of red cells	Hemolysis begins at 0.45% of NaCl and completes at 0.35% of NaCl.

2. Coagulation studies

Bleeding time (Duke method)	1–5 min.
Clotting time (capillary tube method)	2–8 min.
Fibrinogen	200–400 mg%
Fibrin degradation product	10 µg/dl
Activated partial thromboplastin time (APTT)	25–40 sec.
Thrombin time	15–20 sec.
Clot retraction time	50% by 1 h
Whole blood clot lysis time	> 24 h

3. Gases

PO$_2$

Arterial blood (PaO$_2$)	80–100 mmHg
Venous blood	25–40 mmHg

PCO$_2$

Arterial blood (PaCO$_2$)	35–45 mmHg
Venous blood	40–50 mmHg

4. pH
7.35–7.45

B. Serum

Bilirubin

Adult	0.2–0.8 mg %
Newborn	0.5–5 mg %
At 3 days after birth	1–10 mg %
Creatinine	0.6-1.8 mg %
Calcium	9–11 mg/dl
Iron	50–150 µg/dl
Plasma glucose (fasting)	70–110 mg/dl (111–125 mg% is prediabetes)
Plasma glucose (postprandial, 2 hours)	< 140 mg%
Plasma glucose (random)	< 200 mg%

Electrolytes

Sodium	136–145 meq/L
Potassium	3.5–5 meq/L
Chlorides	96–106 meq/L
Phosphorus (inorganic)	2.5–4.5 mg/dl
Cholesterol	120–200 mg/dl
Osmolality	280–295 mosm/kg of water

C. Urine

Glucose

Qualitative	Absent
Quantitative	16–300 mg/24 h

Protein

Qualitative	Absent
Quantitative	10–150 mg/24 h
Bilirubin	Absent
Hemoglobin	Absent
Creatine	0–200 mg in 24 h
Creatinine	15–25 mg/kg body weight/day
Uric acid	250–750 mg/24 h
Urobilinogen	0.05–3.5 mg/24 h
Sodium	40–220 meq/24 h
Potassium	25–125 meq/24 h
Chloride	10–200 mmol/l
Calcium (normal diet)	100 – 300 mg/24 h
Osmolality	100–900 mosm/l
pH	4.6–8.0 (average 6)

D. Cerebrospinal fluid

Glucose	50–70 mg/dl
Protein	10–30 mg/dl
Bilirubin	Absent
Cells	0–5/mm^3 (usually lymphocytes)
Chloride	110–125 mmol/l
Pressure	7–20 cm of water
pH	7.34–7.43

E. Semen

Liquefaction	Completes at 15 min.
Morphology	Minimum 60% normal
Motility	Minimum 75% motile
pH	7.2–8.0
Count	50 million/ml
Volume	2–5 ml

F. Synovial fluid

Cells	200 cells/mm^3
Glucose	Same as serum
Hyaluronic acid	2.5–4 g/dl
Proteins	2.5 g/dl
pH	7.32–7.64
Crystals	Absent

G. Stool

Fat	3–5 g/day
Nitrogen	2.2 g/24 h
Stercobilinogen	40–280 mg/24 h
Corpoporphyrin	15–500 mg/24 h

H. Cardiovascular parameters

Heart rate	: 60 to 100 per min.
Cardiac output	: 5 litres per min (each ventricle)
Systolic BP	: 100–119 mmHg (120–139 mmHg is prehypertension)
Diastolic BP	: 60–79 mmHg (80–89 mmHg is prehypertension)
Pulse pressure	: 20–50 mmHg

Bibliography

Hematology

Bain B, Bates I, Laffan M. 2016. *Dacie and Lewis Practical Hematology*; 12th edition. London: Churchill Livingstone.

Kaushansky K, Litchman MA, Prchal JT, Levi MM, Press OW, Burns LJ, Caliguri MA. 2020. *William's Hematology*; 9th edition. London: McGraw-Hill.

Pal GK and Pal P. 2003. *Textbook of Practical Physiology*; 2nd edition. Hyderabad: Orient Longman Publications.

Renu S, Pati HP, Mahapatra M (eds.). 2018. *de Gruchy's Clinical Hematology in Medical Practice*; 6th edition. London: Science.

Turgeon ML. 2019. *Linne and Ringsrud's Clinical Laboratory Science*; 8th edition. New York: Elsevier.

Human and Clinical Practicals

Bannister R and Mathews CJ (eds.). 2013. *Autonomic Failure: A Textbook of Clinical Disorders of the Autonomic Nervous System*; 5th edition. London: Oxford University Press.

Barett KE, Barman SM, Brooks HL and Yuan J (eds.). 2020. *Ganong's Review of Medical Physiology*; 26th edition. New York: McGraw-Hill.

Glynn M and Drake W (eds.), 2019. *Hutchison's Clinical Methods*; 23rd edition. London: WB Saunders.

Jameson JL, Fauci AS, Kasper DL, Hauser SL, Longo DL, and Loscalzo J (eds.). 2018. *Harrison's Principles of Internal Medicine*; 20th edition. New York: McGraw-Hill.

Johnson EW and Pease WS (eds.). 2015. *Practical Electromyography*; 3rd edition. London: Williams and Wilkins.

Kinirons M and Ellis H (eds.). 2011. *French's Index of Differential Diagnosis*; 15th edition. London: Butterworth-Heinemann.

Koeppen BM, Stanton BA. 2018. *Berne and Levy Physiology*; 7th edition. New York: Elsevier.

Mishra UK and Kalita J. 2019. *Clinical Neurophysiology*; 4th edition, New Delhi: Elsevier.

Narashiman C and Francis J (eds.). 2013. *An Introduction to Electrocardiography*; 8th edition. London: Wiley.

Ogilvie C. 1980. *Chamberlain's Symptoms and Signs in Clinical Medicine*; 10th edition. London: John Wright and Sons Ltd.

Pal GK, Pal P and Nanda N. 2019. *Comprehensive Textbook of Medical Physiology*; 2nd edition, New Delhi: Jaypee Publications.

Pal GK, Pal P and Nanda N. 2019. *Textbook of Medical Physiology*; 3rd edition. New Delhi: Elsevier (India) and Ahuja Publications.

Papadakis MA and Me Phee SJ (eds.). 2020. *Current Medical Diagnosis and Treatment*; 45th edition. New York: McGraw-Hill-Lange.

Sahu D. 1983. Critical Approach to Clinical Medicine. New Delhi: Vikas Publishing House Pvt Ltd.

Experimental Physiology

Bell GH. 1959. *Experimental Physiology*. London: Churchill Livingstone.

Ghosh MN. 2007. *Fundamentals of Experimental Pharmacology*; 3rd edition. Kolkata: Scientific Book Agency.

Levedahl BH, Barber AA and Grinnel A. 1971. *Laboratory Experiments in Physiology*; 8th edition. New York: CV Mosby Co.

Sharpey-Schafer EA. 2012. *Experimental Physiology*. London: Scholar Select Publication.

Tuttle WW and Schottelius BA. 1963. *Physiology Laboratory Manual*. New York: CV Mosby Co.

Index